COMMUNICATIVE DISORDERS RELATED TO CLEFT LIP AND PALATE

COMMUNICATIVE DISORDERS RELATED TO CLEFT LIP AND PALATE

THIRD EDITION

Edited by
KENNETH R. BZOCH, PH.D.

Professor and Chairman, Department of Communicative Disorders,
College of Health Related Professions, University of Florida;
Director, Shands Hospital Communicative Disorders Clinics, Co-Director,
University of Florida Craniofacial Center, Gainesville

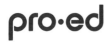

8700 Shoal Creek Boulevard
Austin, Texas 78757

pro·ed

© 1989 by PRO-ED, Inc.
8700 Shoal Creek Boulevard
Austin, Texas 78757-6897

Library of Congress Cataloging-in-Publication Data

Communicative disorders related to cleft lip and palate / edited by
    Kenneth R. Bzoch.—3rd ed.
        p.   cm.
    Reprint. Originally published: 3rd ed. Boston : Little, Brown,
c 1989.   Includes bibliographical references.
    Includes index.
    ISBN 0-89079-315-8
    1. Cleft palate—Complications and sequelae.   2. Cleft lip–
Complications and sequelae.   3. Speech disorders.   4. Speech
disorders in children.   I. Bzoch, Kenneth R.
    [DNLM: 1. Cleft lip.   2. Cleft Palate.   3. Speech Disorders.
WV 440 C734 1989a]
RD525.C66   1991
616.85'5—dc20
DNLM/DLC
for Library of Congress   90-9196
                                                              CIP

Printed in the United States of America

    2   3   4   5   6   7   8   9   10   97   96   95   94

Contents

Contributors

Larry E. Adams, Ph.D.

Associate Professor and Vice-Chairman, Department of Biocommunication, University of Alabama at Birmingham School of Medicine, Birmingham

Doris P. Bradley, Ph.D.

Professor of Speech and Hearing Sciences, University of Southern Mississippi, Hattiesburg

Kenneth R. Bzoch, Ph.D.

Professor and Chairman, Department of Communicative Disorders, College of Health Related Professions, University of Florida; Director, Shands Hospital Communicative Disorders Clinics, Co-Director, University of Florida Craniofacial Center, Gainesville

Edward Clifford, Ph.D.

Professor of Medical Psychology, Departments of Psychology and Surgery, Duke University School of Medicine, Durham, North Carolina

Miriam Clifford, Ph.D.

Research Associate, Department of Psychiatry, Duke University Medical Center, Durham, North Carolina

Virginia L. Dixon–Wood, M.A.

Speech Pathologist, Department of Pediatrics, University of Florida College of Medicine; Coordinator, University of Florida Craniofacial Center, Gainesville

Samuel G. Fletcher, Ph.D.

Professor and Chairman, Department of Biocommunication, University of Alabama at Birmingham School of Medicine, Birmingham

Elise Hahn, Ph.D.

Professor of Speech Pathology (retired), California State University, Los Angeles

F. Joseph Kemker, Ph.D.

Professor, Department of Communicative Disorders, College of Health Related Professions, University of Florida; Chief Audiologist, Shands Hospital Communicative Disorders Clinics, Gainesville

Raymond D. Kent, Ph.D.

Professor of Communicative Disorders, University of Wisconsin — Madison, Madison

Julie M. Liss, M.A.   Department of Communicative Disorders,
                                             University of Wisconsin — Madison, Madison

Martin J. McCutcheon, Ph.D.   Professor of Biomedical Engineering, University
                                             of Alabama at Birmingham, Birmingham

Hughlett L. Morris, Ph.D.   Professor of Speech Pathology, University of
                                             Iowa; Director, Division of Speech and
                                             Hearing, Department of Otolaryngology —
                                             Head and Neck Surgery, University of Iowa
                                             Hospitals and Clinics, Iowa City

John A. Nackashi, M.D.   Associate Professor of Pediatrics, University of
                                             Florida College of Medicine; Clinical Medical
                                             Director, University of Florida Craniofacial
                                             Center, Gainesville

Sally J. Peterson–Falzone, Ph.D.   Clinical Professor, Department of Growth and
                                             Development, University of California School
                                             of Dentistry, San Francisco

Betty Jane Philips, Ed.D.   Professor, Department of Otolaryngology and
                                             Human Communication, Creighton University
                                             School of Medicine; Director, Special Clinical
                                             Programs, Boys' Town National Institute for
                                             Communication Disorders in Children, Omaha

Dennis M. Ruscello, Ph.D.   Professor and Chairman, Department of
                                             Speech Pathology and Audiology, West
                                             Virginia University, Morgantown

Jane Scheuerle, Ed.D.   Professor, Department of Communication
                                             Sciences and Disorders, University of South
                                             Florida, Tampa

Ralph L. Shelton, Ph.D.   Professor, Department of Speech and Hearing
                                             Sciences, University of Arizona, Tucson

Robert J. Shprintzen, Ph.D.   Professor of Plastic Surgery and Otolaryngology,
                                             Albert Einstein College of Medicine of Yeshiva
                                             University; Director, Center for Craniofacial
                                             Disorders, Bronx, New York

Donald W. Warren, D.D.S., Ph.D.   Kenan Professor, University of North Carolina
                                             at Chapel Hill School of Dentistry; Director,
                                             Oral-Facial and Communicative Disorders
                                             Program, University of North Carolina at
                                             Chapel Hill School of Medicine, Chapel Hill

William N. Williams, Ph.D.   Associate Professor, Department of Oral
                                             Biology, University of Florida College of
                                             Dentistry, Gainesville

Deborah R. Zarajczyk, M.A.   Director of Speech Pathology and Audiology,
                                             Easter Seal Society, Daytona Beach, Florida

Preface

The authors of the second edition and I were very gratified at the long and favorable acceptance and adoption of *Communicative Disorders Related to Cleft Lip and Palate* for classroom use. However, due to the rapid accumulation of new, related information it became apparent four years ago that a third edition would soon be needed.

The new information, not available when the second edition was written, included extensive research in genetics and cooperative clinical research from many craniofacial centers on syndromes related to clefting. A generation of experience in craniofacial surgery for many congenital syndromes, such as Apert's and Cruzon's, and many other generally untreatable and untreated syndromes needed to be added. Also, new technological advancements in instrumentation to measure voice and speech behavior and to peer into the body in order to refine clinical diagnostic impressions of velopharyngeal insufficiency for speech, as well as updating of established technologies such as videofluoroscopy, required new chapters. Particularly, for me, the accelerated trend in our profession for early diagnosis, interventional therapy, and treatment of language disorders, which are common in cleft palate sample populations, needed documentation and updating from the introductory treatment in the second edition. A final effort was made to add case study material to better illustrate specific treatment strategies and therapy techniques developed by experienced clinicians for the guidance of future practitioners. As in previous editions, the completion of this book took twice as long as the original time set aside for it.

Since instructors have found the book's structure of three rather than five parts useful for teaching a professional course of study on the subject, the general outline adopted for the second edition has been followed. The book contains more information than can be adequately covered in one semester or quarter of study. However, each chapter constitutes an expert's complete review of a topic area, with an introduction, generally updated review, and extensive bibliography for further study. The instructor is free to assign specific chapters for in-depth discussion, others for topics in term papers, and others for later reference. To make room for new material, several of the former chapters were eliminated or covered more concisely in the introductory chapter.

The goal of this book is to give a complete overview of the nature and management of communicative disorders related to cleft palate, craniofacial disorders, and acquired problems of velopharyngeal insufficiency for speech. This overview is presented with state-of-the-art information in a series of interrelated chapters, by 23 recognized authorities writing in their specialized areas of knowledge for professional students or practitioners. The third edition is intended to be used as a textbook for advanced graduate students or as an updated reference for practitioners in speech pathology or audiology.

Part I, *General Aspects*, includes four chapters. They introduce, review, and update the basic principles, anatomy, velopharyngeal function for speech, classification of clefts, basic concepts in craniofacial anomalies, psychological aspects, and the team approach. This part now includes an entirely new chapter by Sally J. Peterson–Falzone on basic concepts in craniofacial defects. It also includes an updated review of psychological aspects by Edward Clifford; a discussion of a model of transactional teams by a pediatrician, John A. Nackashi; and a description of the training and role of the medical, dental, and health-related profession specialists on a modern cleft palate team by a team coordinator, Virginia Dixon–Wood.

Part II, *Diagnostic Aspects*, is divided into three sections: *Evaluation of the Probable Causes of Related Communicative Disorders, Evaluation of Basic Causes of Related Communicative Disorders,* and *Objectified Instrumental Diagnostic Evaluations.* Unlike the second edition, the section requiring the greatest attention was the last, covering instrumental diagnostic tools. They have literally moved out of speech science laboratories and into the diagnostic center clinics in the past decade. Completely new chapters were written for this section by Robert J. Shprintzen, on nasopharyngoscopy; by Donald W. Warren, on aerodynamic assessment of velopharyngeal function; by Samuel Fletcher, Larry Adams, and Martin McCutcheon, on nasometer oral-nasal measures; and by Raymond Kent, Julie Liss, and Betty Jane Philips, on sonogram acoustic indices of velopharyngeal dysfunction in speech. Former contributors to Part II who updated or completely rewrote their chapters, namely, Doris Bradley, Edward and Miriam Clifford, Hughlett Morris, and William Williams, along with myself, welcome the new authors to the writing team. We also welcome F. Joseph Kemker and Deborah Zarajczyk who contributed a new chapter on audiological testing and management of hearing in cleft palate patients. Without their contributions, it would not have been possible to have up-to-date information on cleft palate diagnostic evaluations.

Part III, *Habilitative and Rehabilitative Aspects*, builds upon the general background science related to cleft lip and palate, craniofacial disorders, and diagnostic tests and procedures. It is the application of the diagnostic information to the therapeutic interactions with clients that constitutes what is called speech and language therapy. The physiological basis for the changes in speech behavior that can and do take place in therapy has its basis in oral sensory and auditory monitoring. This topic is covered in an entirely rewritten chapter on sensory function in speech production and remediation by Ralph Shelton. New chapters by Jane Scheuerle, on stimulating language development in infants and toddlers, and by Dennis Ruscello, on the possibilities of modifying velopharyngeal func-

tion through training procedures, have been added. A former chapter by Elise Hahn, with guidelines for directing a home language stimulation program for families of infants with cleft lip and palate, is repeated, as it anticipated the developments leading to early intervention in problems of delayed speech and language development. This is also the emphasis in my revised chapter, updating rationale, methods, and techniques of cleft palate speech therapy, illustrated with case studies. Early intervention and the possibility of regular prevention of communicative disorders are emphasized throughout this final section.

We are entering what should be an exciting decade of work in our profession. This book presents the highlights of over three decades of productive interdisciplinary clinical and basic research fostered by the team approach in cleft palate management. It seems the critical mass of information coupled with new legislation on preventive community programs for high-risk infants up to 3 years, which is necessary for a general focus on prevention, has only recently been reached. The family-centered focus on early identification and the providing of coordinated services in speech and hearing during the period of the earliest preschool age development is the established norm rather than a dream because of the cleft palate team approach over the past decades. The demonstrated efficacy of this approach to cleft palate treatment provides a model for the new types of cooperative teams needed to help the broader population of children born with environmental and physical disorders other than cleft palate.

K. R. B.

I.

GENERAL ASPECTS

CHAPTER 1

Introduction to Communicative Disorders in Cleft Palate and Related Craniofacial Anomalies

Kenneth R. Bzoch

Unlike the earlier editions of this book, there seems no longer to be any need for apologetics as to why graduate students or practitioners in the fields of speech pathology or audiology should undertake a specific course of study in the area of cleft palate and related craniofacial disorders. The advances over the past decade in both clinical and basic research have been significant. Also, technological and instrumental advances in the assessment of velopharyngeal function have been developed. These diagnostic tools are described in Part II, Section C, along with methods for utilizing them, by experienced clinicians expert in their application in both research and clinical diagnosis.

There seems to me no longer to be sufficient reason on the basis of the birth of a child with an isolated cleft of the lip or palate alone for the continued high probability of sequelae of many years of stigmata from speech and language disorders. However, we now know that some children born with cleft palate really have complex syndromes involving multiple disorders with potential medical and learning problems predisposing to developmental disabilities. Some of these syndromes, which are more frequently studied and managed in the larger craniofacial centers, include the sequelae of general mental retardation or significant hearing impairment. These conditions can cause significant developmental speech and language disorders in addition to the effects of cleft palate. However, even for children presenting with isolated cleft lip and palate, the consequences of early hospitalization and surgery, prolonged feeding difficulties, facial disfigurement, and the altered interpersonal interactions they may engender in the extended family and beyond, present early management problems predisposing toward speech and language disorders. This new edition introduces the reader to the new science and clinical art of syndromology and the related area of congenital craniofacial disorders that were not covered in the earlier editions. Our goal is to present the current state of the art and state of the science of effective management of cleft lip and palate and related craniofacial disorders of oral communication and language skills.

Despite these necessary qualifications, the experience of over three decades of work in this area of communicative disorders indicates that with orientation to the body of knowledge contained in this book, successful management and the frequent prevention of the severe communicative disorder problems encountered in this large population of human beings is possible today.

The early identification of syndromal and environmental factors, which influence the potential outcome of early team management of infants with cleft palate, has become more important due to our increased knowledge base from clinical and genetic research. Of similar importance is the preventive management by audiologists of the usual significant conductive hearing loss in infancy which is common for most children born with cleft palate.

The goal of preventing communicative disorders from developing in the early lives of these in-

sequelae → a pathological condition resulting from a disease. (something that follows
stigmata → mark of indicative of abnormality; a mark of reproach/disgrace

3

fants will always be limited by environmental factors beyond the control of a cleft palate team. Limitations resulting from poor parenting, lack of good nutrition in infancy, poor environmental language stimulation, and even the absence of available medical care for rural families living in poverty frustrate the best efforts at effective early prevention programs. The lack of third-party funding for nonsurgical medical care and for speech and language therapy or needed dental services in many communities can only be overcome by working with state programs for crippled children and exerting influence on state and federal legislatures to provide these services.

Much progress has been made over the past decade in this regard, but the implementation and improvement of exisiting legislative programs has become the exciting challenge of the next decade. The optimistic goal of preventing communicative disorders from developing in the early lives of infants born into this population requires close evaluation and management of three additional areas at this time: (1) identifying and learning to better manage syndromes of multiple disorders and craniofacial disorders, (2) overcoming limiting environmental factors through effective state-wide programs, and (3) better managing significant hearing loss during the development of emergent language skills.

The delivery of health-related services for effective management of congenital velopharyngeal incompetency and facial stigma for infants born with isolated cleft lip with or without cleft palate may be better understood by reviewing the three decades of clinical research reviewed in this text. The effective management of syndromes of multiple disorders with clefts or genetic craniofacial disorders are less well understood.

RATIONALE FOR A COURSE OF STUDY

It appears from the literature that what has been called "cleft palate speech" is based primarily in functional learning disorders in oral expressive language. These compensatory and early identifiable patterns of defective speech production are usually learned and partly habituated in the first years of development, particularly from birth to 3 years of age. Their development can usually be prevented by a coordinated team program focused on early prevention and by a community-based intervention program as will be described.

The main exception to characterizing what has been called cleft palate speech as primarily a functional learned disorder of speech production is the persistence of symptoms of nasalance distortions during speech utterances that are due to remaining or recurring velopharyngeal insufficiency to support normal speech and language development. This condition occurs with some frequency after primary surgical reconstruction. Clinical impressions from behavioral observations and clinical tests can now be more objectively related to the decision that continued velopharyngeal insufficiency to support normal speech and voice production continues after primary surgical reconstruction of clefts of the palate before school age is reached. Diagnostic speech evaluation tests and techniques described in this text can be used for this purpose as early as 2 years of age.

When velopharyngeal insufficiency is evident after primary surgical reconstruction of cleft structures, secondary palate reconstruction rather than functional retraining through speech therapy is usually indicated for correcting continued patterns of velopharyngeal insufficiency–related disorders of speech. Such problems can usually be identified between 2½ and 4 years of age. However, exceptions to this rule can be selected through clinical diagnostic tests, case history reports, and careful observation of inconsistencies in nasalance distortions of individual cases.

Clinical indices which indicate inconsistent problems related to velopharyngeal function for speech provide a fair prognosis for proceeding with a limited period of diagnostic speech therapy or even palatal training procedures. The clinical indices for selecting subjects for early direct therapy training particularly need to be understood by the beginning speech clinician and those entering clinical practice in this area with infants and preschool children.

It should also be noted that persistent distortions of sibilant sound elements related directly to dental or occlusal abnormalities constitute another organic basis for prolonged speech production problems. The speech pathologist therefore needs to know and utilize what the dental specialists can do to remove dental and occlusal hazards to normal speech production. This is especially relevant for the finding from error pattern articulation test data of the development of lateral lisping distortions of sibilant sounds, which can often be related directly to missing lateral incisor teeth or class III malocclusions. The earliest possible correction of dental speech hazards is part of a routine cleft palate team effort. It is often also needed for the effective treatment of some non-cleft clients with similar developing speech articulation problems.

Since these structurally related speech disorders are usually correctable early, they need to be identified by a speech pathologist as causally related to developmental speech disorders needing early referral for physical management before proceeding with extended speech therapy.

If the often lifetime disorder of oral expressive language termed *cleft palate speech* and the handicap it presents for all future interpersonal interactions and education are in fact most often preventable for infants born with clefts of the palate, then this should be our first goal with this large group of clients. Prevention through early intervention will be emphasized in the following.

Unfortunately, isolated and late speech and language therapy services provided through school programs or speech clinicians working in private practice or community clinics too often characterize the speech therapy services available in most communities in the United States today. A basic understanding of the nature of a "cleft palate team approach" is the second emphasis in the following course of study.

Perhaps, with the future implementation of Public Law 99-457 (the Education of the Handicapped Act, amended in 1986 focused on early intervention for all high-risk infant populations from birth to 3 years of age), significant improvements in both special education and health care services will be made available to infants and preschool children with cleft palate. The effective means for preventing handicaps in this high-risk population are better understood through the experience of decades of transdisciplinary clinical team efforts and clinical research focused on effective early intervention. The long-term goal of this new legislation is to establish family-centered programs for all high-risk infants to prevent primary developmental disabilities. Primary speech and language learning disabilities constitute one of the most serious forms of such preventable developmental disabilities in the newborn.

Newborns with other serious environmental and possible physical handicaps for normal development from birth to age 3 (e.g., low birth weight, mother with drug addiction problem, single parent in poverty, etc.) are targeted for new interdisciplinary intervention programs to prepare them for mainstreaming in the public education system. The past success of cleft palate teams, achieved through early interdisciplinary longitudinal evaluations of infants often presenting with these same environmental handicaps in addition to their congenital abnormalities, should provide a model for the kind of interventive programs needed.

Specialization through long clinical or research experience in the fields of speech and language pathology and audiology dictates that no single or small group of practitioners in the cleft palate area today has the expertise to write an introductory text for new or practicing professionals. As with the past editions of this book, experienced practitioners have contributed comprehensive overviews of their areas of expertise. With current references, including a basic and classic bibliography for in-depth study, these chapters form the building blocks of a structured text on the current state of the art in this area, namely, communicative disorders in the cleft palate and related craniofacial disorders population. The book is directed at the level of the beginning clinican and to those without experience in this organic area of clinical practice and research work.

Another goal of this book is to present a clear description of the usual role of the speech pathologist and audiologist along with a description of the training and usual roles of the other team members in the medical, dental, and health-related specialties with whom we should learn to work cooperatively. Clinicians working outside of established cleft palate or craniofacial teams can provide many of the clinical services needed in their communities. These sites are often far from the nearest established cleft palate center.

A review of some established principles from three decades of cleft palate team experience, basic information on formation of the face and palate from embryology, a review of useful and preferred classification systems for clinical practice and research, a review of the anatomy of the velopharyngeal mechanism, and a presentation of the recently developed state-wide guidelines for the delivery of health care services constitute the remaining areas that are covered in this introductory chapter.

SOME PRINCIPLES FOR CONSIDERATION

The following statements of principles are based mainly on empirical grounds, although they seem equally defensible logically and on scientific grounds. They are presented to better relate the information in this limited organic area to the broader area of work in communicative disorders in general as clinician or researcher.

Principle I. Congenital disorders of the speech and hearing mechanisms of the body cause more extensive primary speech and language disabilities than later similar acquired disorders. Figure 1-1 illustrates this basic principle related to all underlying physical causes of developmental communicative disorders. *Congenital disorders, especially those occurring in utero (prenatal shaded area in Fig. 1-1), generally have a broader and a more pervasive effect (crosshatched areas) on the learning of symbolic language and on speech skill development than do similar acquired disorders in later life.*

This principle applies particularly to the speech habilitation of a client who acquires velopharyngeal insufficiencies from trauma or surgical removal of tumors after developing normal speech and language skills. Indeed, speech habilitation for such patients usually involves only the effective restoration of palatal structures through prosthetic or surgical means.

The main point is that the problem of congenital velopharyngeal insufficiency for normal speech and language development coupled with the problem of a basic abnormality of the structure and

Figure 1-1. Principle of broader effects for congenital causes of communicative disorders compared with similar acquired causes.

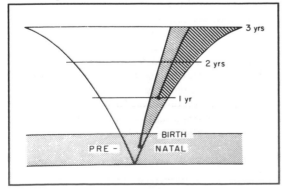

function of the eustachian tube affecting hearing acuity is common to almost all infants born with cleft palate. The effects of these often peripherally limited abnormalities influence the developing fetus even before the early language learning process begins after birth. They are present at birth and adversely affect the earliest stages of emergent language learning skills. They therefore present a generally more significant set of high-risk factors than any form of later acquired velopharyngeal insufficiency.

Cleft palate also usually presents a higher risk for primary language learning disabilities than generally occurs for very low-birth-weight children. Longitudinal studies of this new population of surviving very low-birth-weight infants are being conducted at neonatal facilities in most communities. Many of the lessons learned from effective early management of cleft palate infants through the longitudinal team approach with early involvement of parents and repeated reevaluations in the first years of life seem applicable to the establishment of effective preventive services for these high-risk infants.

The birth of a child with cleft palate poses a higher risk for primary speech and language learning disabilities than many other problems of other groups of high-risk infants. Understanding the basic ingredients required for preventing communicative disorders in this population should provide some established methods for preventing primary developmental disabilities in a much broader population of our clinical concern over the next decade.

This principle also applies to the differences between endogenous central nervous system abnormalities, as compared to exogenous types (i.e., outside the genes), which occur after birth from trauma or disease. The *brain-damaged child* may present at school age with similar levels of mild, moderate, or severe retardation. However, the mongoloid child (i.e., the 1 in 660 newborns with trisomy 21 syndrome) can be predicted to have a much broader extent of retardation and learning disabilities than any peer of similar age, sex, and general IQ who acquired brain damage later in development. Neurogenic velopharyngeal insufficiencies for normal speech development may also underlie the speech problems of either type of retarded child.

The most extreme example probably lies in the area of congenital deafness as contrasted to acquired deafness. The autobiography of Helen Keller [26], and its dramatization in the film *The Mir-*

acle Worker perhaps best illustrates this point. Although Helen Keller became both deaf and blind early in life, hers was not a congenital condition. Rather, she acquired this disability from meningitis at 1 year of age. She had therefore already laid down the basic pattern of oral language, learned in the first year of life. She achieved remarkable language skills through early tactile modality interventive training and long-term motivated practice. When one reads her autobiography, the significance of that first year of language development becomes crystal-clear as Helen Keller remembers rather than learns for the first time the word symbol for *water*. If one also reflects on the extreme differences in language acquisition between children born with isolated deafness and those born only blind, the significance of the first weeks, months, and years of auditory modality–stimulated learning of speech and language skills can best be appreciated.

Principle II. Normal velopharyngeal function is critical to the development of phonological speech sound articulation skills. The role of the palate as a critical part of the normal articulation mechanism for speech has, perhaps, been underemphasized and misunderstood due to the usual focus on the role of the velopharyngeal mechanism in regard to hypernasality, a resonance distortion phenomenon of voice quality. The anatomical name for the soft palate is *velum* (from the Latin for "veil" or "curtain") because it stretches like a curtain across the nasopharynx to seal off the nasal cavities from the oral and pharyngeal cavities throughout most of the temporal sequences in connected speech production.

Failure to seal off the nasopharynx from the oral and pharyngeal cavities allows constant coupling of these resonating cavities during attempts at normal speech production. The result is a hypernasal voice quality and nasal distortions of pressure consonant sounds. This is because the physiologic act of speech co-articulation also requires firm velopharyngeal closure in order to allow for the impounding of breath pressure in the oral cavity for plosive and fricative consonant sound elements, a pneumatic rather than acoustic requirement for articulation of speech sound elements. This pneumatic requirement is affected by even a small degree of incompleteness of the seal in the nasopharynx.

Through the babbling, jargon, and first, single, spoken word stages of emergent language development, an infant strives through successive approximations to produce syllables and, later, words modeled after the speech utterances of their caretakers. The early attempts of cleft palate infants to form such meaningful syllables and words often has very negative effects on articulation skill development, if they are initiated during a period of development with prolonged velopharyngeal insufficiency to impound oral breath pressure for simple initial plosive sounds in first words and early pivot sentences. The open cleft or only partially reconstructed palate of infants born with cleft palate can prevent the production of the usual bilabial or lingua-alveolar plosives like the /p/, /b/, and /d/ sound elements common in early social babbling and later jargon, first word, and sentence utterances.

It appears, therefore, that much more than a voice or resonance disorder of speech is most often introduced during the primary learning period of developing motor speech habits in expressive language development for cleft palate children with uncorrected velopharyngeal incompetence, especially during the second year of life and beyond. Developmental phonological skills in expressive oral language are programmed to emerge in the first 2–3 years of life. These developing skills are often seriously affected due to the frequent need to substitute consonantlike sound elements produced below the level of the velopharyngeal mechanism (i.e., the substitution of glottal stops or velar or pharyngeal fricative sound elements for anterior oral consonants) where air pressure and flow are sufficient to approximate pressure consonant sounds.

This abnormal learning seems often to take place in order for the child to achieve intelligible word utterances in early expressive oral language. The resulting motor substitution gestures of speech production can become well habituated before the third year. They can also last a lifetime if reinforced over time, even after correction of the underlying problem of velopharyngeal insufficiency.

It appears that velopharyngeal insufficiency through infancy predisposes toward the development of such articulatory gross substitution error patterns in early speech efforts rather than causes them. Some children with prolonged velopharyngeal insufficiency for speech do not fall into this developmental trap. However, velopharyngeal insufficiency after 1 year of life strongly predisposes to this atypical sound substitution pattern.

Moving through the normal or usual stages of early emergent language development seems to require the ability to approximately produce intelligible meaningful single words, and usually

To close/obstruct

after 18 months, to progress to intelligible pivot sentences and longer 2- and 3-word utterances. Passing through these stages with understandable speech leads to the development of generative grammar skills, being able to express verb concepts with nouns and later specifying meaning with adjectives and prepositions to carry the intended meaning in expressive language.

The understandable encoding of early oral language attempts at meaningful speech communication in any language depends primarily on the ability of any infant to produce the major vowel-consonant and oral-nasal consonant contrasts in early speech efforts. Children with uncorrected clefts cannot produce these contrasts normally. Cleft palate children with prolonged velopharyngeal insufficiency often develop abnormal articulation. If identified by early articulation screening assessments, correction through direct articulation-centered speech therapy is much easier at 2, 3, or 4 years of age than later in life.

It is generally possible today for plastic surgeons to reconstruct the hard and the soft palate cleft conditions at 6 to 12 months after birth. However, many plastic surgeons prefer to wait longer. The newer practice of early total reconstruction about age 1 appears to be one major factor required to eliminate the past tendency for the development of grossly abnormal articulation habits in speech production. However, early surgical reconstruction alone is not sufficient for the prevention of cleft palate speech disorders. Frequent monitoring of hearing, of language skill development, and of dental treatment needs by a cleft palate team are equally important in the early years. Particularly, routine monitoring of hearing through audiological tests and otological treatment is needed for prevention of speech and language disorder sequelae.

The fact that a palatal cleft has been completely reconstructed surgically early in life does not mean that velopharyngeal competency for speech has been achieved. The reconstructed mechanism still may not provide velopharyngeal competency for normal speech and language development. Reports from cleft palate treatment centers indicate that as many as 15 to 20 percent of primary closures fail to provide velopharyngeal adequacy for speech. When complete palatal closure is postponed to the second, third, or later years of life, an infant's previous speech learning may lead to prolonged nasal distortion or to continued gross sound substitution habits affecting later language skills. This is particularly so when a routine plan for two-stage closures (i.e., closure of the soft palate only with attempts at obturation of the hard palate cleft by dental prosthesis until a later age) is followed. This is because effective obturation of remaining clefts of the hard palate is difficult to maintain over the critical periods of rapid growth and changes in the oral and nasopharyngeal dimensions of the growing child.

If the palate is actually incapable of functioning adequately to support clear speech production after early or comparatively late reconstruction, nasal distortion will persist, even after direct diagnostic speech therapy training. This is often the best indication of postoperative velopharyngeal insufficiency at the early postoperative stage of development. Total early elimination of the articulation problems that were characteristic of past populations of cleft palate individuals requires the differential diagnosis of organic versus functionally based errors of misarticulation in their early speech behavior, often before 3 years of age.

Principle III. When one part of the speech mechanism is congenitally defective, compensatory abnormalities of the function and structure of the remaining parts may develop and become habituated. Although the condition at birth of isolated cleft palate does not involve structural abnormalities of the larynx or the tongue, it appears that it frequently causes later abnormal functioning of these parts [23, 31, 55]. Occasional newly identified syndromes that might initially be considered as isolated cleft palate, such as the Opitz–Frias syndrome [50], do present with malformations of the larynx or tracheo-esophageal fistula, but these are very rare.

For all children, with or without cleft palate, the component parts of the necessary total speech mechanism (i.e., the breathing, phonation, articulation, and resonance mechanisms) must work together as a unit to produce meaningful voice and speech utterances. This oral communication learning begins early through (1) comfort sounds, (2) isolated babbling, (3) social babbling, (4) long jargon utterances mimicking connected speech, and (5) the first true symbolic word stages, all in the first year of life. Coordinated utterances produced by the total speech mechanism of the body increase in the second year through pivot sentences and continued long jargon utterances, often including approximations of true words in correct grammatical syntactic relations to other words in the utterance. The amount of speech used each day usually increases with longer and longer sentences as a child progresses through stages of improved generative grammar skills before the third birthday.

When children with cleft palate pass through these stages of emergent language development and beyond with velopharyngeal incompetency, only a limited set of compensations are available to them to more closely approximate intelligible speech. They may learn to constrict the oropharynx or laryngopharynx below the level of the velopharyngeal mechanism to approximate plosive and fricative consonant sound elements in words. This often leads to abnormal tongue carriage and movement patterns in connected speech. They may learn to initiate or close off syllables with the vocal folds, habituating glottal stop substitutions for most oral consonants. This also causes a lack of normal co-articulation movement patterns of the tongue. They may weaken phonation of the vowel sounds through aspirate phonation to minimize perceived nasal distortion. All of these compensations result in abnormal lingual and laryngeal functions in speech production, although these organs of the speech mechanism are normal in structure and potential function.

The important point is that differences in breathing, phonation, and lingual functions will contribute to the speech defects of many cleft palate clients. Much as the initial laryngeal blocking of secondary stutterers may spread to lingual and even facial tonic or clonic blocks, the tongue and the larynx get involved in the physiological abnormalities of *cleft palate speech.*

Principle IV. Abnormal functions can modify physical structures of the body over time. Although it is the inherited genetic code which predetermines the general size and shape of all structures of the body, abnormal daily functions can also alter and change the size of the developing structures of the speech mechanisms. Sequences leading to structural abnormalities affecting even the facial skeleton can occur in early embryological development where an early abnormality of one organ or structure can cause a series of later-forming structures to develop abnormally. This is particularly true for the position, size, and shape of the bones of the human face surrounding the mouth and orbits of the eyes.

However, even after birth, abnormal or unbalanced muscle forces on the rapidly growing bones of the face can greatly influence and exacerbate facial abnormalities. Clinically documented observations and cephalometric measurements of the developing facies in individuals with cleft lip or palate and animal research provide many examples of such occurrences.

Developmental studies of infants born with the *Pierre Robin sequence* (i.e., a small mandible with a cleft of the secondary palate with an unusual rounded contour) often demonstrate this principle. The condition is believed to be most often due to mechanical restraint of the chin prior to 9 weeks in utero allowing the tongue to be superiorly and posteriorly positioned, thereby impairing closure of the palatal shelves. Pierre Robin sequence may occur in otherwise normal infants who show a remarkable gain in mandibular growth in the first 2 years of life after birth.

Insofar as this explanation fits the majority of the children labeled as having the Pierre Robin sequence at birth, it illustrates the principle that abnormal function (i.e., pressure against the mandible restricting movement functions in utero) may modify other related developing physical structures (the secondary palate). However, more recent clinical research indicates that this sequence may also occur as part of a multiple defect syndrome, such as the *Stickler syndrome,* and with a large number of other disorders with very different prognoses [50, pp. 206–209].

Clefts of the lip, or rather the "primary palate" with or without cleft palate, afford many opportunities for observations of the effects of abnormal muscle forces on the developing facial skeleton. It is instructive to compare infants born with an incomplete cleft of the lip with cleft palate to those whose cleft is unilateral-complete through both the primary and secondary palates. Figure 1-2A and B illustrates these differences. There is regularly a marked difference in the prenatal growth of the facial skeleton. The facial muscles on the side of the unilateral-complete clefts (see Fig. 1-2A) exert an unbalanced force. The stronger, unrestricted force of the muscles on the noncleft side regularly bend the entire premaxillary segment, displacing it forward and laterad from its normal position in the facies. The tip of the nose is carried along with the rotating premaxillary segment, causing the alar cartilage on the cleft side to be elongated and changing its normal crescent shape, making initial nasal reconstruction difficult. This nasal and premaxillary distortion is limited by the small connecting band of tissue across the floor of the nose, resisting somewhat the stronger muscle force on the noncleft side (see Fig. 1-2B).

Blockage of nasal breathing from an overcorrecting pharyngeal flap operation or other obstruction to normal nasal breathing functions presents another illustration of this principle. The resultant "adenoid facies" with flaccid facial muscle

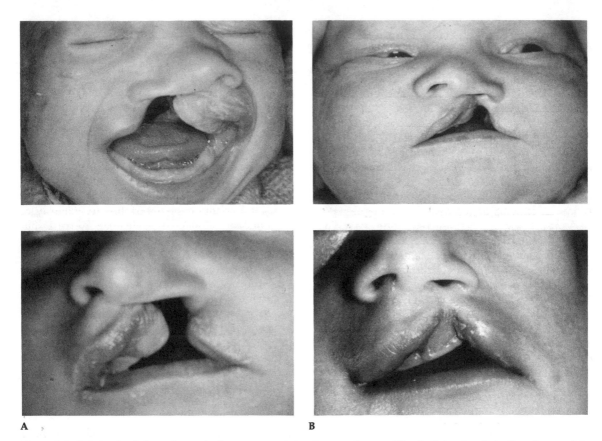

Figure 1-2. Effects of unbalanced muscle forces on nasal structures and premaxilla. A. Extensive distortions in complete clefts of primary and secondary palates. B. Limited distortions in incomplete pre-palate with complete palate clefts.

tone, open mouth for breathing, small underdeveloped nasal capsule, and retarded appearance often results from such early abnormal functional breathing patterns which become habituated.

On a less certain basis, the interest in what is called "tongue thrust," or probably more correctly, abnormal forward tongue carriage, related to breathing, swallowing, and speech functions, may cause serious open-bite malocclusions and even oral-facial skeletal abnormalities over time.

The research literature from cleft palate centers over the past decade frequently focused on the negative effects of oral habits, including speech and deglutition (swallow patterns), on the growth and development of the dental structures, and even the facial skeleton. These considerations include the possible adverse effects which abnormal muscle forces during speech, respiration, deglutition, and oral habits such as prolonged finger-sucking, may have on growing facial bones and dental maloccusions.

The possibly positive side to this principle regarding changes in size and function of structures has also been documented in individual case studies. The fact that muscular function can cause over time an increase in muscle size to achieve functional speech production also needs to be considered. The effectiveness in some cases of speech appliance reduction programs in developing muscle hypertrophy or increased mobility of the velopharyngeal mechanism to the point of adequacy of velopharyngeal function without the prosthesis is reviewed in Part III of this book.

Our center also recently analyzed the compensatory muscle functions developed by a 10-year-old boy whose tongue was removed surgically 6 days after birth. He developed essentially normal phonological (articulatory) oral language skills and intelligible speech by 3 years of age, which he maintained throughout childhood. Videofluoroscopic and direct visual analysis studies revealed that the glossopalatinus muscles running through the anterior pillars of fauces had actually hypertrophied to the point that they regularly moved across the posterior oral cavity to effectively touch each other at midline to produce the /k/ and /g/ speech sound elements in connected speech.

This boy's main remaining facial skeletal abnormality was due to restricted growth of the mandible, which was related to the force of scar contraction in the floor of the mouth. This enabled him to substitute lower lip movements for the normal anterior tongue articulation contacts needed to approximate all bilabial, lingua-dental, and lingua-alveolar consonant sound elements in connected speech with a normal rate and phonological inflection.

This principle, then, emphasizes the importance that speech pathologists should place on the possible effects over time that speech motor patterns and other oral functions can have on normal or acceptable growth and development of the facies and dental arches, and on the compensatory articulation potential for intelligible speech production in the absence of normal speech articulation structures.

Principle V. A functional coordinated team approach is necessary for the regular effective habilitation of infants born with cleft lip, cleft palate, or related craniofacial disorders. The objective of the clinical cleft palate team is to bring the individual child, as early in life as possible, to the point where the child does not differ significantly from his or her peers in health, education, or the ability to interact socially with others [38]. The goals are to provide the surgical, medical, dental, counseling, and interventive therapy services needed to achieve essentially normal speech and language development and skills, facial appearance, dento-occlusal development, and hearing. If any one of these goals is not achieved, it can have a negative effect on the others and make a significant difference in the personal life of the child born with cleft lip or palate. The coordination of services from several health care specialties appears to be the key to reaching these goals.

What the plastic surgeon does to reconstruct the cleft areas will influence the ability of the pedodontist or orthodontist to achieve normal dento-occlusal development. Dental specialists should work closely with the primary surgeon to achieve the best possible results. At what age, by previous training or individual case necessity, the plastic surgeon chooses to complete primary reconstruction of the palate, the timing of the procedure will greatly influence the ability of the

speech pathologist to guide the child through the normal stages of emergent language development without the development of functional cleft palate speech compensations.

For these reasons, the basic cleft palate team is formed around the plastic surgeon, dental specialists, and speech pathologist working cooperatively in a team approach. However, experience has shown that other health care specialists are often needed to achieve team goals. An otherwise complete and coordinated treatment program which ignores the frequent otological complications until school age often fails to achieve the overall goals of the cleft palate team. Today, provision for genetic counseling, audiological testing, pediatric and otological medical care, and psychological counseling services are a usual and important part of the team approach.

Chapter 4 covers the usual roles of the various specialists involved in the craniofacial team. There is general agreement today among medical, other health care, and educational services that the goal of early normalization of this population is most efficiently provided by an individualized treatment program developed and carried out through a coordinated team approach.

RELATED BASIC EMBRYOLOGY

The usual occurrence of clefts of the facies or palate is best understood through a review of the early embryological development of these structures. The preferred classification systems for studying clefts of the primary and secondary palate are based on embryological development. The clinical student should have an understanding of where and why clefts of the face or mouth are most likely to occur, and particularly when in the early calendar of fetal development a particular cleft could have occurred. For a more comprehensive review, the reader is referred to Patten [42] and Millard [34, 36], as well as Zemlin [56] and Crelin [11].

A review of early embryological development indicates that clefts of the face or palate all occur from some disturbance of the usual fusing of processes in the anterior head area in the first 2½ months after conception. This fact often helps in counseling parents who blame themselves for some occurrence which happened in the second or third trimester. A general description of the complex process of the formation of the face and mouth follows.

EARLIEST EMBRYOLOGICAL DEVELOPMENT

An extremely rapid multiplication of similar cells begins in the fallopian tube approximately 24 hours after fertilization of the ovum by a single microscopic sperm. The new potential human individual spends its first days gradually moving through the fallopian tube while its similar unspecialized cells are multiplying. It passes into the uterus as a tiny human seed inside a spherical vesicle of cells. If successfully implanted in the uterine lining, the seed continues to multiply, its cells increasing into a disk shape with two specialized cell layers leading to the differentiation of three types of specialized cells. The berry-shaped cell mass enlarges outward, creating a central depression called a *blastula*. An *inner cell mass*, which is identifiably darker, begins grouping together and through rapid multiplication forms the primitive gut. The blastula continues growing rapidly forming a flattened platelike formation called the *embryonic disk*. By the third week of development, the primitive formation of the *stomodeum*, or mouth area, can be identified surrounded by the developing brain above and heart below, as illustrated in Figure 1-3A. After the third week the embryo already has a functioning body with identifiable head features. After this stage rapid growth occurs with maturation proceeding in a cephalocaudal direction (i.e., the head and its structures are growing much more rapidly and will mature before the trunk and the limbs). By the time the infant is 1 year old the brain has already attained 50 percent of its adult weight.

The stomodeum, or primitive mouth area, initially ends blindly and is not connected to the foregut. As the stomodeal depression is deepened, its ectodermal floor comes to lie against the entodermal lining of the foregut. This two-layered membrane is known as the oral plate or buccopharyngeal membrane (see Fig. 1-3A). In human embryos, it breaks through toward the end of the fourth week (see Fig. 1-3B) to establish the oral opening to the lungs and internal organs.

Three primordial cell layers develop within the embryonic disk. Each will give rise to different types of body structures. From the *ectoderm*, the outermost layer of cells in the embryonic disk, are developed the brain and nervous system, hair and nails, the lining of the oral and nasal cavities, the pharynx, the epidermis, and the dental enamel. The *endoderm* is the innermost cell layer of the embryonic disk. The endoderm gives rise to the esophagus, stomach, intestines, respiratory organs, the tissue covering the larynx, the structures of the middle ear, and the eustachian tube. The *mesoderm* is the middle layer, and gives rise to the bony skeleton and the muscles, blood, cartilage, and connective tissues.

It is in the second month after conception then, between 5½ and 8 weeks of development, that the primary processes forming the face and upper lip come together and fuse. Clefts of the facies, lip, and premaxilla may occur during this period. Between the eighth and ninth week of embryogenesis, the palatal processes forming the roof of the mouth and dividing it from the nose should meet, be penetrated by mesodermal cells, and fuse, forming the primitive hard and soft palates. It is during this early period of uterine development, therefore, that cleft lip and palate occurs for 1 in every 600 to 700 human live births. Our next focus is to review and illustrate some detail of the morphogenesis of the face and mouth from 5½ to 10 weeks after conception.

MORPHOGENESIS OF THE FACE AND MOUTH

The normal development of the face is best basically understood as the final complex process of the merging and fusion of five *processes, prominences, or swellings,* completing the basic formation of structures of the face surrounding the stomodeum or primitive mouth and nasal cavities. These prominences include (1) the frontonasal process, which grows downward from the forebrain; (2) and (3) the two maxillary processes, which grow forward and mediad; and (4) and (5) the two mandibular processes below (2) and (3) which fuse first to form the mandible and lower lip.

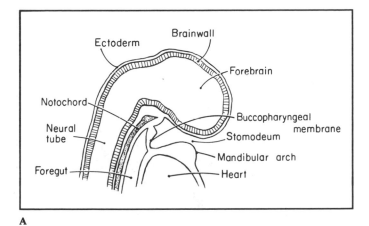

A

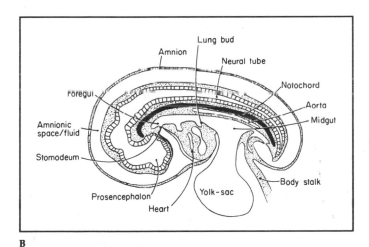

B

Figure 1-3. A. Three-week embryo; buccopharyngeal membrane intact. B. Four-week embryo after rupture of buccopharyngeal membrane.

The frontonasal process as it grows downward gives rise to two specialized patches of widely separated ectodermal cells, which grow into depressions, developing the *olfactory pits.* By the end of the sixth week, as illustrated in Figure 1-4, these circular pits, along with the downward growth of the frontonasal process, cause a division of the frontonasal process into the *median nasal processes* and two *lateral nasal processes* which develop lateral to the olfactory pits. The lateral nasal processes form the alar cartilages of the nose and also must fuse with the two maxillary processes to form part of the infraorbital area of the midface. These processes must fuse with the max-

illary processes, or oblique facial clefts can occur in this area. The median nasal process continues growing downward to form the *globular process,* which forms the remaining structures that originate from the median nasal process, including the primary palate or human premaxillary structures. Cleft lip, or rather clefts of the primary palate, will occur if the globular process fails to fuse with the paired maxillary processes to form the upper middle lip and the entire premaxilla, including the anterior alveolar ridge with its two central and two lateral incisor teeth. Figures 1-4 and 1-5A and B illustrate what fusion processes fail to occur when a cleft lip or cleft of the primary palate presents at birth. Cleft lip predisposes to the formation of cleft palate. Approximately 42 precent of children born with cleft lip also present with cleft palate.

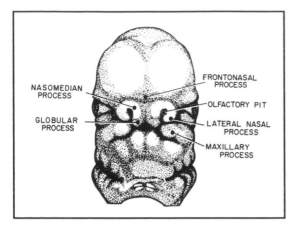

Figure 1-4. Frontal drawing of a 6-week embryo showing formation of the face through fusing of five major processes.

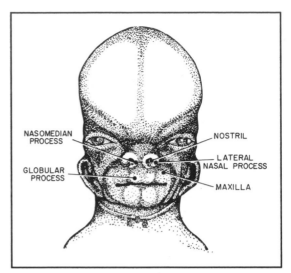

A

FORMATION OF THE SECONDARY PALATE

Following the formation and fusion of the primary palate and mid–upper lip at between 5½ and 8 weeks of gestation, the secondary palate (hard and soft palate structures) forms at between 8 and 10 weeks of gestation, dividing the nasal from the oral structures. These structures are formed from the two palatal processes of the maxillary processes which grow out medially from the inner aspect of the maxillary processes. Until the eighth week of fetal development, these processes, or palatal shelves, lie almost perpendicular to the sides of the tongue, which is carried high in the stomodeum filling the area which will become both the nasal and the oral cavities.

Between the eighth and the ninth week, there is a sudden growth spurt in both the length and the width of the mandible and its neuromotor connections which enables the mandible to swing open. The tongue drops out of the nasal cavity area as rapid differential growth of the palatal shelves bring them into a horizontal position enabling them to touch and fuse starting at the most anterior point behind the primary palate.

Figure 1-6 illustrates the process of normal fusion of the palatal shelves from this anterior contact backward. It also appears necessary that only two, rather than three or more, layers of epithelium have formed on the edges of the palatal shelves and that programmed cell death occurs in the epithelium in order for mesoderm to penetrate and form the joined hard and soft palates. A

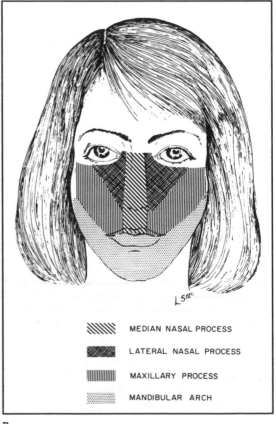

▨	MEDIAN NASAL PROCESS
▨	LATERAL NASAL PROCESS
▥	MAXILLARY PROCESS
░	MANDIBULAR ARCH

B

Figure 1-5. Facial components developed from the five major processes. A. Complete joining of the facial processes at end of 8 weeks. B. Components of the adult face derived from each process.

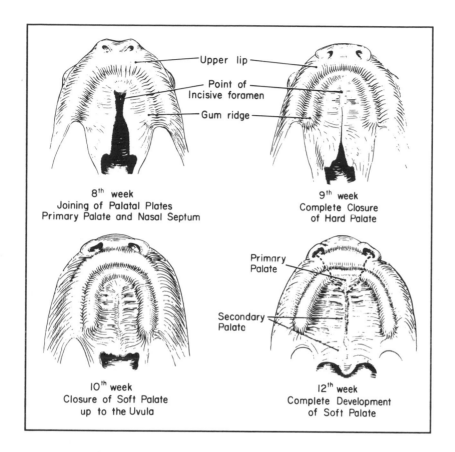

Upper lip

Point of
Incisive foramen

Gum ridge

8th week
Joining of Palatal Plates
Primary Palate and Nasal Septum

9th week
Complete Closure
of Hard Palate

Primary
Palate

Secondary
Palate

10th week
Closure of Soft Palate
up to the Uvula

12th week
Complete Development
of Soft Palate

Figure 1-6. Palatal fusion which takes place as a wedge-shaped closure from front to back.

delay in the timing of contact of the palatal shelves or a lack of mesodermal penetration may cause a failure of the final fusion process, resulting in an isolated cleft of the secondary palate. As the palatal shelves join, they also join and fuse with the inferior edge of the nasal septum which has grown downward to meet them, dividing the right and left nasal cavities. In view of the complexity of these final processes of joining the right and left palatal processes, it seems surprising that more clefts of the secondary palate do not occur, rather than that some do. Clefts of the secondary palate only are sex-linked and occur more frequently in females than in males.

The all-important muscles of the soft palate or velum for speech also evolve from the palatal shelves. This final part of the secondary palatal structures forms beyond the attachment to the nasal septum between the 10th and 12th weeks, also developing from anterior to posterior. Com- plete palatal fusion and the formation of the muscles involved in velopharyngeal functions for later speech development is completed by the 12th week of fetal development.

USEFUL AND PREFERRED CLASSIFICATION SYSTEMS

The following information on classification of cleft lip and cleft palate is drawn mainly from the more extensive review of Berlin [5], who stated in 1979: "A standardized and universally accepted classification of cleft lip and palate does not yet exist." Unfortunately, this is still the case. The process of reaching that goal has become exceedingly more complex through the similar need for an acceptable classification system for related craniofacial disorders and subclassifications for clefts occurring with syndromes. I present here only the most frequently used classification systems found to be most useful at this time along with a bibliography for further reading.

The early classification systems proposed by surgeons and orthodontists tended to emphasize the anatomical areas and structures where clefts and malformations needing surgical or dental reconstruction were found in birth. They often separated clefts of the alveolus from cleft lip, although embryologically these structures derive from the same processes. The early classification system of Dorrance [15], Olin [40], and Davis and Ritchie [12] provided such separate categories for alveolar clefts. The classification systems proposed by interdisciplinary committees of the American Cleft Palate Association (ACPA) in the past and similar groups working on the problem today prefer systems based on embryogenesis as reviewed above.

Current thinking based on more recently identified syndromes with cleft lip and palate also strives to categorize syndromal clefts by their underlying metabolic or sequential etiologies. Craniofacial abnormalities are classified by the areas, structures, or the types of tissues affected.

USEFUL CLINICAL CLASSIFICATION SYSTEMS

It appears at this time that the two most useful short clinical reference systems available are the early short but incomplete identification system proposed by Veau in 1931 [53] and the more complete clinical classification system based on Kernahan and Stark's then (1958) new classification of cleft lip and palate [29] as it has evolved into Kernahan's striped Y system [27, 28], a symbolic recording system is illustrated in Figure 1-7.

Although the Veau system is too incomplete for clinical record use today, it is useful for quick general reference when reviewing the nature of isolated cleft case studies to be evaluated in upcoming clinics. That is, it is easier to note that John S. to be examined or reexamined this week was born with a Veau class III cleft on the left side rather than noting that his original presenting condition involved complete clefts of both the primary and secondary palates, or prepalate and palate, involving the floor of the nose, the lip, and premaxillary structures up to the incisive foramen, and the entire midline of the remaining hard and soft palate structures. The Veau system, which is still used to classify many of the cases presenting to cleft palate teams, is as follows:

Group I. Cleft of the soft palate only
Group II. Cleft of the hard and soft palate to the incisive foramen
Group III. Complete unilateral cleft of the soft and hard palate and of the lip and alveolar ridge on one side
Group IV. Complete bilateral cleft of the soft and hard palate and/or the lip and alveolar ridge on both sides.

The recommended schematic striped Y-system with Elasahy's [16] and Millard's [34] revisions is now more useful, even for routine clinical team classification purposes. It is generally compatible with the basic criterion of being based on the normal pattern of embryogenesis and with the more detailed classification system recommended by the nomenclature committee of the ACPA [24] in 1960 and published in its final version by Harkins et al. in 1962 [25].

Figure 1-7. Kernahan's striped Y for symbolic clinical classification.

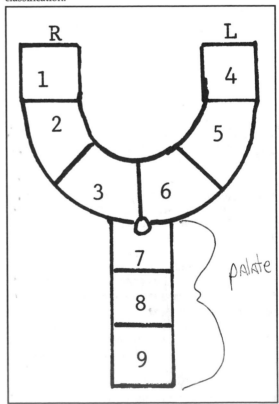

The modified striped Y-system, illustrated in Figure 1-8, is recommended at present for more routine clinical classification purposes. It can be recorded in a corner of the clinic identification form and provides a quick visual reference as well as depicting the original extent of presenting isolated clefts of the primary and secondary palates and combined clefts of the prepalate and palate. It is useful for roughly equating groups of subjects for simple clinical research as well as for clinical reference purposes. The numbering system provides some compatibility for computer storage and retrieval of classification data. As modified by Elasahy's revision [16] and Millard's addition of an inverted triangle, this system has recently been well illustrated [34].

Figure 1-7 illustrates the basic striped Y system proposed by Kernahan in 1973 [28]. In this figure, the stem of the Y represents the palate and the branching arms represent the lip, the alveolar process, and the premaxillary segment on the right and the left sides to the incisive foramen (small circle). The examiner records degrees of clefts within the numbered segments by shading within the basic diagram.

Figure 1 8 illustrates the striped Y as modified by Elasahy [16] and renumbered by him to include 13 sections. He added triangles onto the top of the arms numbered 1 and 5 in this figure to represent each nasal floor. He added a circle between the arms numbered 13 to permit indication of the amount of protrusion of the premaxilla, and he added a circle below the stem numbered 12 to indicate velopharyngeal incompetency. As renumbered, triangles 1 and 5 represent the floor of the nose on the right and left sides; sections 2 and 6 represent the lip; sections 3 and 7 represent the alveolar ridges; and sections 4 and 8, the premaxilla to the incisive foramen (small circle). The stem is numbered 9 and 10 for each half of the hard palate and 11 for the soft palate. The circle number 12 was added to represent those cases presenting with congenital velopharyngeal incompetency without obvious clefts. This figure also includes the inverted triangles at the end of the branching arms, which were added by Millard [34] to indicate distortions of the alar cartilages of the nose. Use of the modified striped Y system eliminates the former differences in terminology for major divisions (i.e., clefts of the primary palate only, clefts of the secondary palate only, and clefts of the primary and secondary palates in the original Kernahan and Stark terminology compared to clefts of the prepalate, clefts of the palate, and clefts of the prepalate and

palate in the ACPA system). The modified striped Y system also provides numerical categories compatible for computer-processed data storage and retrieval, but the necessity of using different lines and shadings to indicate the finer extent of clefts within sections limits its usefulness for research.

PREFERRED CLASSIFICATION SYSTEMS

Specific identifying information on the extent of isolated cleft lip and palate with an added sub-

Figure 1-8. Elasahy's revised striped Y including Millard's inverted triangle.

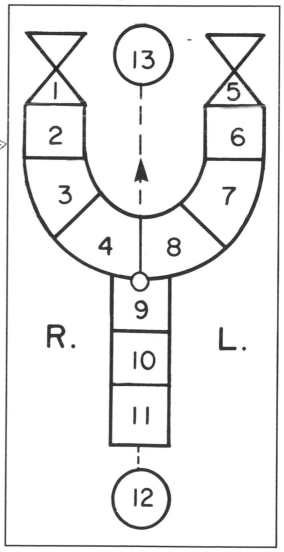

classification by known syndromes with and without clefts, and a basic classification describing the extent of craniofacial malformations documented by pictures and x-ray data as necessary, are needed for controlled clinical research purposes. Therefore, the more detailed system recommended for classifying cleft lip and palate and previously approved by the ACPA [25] is the system generally preferred today. Although it has its deficiencies, it is still the most widely used system for detailed classification of isolated clefts and meets most of the criteria proposed earlier by Pruzansky [44], Koepp–Baker [30], and Berlin [5]. This system is recommended for clinical research purposes in large cleft palate centers.

Pruzansky's description, classification, and analysis of unoperated clefts of the lip and palate, published in 1953 [44], was the direct precursor of present thinking on classification systems. He first proposed using only three major headings as follows: (1) cleft lip, (2) cleft lip and palate, and (3) cleft palate, and considered any separate category for alveolar clefts as unnecessary and misleading. The earlier, classic book by Fogh–Anderson [17] on the inheritance of "harelip" and cleft palate preceded this conceptual change by proposing a single genetic classification for harelip in which associated alveolar clefts that might extend through the premaxillary segments as far as the incisive foramen were included. Genetically, cleft lip of any extent through the primary palate, whether it presents with cleft palate or not, is a separate entity from any isolated cleft of the soft or hard palate. Clefts of the lip or primary palate with or without cleft palate will occur predominantly in males whereas clefts limited to the palate occur predominantly in females.

Based on both genetic and embryological premises, the original Kernahan and Stark recommendations in 1958 [29] followed by the recommendations by Harkins et al. from the ACPA in 1960 [24] and 1962 [25] have been those most frequently adopted in cleft palate centers. They seem to represent today the most useful classification systems for detailing the variations in isolated clefts of the lip and palate. The more detailed ACPA classification is presented in Table 1-1.

More work in this area is needed. Even these recommended classification systems fall short of detailing the differences in width of clefts, availability of muscular velar tags, and other significant variables affecting the outcome of primary palatal surgical reconstruction. Figure 1-9 presents some of the varying configurations of cleft palates affecting the outcome of these procedures. The clefts are all complete to the incisive foramen and fall into the same classification of the ACPA system. However, the extreme width of the upper left primary cleft includes little hard palate bony shelf and no visible nasal septum. Other clefts of the secondary palate do not have this same deficiency of related structures critical for effective reconstruction. Contrast this illustration to the similar classified but pear-shaped cleft in the upper right and to the V-shaped cleft in the lower right. Although these clefts would be classified as similar, their differences could be critical for evaluating the later efficacy of specific primary palatal reconstruction procedures.

The very different clefts illustrated in Figure 1-10 also reveal some unresolved problems of classification for future clinical research. The infant shown in the bottom left and right of the figure had an atypical oral-facial-digital syndrome malformation. There was an almost total absence of muscular tissue where the soft palate tags should be. There was also an occult midline submucous cleft through the hard palate and there were connective tissue bands across the mandibular alveolar ridge and tongue. Despite these unusual malformations, this infant was successfully managed with a speech appliance and developed age-appropriate language skills. The two upper illustrations of overt clefts through the soft and part of the hard palate would be classified similarly by the ACPA classification system, but their obvious differences do present different surgical problems for functional palatal reconstruction.

Chapter 2 provides a detailed discussion with more extensive references in regard to basic concepts in congenital craniofacial disorders. However, Figure 1-11 is presented here as an introduction to current concepts in regard to the classification of congenital or acquired craniofacial disorders. The classification is based both on embryogenesis and on the necessary surgical manipulation required in craniofacial surgery. This figure by Habal [21] includes a drawing of the earlier Tessier anatomical classification of facial, craniofacial, and laterofacial clefts [52].

As discussed by Habal and Maniscalco [21], the conditions leading to *cranial* deformities present mostly from (1) hydrocephalic, large neurocranium conditions or (2) craniosynostosis. *Cranioorbital* deformities may result from (a) hypertelorism (widely separated eyes) related to frontonasal dysplasia, (b) hypotelorism (eyes close together) related to holoprosencephaly, (c) orbital dystopia

**TABLE 1-1. RECORDING FORM FOR USE OF RECOMMENDED
CLASSIFICATION SYSTEM OF THE AMERICAN CLEFT PALATE ASSOCIATION (ACPA)**

CLEFTS OF PREPALATE

Cleft lip
  Unilateral
    Right, left
    Extent in thirds ($\frac{1}{3}$, $\frac{2}{3}$, $\frac{3}{3}$)
  Bilateral
    Right
    Extent in thirds ($\frac{1}{3}$, $\frac{2}{3}$, $\frac{3}{3}$)
    Left
    Extent in thirds ($\frac{1}{3}$, $\frac{2}{3}$, $\frac{3}{3}$)
  Median
    Extent in thirds ($\frac{1}{3}$, $\frac{2}{3}$, $\frac{3}{3}$)
  Prolabium
    Small, medium, large
  Congenital Scar
    Right, left, median
    Extent in thirds ($\frac{1}{3}$, $\frac{2}{3}$, $\frac{3}{3}$)

Cleft of alveolar process
  Unilateral
    Right, left
    Extent in thirds ($\frac{1}{3}$, $\frac{2}{3}$, $\frac{3}{3}$)
  Bilateral
    Right
    Extent in thirds ($\frac{1}{3}$, $\frac{2}{3}$, $\frac{3}{3}$)
    Left
    Extent in thirds ($\frac{1}{3}$, $\frac{2}{3}$, $\frac{3}{3}$)
  Median
    Extent in thirds ($\frac{1}{6}$, $\frac{2}{3}$, $\frac{3}{3}$)
  Submucous
    Right, left, median

Cleft of prepalate
  Any combination of foregoing types
  Prepalate protrusion
  Prepalate rotation
  Prepalate arrest (median cleft)

CLEFTS OF THE PALATE

Clefts of soft palate
  Extent
    Posterior to anterior ($\frac{1}{3}$, $\frac{2}{3}$, $\frac{3}{3}$)
    Width (maximum in millimeters)
  Palatal shortness
    None, slight, moderate, marked
  Submucous cleft
    Extent ($\frac{1}{3}$, $\frac{2}{3}$, $\frac{3}{3}$)

Cleft of hard palate
  Extent
    Posterior to anterior ($\frac{1}{3}$, $\frac{2}{3}$, $\frac{3}{3}$)
    Width (maximum in millimeters)
  Vomer attachment
    Right, left, absent
  Submucous cleft
    Extent ($\frac{1}{3}$, $\frac{2}{3}$, $\frac{3}{3}$)

CLEFTS OF PREPALATE AND PALATE

Any combination of clefts described above under
clefts of prepalate and clefts of palate

**FACIAL CLEFTS OTHER THAN PREPALATE
AND PALATE**

Yes, no*
If yes, use also velopharyngeal classification form
and/or syndrome description in basic records.*

* Added to basic ACPA classification for recording form.

(eyes on different horizontal planes), or (d) exorbitism (retroposed eye sockets) as may be present in untreated Apert and Crouzon syndromes.

Craniomaxillofacial deformities include (a) Apert syndrome, (b) Crouzon syndrome, (c) Pfeiffer syndrome, and (d) Carpenter syndrome. *Craniomandibulofacial bilateral* deformities are mainly cases presenting with Treacher Collins syndrome and *Craniomandibulofacial unilateral* deformities which compose varying degrees of hemifacial microsomia and Goldenhar syndrome.

Craniofacial cleft deformities (Tessier clefts) may be (a) midline clefts from frontonasal dysplasia, (b) oblique clefts, or (c) transverse clefts. *Cleft lip deformities,* shown in Figure 1-6, refer to (a) early or (b) late sequelae of midface growth arrest following surgery for cleft lip and palate and usually requiring orthognathic surgery. *Mandibular deformities* include (a) prognathism (forward-jutting

mandible) and (b) segmental deformities of the mandible from various causes requiring surgical reconstruction of the mandible. In his discussion of craniofacial deformities Habal [21] also felt there was a need to include a category for unspecified craniofacial clefts and categories for traumatic deformities and deformities secondary to tumor resection.

The above review of the literature indicates that, as in the past, the struggle for an ideal solution to standardized reporting is far from resolved. Some useful and even preferred classification systems have been presented for the reader's information and initial use in the cleft palate and craniofacial disorders area. Many valid criticisms of the presently available classification systems have been and should be raised. There is a continuing need for a more complete classification of neurogenic velopharyngeal incompetency prob-

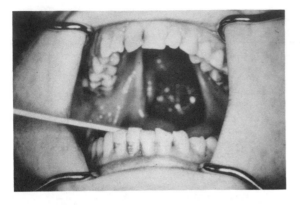
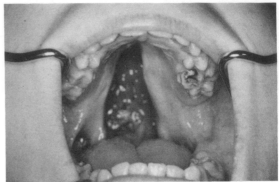
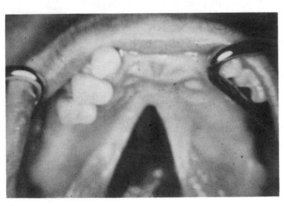
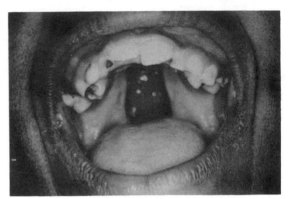

Figure 1-9. Variations in clefts of the hard and soft palates which are not accounted for by present classification systems.

lems and a less redundant classification of craniofacial and syndromal disorders.

RELATED BASIC ANATOMY OF VELOPHARYNGEAL FUNCTIONS FOR SPEECH

Our purpose here is to relate the several paired muscles of the velum which accomplish the rapid velopharyngeal functions underlying normal speech production in such a way as to enhance later clinical observations or research investigations related to cleft palate speech disorders. Descriptions of the paired muscles and the structures of and surrounding the velopharyngeal mechanism that are critical for normal speech

production are introduced under the subheadings *On Veils and Curtains, On Slings and Arrows, On Sphincters and Pads, On Hearing and Movement,* and *On Age and Sex* to aid in the understanding of related concepts which assist in later recall of specific muscles and related structures.

The reader is encouraged to consult additional sources for further detailed illustrations while studying the muscles and anatomical structures described here. Basic anatomy texts such as *Gray's Anatomy* [19], *Morris' Human Anatomy* [1], *Cunningham's Manual of Practical Anatomy* [6], and *Oral Anatomy* [49] are useful for reviewing the normal anatomy of the bones and muscles of the face and velopharyngeal mechanism for speech. The finer details of the anatomy and physiology of the velopharyngeal mechanism as a functional part of the entire speech mechanism is well covered in the 1982 text by Dickson and Maue–Dickson [14]. We review here only the normal structures and muscles of the velopharyngeal mechanism.

While it is considered important to know the normal anatomy and physiology of the velophar-

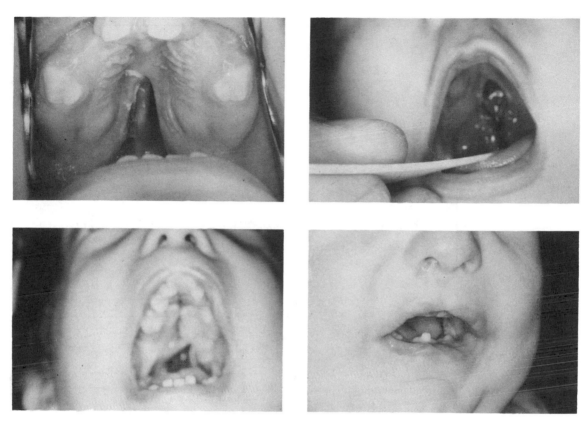

Figure 1-10. Syndromal clefts and incomplete clefts of the palate not completely fitting standard classifications.

yngeal mechanism before undertaking work in this area, it is perhaps more important to learn and understand that the muscle attachments adjacent to congenital clefts of the primary or the secondary palates are abnormal. Their surgical repositioning during reconstruction is usually necessary in order to obtain normal function of the lip and soft palate for speech. An excellent illustrated review of the abnormal insertion of facial lip muscles can be found in Millard's *Cleft Craft*: see Volume 1 [34] for unilateral cleft lip deformities, Volume 2 [35] for the more severe differences found in bilateral complete clefts of the primary palate, and Volume 3 [36] for the abnormalities usually found in palatal muscles with cleft palate. The following more specific references are also recommended for their more detailed discussions and illustrations of the normal and abnormal anatomy of the velopharyngeal mechanism as related to cleft lip and palate: Maue–Dickson [33], Dickson et al. [13], Ross and Johnson [46], Brescia [7], Fritzel [18], Bzoch [9], and Shearer [48].

ON VEILS AND CURTAINS: STRETCH, SEAL, AND COUPLING

The proper name in gross anatomy for the muscular structure called the soft palate is *velum.* If you are a neophyte in the study of anatomy of the speech mechanisms, it is good to learn at the outset that most scientific-sounding anatomical terms are simply Latin or Greek words used by early anatomists to describe structures. Anatomical terms almost always describe either the apparent (1) function, (2) shape, (3) location in the body, or (4) specific points of origin and insertion of muscles. The selection of the word *velum* ("veil" or "curtain") to describe the main function of the soft palate appears to have been a very insightful one, since its functions in speech and deglutition are hidden from the unaided eyes of the observer. Both the Latin and the Greek meanings for velum refer to its having a function similar to that of a curtain or veil. Today, speech pathologists can observe and even measure in detailed videofluoroscopic speech studies the normal and abnormal

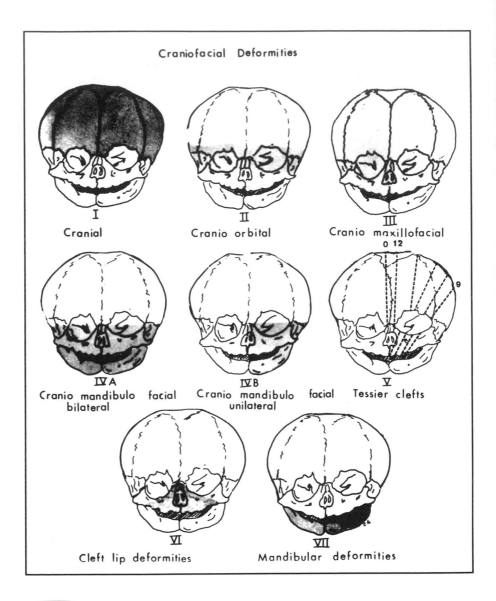

Craniofacial Deformities

I Cranial

II Cranio orbital

III Cranio maxillofacial

IV A Cranio mandibulo facial bilateral

IV B Cranio mandibulo facial unilateral

V Tessier clefts

VI Cleft lip deformities

VII Mandibular deformities

Figure 1-11. Categorization schema of craniofacial deformities by Habal [21, 22].

functions of the velum as it stretches like a curtain or veil across the nasopharynx.

Figure 1-12 illustrates the extent of activity of the velum of an adult during speech production. It illustrates the contrasting positions, length, and shape of this muscular organ as observed and measured from standardized lateral cephalometric x-ray images — at rest and during the production of different types of repeated syllables in speech samples.

The phenomenon referred to as *stretch* of the velum during function for speech can be visualized by comparing the length of the outline of the soft palate at rest with the configurations found for it during syllables initiated by /p/, /b/, /f/,

or /w/. The phenomenon referred to as *seal* of the nasopharynx by the velum (required for the production of nonnasal syllables) can be partly visualized in two dimensions by the firm area of contact of the velum with the posterior nasopharyngeal wall beginning at point Q3, which is three-fourths of the full length of the soft palate in function for speech. The limited extent of velar downward movement required for *coupling* the nasal cavities with the pharyngeal and oral cavities for the production of nasal consonants can be seen by comparing the outlines of the stretched and sealed

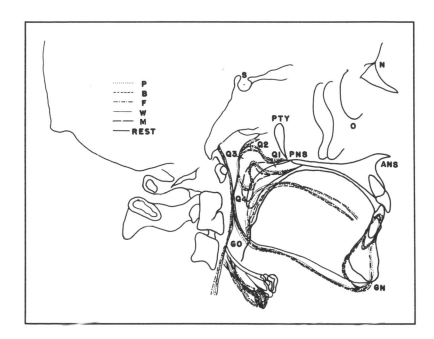

Figure 1-12. The stretch, seal, and coupling phenomena of normal velopharyngeal functions for speech. Q1 through Q4 = 1st through 4th quarters from hard palate to end of soft palate.

velum for the oral consonant syllables with the more central position in the nasopharynx of the velum during the production syllables initiated by /m/.

Figure 1-12 is taken from a report of a biometric cephalometric analysis of records from 44 normal-speaking young adults by Graber et al. [20]. The grouped analysis indicated that the velum, as seen in the lateral view, consistently increases in length from rest to a functional speech position. Other conclusions were that the velum contacts the back wall of the pharynx between the midpoint and the third quadrant (that portion of the soft palate three-fourths distant from the hard palate attachment). This is the usual effective velopharyngeal closure area for normal-speaking young adults. For all subjects, the velum always made a firm closure for repeated oral syllables. It was observed and reported further that the nasopharynx remained only partly open as compared to the rest position during repeated nasal syllable productions. It appears that two paired muscles in particular account for the observed phenomena of the usual normal functioning of the velopharyngeal mechanism for speech.

ON SLINGS AND ARROWS

Most investigators agree that it is the *levator palati* paired muscles and the *palatopharyngeus* whose right and left muscle bundles join at midline in the soft palate to form two interdigitating, strong muscle *slings* which largely account for the stretch, seal, and coupling articulation phenomena necessary for normal speech production. The anatomical positions of these muscle slings and their resultant force on, and direction of movement of, the velum are indicated by the *arrows* in Figure 1-13A and B. A description of these muscles for velopharyngeal valving, and illustrations showing their relations to the other muscles of the velopharyngeal mechanism for speech, are presented below.

The levator palati is illustrated in Figure 1-14 as it might be viewed from a superior and partly lateral-posterior view. It is a strong paired muscle of even dimensions that arises at the base of the skull from a small area on the lower surface of the petrus portion of the temporal bone. It descends in a frontomedial direction along the posterior and inferior border of the eustachian tube. It inserts into the middle third of the soft palate (velum). Within the velum, its fibers spread, interlace with other palatal muscles, and join at midline with the levator fibers from the other side of the palate to form a strong muscle sling superiorly based from points of origin above, lateral to, and behind the velum.

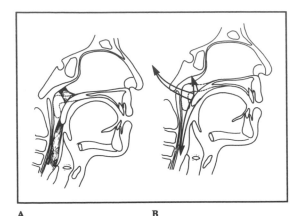

A   **B**

Figure 1-13. A. Relative positions of the paired muscular slings of the levator palati and the palatopharyngeus at rest. B. Arrows indicate the resultant upward and backward force of their simultaneous contractions.

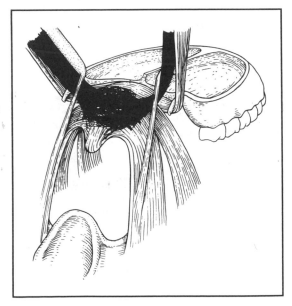

Figure 1-14. Position of the levator veli palatini muscles in relation to the other muscles of the velopharyngeal mechanism.

The levator palati muscle is innervated by the pharyngeal plexus which also supplies innervation to all the other muscles of the velopharyngeal mechanism except the *tensor palati* and the *musculus uvulae*. This plexus is composed of branches of four cranial nerves which indicates its high priority in human anatomy, as the velopharyngeal mechanism is intimately involved in respiration and deglutition as well as in the uniquely human evolu-

tionary function of speech. Branches of the glossopharynegeus, the vagus, the sympathetic, and the cranial portions of the accessory nerves constitute this plexus. Research reported by Nishio et al. [39] also indicates that the levator palati, the musculus uvulae, and the superior constrictor muscles of the velopharyngeal mechanism receive an additional motor innervation from the facial nerve.

It appears from electromyographic (EMG) research studies that it is the levator palati muscles which contribute the major upward and backward force on the velum. This accomplishes its necessary stretch, elevation, and sealing-off of the nasopharynx to enable oral speech production. This muscle is often considered the primary muscle for oral speech production [3, 4, 18]. The levator may also assist in eustachian tube functions of regulating air pressure in the middle ear that is so important for the high level of acuity requisite for the early development of speech and language skills. Abnormal function of this muscle has recently been related to blockage of eustachian tube function. However, if you look closely at the attachments and insertion of this muscle sling, it is apparent that its effects on the eustachian tubes is usually indirect rather than direct. The normal midline insertions of this muscle sling are obviously absent in a child born with cleft palate. The paired muscles with clefts of the palate actually insert forward in a direct or indirect attachment to the posterior and lateral margins of the cleft hard palate. This abnormal insertion obviously interrupts the sling action of the paired levator muscles which should lift the repaired velum upward and backward to accomplish velopharyngeal valving requisite for normal speech production. Modern reconstructive surgery techniques, which are most successful, consider this need and provide for the retropositioning of the levator sling (a technique called intervelar veloplasties) to enhance the "batting average" of successful primary reconstructions of the soft palate.

The second most important muscular sling is formed by the paired *palatopharyngeus muscles* which originate from a wide area on the posterior border of the thyroid cartilage and the aponeurosis of the side and back walls of the laryngopharynx. This muscle sling is illustrated in Figure 1-15 as it relates to the levator sling and other muscles of the velopharyngeal mechanism for speech. Its muscle fibers are generally oriented vertically from these points of origin to run upward and forward in the lateral laryngeal and oral pharynx,

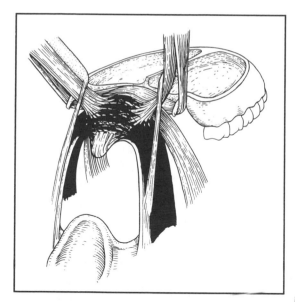

Figure 1-15. Position of the palatopharyngeus muscles in relation to the other muscles of the velopharyngeal mechanism.

converging in the side walls of the velum, and meeting in midline in the velum.

These muscle fibers interdigitate with those of the levator palati to form most of the muscular components of the midsections of the soft palate. The paired right and left muscle bundles meet and join at midline in the velum forming another sling pulling downward and backward on the velum. This apparently helps to stretch the velum across the nasopharynx during speech.

The palatopharyngeus muscle runs through the posterior pillars of fauces, just behind the tonsils, which fold marks the accepted division of the oral cavity from the pharynx. They are usually easily observed in an interoral examination of the speech mechanism which should be a part of any speech pathology evaluation.

Figure 1-13A illustrates the relative positions of these two muscle slings in lateral view within the supralaryngeal organs of the speech mechanism. The resultant lifting and stretching force of these two muscle slings indicated by the arrows in Figure 1-13B illustrates how the physiologist Podvinek [43] originally conceived of how their interaction helped to accomplish the movements of the velum observed in speech. This description remains the best account of the usual stretching and elevation movements of the velum required for normal voice and speech production.

ON SPHINCTERS AND PADS

The early concept of a simple trap door–like movement of the soft palate, as seen from the lateral view and described in the early research literature on velopharyngeal valving for speech, is incomplete. When viewed in three dimensions, velopharyngeal valving function can be seen to involve rather a *sphincterlike* closure movement pattern. A more recent theory of how the relationship of the muscles and structures surrounding the velopharyngeal mechanism accomplish velopharyngeal functions for speech properly considers this function in three dimensions rather than two dimensions. As can now be observed through cine- or videofluoroscopy or nasopharyngoscopy, as described in Chapters 11 and 12, respectively, the velopharyngeal mechanism functioning for speech actually closes and seals through a sphincteric closure pattern.

As velopharyngeal closure for speech occurs, the velum not only moves upward and backward to accomplish seal, but the side walls of the nasopharynx also move medially, often very extensively, contributing to closure. Occasionally, the back wall of the nasopharynx also moves forward creating a bulge at the point of closure or below. This is referred to as *Passavant's pad*, although it is a muscular bulge rather than a permanent pad in the nasopharynx. Also, the *adenoid pad*, which develops in early childhood above and behind the velum to become a semipermanent pad contributing to velopharyngeal closure and seal in children and young adults, provides a forward bulge aiding in firm closure, especially for postoperative cleft palate subjects. The manner in which these two pads may assist in achieving velopharyngeal closure for speech is illustrated in Figure 1-16A and B.

The muscle which could account for this sphincteric closure movement pattern as well as the occasional forward bulge of a Passavant's pad is the *superior pharyngeal constrictor*. Some investigators have also listed the *salpingopharyngeal muscles* as possibly assisting in the mesial movement of the lateral nasopharyngeal walls assisting in velopharyngeal closure. There is usually marked mesial movement of the lateral pharyngeal walls but seldom significant forward movement of the posterior wall of the nasopharynx to assist in effective velopharyngeal closure.

Dickson and Maue–Dickson [14], however, state from numerous dissections that the salpingopha-

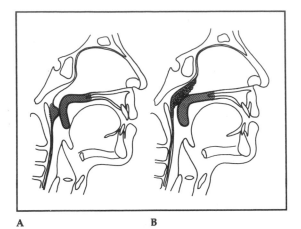

Figure 1-16. The two "pads" which may affect velopharyngeal valving. A. Anterior prominence of an actual Passavant's pad from cephalometric tracing. B. Usual position of the adenoid pad.

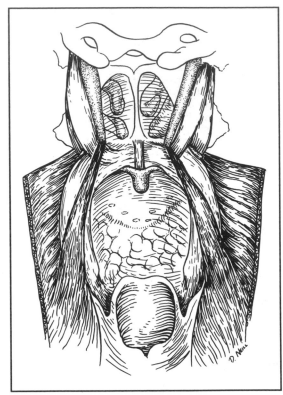

Figure 1-17. Posterior-superior view of nasopharynx; superior pharyngeal constrictor divided and spread laterally, revealing relative positions of several muscles of velopharyngeal mechanism.

ryngeus fold seems to contain few muscle fibers. It is also often absent of muscle in human subjects, composed primarily of glandular tissues. The other muscle probably involved in this sphincteric movement pattern (i.e., the superior pharyngeal constrictor) is able to account for the frequently observed sphincteric closure phenomenon described below.

The superior pharyngeal constrictor muscle illustrated in Figure 1-17 constitutes most of the muscular wall of the upper pharynx. Its fibers generally form a broad-band loop which is open anteriorly from its points of origin from bone or connective tissue except for one portion which originates from the muscles of the soft palate, and the most inferior section which originates from the back portion of the tongue.

These two complete muscular rings of the superior pharyngeal constrictor muscular fibers seem to be capable of true sphincteric closures at these points of origin. The broad anterior points of origin of this muscle include (1) the hamulus process and adjacent portions of the lower half of the medial pterygoid plates of the sphenoid bone of the skull, (2) the velum, (3) the pterygomandibular raphe, (4) the posterior end of the mylohyoid line on the inner aspect of the mandible, and (5) the posterior and inferior portion of the tongue. From these sites of origin, the muscle fibers curve backward, first laterally and then medially, in a mainly horizontal direction to insert into a median fibrous raphe in the posterior midline of the upper pharynx. The lower part of the superior

pharyngeal constrictor is overlapped by fibers of the medial pharyngeal constrictor which also inserts into a medial raphe or connected tissue which extends downward through the pharynx. This muscle in turn is overlapped by the inferior pharyngeal constrictor which completes the muscular lining of the entire pharynx.

Contraction of the superior constrictor muscles would obviously constitute the main possible muscle contraction to explain the regularly observed narrowing and lateral movement of the upper pharyngeal area during velopharyngeal valving for speech. The most effective movement would be in the lateral nasopharyngeal walls due to the insertion of the the muscle fibers into an immobile median raphe on the posterior wall. However, the inconsistent occurrence of a Passavant's pad [41] with marked forward movement of the posterior wall must also be accomplished by the superior constrictor. The forward bulge of the Passavant's pad, when it occurs, appears to be due to those complete circular muscle fibers of the superior constrictor which originate in the velum and form a true sphincter.

The *salpingopharyngeus muscle* may also contribute to the lateral wall movement in the nasopharynx during velopharyngeal valving for speech. Indeed, a distinct salpingopharyngeal fold is often clearly indented in prosthetic speech appliance bulbs inserted in the nasopharynx to correct gross velopharyngeal incompetency when this method of correction is utilized rather than secondary surgical reconstruction of the velopharyngeal mechanism. The relative position of this muscle when present is illustrated in Figure 1-18. It can be seen in this figure that the salpingopharyngeus branches off from the palatopharyngeus in the oropharynx to insert into the cartilaginous wall of the eustachian tubes.

Considered as a separate muscle, the salpingopharyngeus originates on the posterior-lateral walls of the laryngopharynx. Its fibers are vertically oriented medial to the generally horizontally oriented fibers of the three pharyngeal constrictor muscles surrounding the pharynx. From this area of origin this paired muscle courses upward in the lateral walls of the pharynx to insert into the tip of the medial cartilaginous wall of the eustachian tubes. These muscles often produce a sharp narrow ridge, termed the salpingopharyngeal fold, on the lateral wall of the nasopharynx just below and behind the eustachian tube orifices. On con-

striction, this muscle could assist in narrowing the lateral nasopharyngeal walls as well as in opening the inferior end of the eustachian tube during swallow and other functions to balance air pressure in the middle ear cavity.

The adenoid pad illustrated in Figure 1-16B is of special interest in our review of velopharyngeal function for speech. It is a usually developing mass of lymphatic tissue related to the tonsils which develops in the upper posterior nasopharynx and is known as the *adenoid.* The adenoid pad, also called the pharyngeal tonsil, develops in early childhood on the posterior wall of the nasopharynx, mainly between the openings of the eustachian tubes.

The adenoid or pharyngeal tonsil has a physiological purpose similar to the *palatine tonsils*, mainly, to limit and control the frequent upper respiratory infections which occur for most human beings in childhood and adolescence. It allows the body to develop antibodies to the most frequent strains of infectious bacteria that invade the body through the upper respiratory tract.

The *tonsils* (i.e., palatine tonsils) can be seen during intraoral speech evaluations between the anterior and posterior pillars of fauces. Hypertrophy of the tonsils appears to have a negative effect on velopharyngeal competency for speech.

The adenoid pad, on the other hand, may greatly facilitate velopharyngeal closure for the many borderline cases of velopharyngeal competency following primary surgical reconstruction of a cleft palate. That is, the palatine tonsils when hypertrophied tend to inhibit velar elevation required to obtain closure and seal in the nasopharynx from a soft palate shortened by scars and underdevelopment due to a congenital cleft and surgical reconstruction. In contrast, the adenoids, which are present as a mass of soft tissue creating a forward bulge on the posterior nasopharynx at about the usual site of velopharyngeal closure for speech, clearly aid in achieving velopharyngeal closure for speech. The adenoid pad can best be visualized from lateral head x-ray or fluoroscopic images or through nasoendoscopy. On x-ray images the pad often appears as a forward bulge on the posterior nasopharynx with an indentation which coincides with the area of closure of the velopharyngeal mechanism. Removal of adenoid tissue in an effort to control chronic or recurrent upper respiratory infections may result in velopharyngeal insufficiency to support nonnasal speech production, particularly in cases of postoperative cleft palate or submucous clefts of the

Figure 1-18. Position of salpingo pharyngeus (when present) in relation to other muscles of velopharyngeal mechanism.

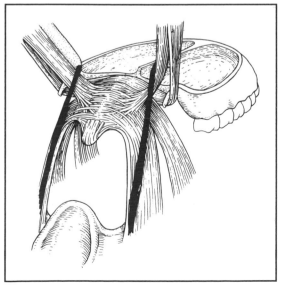

velum which present with borderline adequacy for speech.

While the adenoid pad most often assists in attaining and maintaining velopharyngeal adequacy for speech, it may also hypertrophy to the extent of blocking the nasopharynx, causing hyponasality or denasality of voice quality and possible obstruction of the function of the eustachian tubes. The speech pathologist trained in the cleft palate area is often consulted by otolaryngologists or plastic surgeons regarding the advisability and probable effects of tonsil and adenoid surgery on voice quality and speech production. The conditions of hypernasal distortion of voice quality versus hyponasal distortion related to adenoid hypertrophy are often confused by medical specialists. A battery of clinical tests and objective instrumental studies of the effects of adenoid and tonsillar hypertrophy described in this book should be employed when consulting in this regard.

A seminal study by Subtelny and Baker [51] has shown that the adenoid pad has a growth and recession pattern which reaches a peak in the early school years followed by a period of receding to disappearance by early adult life.

ON HEARING AND MOVEMENT

Two of the muscles of the velopharyngeal mechanism already described are often considered to be related to hearing because of their possible effects on eustachian tube function. These are the levator palati and the salpingopharyngeus which insert around the eustachian tube openings in the nasopharynx. However, the levator palati muscles do not have a direct attachment to the cartilages at the eustachian orifices. The salpingopharyngeus muscles, which may be so attached, are often inconsistent in human anatomy and their effect on the opening of the tubes, if present, is limited. Research indicates that it is rather the *tensor palati* muscles that are primarily involved in the hearing-related task [47]. The relative position of the two bellies of this muscle as it relates to the other muscles of the soft palate is illustrated in Figure 1-19.

The detailed anatomy of the muscles in the eustachian tube area indicates that the lateral belly of the tensor palati actually connects with the *tensor tympani* of the middle ear. These muscles are positioned best for the primary task of balancing

air pressure in the middle ear by opening the eustachian tube during physiological functions including swallowing and speech.

The tensor palati muscles are illustrated in Figure 1-19 and in Figure 1-20A. It can be seen from these figures that this muscle has both a medial and a lateral muscle belly. These are connected by a tendon which swings around the hamular process of the pterygoid plates of the sphenoid bone, as illustrated in Figure 1-19. The lateral belly of this muscle is a flat, triangular muscle bundle with its base along the anterior wall of the cartilagi-

Figure 1-19. Position of the two bellies of tensor palatini in relation to other muscles of velopharyngeal mechanism.

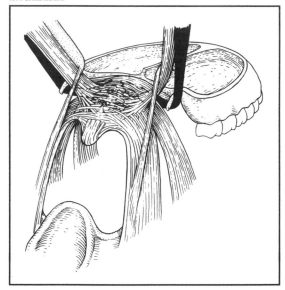

Figure 1-20. Muscles affecting hearing and movement. A. Tensor palatini and its relation to the levator (partly resected on right). B. Relative positions of levator and its possible antagonist, the glossopalatini.

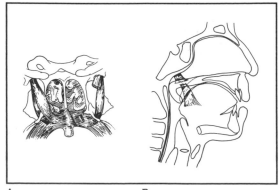

A   B

nous eustachian tube, the spina angularis of the sphenoid, and the scaphoid fossa at the base of the medial pterygoid plate. Its apex forms a tendon which makes a right-angle turn around the hamulus. From this tendon the medial belly passes mediad and is inserted into the most anterior portion of the palatine aponeurosis, to which the other soft palate muscles also attach.

Unlike the other palatal muscles, the tensor palati gains its efferent motor innervation from the mandibular branch of the trigeminal nerve. This suggests that it has an evolved purpose different form the other muscles of the velopharyngeal mechanism. Since the lateral belly of the tensor has a muscular connection with the tensor tympani in the middle ear [37], this purpose appears to be primarily for opening the eustachian tube to balance air pressure in the middle ear, which is essential for normal hearing function.

In addition to this primary function, the medial belly of this muscle appears to tense and somewhat depress the anterior protion of the soft palate during acts of swallowing [47, 54] It is during acts of swallowing that air pressure normally passes air to the middle ear to maintain a balance of pressure behind and in front of the tympanic membrane or eardrum.

Although the medial belly of the tensor palati may tend to lower and tense the anterior portion of the velum during swallow, the most likely muscle responsible for the rapid downward movement of the velum during the co-articulation movement patterns observed during speech is the *glossopalatinus muscle,* which is described below under its alias as the *musculus palatoglossus.*

This muscle is illustrated in Figure 1-20B as it relates as an antagonist to the levator palati, and in Figure 1-21 as it relates to the other muscles of the velopharyngeal mechanism. It arises from transverse fibers of the tongue in the posterior oral cavity. Its fibers ascend both upward and backward to form the anterior pillar. The superior fibers of this paired muscle insert into the soft palate on the lower side of the palatal aponeurosis.

When the palatoglossal muscles contract, their force on the elevated velum could pull it downward and somewhat forward. However, if the upward force of the antagonistic levators is stronger, contraction of the palatoglossus muscles might rather raise the back portion of the tongue as required for articulation of the /k/ and /g/ consonant sound elements and for production of back vowel resonance tones in connected speech. It is unclear as to whether the palatoglossus regularly

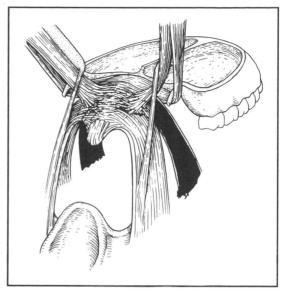

Figure 1-21. Position of the glossopalatini muscles in relation to other muscles of the velopharyngeal mechanism.

functions as an antagonist to the levator to accomplish the rapid opening and closing of the velopharyngeal port to produce the required consecutive oral and nasal syllables. However, this rapid movement does occur in normal speech production within milliseconds and Fritzel [18] has presented some EMG evidence that contraction of the glossopalatini timed with the relaxation of the levator accomplishes this rapid co-articulation movement.

ON AGE AND SEX

There are two usual variances from the typical configuration of velopharyngeal valving for speech that should be known and anticipated by the clinical student. The first is related to age, as illustrated in Figure 1-22. There is, particularly, a large difference in lateral configuration of the palate during speech, in the area of closure and seal, and in the depth of the nasopharynx, which has to be bridged by the velum between infants or toddlers and adult speakers.

The second distinctive difference in palatopharyngeal function patterns is related to the sex of adult speakers, as illustrated in Figure 1-23A and B. Research investigations have described three usual distinct differences in the pattern of velo-

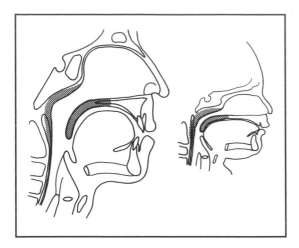

Figure 1-22. Comparison of the relative positions of velum to cranial base in adults (A) and infants (B).

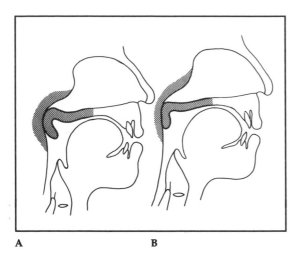

A   B

Figure 1-23. Comparison of velar configuration during speech, found in normal adult male (A) and female (B) speakers.

pharyngeal valving for speech between male and female subjects. These need to be considered for prosthetic or secondary surgical procedures often used to correct velopharyngeal inadequacies found in adult subjects.

The difference between infants and adults is explainable by the patterns of facial growth in human beings. There is regularly a marked downward and forward growth pattern of the maxilla and midface away from the cranial base during childhood and adolescence. That portion of the skeleton of the skull which forms the framework within which the velopharyngeal mechanism must perform its required movements to maintain velo-

pharyngeal adequacy to support normal speech becomes larger with growth. It moves further away from both the cranial base and the back portion of the nasopharynx. Comparison of even the 1-year Bolton standard tracings of the head with the average tracings of 3-year-old subjects in the growth norms developed by Broadbent et al. [8] reveals how extensive the growth in this area is, particularly in early childhood. If one likens this surrounding bony structure to a door frame, it is obvious that it will take a larger door (velum) to fit the frame and provide closure over this period of growth. The comparison of the sagittal section of the head of an infant with that of an adult, as illustrated in Figure 1-22A and B, shows the total extent of difference in the surrounding framework which accounts for the necessary change in the pattern of velopharyngeal valving for speech between infants and adults. As a consequence of this change, there is regularly a higher and more forward position for the area of velopharyngeal closure for speech in young children when compared to adults. Calnan [10] first described this "infantile" position for velopharyngeal closure as being level with the base of the basisphenoid. Aram and Subtelny [2] later also described a comparatively more forward and higher position for velopharyngeal closure in young children. They related this finding to the fact that the hard palate in young children is closer to the upper limit of the nasopharynx. The relatively greater forward inclination of the posterior pharyngeal wall in infancy, along with the changing dimensions of resting palatal length as well as increased depth to the nasopharynx, then account for these differences.

Since the resting palatal length of the velum also increases with age, it appears that the final muscle of the palate to be described here, the *musculus uvulae*, must increase in length considerably from infancy to adult life. This muscle was formerly often slighted as not having any important function in relation to velopharyngeal valving for speech. Recent clinical research now indicates that even slight deficiencies in the bulk of this midline muscle have adverse effects on velopharyngeal adequacy for speech. This muscle is illustrated in its superior relationship to the other muscles of the velum in Figure 1-24.

The musculus uvulae is a slender paired muscle running in an anterior-posterior direction over the superior midline margin of the soft palate. It arises from the aponeurosis at the back of the hard palate and courses over the other muscles

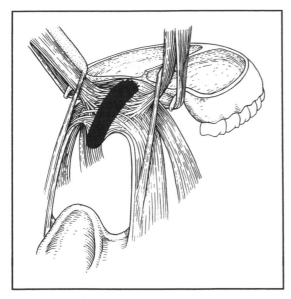

Figure 1-24. Superior position of the musculus uvulae to all other muscles of velopharyngeal mechanism.

described above to insert into the tip of the uvula. Its fibers generally overlie those of the other palatal muscles with the possible exception of some of the fibers of the palatopharyngeus. Its muscle bulk therefore contributes to the general convex shape of the superior border of the velum, the surface which must fit against the generally concave surface of the posterior nasopharynx to provide a complete seal in the nasopharynx. For this reason, it is now considered to be a very important muscle related to velopharyngeal valving for speech. A lack of muscle bulk in the midline of the posterior margin of the velum may cause a leak in the velopharyngeal mechanism significant enough to adversely affect speech.

The uvular muscle derives its neural innervation from the lesser palatine nerves of the facial nerve. Also, contraction of this muscle, like all muscles, would tend to shorten its length. The palate stretches rather than shortens at midline during velopharyngeal valving for speech. These facts suggest that the purpose of this muscle may be more related to deglutition than directly to velopharyngeal valving for speech. Be that as it may, a midline deficiency of the bulk of this muscle has been shown to adversely affect velopharyngeal seal necessary for speech. The stronger contraction of the uvular end of this muscle in adult males may help to account for the sex differences in the velar configuration of normal adult subjects.

It seems appropriate at the end of a lengthy review of velopharyngeal anatomy to attempt to recover the reader's interest by discussing the topic of sex. I can only trust that my fellow feminists will forgive me for continuing to use the more evocative word "sex," which still engenders more meaning than the word gender preferred by some today. Sex, like age, appears to have a basic influence on patterns of velopharyngeal valving for speech as well as patterns for life.

McKerns and Bzoch [32] reported a fundamental difference between male and female adult speakers in several aspects of velopharyngeal valving for speech. Those differences can be seen in Figure 1-23 by comparing A with B. Firstly, it can be seen that the basic orientation of the velum to the posterior wall forms an acute angle in male subjects whereas it forms a right angle in females. Secondly, the extent of the area of seal during velopharyngeal closure for speech is much greater for females than for males. Thirdly, the midpoint of closure in the nasopharynx is above the palatal plane in males and below the palatal plane in females. Although the palate is generally longer at both rest and function in males and it lifts higher above the palatal plane at its highest point of elevation, the differences cited could not be explained on the basis of the ratio of velar length to nasopharyngeal depth. The authors suggested the possibility that the relative areas of muscle insertions, particularly of the slings of the levator and palatopharyngeus, may differ between the sexes. It is still not known if these differences are the result of secondary sex changes in puberty or if they also exist in early childhood as the study has not been duplicated during childhood to date.

GUIDELINES FOR THE CARE AND TREATMENT OF CHILDREN WITH CLEFT LIP, CLEFT PALATE, AND CRANIOFACIAL ANOMALIES

For many years, there has been a need for general guidelines on the team management of children born with cleft lip with or without cleft palate.

Particularly, directors of state service programs for crippled children, now usually more properly referred to as divisions of children's medical services, required such guidelines. Also, third-party providers of services need such guidelines. Who should consititute a cleft palate team? What services should be provided? And what services should be compensated for by third-party providers? On the national level the ACPA has a committee working on developing such guidelines for national health delivery service programs. However, since care for all congenitally handicapped children must be provided in our democratic society through resources generated within state boundaries, such guidelines for the future must be generated and approved by states to be implemented. Several states are presently developing their own guidelines to assure the future quality of state-supported services by such interdisciplinary teams.

Starting in 1982, legislation in the State of Florida provided funds for establishing an advisory committee to develop such initial guidelines with consultation and assistance from the Florida Cleft Palate Association and all existing providers of health-related services previously approved by the state for compensation for their professional services. These guidelines presently require that speech pathology and audiology services be provided by clinicians certified in their professions and licensed by the state for providing such services through district cleft palate teams or in private practice. These guidelines, as revised in 1987, provide valuable educational information regarding the cleft palate team approach and effective early intervention management procedures that have evolved over time and which include the important potential role of the clinical fields of speech and language pathology and audiology. Those portions of the recent in-state publication entitled *The Florida Cleft Lip, Cleft Palate and Craniofacial Anomalies Program* most relevant to this course of study are paraphrased below with the permission of the present director of the Division of Children's Medical Services, Florida Department of Health and Rehabilitation Services program.

It was agreed that the minimal number of specialty representatives for approved district area cleft palate teams needed to address the medical, surgical, dental, and communicative needs of children born with cleft lip and palate should include but not be limited to a board-certified (1) pediatrician, (2) plastic surgeon, (3) orthodontist, (4) speech and language pathologist, (5) audiologist,

(6) nurse, and (7) social worker or other coordinator to help provide health care and psychosocial services to the patient and family to assist in case management and coordination of needed services. These health providers should provide their services as a part of a functional team approach. They should ideally all participate in each face-to-face cleft palate clinical conference.

The other clinical specialists considered as being valuable as consultants or regular team members include a (1) psychologist, (2) pediatric dentist, (3) radiologist, (4) otolaryngologist, (5) prosthodontist, (6) geneticist, (7) anesthesiologist, (8) neurosurgeon, (9) ophthalmologist, (10) oral and maxillofacial surgeon, (11) nutritionist, and (12) special education representative. These specialties are particularly needed in large craniofacial center team programs. The usual roles and backgrounds of these frequent and occasional cleft palate team members are described in Chapter 4.

The present guidelines propose that cleft palate teams for local areas should meet together for a minimum of 10 yearly clinics. They should also refer more complex syndromal or craniofacial disorder cases to a state-approved craniofacial center for initial comprehensive evaluation and specialized craniofacial surgical treatment if indicated. For the management of the speech, language, and hearing disorders often consequent to the birth of a child born with cleft lip or palate, the present guidelines recommend that the team speech pathologist and audiologist provide for a screening of prespeech interactive communication with parents and for longitudinal, speech, language, and hearing developmental assessments within a team setting format. These should be focused on factors of auditory function, resonance, phonatory voice quality, age-appropriate articulation skills, and both receptive and expressive age-appropriate language skills.

Communication disorder evaluations should usually include (1) review of the individual case history, (2) evaluation of the home environment, (3) assessment of middle ear function and hearing acuity, (4) direct test response observation and test response data on nasal air emission, hypernasality, or hyponasality during speech efforts, (5) assessment of vocal quality of laryngeal functions, being especially aware of the development of atypical aspirate or hoarse voice quality, (6) assessment of an age-appropriate standardized screening articulation test, and (7) assessment of language skills for both receptive and expressive language as appropriate for the child's age and condition.

A minimum of 6-month intervals for screening speech, language, and hearing reevaluations followed by referral for treatment deemed necessary is advised for cleft palate team management up to 6 years of age. At least annual evaluations after that age are recommended to be carried out by the entire cleft palate team, depending on the outcome of early treatment.

TREATMENT PROTOCOLS FOR OPTIMAL STANDARDS OF CLEFT PALATE CARE

SHORTLY AFTER BIRTH

Parents should be counseled by team members prior to hospital discharge regarding feeding, needed surgical correction of defects, and the importance of prelanguage stimulation.

FIRST YEAR

Surgery to correct any clefts of the primary palate (cleft lip) should be performed, usually at 2 to 3 months of age.

Referral of complex cases to a complete craniofacial center for initial comprehensive evaluation and recommendations.

Early evaluation by a cleft palate team with recording of basic information, including details of the extent and classification of congenital abnormalities. Collection of pertinent baseline records.

Family genetic counseling.

Audiometric evaluations with referrals for otologic treatment and/or amplification and auditory training as indicated.

Counseling of parents on the basics of pragmatic language stimulation techniques and the norms of early speech and language development skills.

Pediatric dental evaluation with instruction in dental hygiene and treatment, including presurgical maxillary orthopedic appliances coordinated with initial lip cleft closure procedures in selected cases (usually combined clefts of both the primary and secondary palates).

Team reevaluations followed by recommended treatment at or before 6 months and 12 months of age.

SECOND YEAR

12–18 MONTHS

Complete closure of both the hard and soft palate structures by 12 months of age if possible. Recent extensive cephalometric research by Ross [45] indicates that early complete palatal closures of unilateral complete clefts (repair prior to 12 months of age) result in better facial growth patterns than later complete closures.

Assessment of the adequacy of velopharyngeal functions for speech from clinical behavioral observational tests and parental history and any possible instrumental tests by the speech and language pathologist over the first year following surgery.

Family counseling, as appropriate, relative to the patient's plan of treatment.

Audiological and otological monitoring of middle ear functioning and the presence of disease.

Development of a home-based speech and language stimulation program, if indicated during routine reevaluation team clinics.

Team reevaluation at approximately 18 months of age.

Dental evaluation, with instruction and treatment as indicated.

18–24 MONTHS

This is considered to be the most critical and rapid period of motor speech and expressive language skill development. Speech and language skill acquisition should be monitored as regularly as possible, but at a minimum of 6-month intervals; a direct speech and language therapy program is established as indicated.

Audiological monitoring with otological treatment as needed.

THIRD YEAR

Usual respite from secondary surgical intervention.

Speech and language reevaluations with recommendations for further diagnostic therapy to determine velopharyngeal adequacy to support further speech and language development or modify cleft palate speech gross substitution error patterns.

Audiological and otological examinations and treatment as needed.

Two complete team reevaluations, including planning for implementation of possible dental, orthodontic, or secondary surgical palatal reconstruction.

Referral to an early educational setting outside the home (i.e., Head Start, pre-kindergarten, or day care centers) as deemed appropriate.

FOURTH YEAR

Patients identified as having had complete primary reconstruction of palatal clefts with persistent clinical evidence of persistent velopharyngeal insufficiency for normal speech and language development from repeated clinical tests and developmental histories should usually be referred for secondary palatal reconstructive surgery or for a limited period of prosthetic speech appliance management. Cine- or videofluoroscopy and/or nasoendoscopy are advisable before proceeding with recommendations for secondary surgical or prosthetic correction of velopharyngeal insufficiency. Correction of velopharyngeal insufficiency for normal speech development should be identified and verified through objective instrumental means as early as possible.

Speech and language skill reevaluations and implementation of speech and language therapy as needed.

Two team evaluations with implementation of the surgical, dental, hearing, and psychosocial and economic needs of the family and child should be provided.

FIFTH YEAR

Team visit and reevaluation at 6-month intervals.

Pediatric health care review with dental evaluation and treatment, possible first-phase orthodontic treatment or planning, speech and language evaluation and treatment as indicated, and correction of velopharyngeal insufficiency as needed.

SIXTH YEAR

Speech and language therapy as required for each patient.

Pediatric dental evaluation and treatment.

Orthodontic casts, photographs, or cephalometric x-rays deemed necessary for evaluation and treatment planning or the efficacy of new surgical intervention procedures for complex or congenital craniofacial disorders.

Audiological and otological monitoring and treatment as needed.

Complete team reevaluations at 6-month intervals for unresolved, more complex case studies.

EARLY SCHOOL AGE

Initial treatment should be completed (i.e., basic surgical, dental, pediatric medical care, and developmental speech and language and hearing problems should be eliminated or modified as possible).

Orthodontic and surgical treatment procedures are required, most often bone graft reconstructions of alveolar area clefts through bone grafts after two-third eruption of the permanent cuspids.

EARLY ADOLESCENCE

Treatment services may include lip revisions, rhinoplasties, alveoloplasties with bone grafts, routine speech and language reevaluations with therapy as indicated, routine dental care, and mixed dentition orthodontic treatment as indicated by team evaluations.

Psychosocial counseling of each child born with cleft palate should be provided, as indicated by team clinic evaluations.

REFERENCES

1. Anson, B. (Ed.). *Morris' Human Anatomy* (12th ed.). New York: McGraw-Hill, 1966.
2. Aram, A., and Subtelny, J. Velopharyngeal function and cleft palate prostheses. *J. Prosthet. Dent.* 9:149–158, 1959.
3. Bell–Berti, F. The Velopharyngeal Mechanism: An Electromyographic Study. In Haskins Laboratories, *Status Report on Speech Research* (Suppl.). 1973.
4. Bell–Berti, F. Control of pharyngeal cavity size for English voiced and voiceless stops. *J. Acoust. Soc. Am.* 57:456–461, 1975.

5. Berlin, A. J. Classification of Cleft Lip and Palate and Related Craniofacial Disorders. In K. R. Bzoch (Ed.), *Communicative Disorders Related to Cleft Lip and Palate* (2nd ed.). Boston: Little, Brown, 1979. Chap. 2, Pp. 20–36.

6. Brash, J. *Cunningham's Manual of Practical Anatomy* (12th ed.). Vol. 3, *Head and Neck: Brain.* New York: Oxford University Press, 1958.

7. Brescia, N. Anatomy of the Lip and Palate. In W. C. Grabb, S. W. Rosenstein, and K. R. Bzoch (Eds.), *Cleft Lip and Palate.* Boston: Little, Brown, 1971. Chap. 1, Pp. 3–20.

8. Broadbent, B., Sr., Broadbent, B., Jr., and Golden, W. *Bolton Standards of Dentofacial Development and Growth.* St. Louis: Mosby, 1975.

9. Bzoch, K. R. *Assessment: Radiographic Techniques. Speech and the Dentofacial Complex: The State of the Art. ASHA Reports* No. 5. Washington, D.C.: American Speech and Hearing Association, 1970. Pp. 248–270.

10. Calnan, J. Diagnosis, prognosis, and treatment of "palatopharyngeal incompetency" with special reference to radiographic investigations. *Br. J. Plast. Surg.* 8:265–282, 1955.

11. Crelin, E. *Development of the upper respiratory system. Ciba Found. Symp.* 28:3, 1976.

12. Davis, J. S., and Ritchie, H. P. Classification of congenital clefts of the lip and palate. *JAMA* 79:1323, 1922.

13. Dickson, D., Grant, J., Sicker, H., and Du Brul, E. Status of research in cleft palate anatomy and physiology, July, 1973. *Cleft Palate J.* 11:471–486, 1974.

14. Dickson, D. R., and Maue–Dickson, W. *Anatomical and Physiological Basis of Speech.* Boston: Little, Brown, 1982.

15. Dorrance, G. M. *The Operative Story of Cleft Palate.* Philadelphia: Saunders, 1933.

16. Elasahy, N. The modified striped Y: A systematic classification for cleft lip and palate. *Cleft Palate J.* 10:247, 1973.

17. Fogh–Anderson, P. *Inheritance of Hairlip and Cleft Palate.* Copenhagen: Nyt Nordisk Forlag–Arnold Busck, 1942.

18. Fritzel, B. The velopharyngeal muscles in speech. *Acta Otolaryngol.* Goteborg (Suppl.), 250:5–81, 1969.

19. Goss, C. (Ed.). *Gray's Anatomy* (25th ed.). Philadelphia: Lea & Febiger, 1950.

20. Graber, T., Bzoch, K., and Aoba, T. A functional study of the palatal and pharyngeal structures. *Angle Orthod.* 29:30–40, 1959.

21. Habal, M. B., and Maniscalco, J. E. Categorization of craniofacial deformities based on our experience with surgical manipulation. *Ann. Plast. Surg.* 6:6, 1981.

22. Habal, M. B., and Maniscalco, J. E. Categorization of Craniofacial Deformities. In *Advances in Plastic Surgery* 1:24, Chicago, Yearbook Medical Book Co., 1984.

23. Hamlet, S. Vocal compensation: An ultrasonic study of vocal fold vibration in normal and nasal vowels. *Cleft Palate J.* 10:267–285, 1973.

24. Harkins, C. S., Berlin, A., Harding, R., Longacre, J., and Snodgrasse, R. Report of the nomenclature committee. *Cleft Palate Bull.* 10:11, 1960.

25. Harkins, C. S., Berlin, A., Harding, R., Longacre, J., and Snodgrasse, R. A classification of cleft lip and cleft palate. *Plast. Reconstr. Surg.* 29:31, 1962.

26. Keller, H. *The Story of My Life.* New York: Lancer Books, 1968.

27. Kernahan, D. A. The striped Y: A symbolic classification for cleft lip and cleft palate. *Plast. Reconstr. Surg.* 47:469, 1971.

28. Kernahan, D. A. Letter to the editor. *Plast. Reconstr. Surg.* 51:578, 1973.

29. Kernahan, D. A., and Stark, R. B. A new classification for cleft lip and cleft palate. *Plast. Reconstr. Surg.* 22:435, 1958.

30. Koepp–Baker, H. Pathomorphology of Cleft Palate and Lip. In S. Travis (Ed.), *Handbook of Speech Pathology.* New York: Appleton-Century-Crofts, 1957.

31. McWilliams, B., Lavorato, A., and Bluestone, C. Vocal cord abnormalities in children with velopharyngeal valving problems. *Laryngoscope* 83:1745–1753, 1973.

32. McKerns, D., and Bzoch, K. Variations in velopharyngeal valving: The factor of sex. *Cleft Palate J.* 7:652–662, 1970.

33. Maue–Dickson, W. Section II, Anatomy and physiology, cleft lip and palate research: An updated state of the art. *Cleft Palate J.* 14:270–276, 1977.

34. Millard, D., Jr. *Cleft Craft: The Evolution of Its Surgery.* Vol. 1, *The Unilateral Deformity.* Boston: Little, Brown, 1976.

35. Millard, D., Jr. *Cleft Craft: The Evolution of Its Surgery.* Vol. 2, *Bilateral and Rare Deformities.* Boston: Little, Brown, 1977.

36. Millard, D., Jr. *Cleft Craft: The Evolution of Its Surgery.* Vol. 3, *Alveolar and Palatal Deformities.* Boston: Little, Brown, 1980.

37. Misarya, V. Functional anatomy of tensor palati and levator palati muscles. *Arch. Otolaryngol.* 102:265–270, 1976.

38. Morris, H., Jakobi, M., and Harrington, D. Objectives and criteria for the management of cleft lip and palate and the delivery of management services. *Cleft Palate J.* 15:1, 1978.

39. Nishio, J., Matsuza, T., Ibuki, K., and Miyazaki, T. Roles of the facial glossopharyngeal and vagus nerves in velopharyngeal movement. *Cleft Palate J.* 13:201–214, 1976.

40. Olin, W. H. *Cleft Lip and Palate Rehabilitation.* Springfield, Ill.: Thomas, 1960.

41. Passavant, G. Ueber die Verschliessung des Schlundes Beim Sprechen. *Arch. Pathol. Anat. Physiol.* 46:1, 1886.

42. Patten, B. Embryology of the Palate and the Maxillofacial Region. In W. B. Grabb, S. Rosenstein, and K. Bzoch (Eds.), *Cleft Lip and Palate.* Boston: Little, Brown, 1971.

43. Podvinik, S. The physiology of the soft palate. *J. Laryngol. Otol.* 66:452, 1952.

44. Pruzansky, S. Description, classification, and analysis of unoperated clefts of the lip and palate. *Am. J. Orthod.* 41:590, 1953.

45. Ross, R. B. Treatment variables affecting facial growth in complete unilateral cleft lip and palate. *Cleft Palate J.* 24:3–77, 1987.

46. Ross, R., and Johnson, M. *Cleft Lip and Palate.* Baltimore: Williams and Wilkins, 1972.

47. Rich, A. A physiological study of the eustachian tube and its related muscles. *Johns Hopkins Hosp. Bull.* 31:206, 1920.

48. Shearer, W. *Illustrated Speech Anatomy* (2nd ed.). Springfield, Ill.: Thomas, 1968. Pp. 66–72.

49. Sicher, H., and Du Brul, E. *Oral Anatomy* (5th ed.). St. Louis: Mosby, 1970.

50. Smith, D. *Recognizable Patterns of Human Malformation* (3rd ed.). Philadelphia: Saunders, 1982.

51. Subtelny, J., and Baker, H. The significance of adenoid tissue in velopharyngeal function. *Plast. Reconstr. Surg.* 17:235, 1951.

52. Tessier, P. Anatomical classification of craniofacial and laterofacial clefts. *J. Maxillofac. Surg.* 4:69, 1976.

53. Veau, V. *Division Palatine.* Paris: Masson, 1931.
54. Wardill, W., and Shillis, J. Movements of the soft palate, with special reference to the function of the tensor palati muscle. *Surg. Gynecol. Obstet.* 62:836, 1936.
55. Williams, W. *Deviant Lingual Patterns of Cleft Speakers.* Dissertation, University of Florida, Gainesville, 1969.
56. Zemlin, W. *Speech and Hearing Science: Anatomy and Physiology.* Englewood Cliffs, N.J.: Prentice-Hall, 1968.

CHAPTER 2

Basic Concepts in Congenital Craniofacial Defects

Sally J. Peterson-Falzone

From conception to birth, the developing human is vulnerable to more literal threats to life and limb than at any other time until old age. Fully one half of all fertilized human eggs die before birth: approximately 30 percent in early embryogenesis, 20 percent later in pregnancy [29]. Of those babies who do survive the perilous prenatal period and the trauma of birth, about 5 to 6 percent exhibit congenital malformations recognizable at birth. In another 9 to 10 percent, defects present at birth are not detected or do not become manifest until later in life [29]. In the United States, about 1 in 600 newborns presents with craniofacial malformations [29]. A large percentage of the individuals affected by these defects require the services of specialists in communicative disorders, and understanding the etiology and complexity of these anatomical and physiological differences requires understanding a number of concepts which do not ordinarily pertain to other communicative disorders.

Cleft lip and palate provides an excellent teaching example for consideration of how concepts have changed over the past decade regarding (1) the frequency with which birth defects occur *in combination* rather than in isolation, and (2) how the presence of concurrent defects changes our understanding of the etiology of the cleft or other defects. The frequency with which clefts occur in combination with other birth defects is known to have been seriously underestimated in the majority of the earlier literature. For example, MacMahon and McKeown [18] reported a frequency of associated malformations in 9.1 percent of cases

of cleft lip, 14.9 percent of cleft palate, and 21.0 percent of cleft lip and palate as recorded on hospital records. Greene and co-workers [14] used birth certificate data to report a frequency of associated defects of 7 percent of cleft lip infants, 24 percent of cleft palate, and 14 percent of cleft lip and palate. Meskin and Pruzansky [21] reported similar numbers: 5.6 percent of cleft lip cases, 17.8 percent of cleft lip, and 10.3 percent of cleft lip and palate. However, in one early study [31] in which the individuals were actually *examined* for associated defects, the frequency was 16 percent in cleft lip with or without cleft palate and 51 percent in cleft palate alone.* The majority of studies have agreed on a higher occurrence of such defects in cleft palate alone rather than cleft lip with or without cleft palate [1, 6–10, 13, 15, 17, 31, 34], the figures of MacMahon and McKeown [18] being an exception. Beder et al. [1] reported that the more extensive clefts had the greatest number of associated anomalies, and Green et al. [14] found more associated malformations in bilateral than unilateral clefts.

Recent studies have shown just how seriously underreported associated defects have been: Rollnick and Pruzansky [25] reported that 44 percent of 2,512 cases of all types of clefts had associated malformations, and Jones [16] found an incidence of 17/30 (56.6%) among children with isolated cleft palate. In a study of 1,000 cases with clefts, Shprintzen et al. [26] reported that at least one minor or one major associated anomaly was found in 44.6 percent of those with cleft lip, 50.3 percent of those with cleft lip and cleft palate,

---

*The terms "cleft palate alone" or "isolated cleft palate" are usually used to refer to cleft palate in the absence of cleft lip. These terms can become confusing when dysmorphologists use "isolated cleft" to refer to clefting (of lip and/or palate) in the absence of any other associated anomalies.

and 56.2 percent of those with clefts of the secondary palate alone (including submucous clefts). Associated anomalies occurred in a total of 53.4 percent of their sample. These included an identified syndrome, sequence, or association in 31 percent, and "provisionally unique pattern syndromes" in another 22 percent. In about 11 percent, minor findings occurred which were either not part of an anomaly pattern or were familial characteristics. Discounting these, Shprintzen et al. [26] concluded that only 47 percent of their sample had "clefts in isolation." Interestingly, Cohen concluded in 1978 [5] that there were 154 syndromes which included cleft lip and/or palate as one feature. In less than one decade, Shprintzen [27] estimated the number of such syndromes to be well over 300.

Failure to recognize all findings associated with a cleft or other birth defect has serious consequences. First, the associated findings may signal the presence of an entirely different etiology. A classic example is Van der Woude syndrome (Fig. 2-1), in which the presence of lower paramedian lip pits in an individual with or without a cleft signals the presence of an autosomal dominant disorder, vastly changing the recurrence risks over what they would otherwise be for cleft alone. Another example is cleft palate occurring as part of the Pierre Robin sequence (Fig. 2-2A and B). The recurrence risks are far lower than in cleft palate with no other associated defects. Conversely, the Pierre Robin sequence may be part of the broader Stickler syndrome, another autosomal dominant disorder which automatically means a 50% recurrence risk for offspring of affected individuals. Second, inaccurate or incomplete diagnosis typically leads to naive treatment planning, in both physical and behavioral aspects. For example, pharyngeal flaps can be life-threatening in syndromes such as mandibulofacial dysostosis in which the nasopharyngeal airway is inherently small, and several of these syndromes are so variable in severity that the surgeon may easily miss the mildly affected cases. Similarly, expected patterns of mandibular growth vary significantly in various forms of "micrognathia," and failure to accurately discriminate the many disorders in which this is one feature can lead to erroneous treatment plans. Finally, speech pathologists must obviously adjust treatment plans when, for example, a child is referred for therapy with a diagnosis of "cleft palate" but turns out to have some multiple-anomaly syndrome.

Figure 2-2. Child with Pierre Robin sequence at the ages of 5 months (A) and 2 years (B). Tracheostomy was necessitated by airway obstruction, which did not resolve with more conservative management.

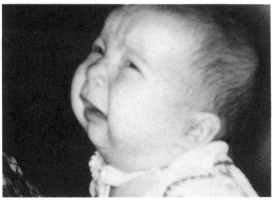

A

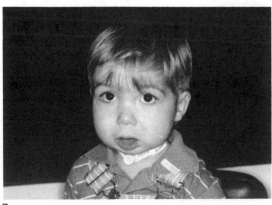

B

Figure 2-1. Paramedian lower lip pits with cleft lip and palate in an infant with Van der Woude syndrome.

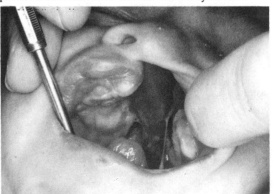

TERMINOLOGY

Study of the causation of birth defects involves three somewhat overlapping areas of investigation:

1. *Epidemiology* — the science dealing with relationships of the various factors which determine the frequency and distribution of a disease or disorder in a population. This topic thus encompasses, in theory, both incidence and everything related to causation.
2. *Etiology* — the factors or study of factors that cause disease; the sum of knowledge regarding causes.
3. *Pathogenesis* — the development of morbid conditions or disease. Pathogenesis describes what goes wrong (in this case, during prenatal development), and etiology indicates the cause. Unfortunately, use of these two terms is not clearly differentiated in the literature. For example, lack of tongue withdrawal from between the palatal shelves, which is itself a result of preceding events, is treated as a causal factor under "etiology" by some authors but merely as a step in pathogenesis by others.

Two other commonly confused terms are "congenital" and "genetic." The term *congenital* simply means "existing at birth," and does not imply what actually caused the trait or disorder to occur. The causes of congenital disorders generally fall into the categories of genetic, chromosomal, multifactorial, environmental, and "unknown." The term *genetic* means "determined by properties of the genes." Some genetic disorders, such as Huntington's chorea, do not become manifest until many years after birth and are thus not considered by some geneticists to be truly congenital,* although the underlying pathology (a defective gene) is present from the time of conception. Genetic disorders may be subdivided into (1) "inherited," meaning that the abnormal genes were passed from one or both parents to the child, and (2) "acquired," meaning that the abnormal genetic material was not present in either parent but rather resulted from a change or "mutation" in the material at the time of conception [12]. Within a given family, a genetic disorder may pass from the "acquired" to the "inherited" subdivision. Gard-

ner [12] cites the example of neurofibromatosis: The vast majority of cases of this disease are the result of genetic mutation, but if the affected individual reproduces, he or she has a 50 percent chance of passing the altered gene on to his or her children. Consequently, what was originally a sporadic or "acquired" gene disorder becomes in the next generation an inherited disorder.

Genetic disorders may also be labeled *monogenic* or *polygenic*. The former term means that a single defective gene causes the defect to occur, the latter that several defective genes must act in combination to produce the defect.

The term *chromosomal* means "pertaining to chromosomes." Although chromosomes are composed of genes, "chromosomal" is not synonymous with "genetic." The former term means only that, with existing techniques, geneticists are able to identify changes in chromosome number or structure or both. Chromosomal disorders, like genetic disorders, may be subdivided into "inherited" (the chromosomal abnormality is also found in the somatic cells of one of the parents) and "acquired" (the abnormality is the result of a change taking place at the time of formation of the sperm or ovum). Most people with a chromosomal abnormality, however, are not reproductively fit, and consequently a child born with a chromosomal disorder usually represents a new mutation [12]. (See An Introduction to Human Genetics below.)

Many traits or defects are thought to be *multifactorial* in origin, meaning that they are caused by multiple factors, genetic and possibly also environmental, each with only a minor effect [33]. These traits appear in the individual only when a sufficient number of causative factors (genes with or without environmental factors) are present to reach a critical *threshold*.

Traits or defects may also be labeled as "familial" or "sporadic." The term *familial* means "characteristic of a family," that is, more common in relatives of an affected individual than in the general population. This term makes no presumption regarding *why* the trait or defect has occurred previously. Generally the cause is monogenic or polygenic, due to the reduced ability of people with chromosomal disorders to reproduce, but the genetic basis may be of several different types or may in fact be unknown. Some "familial" traits may actually be environmental, such as developmental delay related to depressed socioeconomic status. *Sporadic* means "occurring occasionally,

*This is, however, a point of some dissent.

singly, or in scattered instances." Again, no assumption is made with regard to cause.

Known *environmental* causes of birth defects include various kinds of drugs, radiation, and viruses. The most well-known drug-induced defect is the thalidomide syndrome. Very few environmental agents have actually been proved to cause defects in humans, partially because human beings cannot be experimentally "dosed" as can laboratory animals. For this reason, some agents which have been suspected to cause birth defects can only be said to be "linked" to or associated with those defects in epidemiological studies. When an agent or event is proved to cause a defect or to raise the incidence of a defect, it is termed a *teratogen*. In the 1960s, a link was suspected between diazepam (Valium) and cleft lip, but no rigorous studies have emerged proving causation. As of this writing, the only drug which has been proved to raise the incidence of clefting in humans is phenytoin (Dilantin), although it has been difficult for epidemiologists to segregate the effect of the drug from the effect of the seizure disorder itself on the developing fetus.*

By far the majority of craniofacial defects are truly *malformations*, that is, they are defects caused by an error in the earliest stages of tissue formation or "morphogenesis." By contrast, a congenital *deformation* is a structural defect due to the action of unusual mechanical forces on normally developing tissue. The abnormal mechanical influences may be due to abnormalities of the uter-us, or to problems within the fetus itself such as myopathy or a neurological condition affecting fetal position and movements. Some cranial, ear, and limb abnormalities, among others, are actually deformations rather than malformations. A *disruption* is a defect resulting from a breakdown of, or interference with, an originally normal developmental process. Examples include abnormalities resulting from amniotic bands, and limb reduction defects caused by vascular anomalies [33].

It is also necessary to understand that multiple birth defects occurring in a single infant are related in different ways. The term *syndrome* is used only when multiple structural defects cannot be explained on the basis of a single defect in the formation of embryonic tissue but rather appear to be the consequence of multiple defects in one or more tissues, although each of the independent defects is thought to be due to a single cause (a gene defect, chromosomal abnormality, or teratogen). Examples of syndromes affecting the craniofacial complex include Van der Woude syndrome; Apert syndrome; mandibulofacial dysostosis, also called Treacher Collins syndrome (Fig. 2-3A and B); and many more. The term *sequence* is used if all the anomalies can be explained on the basis of a single structural or mechanical problem leading to a "cascade" of subsequent defects [30]. The best known example in craniofacial defects is the Pierre Robin sequence (see Fig. 2-2A and B), which most current literature still mistakenly terms a "syndrome." Finally, the term *association* is

Figure 2-3. Characteristic features of mandibulofacial dysostosis (Treacher Collins syndrome), including antimongoloid slant of the palpebral fissures, colobomata, defects of the lower lashes, maxillary and mandibular hypoplasia, and bilateral defects of the auricles (and middle ears) with conductive hearing loss.

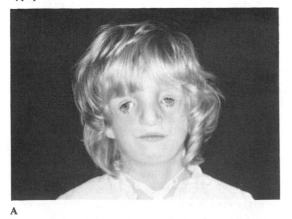

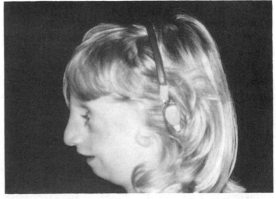

A   B

*Acutane (isotretinoin), a currently popular drug for treating acne, causes multiple birth defects, including ear anomalies but not clefting. The implications for teenage pregnancies are obvious.

used when a pattern of anomalies occurs in patients or at frequencies higher than would be expected by chance alone and the pattern has not yet been identified as a sequence or syndrome. (For further discussion, see Cohen and Stool [4], Smith [30], and Thompson and Thompson [33].) Some dysmorphologists add the modifier of "provisionally unique" when discussing a suspected syndrome, sequence, or association not yet described in other patients.

AN INTRODUCTION TO HUMAN GENETICS

The nucleus of each somatic* cell in the human body contains 46 chromosomes which consist of intertwined strands of proteins that carry all the genetic information coding the development of that body. Half of that information is contained on the 23 chromosomes contributed by the individual's mother, half on the 23 contributed by the father. The chromosomes come in "pairs," there being 22 pairs of *autosomes* or non–sex chromosomes, and one pair of sex chromosomes. In normal females, the pair of *sex chromosomes* consists of two X chromosomes; in males, one X chromosome is contributed by the mother and a Y chromosome is contributed by the father. The normal ovum formed by the female and the sperm formed by the male, both known as *gametes*, contain only one-half the number of chromosomes (or *haploid number*) found in other cells of the body so that, when they unite in conception, the conceptus or *zygote* has the correct number of 46. Each ovum contains 22 autosomes and an X sex chromosome; each sperm, 22 autosomes and either an X, meaning the newly conceived individual will be a female, or a Y sex chromosome, meaning the zygote will be a male.

The process by which ova and sperm are formed is known as *gametogenesis*. This process consists primarily of a special type of cell division known as *meiosis* which eventually provides an appropriate number of chromosomes in each mature gamete. The primordial genetic material in the female is termed an *oogonium*, which matures into an *oocyte*, which becomes the mature *ovum*.† The comparable stages in the male gamete are *spermatogonium, spermatocyte,* and *sperm,* respectively. The duplication ("copying") and segregation of chromosomal material during gametogenesis is a rather delicate process, and vulnerable to errors resulting in abnormalities in the number or structure of chromosomes in the sperm or ovum. The most familiar example is known as trisomy 21, or Down syndrome. Individuals with this syndrome have three of the chromosomes known as 21, instead of two. In most cases, this is due to failure of the copies of the 21st chromosome to segregate properly during the process of *oogenesis* in the mother, so that the ovum carries two instead of just one such chromosome. When that ovum unites with a sperm also carrying a copy of each of the 22 autosomes plus a sex chromosome, the resulting conceptus is then *trisomic* for chromosome 21.

Trisomies such as Down syndrome‡ constitute one type of error in chromosome number, and result in serious phenotypical disorders.§ Monosomies, in which only one member of a given chromosome pair is present, are extremely rare except for monosomy X (Turner syndrome).

In the rather complex process by which chromosomal material is duplicated and segregated to produce gametes, errors can also occur in chromosome structure. With the exception of the Y sex chromosome, chromosomes are normally shaped something like an X, with the upper arms being shorter than the lower arms. In genetic shorthand, the upper arms are termed *p* and the lower arms *q*. (The central part of the X is termed the *centromere*.) Breakage can occur in the arms, resulting in duplications, inversions, deletions, or translocations in the daughter cells. According to Thompson and Thompson [33], small *duplications* are fairly common and much less harmful than *deletions*. In the latter, the loss of genetic material

---

* The term *somatic* means "body." The term *somatic cell* is used to refer to cells of the structure of the body, as opposed to those of the viscera.

† A woman is born with all the oocytes, already matured from oogonia, that she will ever produce. That is one reason why the incidence of many birth defects goes up with maternal age: The genetic material contributed by the mother is as old as she is. Men, on the other hand, form sperm anew throughout their reproductive lives.

‡ In about 4 percent of cases, Down syndrome is not due to a pure trisomy but to a translocation.

§ *Phenotype* refers to the observable characteristics of the individual. *Genotype* refers to genetic constitution. *Karyotype* refers to the chromosome set, and is often used to refer to a "picture" of the chromosomes of an individual arranged in homologous pairs. The normal karyotype for a male is designated "46,XY" and that for a female "46,XX."

generally has serious consequences. A classic example is the cri-du-chat syndrome, otherwise known as the "5p-" or "5p deletion" syndrome, in which deletion of a portion of the short arm of chromosome 5 causes physical abnormalities and severe developmental disability. *Inversions* involve rearrangement of genetic material on a single chromosome as a result of breakage and reconstitution. *Translocations* involve exchange of genetic material between nonhomologous chromosomes (chromosomes belonging to different pairs). Individuals whose karyotypes show either inversions or translocations *may* be phenotypically normal. However, when copies of the abnormal chromosomes are formed in the process of gametogenesis, the result can be gametes with unbalanced amounts of genetic material. (See Stern [32] or Thompson and Thompson [33] for full explanations of both the normal process of gametogenesis and the process by which chromosomal abnormalities occur.)

As noted previously, chromosomes are composed of thousands of genes. Each gene occupies a *locus* on its chromosome, and has a counterpart gene occupying the counterpart locus on the paired chromosome, the exception being genes located on the sex chromosomes, since the latter are not truly paired. The two counterpart genes are called *alleles*. One member of each allelic pair is contributed by the mother, one by the father. If the two alleles are identical, the individual is said to be *homozygous* for that gene or the trait it produces. If the alleles are different, the individual is *heterozygous*. In birth defects, the alleles or genes are typically termed normal or abnormal.

In general, there are four factors affecting how a gene will act in determining a trait of the individual: (1) the basic pattern of transmission of the trait (autosomal dominant, autosomal recessive, X-linked, multifactorial); (2) sex limitation or sex influence of certain, but not all, traits; (3) penetrance; and (4) expressivity.

The term *autosomal dominant* means that the trait is transmitted by just one (abnormal) allele occurring on one of a pair of autosomes (see Fig. 2-4). If a trait is *autosomal recessive*, both of the alleles must be abnormal for the individual to be clinically affected. That is, one abnormal gene was contributed both by the mother and by the father. If an individual is heterozygous for an abnormal recessive gene, he or she is typically termed a *carrier* or *heterozygous carrier*. There are some recessive diseases and disorders in which the heterozygous carrier, while not clinically affected or showing

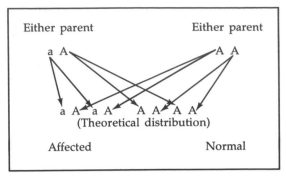

A

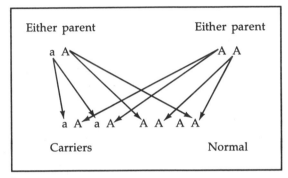

B

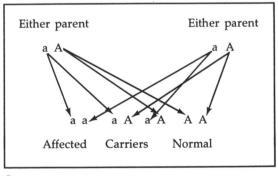

C

Figure 2-4. Theoretical distribution of genes to offspring in autosomal dominant and autosomal recessive inheritance. A. Autosomal dominant inheritance, one parent affected. a = abnormal gene, A = normal gene. One-half of the offspring will be affected: one-half will be normal with no possibility of transmitting the disorder. B. Autosomal recessive inheritance, one parent carrying the mutant gene. One-half of the offspring will be carriers, but not affected unless there is some minor defect in the heterozygote. C. Autosomal recessive inheritance, both parents carrying the mutant gene. Note: In some recessive disorders, the a a homozygous condition is lethal. Thus, of the *liveborn* children, two-thirds will be carriers and one-third will be normal.

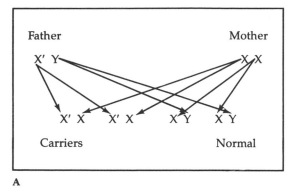

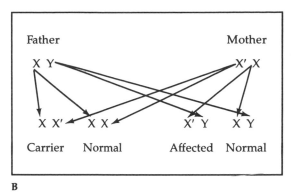

Figure 2-5. Theoretical distribution in X-linked inheritance. A. X-linked inheritance, father affected (X' = X carrying the abnormal gene). All the daughters will be carriers, all the sons will be normal, with no possibility of transmitting the disorder to their offspring. B. X-linked inheritance, mother as carrier. One-half of daughters will be carriers; like their mothers, one-half will be normal. One-half of sons will be affected, and one-half will be normal.

the complete form of the trait, exhibits some minor but significant phenotypical differences. (See Smith [30] for a discussion of this seeming paradox.) In general, recessive disorders are much more severe than dominant disorders. *X-linked* traits are transmitted on the X chromosome as illustrated in Figure 2-5. *X-linked recessive traits are expressed, with rare exceptions, only in the male:* He has no counteracting "normal gene" on a paired chromosome,* and thus expresses the trait with only a "single dose." An X-linked recessive trait observed in 1 in 1,000 males in a given population would, in theory occur in 1/1,000 × 1/1,000 or 1/1,000,000 females since they would require a "double dose." *X-linked dominant* disorders are expressed in the XX female but usually with a less severe effect than in the XY male.

Multifactorial inheritance has already been discussed and is not, strictly speaking, a purely genetic inheritance pattern but may still have significant recurrence risks.

Traits which are transmitted on the autosomes should appear in equal numbers in both sexes. However, some can be expressed in only one sex, and are termed *sex-limited*. Examples include uterine and prostate cancer. Traits which are expressed in both sexes but in widely different frequencies are said to be *sex-influenced*. A classic example is baldness.

Two critical concepts in understanding the action of genes are *penetrance* and *expressivity*. In theory, we would expect a trait to be expressed 100 percent of the time that a given gene is present in the individual. However, this is not the case. For example, when a trait which is known to be autosomal dominant occurs in a grandparent and grandchild, but not in the intervening parent, the gene is present in the parent but has not penetrated. The trait is then said to have shown *reduced penetrance*. Penetrance is an all-or-none phenomenon, and is expressed mathematically as the percentage of individuals who have the gene for a condition who actually show the trait [33]. Traits also vary in the degree to which they are *expressed*. Roughly speaking, we may equate expressivity with severity. However, the trait may be expressed in a different form, for example, a submucous cleft without lip pits in one member of a kindred with Van der Woude syndrome, lip pits without a cleft in another. Expressivity, as opposed to penetrance, is a matter of degree. Clearly, when the expression of a disorder is very mild, it may be missed altogether by all but the most astute clinician.

Geneticists predict the likelihood of occurrence of a trait or disorder in a population, or recurrence within a given family, based on observations of its inheritance pattern. The calculations are rarely as simple as portrayed in Figures 2-4 and 2-5 because of the variables of sex limitation, sex influence, and penetrance. When a trait is transmitted via multifactorial inheritance, calculation of recurrence risks is even more tedious. The most popular theory regarding the genetics of clefting, exclusive of its occurrence in syndromes, sequences, or associations, has been the "polygenic, multifactorial" threshold concept. However, some geneticists have felt a more appropriate model to

---

* The Y chromosome is very small and not truly a "counterpart" for the X chromosome. While its presence is essential for determination of the male sex, very few other traits have been shown to be transmitted on it (e.g., "hairy ears").

be a "single mutant (autosomal dominant) gene" with "allelic restriction"* [3, 11, 19, 20]. A number of authors have stressed the etiological heterogeneity for both cleft lip with or without cleft palate and isolated cleft of the secondary palate, which are separate genetic entities, in part because of the large number of syndromes, sequences, and associations in which clefting occurs [2, 20].

EXAMPLES OF CRANIOFACIAL DEFECTS

Possibly the majority of congenital defects affecting the craniofacial complex and thus the functions of speech and hearing are transmitted as autosomal dominant traits. These include achondroplasia, Van der Woude syndrome, Apert syndrome (acrocephalosyndactyly type I) (Fig. 2-6A and B), Crouzon disease (craniofacial dysostosis), Pfeiffer syndrome, Treacher Collins syndrome (see Fig. 2-3A and B), also known as mandibulofacial dysostosis, the velocardiofacial syndrome, Stickler syndrome, the ectrodactyly-ectodermal dysplasia-cleft (EEC) syndrome, the oral-facial-digital syndrome (OFD, type I; autosomal dominant but lethal in the XY male so all cases are female), Freeman-Sheldon syndrome, Melnick-Fraser syndrome (branchio-oto-renal or BOR syndrome), Waardenburg syndrome, Sae-

thre-Chotzen syndrome, and many others. (For information on the features of these syndromes and their effect on communication skills, see Peterson-Falzone [22–24] and Siegal-Sadewitz and Shprintzen [28].)

Examples of disorders for which there is evidence of autosomal recessive inheritance include Bloom syndrome, Dubowitz syndrome, Johanson-Blizzard syndrome, Seckel syndrome, Smith-Lemli-Opitz syndrome, Carpenter syndrome, Cockayne syndrome, Ellis-Van Creveld syndrome, Laurence-Moon-Beidl syndrome, Hurler syndrome, Mohr syndrome (oral-facial-digital syndrome, type II), Morquio syndrome, and Werner syndrome [30].

Chromosomal disorders are generally so severe that communication skills are limited by reduced intellectual development, in addition to the possibility of clefting and other physical alterations of the speech or hearing mechanisms. Examples include Down syndrome (trisomy 21), trisomy 18 (10% survival rate), trisomy 13 (18% survival rate), trisomy 8, trisomy 9 mosaic† syndrome, 4p– (4p deletion) syndrome, 5p– (cri-du-chat) syndrome, 9p– syndrome, 13q–syndrome, 18p– syndrome, 18q– syndrome, and many other rare but devastating disorders. Some disorders of chromosomal distribution involve more moderate developmental disorders, such as Klinefelter syndrome (XXY in males) and Turner syndrome (XO females).

X-linked inheritance has been documented in Aarskog syndrome (X-linked semidominant with

Figure 2-6. Two-month-old infant with Apert syndrome. Note abnormal cranial configuration, severe midface retrusion, and proptosis.

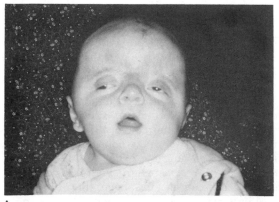 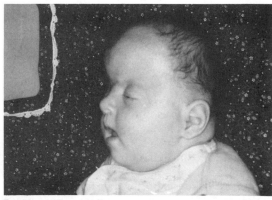

A   B

* *Allelic restriction* means segregation of two alternative alleles at a single locus.
† *Mosaicism* means that only a portion of the somatic cells are affected by the alteration in chromosomes. The severity of the disorder is generally determined by the proportion of altered cells.

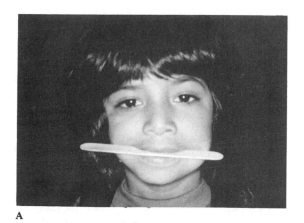 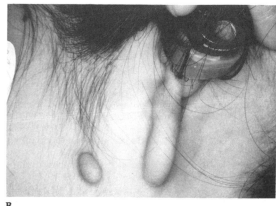

A   B

Figure 2-7. Eight-year-old child with hemifacial microsomia exhibiting relatively mild facial asymmetry (A) but a severe deformity of the auricle (B).

carrier females showing some minor expression); Gillian-Turner-type X-linked mental deficiency syndrome; the Martin-Bell (fragile X) syndrome (although the precise X-linked inheritance pattern is unclear); the otopalatodigital syndrome (also semidominant), Hunter syndrome, and Coffin-Lowry syndrome (semidominant) among others.

A frustratingly large number of congenital defects involving the craniofacial complex are sporadic in occurrence, with no certain inheritance pattern. These include Cornelia de Lange syndrome, Rubinstein-Taybi syndrome, the Pierre Robin sequence, the variable forms of hemifacial microsomia (Fig. 2-7A and B) (also known by a host of other names; see Peterson-Falzone [24]), Russell-Silver dwarfism, Williams syndrome, progeria syndrome, Beckwith-Wiedemann syndrome; Prader-Willi syndrome, Moebius sequence, and Nager syndrome (which closely resembles Treacher-Collins syndrome). For others, etiological heterogeneity has been suggested by the fact that different patterns of occurrence have been found. Examples include Robinow syndrome, Noonan syndrome (some sporadic, some dominant), Coffin-Siris syndrome, and Optiz syndrome, among others [30].

While definitive genetic diagnosis is not the responsibility of the speech-language pathologist,* the danger of failing to recognize significant physical differences in the craniofacial complex and thus failing to make appropriate referrals is very real. It is recommended that professionals in clinical practice, particularly those working with young children, avail themselves of a reasonable library where illustrated references on birth defects are maintained on a current basis. It is also recommended that professionals acquire and maintain a listing of birth defects or craniofacial teams and clinics in their geographical area.

REFERENCES

1. Beder, O., Coe, H., Braafladt, R., and Houle, R. Factors associated with congenital cleft lip and cleft palate in the Pacific Northwest. *Oral Surg.* 9:1267, 1956.
2. Bixler, D. Genetics and clefting. *Cleft Palate J.* 18:10, 1981.
3. Coccia, C., Bixler, D., and Conneally, P. Cleft lip and cleft palate: A genetic study. *Cleft Palate J.* 6:323, 1969.
4. Cohen, M., and Stool, S. Craniofacial Anomalies and Syndromes. In C. Bluestone and S. Stool (Eds.), *Pediatric Otolaryngology.* Philadelphia: Saunders, 1983. Vol. 1.
5. Cohen, M. Syndromes with cleft lip and cleft palate. *Cleft Palate J.* 15:306, 1978.
6. Conway, H., and Wagner, K. Congenital anomalies of the head and neck: As reported on birth certificates in New York City, 1952 to 1962 (inclusive). *Plast. Reconstr. Surg.* 36:71, 1965.
7. Conway, H., and Wagner, K. Incidence of clefts in New York City. *Cleft Palate J.* 3:284, 1966.
8. Curtis, E. Genetical and environmental factors in the etiology of cleft lip and cleft palate. *J. Can. Dent. Assoc.* 23:576, 1957.
9. Czeizel, A., and Tusnadi, G. An epidemiologic study of cleft lip with or without cleft palate and posterior cleft palate in Hungary. *Hum. Hered.* 21:17, 1971.
10. Fraser, G., and Calnan, G. Cleft lip and palate: Seasonal incidence, birth weight, birth rank, sex, site, associated malformations and parental age. *Arch. Dis. Child.* 36:420, 1961.

* A working knowledge of genetics, however, is *not* beyond the grasp of speech-language pathologists. Excellent texts are available, such as Stern [32] and Thompson and Thompson [33].

11. Fukuhara, T., New method and approach to the genetics of cleft lip and palate. *J. Dent. Res.* 44:259, 1965.

12. Gardner, H. What is congenital disease? *Otolaryngol. Clin. North Am.* 14:3, 1981.

13. Gilmore, S., and Hofman, S. Clefts in Wisconsin: Incidence and related factors. *Cleft Palate J.* 3:186, 1966.

14. Greene, J., Vermillion, J., Hay, S., Biggens, S., and Kerschbaum, S. Epidemiologic study of cleft lip and cleft palate in four states. *J. Am. Dent. Assoc.* 68:73, 1964.

15. Ingalls, T., Taube, I., and Klingberg, M. Cleft lip and cleft palate: Epidemiologic considerations. *Plast. Reconstr. Surg.* 34:1, 1964.

16. Jones, M. Etiology of facial clefts: Prospective evaluation of 428 patients. *Cleft Palate J.* 25:16, 1988.

17. Knox, G., and Braithwaite, F. Cleft lips and palates in Northumberland and Durham. *Arch. Dis. Child.* 38:66, 1963.

18. MacMahon, B., and McKeown, T. The incidence of harelip and cleft palate related to birth rank and maternal age. *Am. J. Hum. Genet.* 5:176, 1953.

19. Melnick, M., and Shields, E. Allelic restriction: A biologic alternative to multifactorial threshold inheritance. *Lancet* 1:176, 1976.

20. Melnick, M., Bixler, D., Fogh-Andersen, F., and Conneally, P. Cleft lip +/− cleft palate: An oveview of the literature and an analysis of Danish cases born between 1941 and 1968. *Am. J. Med. Genet.* 6:83, 1980.

21. Meskin, L., and Pruzansky, S. A malformation profile of facial cleft patients and their siblings. *Cleft Palate J.* 6:309, 1969.

22. Peterson-Falzone, S. Articulation Disorders in Orofacial Anomalies. In N. Lass et al. (Eds.), *Speech, Language and Hearing.* Philadelphia: Saunders, 1981. Vol. 2.

23. Peterson-Falzone, S. Resonance Disorders in Structural Defects. In N. Lass et al. (Eds.), *Speech, Language and Hearing.* Philadelphia: Saunders, 1981. Vol. 2.

24. Peterson-Falzone, S. Speech Disorders Related to Craniofacial Defects, Parts I and II. In N. Lass et al. (Eds.), *Handbook of Speech-Language Pathology and Audiology.* Toronto: Decker, 1988.

25. Rollnick, B., and Pruzansky, S. Genetic services at a center for craniofacial anomalies. *Cleft Palate J.* 18:304, 1981.

26. Shprintzen, R., Siegel-Sadewitz, A., Amato, J., and Goldberg, R. Anomalies associated with cleft lip, cleft palate, or both. *Am. J. Med. Genet.* 20:585, 1985.

27. Shprintzen, R. Syndromic cleft lip and palate. Presented in the Symposium on the Etiologic Heterogeneity of Cleft Lip and Palate. American Cleft Palate Association, San Antonio, Texas, May 10, 1987.

28. Siegel-Sadewitz, V., and Shprintzen, R. The relationship of communication disorders to syndrome identification. *J. Speech Hear. Disord.* 47:338, 1982.

29. Slavkin, H. *Developmental Craniofacial Biology.* Philadelphia: Lea & Febiger, 1979.

30. Smith,D. *Recognizable Patterns of Human Malformation* (3rd ed.). Philadelphia: Saunders, 1982.

31. Spriesterbach, D., Spriesterbch, B., and Moll, K. Incidence of clefts of the lip and palate in families with clefts and families with children without clefts. *Plast. Reconstr. Surg.* 29:392, 1962.

32. Stern, C. *Principles of Human Genetics* (2nd ed.). San Francisco: Freeman, 1960.

33. Thompson, J., and Thompson, M. *Genetics in Medicine* (4th ed.). Philadelphia: Saunders, 1986.

34. Wilson, M. A ten-year survey of cleft lip and cleft palate in the southwest region. *Br. J. Plast. Surg.* 25:224, 1972.

CHAPTER 3

Psychological Aspects of Cleft Lip and Palate

Edward Clifford

To understand the psychosocial consequences of clefting, it is important to place this condition within an appropriate frame of reference. We shall consider it within the context of a number of craniofacial malformations and then within the context of all malformations and functional limitations. By contrasting behaviors of people with clefts and other craniofacial malformations with those who have other anomalies, it should become possible to delineate the specific behavioral effects of having a cleft as opposed to the behavioral effects of having any nonspecified defect or functional limitation. We can ask if the behavior in question is a function of having a cleft or would, in general, be a function of having any malformation or disability. In this chapter we refer to all clefts by the generic term *cleft(s)*, unless it is necessary to refer to a specific cleft type.

A basic tenet of personality theory is that early developmental experiences influence later behavior. Consistent with that tenet, emergent psychological processes and experiences may be affected by a number of conditions associated with having a cleft. A cleft, depending on type and severity, is a birth defect having implications for the future growth and development of the child born with it. Functional limitations in the areas of speech, hearing, and dentition are often concomitants of the cleft condition. If the child develops a functional limitation such as poor hearing or poor speech, the child's interactions with others may be affected.

Other sequelae of psychological importance may be present early in life. The fact that some children with clefts of the palate are neither breast-fed nor bottle-fed may have important implications for the mother-child relationship. Problems associated with care and feeding of these children may modify child rearing in significant ways.

The infant with a cleft also faces the prospect of repeated visits to hospitals, clinics, and cleft palate teams for long-term treatment and evaluation. These efforts take place through the formative years and require the child's accommodation to the experiences and to the resulting change in appearance and function.

Finally it should be kept in mind that the experience of having a cleft is but one of many for the person involved. It may merge with other experiences or become particularly salient. Reactions to clefts take place simultaneously with other behaviors. Any descripton reflects the necessary simplification of specific behavioral and social processes.

In this chapter the literature related to psychological and social aspects of development are reviewed within the context of craniofacial malformations and disability in general. Four aspects are considered: (1) early parent-child behaviors and clefts; (2) effects of clefts on personality; (3) effects of clefts on achievement and competency; and (4) the adult status of those born with clefts.

EARLY PARENT-CHILD BEHAVIORS

Much of the research seeking to demonstrate the influence of early experience on the subsequent behaviors of children has focused on the effects of the caretaker on the child. The mother's interactions with her child have been emphasized. Our examination of the effects on mother-child relationships can begin with the birth of the child. Attention has been focused here because the birth of a child with a cleft is perceived as inducing a crisis having significant consequences for later relationships. Because parents want to give birth to a normal, healthy infant, and because they are not prepared for a baby with a defect, the birth precipitates a variety of reactions having shocklike characteristics. These reactions, particularly in the mother, are the concern of much of the literature about birth defects in general and clefts in particular.

EFFECT OF THE BIRTH OF A CHILD WITH A CLEFT

There is little reason to doubt that giving birth to a baby with a birth defect initially evokes a variety of negative feelings. Parents of infants with birth defects have had a number of differing negative affective states attributed to them, including feelings of anxiety, confusion, depression, disappointment, disbelief, frustration, grief, guilt, hurt, inadequacy, rejection, resentment, shock, stigmatization, and withdrawal [4, 15, 27, 29, 33, 49, 87, 88]. The negative feelings reported are not solely associated with clefts but appear to be general reactions to giving birth to infants with any defect present at birth.

The initial negative feelings and their expressed intensity are important because they provide part of the environment in which the child with the defect lives. Negative feelings about the defect may ultimately affect the child. Since intense negative affect is usually present, and since strong emotions may be disorganizing, the resultant effects are perceived to be disintegrative in nature. In such cases, the birth may be experienced as a severe disruption of familial patterns leading toward family disintegration. It should be pointed out that these very strong negative reactions primarily have been identified with giving birth to children with any severe birth defect. For example, more than 20 years ago Winick [99] reported a breakup in more than 50 percent of the families in a study of the effects of giving birth to children with severe cerebral palsy. Similarly, the birth of severely mentally retarded children markedly increased tendencies toward family disintegration [31, 32].

Less severe conditions, however, do not elicit such strong reactions. Pless and Roghmann [65], in a large-scale study of chronically ill children, reported a low rate of family disintegration. Clifford [17] and Clifford and Crocker [23] presented evidence suggesting the birth of a baby with a cleft may have integrative rather than disintegrative effects. Husbands and wives independently reported increases in marital satisfaction. These couples also reported positive changes in themselves following the births of their affected infants. Two other studies report similar findings. Slutsky [87] found that closer husband-wife relationships were reported by 32 percent of the mothers of infants with cleft lip and palate. Similarly, Spriesterbach [88] reported that 34 percent of the mothers and 25 percent of the fathers of children with clefts believed improvements in their marriage had taken place. Relatively few parents (10% of the mothers, 7% of the fathers) indicated that the marital relationship had been adversely affected. It seems reasonable therefore to expect an initial expression of negative feelings without implications for family disintegration. In the case of less severe birth defects the evidence suggests that family integration is not adversely affected in most cases.

There is an implication in several studies that the original negative effects following the birth of the baby with a defect may continue unabated for an unstated, but lengthy periods of time [12, 31, 60]. However, several investigators stressed that the first distressful feelings gave way to efforts to cope with the situation. Koch-Schulte [49] found that feelings of depression lasted up to 4 days in her studies of 13 sets of parents of babies with cleft lip and palate. Using clinical evidence Tisza and Gumpertz [89] reported that expressions of love and compassion emerged once mothers of infants with clefts overcame the original feelings and mastered their painful emotions. Clifford [17] reported that the effects of the original shock dissipated before the mother and infant were discharged from the hospital; and in a study of mothers of infants with cleft lip and palate Slutsky [87] reported that within a short time mothers recovered from their painful reactions to the birth.

One aspect of cleft palate, in contrast to other birth defects, needs to be emphasized. When mental retardation or severe cerebral palsy is apparent at birth, a high degree of uncertainty about the future of the infant is involved. Parents may be advised that only time will reveal the ultimate capabilities of their children. In contrast, a cleft is often pointed out as a structural defect capable of being repaired very early in the life of the child. Where a cleft lip is involved, for example, surgical repair can be anticipated within several weeks of the birth, while clefts of the palate may be closed before the child's first birthday. The expectation of early intervention, characteristic of the surgical treatment of clefts, in sharp contrast to other anomalies where parents must wait for the unfolding of the infant's status, may account for the comparatively benign reactions reported and for the seemingly rapid dissipation of the effects of the birth on the parents.

We cannot take a simplistic approach to these recalled reactions. In all probability they are not only a function of the birth defect itself. While it is reasonable to expect expressions of negative feelings, the resolution of the crisis present at birth is more likely to be related to the strengths and weaknesses of the parents, their abilities to cope with unexpected situations, their unique personal histories, and the state of their marriage.

THE HOSPITAL ENVIRONMENT

Parents remember and recall many details about the birth of a baby with a cleft and what happened to them in the hospital that may be affected by the hospital environment. For example, after being informed about their infant's condition, mothers indicated that the sight of the child was less disturbing to them than receiving the information that something was wrong with it. Parents find it difficult to tolerate the interval between being informed about the defect and seeing the baby. Because of the uncertainty involved, it is not unusual for parents to have disturbing fantasies about what is wrong which may not be specifically related to the defect itself [28].

While hospitals are well equipped for meeting crises associated with the maintenance of life, they are often not well equipped to handle emotional crises. Spriesterbach [88] stated that both paraprofessionals and professionals involved in the delivery were shocked when a baby with a cleft was born. Hospital personnel, if not trained to cope with either their own feelings about babies with defects or with feelings of parents, may upset parents who seek their help [68]. Mothers have reported evasiveness or abruptness on the part of professionals giving them information about the baby [28, 31]. In one study, it was found that 26 percent of the mothers and 28 percent of the fathers were not told about the baby's cleft by the physician [88]. In many cases there was a delay in telling the mother about her baby [23, 87 ,88]. Clif-

ford and Crocker [23] reported that the longer the delay in telling the mother about her baby or in showing the baby to her for the first time, the greater was the recalled impact. Delay had other effects: the longer the interval during which the mother did not see her baby, the greater was the recall of unhappy feelings on first seeing the baby.

CHILD-REARING ATMOSPHERES

Most reports imply that children with clefts are reared in socially restrictive atmospheres. On the basis of clinical experience, Castellanos and Stewart [15] believe that parents of children with clefts avoid social contacts because of the appearance of their children. In general, physically handicapped children are seen as having fewer interpersonal and social experiences and are less likely to be taken out on social occasions than normal children [68, 69].

Parents of children with craniofacial malformations have been reported as vacillating between expressing approval and warmth and expressing rejection and hostility, setting the scene for the display of oversolicitous and overprotective maternal behaviors [53]. Children with clefts, or other physical handicaps, may have parents who deal with them in a loving manner yet who tend to be arbitrary with them. There is some evidence that the affected child is given no voice in family matters; parents and children rarely talk about the defect; the child's questions are discouraged; and the affected child is given less responsibility than that given to a normal child [68, 69, 99].

An extensive interview study, however, casts doubt on the assumption that such an atmosphere generally exists in the case of cleft palate. Spriesterbach [88] interviewed 174 mothers and 167 fathers of children with clefts and 175 mothers and 170 fathers of children without clefts. Questions were asked about the extent of familial social life and the kinds of recreation and entertainment patterns. No significant differences were obtained between those two groups of parents.

If parents of children with clefts are overly solicitous or overprotective, some indication should exist in the personality profiles of the parents and in the behavior of the children. Using the Minnesota Multiphasic Personality Inventory, Goodstein [36] compared the personality profiles of 170 mothers and 157 fathers of children with clefts with profiles of 100 mothers and 100 fathers of normal children. No significant differences between the two groups of parents were found.

It seems clear that the clinical speculations about the effects of a cleft on caretakers have not been substantiated. Other than the fact that the child does have a cleft, the atmosphere in which the child is raised appears to be very little different than the environment in which children without a cleft are raised.

EARLY CHILD-REARING BEHAVIORS

Babies are expected to be completely dependent on their primary caregivers, their mothers, who provide life support, protection, love, and care [6]. Babies are expected to signal distress through crying and irritability to which mothers are expected to be responsive through appropriate caretaking activities. Babies have input into this social situation by being socially oriented, by attending to maternal behaviors, and by soliciting maternal behaviors that go beyond routine care [66].

In the usual, unidirectional socialization model, stress is usually placed on the role of powerful parents who control the environment and dominate all input to the baby. In this way they, presumably, directly shape and modify babies' behaviors. Babies are thus passively manipulated by their parents who are assumed to have a number of child-rearing skills with which they influence development.

However, recent formulations emphasize an active role for infants; they are not manipulated passive objects; infant reactions influence and modify parental behaviors, interactions, and ultimately their own socialization. Parents are influenced by the presence of a malformation, the baby's activity level, and by the baby's temperament [47]. Babies, in turn, are influenced by characteristics of parents including the sensitivity of parents to infant signals, the degree to which they are controlled, and expressed parental feelings of acceptance-rejection. Thus, a dynamic interaction exists between babies (care receivers) and parents (caregivers).

One of the earliest interactions between mother and child centers about feeding the baby. Information about the prevalence and severity of feeding difficulties encountered and their effects on the infant and mother is lacking. Prospective studies examining the child-rearing behavior of mothers of infants and young children are conspicuous by their absence.

Although it is known that a high proportion of the population with palatal clefts have feeding difficulties — 73 percent of 124 such infants had severe or moderate difficulties [88] — and although psychoanalytic theory in particular posits a relationship between early feeding and nurturing experiences and later personality development [67], few studies have taken advantage of this experiment of nature that cleft palate provides.

Feeding the child with a palatal cleft may result in dissatisfaction for mother and child because it can be slow and frequently interrupted. This atmosphere could interfere with one of the primary early satisfactions of mothering for both infant and mother. There may be a lack of adequate sucking opportunity, further contributing to possible frustration and perhaps leading to personality disturbances that are evidenced later in life [3, 89, 92].

Spriesterbach [88] reports that 85 percent of the mothers of children with clefts recalled some feeding problems with the children. In contrast, however, Tisza, Irwin, and Scheide [90] claim that mothers of such infants minimize the feeding difficulties when they recall their experiences. An intimate relationship exists between how babies with clefts were actually fed and reactions by mothers to the feeding situation. While the type of cleft influenced how mothers could feed their babies — bottle, breast, special means — the means used influenced whether mothers experienced strain in the feeding situation. The combination of cleft type and means of feeding influenced the recall of satisfaction or dissatisfaction with feeding several years later [22].

Children were affected by feelings mothers expressed about feeding. The recall of maternal satisfaction in the feeding of their children was related to the children's perception of parental nurturance and punitiveness, as shown by a story completion task. Mothers who were dissatisfied with feeding tended to have children whose stories characterized parents as being relatively low in nurturance and high in punitiveness [25].

Feeding methods did not seem to affect the amount of nonnutritive sucking infants displayed later on. Children fed by bottle or breast did not differ in the extent of nonnutritive sucking from children with clefts who were fed by other means. Furthermore, children with palatal clefts were not reported to differ in extent of nonnutritive sucking from children with cleft lips only [25]. Tisza, Irwin, and Zabarenko [91], however, found themes of oral aggression in the dramatic play of preschool children with clefts. These investigators related these themes to the violation of the child's body through surgical procedures, however, rather than to the feeding experience.

The early mother-child experiences, particularly as they related to the management of the cleft, are seen to have effects on the subsequent behavior of the child. In psychiatric interviews, Tisza et al. [90] observed what they felt to be a remarkable degree of passivity in the children with clefts. Tisza and her co-workers took the position that such children are forced into passivity because their mothers could not protect them from potentially traumatic events. These events include surgical experiences that are essentially inexplicable to young children, hospitalizations with enforced separations from the mother, and periodic examinations at a cleft palate center where the mother participates only as an onlooker.

Little is truly known about early mother-child experiences from the point of view of the child with a cleft. Most of the available information comes from psychiatrically oriented interviews or from parents who are asked to recall their experiences. Neither observational studies nor prospective studies are currently available. The limited evidence that exists allows for no definitive conclusions about this period of development. The home environments of children born with clefts have not been explored adequately, and information about the nature of parent-child interactions is essentially nonexistent.

PERSONALITY CORRELATES

A major focus of research into the psychosocial aspects of clefts has been on the personality of the affected person. Underlying most psychosocial research are assumptions about the effect of the social and cultural milieu on the individual. One set of assumptions has to do with the role of physical attractiveness and physical deviance in society.

PHYSICAL ATTRACTIVENESS

Society is oriented toward the physically attractive, and those who fail to achieve minimal acceptability may suffer rejection or be the objects of subtle prejudice. It has been shown, for example, that unattractive nursery school children were rated by their classmates as being less independent than attractive children and that adult ratings of children were affected by the attractiveness of the children [7]. Adults whose facial features are out of proportion may have negative personality characteristics or low intelligence attributed to them [26, 83].

Recent research has demonstrated that persons born with clefts are affected by the existing social stereotype. Schneidermann and Harding [81] had school children rate photographs of children with bilateral clefts, unilateral clefts, and children without clefts and found that children with clefts were rated negatively. The bilateral cleft photographs were reacted to more severely than the unilateral cleft photographs. Tobiasen [93] prepared two sets of photographs of the same individuals. One set contained photographs with clefts; the other set contained photographs corrected to remove the cleft. The photographs were then rated by school children in the 3rd, 6th, 8th, and 10th grades. Faces with clefts had significantly poorer ratings. They were rated as less good-looking, less popular, less likely to be chosen as friends, and less popular than faces without clefts. In addition, when the gender of the photographs was taken into account, girls with clefts were judged more negatively than boys with clefts. Age of the raters did not play a significant role.

Failure to measure up to a societal norm of attractiveness or of adequate functioning may result in a person's becoming stigmatized. Stigmatization creates persons who in the eyes of society are tainted or discounted and who have a "spoiled identity" calling forth behaviors in observers that are independent of the personal identities of the affected persons [35]. There are negative reactions in those seeing a severely deformed person [43, 54]. Those with facial paralysis or craniofacial malformations believe themselves to be socially inferior, attributing marginal status to themselves [43, 55]. Some individuals with facial disfigurements may believe they have no free choice in their relationships with members of the opposite sex and that they have to content themselves with any willing partner [14].

CLEFTS AND PERSONALITY

A number of very early studies examined the social and psychological adjustment of children with clefts. No differences were found by Watson [97] in study comparing 34 boys with cleft lip and palate, 19 physically handicapped boys, and 40 normal boys. Sidney and Matthews [84] contrasted the social adjustment of 21 children with clefts with two control groups and concluded that inferior social adjustment could not be attributed to the cleft. Billig [8] found normal or better adjustment in most of the 60 patients with cleft lip and palate that he examined; only three (5%) of these patients had unsatisfactory adjustment. Attacking the problem from a different point of view Birch [9] found no children with clefts among the 600 most severely maladjusted children in Pittsburgh public schools.

In only one study has any hint of maladjustment been found. Gluck et al. [34], in comparing the closed records of 292 patients seen for child guidance with the behaviors reported for 50 children with clefts, found that children with clefts demonstrated a higher proportion of enuresis and shyness than the child guidance cases. In general, however, the weight of the evidence indicates that the presence of a defect does not necessarily imply the presence of a personality disturbance. A relatively recent interview by McWilliams [58] stated that there was no compelling evidence that children with clefts differed in major ways from their nonaffected peers or that people with clefts were seriously disturbed.

CLEFTS AND SPECIFIC PERSONALITY CHARACTERISTICS

One group of characteristics, shyness, social inhibition, and passivity, presumably as defensive reactions to earlier negatively experienced social interactions, have been identified with clefts and craniofacial malformations. McWilliams [57] described children with clefts as compliant, passive, and somewhat self-effacing. In seeming contrast, however, a recent study found that children with clefts and associated congenital malformations tended to be noncompliant to parental discipline [95]. Epsteen [30], on the basis of clinical impressions, stated that those with facial disfigurements were somewhat inhibited in social expression.

The parents of children with craniofacial malformations interviewed by Lauer [53] characterized their children as shy, quiet, and uncomfortable in the presence of strangers. Yet, parents also saw their children with clefts and associated malformations to have conduct problems [95], although the frequency of such problems did not differ significantly from a control sample [94]. It is interesting to note that teachers rated children with clefts as being more socially inhibited in school, while parents did not view their children as socially inhibited at home [71].

Spriesterbach [88], using questionnaire interviews, described children with clefts in his sample as less gregarious, less confident, less aggressive, less mature, and more dependent than children in his control sample, although the obtained differences were not tested for statistical significance. In psychiatric interviews, a remarkable degree of passivity was noted in children with clefts [90]. Finally, young adults were characterized as observers rather than participants in social activities [96].

The lack of requisite social skills by the affected children could lead to patterns of withdrawal and inhibition according to Kapp-Simon [46]. Based on teacher ratings and self-appraisals, Richman and his colleagues have emphasized the presence of impulse inhibition (viewed as a conduct disorder) in children and adolescents with clefts [40, 41, 70]. In a subsequent study Richman [72] reported that although group scores for those with clefts indicated good adjustment, a number of adolescents had poor self-perceived social adjustment scores. He concluded that social introversion was related more to appearance factors than to speech factors in this group of adolescents. The argument raised is an important one. While the global adjustment scores of persons with clefts are equivalent to those of the noncleft population, a proportion of those with clefts remain adversely affected; for example, the psychological functioning of 10 percent of young adults was found to be clearly inadequate and an additional 23 percent was characterized as clearly inadequate [42]. One cannot conclude that all children with clefts are normal or that they remain unaffected by having been born with a cleft. McWilliams [58] points out that children with clefts and their parents may pay a high price for the adjustments and accommodations that have to be made.

Several studies, conducted between 1951 and 1971, examined the effect of clefts on personality patterns reflected in personality tests. Group comparisons between those with clefts and their nonaffected peers reveal global similarities rather than differences. For example, Rorschach responses did not differentiate people with clefts from normal subjects [39, 101]. Wirls and Plotkin [101], using an extensive battery of structured and unstructured personality tests, examined the responses of 66 children with cleft lip and palate and an equal number of their siblings and found no significant differences between the two samples of children. No significant differences were found when "cleft" and "normal" samples were compared by Schweckendiek and Danzer [82]. Finally, a number of reviews have concluded there is no evidence in the literature to support the existence of a "cleft palate personality," although some question remains about the prevalence of social inhibition and shyness [19, 20, 38, 58, 78, 101].

Observational studies of children with clefts at home, in school, and in the presence of strangers can serve to clarify in situ behaviors. It would be crucial as well to delineate aspects of the interactions of the affected child with others to determine the conditions under which shyness, withdrawn behavior, and social inhibition become prominent.

SELF-CONCEPT AND BODY IMAGE

The development of a child takes place within a context of interactions with others. During early phases of development these interactions occur within the family unit, and family members, acting as social mirrors, provide children with information about themselves. Perceptions of being valued and accepted, as well as perceptions of attitudes expressed toward them, affect the children's emerging concepts about themselves and their bodies. During later development children are exposed to greater numbers of people, who provide them with further information about themselves. It is when children are involved in interactions with others that they become aware of the effect of their appearance on others. Informal observations indicate that children with facial disfigurements do not perceive themselves as different from physically intact children until the age of 4 or 5 [44, 48]. It is believed that increased contact with a large number of children in preschool,

kindergarten, or first grade, results in their becoming stigmatized [37, 44, 53].

Children also integrate into their self-systems a variety of attitudes toward the body and its functioning. Since initial mother-child relationships involve a high degree of physical contact, mothers convey to their children some of their attitudes toward the body. Those attitudes may be reinforced verbally. In this sense children's body concepts are reflective of the significant people around them [98]. The totality of children's attitudes, their body images, are presumed to be relatively stable, particularly at older ages, although they can be influenced by needs and wishes arising from the unconscious [80]. A discrepancy may arise between persons' true appearances and their body concepts, because their body images fail to correspond to reality.

Several studies have examined body image using the Draw-A-Person technique. The assumption is that the drawings represent unconscious aspects of the personality and are therefore projections of the body image [56]. Interpretations lean heavily on the presence as well as the absence of a variety of body parts depicted in the drawings. Unfortunately, not only do many of the studies suffer from poor experimental design, the validity of the Draw-A-Person as a body image measure is also questionable.

No evidence of facial distortion appeared in the drawings of 12 children with clefts which were compared to those of an equal number of controls [27]. Nor were differences obtained in the Ruess [77] study comparing the drawings of children with clefts with those of their siblings. Ruess first believed that differences would have been obtained had the drawing been confined to the face or the head. In a later study, however, Ruess and Lis [79] found no significant differences among children with clefts, their siblings, and normal controls when facial drawings were compared. Palmer and Adams [61] collected facial and full-figure drawings from 20 children with cleft lip and palate and two control samples of physically normal children and found no significant differences among the groups.

Abel [1] and Abel and Weissman [2] obtained figure drawings from 45 adult patients with craniofacial distortions and other facial anomalies. The absence of facial distortions in the drawings was apparent. The patients were divided into two groups on the basis of their actual appearance — mildly distorted and severely distorted. Since a greater proportion of adults in the severe group (42%) than adults in the mild group (19%) produced drawings with some evidence of facial distortion, the investigators concluded that those with the more severe facial disfigurements were more realistic about themselves than those with mild disfigurements. These conclusions, however, are reached on rather tenuous grounds. The criteria for the presence or absence of a realistic body image are not made clear. The absence of facial distortion in a drawing could as well be called denial, and the presence of distortion deemed an indication of an impoverished or poor body image.

The body satisfactions expressed by a group of 98 adults with clefts were evaluated by Clifford, Crocker, and Pope [24]. Compared to a control sample, body satisfaction levels of the patients with clefts were found to be high, a finding also reported by Bjornsson and Agustsdottir [11]. Although those results seemed to indicate little or no concern with the body, a subsequent analysis revealed that having a cleft did influence the relative satisfaction ratings of specific body parts and functions. When satisfaction levels attributed to each body part or function were ranked, those with cleft of the lip, with or without cleft palate, were less satisfied with speech functions than patients with cleft lip only. Compared to normal subjects, all those with cleft palate were less satisfied with their mouths, teeth, lips, voices, talking, and speech [86].

Brantley and Clifford [13] experimentally examined cognitive organization, self-concept, and body image in 51 patients with clefts, 22 hospitalized obese patients, and 100 normal controls ranging in age between 11 and 18 years. Eighteen different body image variables were involved, including measures of ease of body functioning, appearance, body satisfaction, and concern about physical health. All body image measures had scores derived from a factor analysis of each test. These factor scores were then entered into a discriminant function analysis to determine the best linear combination of body image scores to differentiate among the three groups of adolescents. A linear combination of 11 of 18 body image variables was discriminating. The discriminant function analysis classified normals and subjects with clefts with 72.7 percent accuracy, with subjects with clefts frequently falling into the normal category. When obese adolescents and adolescents with clefts were compared, the function classified 95.9 percent accurately. The investigators

concluded that body image variables seemed to differentiate obese subjects from the other groups but did not seem to play a significant role in cleft palate.

There have been a variety of studies examining the effect of clefts on the self. Some researchers, on the basis of informal and clinical observations, believe that the devalued status of handicapped persons is reflected in self-depreciation and low self-esteem [68, 69]. According to Castellanos and Stewart [15] hypersensitivity and increased demands for personal attention are rooted in strong fears of rejection experienced by the facially disfigured. Other reactions attributed to this group of patients include coping with anxiety through the use of repression, constriction, or depression [5]; feeling of shame and inferiority, and antisocial tendencies [30]; and tendencies toward paranoid ideation [43].

Kapp [45] found that the global self-concept scores (Piers-Harris) of children with clefts and nonaffected peers were similar, while Clifford [18] reported similar findings with adolescents. In addition, self-satisfaction levels in adults with clefts were also found to be relatively high [24]. However, Kapp did find that children with clefts had significantly lower global happiness and satisfaction scores. In a subsequent study with older children, using a different self-concept measure administered by teachers, Kapp [46] examined the self-concepts of primary school–age children and found that children with clefts had poorer global self-concept scores. They viewed themselves as more frequently sad and angry and less socially adept than their peers.

Using a semantic differential approach, the meaning of clefts to adolescents was examined [16]. They considered the concepts of *cleft lip* and *cleft palate* to be relatively benign, closer in meaning to *headache* than to *illness* or *death*.

Despite high levels of self-satisfaction, adolescents with clefts had lower perceived parental acceptance scores than asthmatic adolescents with whom they were compared on the When I was Born test [18]. This test asked respondents to imagine what it was like at the time of their births and assumed that current feelings were projected as perceptions of what happened at birth. A subsequent study obtained responses on this test from 114 adolescents with cleft lip and palate, 11 craniofacial surgical patients, 73 asthmatic patients, 24 hospitalized obese patients, and 140 normal adolescent and young adult controls. In contrast to the other groups, adolescents with clefts perceived their parents to have predominantly negative emotions, imagined a higher degree of parental apprehension, and felt their parents had less pride in them and did not care to nurture them [21].

The Brantley and Clifford study [13] also included 15 self-concept variables, including the When I Was Born test and a variety of self-rating measures. Other than the responses on When I Was Born, which were lower for adolescents with clefts than for obese or normal adolescents, response patterns on self-concept measures demonstrated high self-evaluations for adolescents with clefts as compared to other subjects. Using the pattern of low scores on When I Was Born and higher scores on other self-concept measures, adolescents with clefts were discriminated with 83.4 percent accuracy from normal adolescents and with 90.4 percent accuracy from obese adolescents [13].

In a departure from the usual comparisons of children with clefts and normal peers, Richman, Holmes, and Eliason [76] compared well-adjusted and poorly adjusted adolescents with cleft lip and palate, based on parent reports. They found that the well-adjusted group had more realistic perceptions of their appearance, and viewed their behaviors as being more socially acceptable than the poorly adjusted group. Interestingly, the self-perceptions of the well-adjusted adolescents were similar to the perceptions their parents had about them.

Despite occasional findings indicating that the self-concepts of persons with clefts have been affected, Richman and Eliason [73] concluded that the overall self-concepts of children with clefts were relatively good, although there appeared to be situational concerns related to appearance. Prevailing generalizations and expectations emphasize a persistent belief that having a cleft can only have adverse effects on self-concept. However, the weight of the evidence seems to indicate that having a cleft has subtle rather than gross effects. Self-concept measures do not reveal depressed overall self-evaluations. Body image measures, in general, give no indication that gross distortions are present. The responses to the When I Was Born test seem to indicate that patients with clefts have an awareness that their deformity at birth influenced their parents in negative ways, but their attitudes about themselves are toward the positive end of the scale. Adolescents and adults with clefts tend to be less satisfied with those aspects of themselves and their bodies that are specifically related to having a cleft, namely, parts of the face that are involved with the cleft and aspects of the communication process centering about voice and speech.

ACHIEVEMENT AND COMPETENCY

Our attention up to this point has been focused on personal competency as reflected in personality characteristics of those with clefts. The potential effects of clefts in the attainment of competencies in the areas of social development, visual-motor performance, and intelligence will be discussed now.

SOCIAL DEVELOPMENT

In one of the few studies examining social competency of children with clefts, Goodstein [37] had 139 mothers of children with clefts and 174 mothers of normal children complete the Vineland Social Maturity Scale. Through interviews and direct observations the ability of the child to perform selected social tasks was assessed and the obtained social quotient (SQ), believed to be similar to the IQ concept, was regarded as an index of social maturation. Children with clefts obtained a mean SQ of 99.8, while the normal controls had a mean SQ of 103.5. The difference in means of 3.7 SQ points was statistically significant. On further analysis of the data it was found that most of the difference could be attributed to the lower scores obtained by the young children with clefts (mean SQ = 96.7) and the somewhat higher scores obtained by the normal controls (mean SQ = 108.5). Such emphasis on the relatively small differences found, however, seems questionable, and scores of 96.7 or 99.8 can hardly be classified as reflecting social retardation as suggested by Wirls [100]. The Vineland Social Maturity Scale was also used in another study, in which children with clefts were not found to be significantly different from normal children in levels of social maturity [84].

Another index of social development in our culture is the age of entrance into first grade. In most communities this is determined by birth date and usually occurs when the child is 6 years of age. Spriesterbach [88] reported that the average age on school entrance of children with clefts was 76.0 months, compared to an average age of 75.7 months for the normal control children. At the same time he reported a tendency for children with clefts to be delayed on entering school. When the data are examined for a large number of cases, however, it is found that the delay is caused by the birth date being out of phase with school admission policy, which can hardly be related to the presence of a cleft. Only nine (11%) of the 81 children with clefts and three (3%) of the 89 normal children actually experienced a delayed school entrance.

The amount of information available about the social maturation of children with clefts during the first 6 years of life is very limited. There seems to be little effect of a cleft on aspects of social maturation as they are measured by the Vineland scale or indicated by the age of entrance into school. Children with clefts appear to be operating within normal limits.

It is commonly believed that sensitivities to appearance and function are heightened during adolescence and that those with clefts may be particularly affected. Although the general adjustment of adolescents with clefts appear to be in the normal range, Richman [72] states that affected adolescents have concerns about social interactions specifically related to their feelings about their appearance, while Birch and Lindsay [10] suggest that heterosexual conflicts intensify during this period. There is a strong belief that adolescents with clefts develop defensive patterns because they are vulnerable to any criticism by their peers and do not want to jeopardize interpersonal relationships [85]. Quite obviously, much more needs to be known about social relationships in interaction with having a cleft during adolescence and early adulthood.

VISUAL-MOTOR PERFORMANCE

The question can be raised as to whether there is a neurological substrate associated with clefting, since a relatively high incidence of other associated physical anomalies has been observed. In addition, it has been observed that children with clefts have difficulties in perceptual motor tasks that are not reflected in their overall IQ scores [92].

Ruess analyzed the performance of 49 children with clefts and their siblings on the Bender Visual Motor Gestalt Test and found no discernible pathological condition in either sibling or cleft groupings [77]. In a later study, Ruess and Lis [79] included the Bender in a battery of tests. They compared 97 children with clefts, 237 of their siblings, and 145 normal control children between the ages of 5 and 18. No differences were obtained between the children with clefts and their nonaffected peers.

In a slightly different approach, Lamb, Wilson, and Leeper [50] examined perceptual organizations of 26 children with clefts and 26 sibling controls. They defined a perceptual organization factor as an average of the Block Design and Object Assembly subtest scores of the Wechsler Intelligence Scale for Children (WISC). Scores on this factor for the sample of children with clefts was not significantly different from the scores of their siblings. An examination of the scaled scores obtained reveals that both samples of children were operating within normal limits.

Two recent studies are of particular interest. Richman and Eliason [74] found that children with cleft palate only contrasted to those with combined clefts of the lip and palate on measures of reading disability demonstrated higher levels of reading disabilities and concluded that those with cleft palate only constituted a language disorder group. In a subsequent study Richman, Eliason, and Lindgren [75] compared elementary school children with cleft palate only to those with cleft lip and palate. The incidence of reading disability in the cleft lip and palate group approximated the rate in the normal population (17%), while the reading disability rate in the cleft-palate-only group was significantly higher (33%). One may speculate whether or not this is an argument for the presence of a neural substrate in children with cleft palate only.

The cited studies, however, revealed no evidence of a pathological condition. No reason has been found thus far to expect children with clefts to perform at levels that indicate difficulties with perceptual motor organization, other than that involved in the reading process. In this area of competency, also, they appear to be operating within normal limits.

INTELLIGENCE

Considerable attention has been paid to intelligence levels achieved by children with cleft palate. In part the focus on intelligence testing may be a function of the state of psychometric testing. Standardized tests are readily available and have demonstrable validity and reliability, particularly individually administered tests. Another salient reason for the emphasis on intelligence testing has been the separate Verbal Performance and Full Scale IQs, which have facilitated the examination of intellectual functioning of children with clefts in whom speech disorders and communication difficulties are frequently found.

Subjects with clefts obtain IQ scores *within the test norms for the normal range of intelligence.* The average Full Scale IQ scores reported for cleft palate samples range from 94.0 to 102.6, and the range for the control samples is from 103.8 to 111.3. Reported mean verbal IQ scores for children with clefts ranged between 91.5 and 99.66, while the range for controls varied between 102.6 and 109.4. Finally, Performance IQ scores ranged between 97.9 and 106.9 for subjects with clefts and from 105.2 to 111.4 for control subjects [37, 51, 73, 77, 79, 100].

It can be seen that the ranges reported for children with clefts were slightly lower than the ranges reported for the control children. In some studies, particularly the earlier ones, the difference was statistically significant. It can also be seen that the reported Verbal IQ scores tended to be lower than Performance IQ scores for subjects with clefts; those differences tended to be significant.

While lower IQ scores are sometimes attributed to having a cleft, other, uncontrolled factors may also account for the obtained differences. Such factors may include socioeconomic status and the intellectual level of the parents. Ruess and Lis [79] approached the assessment of intelligence in a more sophisticated fashion. They reasoned there were a number of factors influencing the expression of intelligence, including sex, age, the hearing status of the child, and parental IQ. Each of these variables were systematically controlled, primarily through the use of covariate techniques. Ruess and Lis also used entire families as their subjects. Information was obtained from 97 families in which there were children with clefts. Those families contained 237 siblings. Forty-seven families containing 145 children served as normal controls. The analysis of covariance, adjusting for age, sex, the father's Full Scale IQ, the mother's Full Scale IQ, the child's hearing status, and the child's frequency of ear infections, revealed no statistically significant differences among the groups of children with clefts, siblings, and control subjects. No significant differences could be attributed to cleft

lip only, cleft palate only, or combined clefts of the lip and palate. Ruess and Lis concluded that children with clefts demonstrated no unusual or remarkable deviations from their nonaffected peers [79].

Lamb et al. [50], in a study of 26 children with clefts and an equal number of their siblings, examined the relationship of WISC Verbal, Performance, and Full Scale IQ scores to hearing acuity. Verbal IQ scores for the group with clefts were significantly depressed even when hearing sensitivity was within normal limits. In a later study those investigators used the WISC to examine 73 children with cleft palate to ascertain the effects of cleft type and sex on IQ. No significant differences were found when subjects with cleft palate only and subjects with cleft lip and palate were compared [51].

There appears to be consensual validation in the literature that there are discrepancies between Verbal IQ and Performance IQ levels. Before we can attribute these differences to the presence of the cleft, it is necessary to control a number of factors. Finally, it is appropriate to point out that exclusive attention has been paid to intellectual levels as reflected in IQ scores, while there are no published studies to date of cognitive growth in cleft palate children or their cognitive processing or problem solving behaviors.

ADULT STATUS

The ultimate purpose of cleft palate management is to make it easier for the person born with clefts to take on normal and appropriate roles as an adult. Studies have examined the status of adults with clefts for their educational, vocational, and social achievements. More specifically, attempts were made to determine whether their functioning in these areas was impaired.

EDUCATIONAL STATUS

One measure of educational attainment, or the lack of it, is reflected in the rate at which persons with clefts drop out of high school. This rate has been reported as ranging from 20 to 27 percent of the "cleft" samples assessed [24, 59, 63]. With one exception, the dropout rate reported for those with clefts was not significantly different from the dropout rate of their siblings [59]. In a study of Finnish cleft lip and palate subjects, Latti, Rintala, and Soivio [52] also found no significant differences in dropout rate between the affected subjects and their siblings. Peter and Chinsky [63] also found the dropout rate for their subjects with clefts did not significantly differ from the rate for normal controls or from the 30 percent rate indicated by the U.S. Census.

The obverse of the dropout rate is the educational level achieved. A high proportion of subjects with clefts (73–80%) finished high school or went beyond it. Differences in educational achievement levels between subjects with cleft palate and siblings were not significant [59, 63]. A generational trend analysis in which the educational level of the subjects was compared to parental educational levels, reveals that all subjects had significantly higher educational levels than their parents, as is true nationally. There were no statistically significant differences in generational trends when subjects with clefts, siblings, and normal controls were compared [59, 63]. The data do not indicate that the educational levels achieved by persons with clefts are in any way different from those of the rest of the population.

VOCATIONAL STATUS

Peter, Chinsky, and Fisher [64] examined the vocational and economic status of 196 adult subjects with clefts, 190 siblings of those subjects, and 209 random controls and concluded that adults with clefts functioned within normal limits in terms of employment. The McWilliams and Paradise [59] study of 115 adult patients with clefts similarly revealed no significant differences in occupational levels of the patients, their siblings, and their fathers. Clifford, Crocker, and Pope [24] examined the socioeconomic status levels of 98 adult patients with clefts, comparing the obtained levels to those expected on the Minnesota Scale of Parental Occupations, and found a higher distribution of adults with clefts at upper socioeconomic levels than expected. Similarly, more than half the subjects in a Canadian study were in professional or white collar occupations [42]. No such socioeconomic differences, however, were found in the study by Peter and his colleagues [64].

No differences between adults with clefts and control groups have been obtained for employ-

ment stability or satisfaction, although those with clefts tended to feel less secure in their employment. When unemployed, the subjects with clefts tended to be out of work more frequently and for longer periods of time than normal controls but not as compared to their siblings [64]. Heller, Tidmarsh, and Pless [42] reported that 30 percent of their sample had some difficulty finding employment, and 45 percent were enthusiastic about the positions they currently held.

SOCIAL STATUS

Studies of the social status of adults with clefts primarily have been concerned with marital status. Many persons with craniofacial malformations believe they have no free choice in their heterosexual relationships and that they have to content themselves with any willing partner.

In one study, however, adults with clefts indicated that having a cleft had little influence on their dating behavior during adolescence. They also indicated that they were satisfied with their sexual experiences and with their marriages [24].

On the other hand, two studies agreed that persons with clefts married at significantly lower rates than their siblings [59, 62]. Peter and Chinsky [62] used questionnaires to examine aspects of marital status for subjects with clefts, their siblings, and random controls. Approximately 26 percent of the subjects with clefts never married, in contrast to the approximate 8 percent rate for the other groups. When subjects with clefts married, they were significantly older (a mean difference of approximately 2½ years) than their siblings or than random controls. The type of cleft the person had was not related to marital age [59].

The divorce rate of adults with cleft palate was similar to that for siblings and normal controls. It was found that more marriages were childless, that adults with clefts tended to have fewer children per marriage, and that they had fewer children per years married [62].

Actuarial rates demonstrate that there are effects of clefts on marriage and decisions to have children. Investigations are needed to examine the attitudes and feelings adolescents and adults with clefts have toward marriage that account for these rather subtle differences. It is clear, however, that the drastic effects on heterosexual relationships put forth by Byrt [14] for patients with craniofacial anomalies do not apply to subjects with clefts.

DISCUSSION

In this chapter the literature related to psychological and social aspects of clefts has been reviewed. Four aspects were considered: (1) early parent-child behaviors, (2) personality correlates, (3) achievement and competency, and (4) the status of adults.

The shocklike reactions parents have when a baby with a cleft is born does not in most cases adversely affect family integration. Initial expressions of negative feelings are to be expected, but most frequently these soon give way to efforts to cope with the situation. In part, the benign reactions reported may be a function of the cleft, which is a remedial structural defect. The availability of rehabilitative procedures may tend to reduce the stress and parental anxiety. Parents of children with clefts are not so affected that they provide either overly solicitous or socially restrictive home environments. While early parent-child relationships have to take the sequelae of the cleft condition into account, the coping ability of these parents seems to come to the fore.

The weight of the evidence seems to indicate subtle rather than gross effects on the personality of children with clefts. No evidence of psychopathological conditions or of a persistent personality profile exists. Some degree of consensual validation exists which indicates that children with clefts are shy and withdrawn. However, self-concept measures do not reveal depressed self-evaluations for adolescents with clefts and there is no indication that the overall body image of adolescents with clefts is affected. Aspects of their appearance and functioning may lead to heightened sensitivity in interpersonal relationships. These adolescents do tend to be less satisfied with those aspects of themselves and their bodies that are directly related to having a cleft; they are especially aware of their speech as well as of their lips and their teeth.

The achievements and competencies of children with clefts also appear to be within normal limits. Persistently, however, small but significant differences emerge. The obtained differences are uniformly in the direction of poorer performance for the child with a cleft. There is some indication that when a number of environmental factors are controlled, such as parental intelligence, the reported differences tend to disappear. Information is lacking, however, about details of the cognitive functioning of the affected children. Almost exclusively, attention has been paid to IQ scores, while problem solving or cognitive processing variables have been ignored.

When cleft palate is placed within the context of all craniofacial malformations and is contrasted with a number of other congenital defects as well, the potential modification of the cleft condition becomes apparent. Parental reactions to the child's birth, the absence of familial disintegration following the birth, and the absence of severe personality disturbances in children with clefts may indicate that cleft palate is more benign than other craniofacial anomalies or other birth defects such as severe cerebral palsy or retardation.

Finally, it is clear that these persons, as adults, assume reasonable positions in society and do not appear to be remarkably different from others. Their educational attainments are fairly typical of adults in our society. Occupational levels do not appear to be affected by clefts, although affected adults may feel less secure in their jobs, possibly because they tended to be out of work more frequently and for longer periods of time than adults with whom they were compared. Although fewer cleft palate adults marry, their marriages tend to be stable. They do tend to marry later and have fewer children than the general population. Nevertheless, it can be concluded that a cleft has no drastic effect on marriage. It would seem reasonable to conclude that the cleft palate experience did not prevent the persons having it from assuming adequate places in our society.

REFERENCES

1. Abel, T. M. Figure drawings and facial disfigurement. *Am. J. Orthopsychiatry* 23:253, 1953.
2. Abel, T. M., and Weissman, S. Psychological Aspects. In F. C. Macgregor, T. M. Abel, A. Byrt, E. Lauer, and S. Weissman (Eds.), *Facial Deformities and Plastic Surgery.* Springfield, Il.: Thomas, 1953, Pp. 130–165.
3. Alpert, A. Notes on the effect of a birth defect on the pregenital psychosexual development of a boy. *Am. J. Orthopsychiatry* 29:186, 1959.
4. Barker, R. G. The social psychology of physical disability. *J. Soc. Issues* 4:29, 1948.
5. Barron, J. Physical handicap and personality: A study of seen versus unseen disabilities. *Arch. Phys. Med.* 36:639, 1955.
6. Bell, R. Q. Contributions of Infants to Caregiving and Social Interactions. In M. Lewis and A. Rosenblum (Eds.), *The Effect of the Infant on His Caregiver.* New York: Wiley, 1974, Pp. 1–19.
7. Berscheid, E., and Walster, E. Beauty and the beast. *Psy-*

chol. Today 5:42, 1972.

8. Billig, A. L. A psychological appraisal of cleft palate patients. *Proc. Pa. Acad. Sci.* 25:29, 1951.

9. Birch, J. Personality characteristics of individuals with cleft palate: Research needs. *Cleft Palate Bull.* 2:5, 1952.

10. Birch, J. R., and Lindsay, W. K. An evaluation of adults with repaired bilateral cleft lips and palates. *Plast. Reconstr. Surg.* 48:457, 1971.

11. Bjornsson, A., and Agustsdottir, S. A psychosocial study of Icelandic individuals with cleft lip or cleft lip and palate. *Cleft Palate J.* 24:152, 1987.

12. Boles, G. Personality factors in mothers of cerebral palsied children. *Gen. Psychol. Monogr.* 59:159, 1959.

13. Brantley, H. T., and Clifford, E. Cognitive, self-concept and body image measures of normal, cleft palate and obese adolescents. Paper presented at meeting of American Cleft Palate Association, San Francisco, 1976.

14. Bryt, A. Psychiatric Aspects. In F. C. Macgregor, T. M. Abel, A. Bryt, E. Lauer, and S. Weissman (Eds.), *Facial Deformities and Plastic Surgery.* Springfield, Il.: Thomas, 1953, Pp. 166–207.

15. Castellanos, M. C., and Stewart, M. Psychosocial Implications in Plastic Surgery. In J. M. Converse (Ed.), *Reconstructive Plastic Surgery.* Philadelphia: Saunders, 1964, Pp. 384–393.

16. Clifford, E. Connotative meaning of concepts related to cleft lip and palate. *Cleft Palate J.* 4:165, 1967.

17. Clifford, E. Effects of giving birth to a cleft lip-palate baby. Paper presented at Plastic Surgery Research Council, Durham, N.C., 1968.

18. Clifford, E. The impact of symptom: A preliminary comparison of cleft lip-palate and asthmatic children. *Cleft Palate J.* 6:221, 1969.

19. Clifford, E. Psychosocial Aspects of Orofacial Anomalies: Speculations in Search of Data. In R. T. Wentz (Ed.), *Orofacial Anomalies: Clinical and Research Implications. ASHA Reports* No. 8. Washington, D.C.: American Speech and Hearing Association, 1973.

20. Clifford, E. *The Cleft Palate Experience: New Perspectives on Management.* Springfield, Il.: Thomas, 1987.

21. Clifford, E., and Bentz, E. When I Was Born: A comparative study of normal and clinical samples. Paper presented at American Cleft Palate Association meeting, New Orleans, February 1975.

22. Clifford, E., and Clifford, M. The cleft palate child's perception of parental nurturance and punitiveness. Paper presented at American Cleft Palate Association meeting, San Diego, February 1979.

23. Clifford, E., and Crocker, E. C. Maternal responses: The birth of a normal child as compared to the birth of a child with a defect. *Cleft Palate J.* 8:298, 1971.

24. Clifford, E., Crocker, E. C., and Pope, B. A. Psychological findings in the adulthood of 98 cleft lip-palate children. *Plast. Reconstr. Surg.* 50:234, 1972.

25. Clifford, E., and Sinicrope, P. E. *Feeding History and Father Participation in the Care of Children with Clefts: Effects on the Child's Perception of Parental Roles.* Durham, N.C.: Child Psychiatry Research Laboratory, 1972.

26. Cook, S. W. The judgment of intelligence from photographs. *J. Abnorm. Soc. Psychol.* 34:384, 1939.

27. Corah, N. L., and Corah, P. L. A study of body image in children with cleft palate and cleft lip. *J. Gen. Psychol.* 103:133, 1963.

28. D'Arcy, E. Congenital defects: Mothers' reactions to the first information. *Br. Med. J.* 3:796, 1968.

28b. Drotar S., et al. The adaptation of parents to the birth of an infant with congenital malformation: A hypothetical model. *Pediatrics* 56:710, 1975.

29. Easson, W. M. Psychopathological environment reaction to congenital defect. *J. Nerv. Ment. Dis.* 142:453, 1966.

30. Epsteen, C. M. Psychological impact of facial deformities. *Am. J. Surg.* 96:745, 1958.

31. Farber, B. Family organization and crisis: Maintenance of integration in families with a severely mentally retarded child. *Monogr. Soc. Res. Child Dev.* 25, 1960.

32. Farber, B., and Jenne, W. C. Family organization and parent-child communication: Parents and siblings of a retarded child. *Monogr. Soc. Res. Child Dev.* 28, 1963.

33. Fishman, C. A., and Fishman, D. B. Maternal correlates of self-esteem and overall adjustment in children with birth defects. *Child Psychiatry Hum. Dev.* 1:255, 1971.

34. Gluck, M. R., McWilliams, B. J., Wylie, H. L., and Conkwright, E. A. Comparison of clinical characteristics of children with cleft palates and children in a child guidance clinic. *Percept. Mot. Skills* 21:806, 1965.

35. Goffman, E. *Stigma.* Englewood Cliffs, N.J.: Prentice-Hall, 1963.

36. Goodstein, L. D. MMPI differences between parents of physically normal children. *J. Speech Hear. Res.* 3:31, 1960.

37. Goodstein, L. D. Intellectual impairment in children with cleft palate. *J. Speech Hear. Res.* 4:287, 1961.

38. Goodstein, L. D. Psychosocial Aspect of Cleft Palate. In D. C. Spriestersbach (Ed.), *Cleft Palate and Communication.* New York: Academic Press, 1968. Pp. 201–204.

39. Hackbush, F. Psychological studies of cleft palate patients. *Cleft Palate Bull.* 1:7, 1951.

40. Harper, D. C., and Richman, L. C. Personality profiles of physically impaired adolescents. *J. Clin. Psychol.* 34:636, 1978.

41. Harper, D. C., Richman, L. C., and Snider, B. School adjustment and degree of physical impairment. *J. Pediatr. Psychol.* 5:377, 1980.

42. Heller, A., Tidmarsh, W., and Pless, B. The psychosocial functioning of young adults born with cleft lip or palate. *Clin. Pediatr.* 20:459, 1981.

43. Hirschenfang, S., Goldberg, M. J., and Benton, J. G. Psychological aspects of patients with facial paralysis. *Dis. Nerv. Syst.* 30:257, 1969.

44. Jabaley, M. E., Hoopes, J. E., Knorr, N. J., and Meyer, E. The Burned Child. In M. Debuskey (Ed.), *The Chronically Ill Child and His Family.* Springfield, Il.: Thomas, 1970.

45. Kapp, K. Self-concept of the cleft lip and/or palate child. *Cleft Palate J.* 16:171, 1979.

46. Kapp-Simon, K. Self-concept of primary-school-age children with cleft lip, cleft palate, or both. *Cleft Palate J.* 23:24, 1986.

47. Kearsley, R. B. Iatrogenic Retardation: A Syndrome of Learned Incompetence. In R. B. Kearsley and I. E. Sigel (Eds.), *Infants at Risk: Assessment of Cognitive Functioning.* New York: Wiley, 1979, Pp. 153–180.

48. Knorr, N. J., Hoopes, J. E., and Edgerton, M. T. Psychiatric-surgical approach to adolescent disturbance in self image. *Plast. Reconstr. Surg.* 41:248, 1968.

49. Koch-Schulte, R. Family adjustment to the newborn with cleft lip and palate. Paper presented at the American Cleft Palate Association, Miami Beach, 1968.

50. Lamb, M. M., Wilson, F. B., and Leeper, H. A. A comparison of selected cleft palate children and their sib-

lings on the variables of intelligence, hearing loss and visual-perceptual-motor abilities. *Cleft Palate J.* 9:218, 1972.

51. Lamb, M. M., Wilson, F. B., and Leeper, H. A. The intellectual function of cleft palate compared on the basis of cleft type and sex. *Cleft Palate J.* 10:367, 1973.

52. Latti, A., Rintala, A., and Soivio, A. I. Educational levels of patients with cleft lip and palate. *Cleft Palate J.* 11:36, 1974.

53. Lauer, E. The Family. In F. C. Macgregor, T. M. Abel, A. Bryt, E. Lauer, and S. Weissman (Eds.), *Facial Deformities and Plastic Surgery.* Springfield, Il.: Thomas, 1953, Pp. 103–129.

54. Macgregor, F. C. Social and psychological implications of dentofacial disfigurement. *Angle Orthodont.* 40:231, 1970.

55. Macgregor, F. C., Abel, T. M., Byrt, A., Lauer, E., and Weissman, S. *Facial Disfigurement and Plastic Surgery: A Psychosocial Study.* Springfield, Il.: Thomas, 1953.

56. Machover, K. *Personality Projection in the Drawing of the Human Figure.* Springfield, Il.: Thomas, 1949.

57. McWilliams, B. J. Speech and language problems in children with cleft palate. *Am. Med. Wom. Assoc.* 21:1005, 1966.

58. McWilliams, B. J. Social and psychological problems associated with cleft palate. *Clin. Plast. Surg.* 9:317, 1982.

59. McWilliams, B. J., and Paradise, L. P. Educational, occupational and marital status of cleft palate adults. *Cleft Palate J.* 10:223, 1973.

60. Norval, M., Larson, T., and Parshall, P. *The Impact of the Cleft Lip and Palate Child on the Family: A Preliminary Survey.* Minneapolis: Crippled Children Services, 1964.

61. Palmer, J. M., and Adams, M. The oral image of children with cleft lip and palates. *Cleft Palate Bull.* 12:72, 1962.

62. Peter, J. P., and Chinsky, R. R. Sociological aspects of cleft palate adults I. Marriage. *Cleft Palate J.* 11:295, 1974.

63. Peter, J. P., and Chinsky, R. R. Sociological aspects of cleft palate adults II. Education. *Cleft Palate J.* 11:443, 1974.

64. Peter, J. P., Chinsky, R. R., and Fisher, M. J. Sociological aspects of cleft palate adults III. Vocational and economic aspects. *Cleft Palate J.* 12:193, 1975.

65. Pless, I. B., and Roghmann, K. J. Chronic illness and its consequences: Observations based on three epidemiologic surveys. *J. Pediatr.* 79:351, 1971.

66. Rheingold, H. L. The Social and Socializing Infant. In D. A. Goslin (Ed.), *The Handbook of Socialization Theory and Research.* Chicago: Rand-McNally, 1969.

67. Ribble, M. A. Infantile Experience in Relationship to Personality Development. In J. McV. Hunt (Ed.), *Personality and the Behavior Disorders.* New York: Ronald Press, 1944. Vol. 2.

68. Richardson, S. A. The Effects of Physical Disability on the Specialization of the Child. In D. A. Goslin and D. C. Grass (Eds.), *The Handbook of Socialization Theory.* New York: Rand McNally, 1969. Pp. 1047–1064.

69. Richardson, S. A., Hastorf, A. H., and Dornbusch, S. M. Effects of physical disability on a child's description of himself. *Child Dev.* 35:893, 1964.

70. Richman, L. C. Behavior and achievement of the cleft palate child. *Cleft Palate J.* 13:4, 1976.

71. Richman, L. C. Parents and teachers: Differing views of behavior of cleft palate children. *Cleft Palate J.* 15:360, 1978.

72. Richman, L. C. Self-reported social, speech, and facial concerns and personality adjustment of adolescents with cleft lip and palate. *Cleft Palate J.* 20:108, 1983.

73. Richman, L. C., and Eliason, M. Psychological characteristics of cleft lip and palate children: Intellectual, achievement, behavioral and personality variables. *Cleft Palate J.* 19:249, 1982.

74. Richman, L. C., and Eliason, M. Type of reading disability related to cleft type and neuropsychological patterns. *Cleft Palate J.* 21:1, 1984.

74. Richman, L. C., Eliason, M., and Lindgren, S. C. Reading disability in children with clefts. *Cleft Palate J.* 25:21, 1988.

76. Richman, L. C., Holmes, C. S., and Eliason, M. J. Adolescents with cleft lip and palate: Self-perceptions of appearance and behavior related to personality adjustment. *Cleft Palate J.* 22:93, 1985.

77. Ruess, A. L. A comparative study of cleft palate children and their siblings. *J. Clin. Psychol.* 21:354, 1965.

78. Ruess, A. L. Convergent Psychosocial Factors in the Cleft Palate Clinic. In R. M. Lencione (Ed.), *Cleft Palate Habilitation.* New York: Syracuse University Press, 1967. Pp. 51–70.

79. Ruess, A. L., and Lis, E. F. A multidimensional study of handicapped children. Final report to Maternal and Child Health Services, Health Services, and Mental Health Administration v.s. Dept. of Health, Education, and Welfare, Grant No. MC-R-170007-04-0, 1973.

80. Schilder, P. *The Image and Appearance of the Human Body.* New York: International Universities Press, 1950.

81. Schneiderman, C. R., and Harding, J. B. Social ratings of children with cleft lip by school peers. *Cleft Palate J.* 21:219, 1984.

82. Schweckendiek, W., and Danzer, C. Psychological studies in patients with clefts. *Cleft Palate J.* 7:533, 1970.

83. Secord, P. F. Facial Features and Inference Processes in Interpersonal Perception. In R. Tagiuri and L. Petrullo (Eds.), *Person Perception and Interpersonal Behavior.* Stanford, Calif.: Stanford University Press, 1958.

84. Sidney, R. A., and Matthews, J. An evaluation of the social adjustment of a group of cleft palate children. *Cleft Palate Bull.* 6:10, 1956.

85. Simonds, J. F., and Heimburger, R. E. Psychiatric evaluation of youth with cleft lip-palate matched with a control group. *Cleft Palate J.* 15:193, 1978.

86. Sincirope, P. E., and Clifford, E. Effects of cleft lip-palate on body satisfaction. Paper presented at meeting of American Cleft Palate Association, Oklahoma City, 1973.

87. Slutsky, H. Maternal reaction and adjustment to birth and care of cleft palate child. *Cleft Palate J.* 6:425, 1969.

88. Spriestersbach, D. C. *Psychosocial Aspects of the "Cleft Palate Problem."* Iowa City: University of Iowa Press, 1973.

89. Tisza, V. B., and Gumpertz, E. The parents' reaction to the birth and early care of children with cleft palate. *Pediatrics* 30:86, 1962.

90. Tisza, V. B., Irwin, E., and Scheide, E. Children with oral-facial clefts. *J. Am. Acad. Child Psychiatry.* 12:292, 1973.

91. Tisza, V. B., Irwin, E., and Zabarenko, L. A psychiatric interpretation of children's creative dramatic stories. *Cleft Palate J.* 6:228, 1969.

92. Tisza, V. B., Silvertone, B., Rosenblum, O., and Hanlon, N. Psychiatric observations of children with cleft palates. *Am. J. Orthopsychiatry* 28:416, 1958.

93. Tobiasen, J. M. Social judgments of facial deformity.

Cleft Palate J. 24:323, 1987.

94. Tobiasen, J. M., and Hiebert, J. M. Parents' tolerance for the conduct problems of the child with cleft lip and palate. Cleft Palate J. 21:82, 1984.

95. Tobiasen, J. M., Levy, J., Carpenter, M. A., and Hiebert, J. M. Type of facial cleft, associated congenital malformations and parents' ratings of school and conduct problems. Cleft Palate J. 24:209, 1987.

96. Van Demark, R. R., and Van Demark, A. A. Speech and sociovocational aspects of individuals with cleft palate. Cleft Palate J. 7:284, 1970.

97. Watson, C. G. Personality adjustment in boys with cleft lips and palates. Cleft Palate J. 1:130, 1964.

98. Watson, E. J., and Johnson, A. M. The emotional significance of acquired physical disfigurement in children. Am. J. Orthopsychiatry 28:85, 1958.

99. Winick, M. Comprehensive approach to a child with a birth defect. Bull. N. Y. Acad. Med. 43:819, 1967.

100. Wirls, C. J. Psycho-social Aspects of Cleft Lip and Palate. In W. C. Grabb, S. W. Rosenstein, and K. B. Bzoch (Eds.), Cleft Lip and Palate: Surgical, Dental, and Speech Aspects. Boston: Little, Brown, 1971. Pp. 119–129.

101. Wirls, C. J., and Plotkin, R. R. A comparison of children with cleft palate and their siblings on projective test personality factors. Cleft Palate J. 8:399, 1971.

CHAPTER 4

The Craniofacial Team: Medical Supervision and Coordination

John A. Nackashi • Virginia L. Dixon-Wood

THE CRANIOFACIAL TEAM

The professionals representing numerous disciplines are recognizing that the present age of information is making available an enormous database in the areas of health, business, industry and technology, and government. This ever-expanding database in each discipline is a driving force for increased specialization, as the professionals attempt to maintain competency in their areas of expertise. Concurrently, as the sum of knowledge grows, new and increasingly complex problems are arising which cross the boundaries of professional disciplines, requiring new collaborative strategies. This expanding database and the need to solve increasingly complicated problems are trends requiring the increased interaction of the professionals representing specific disciplines (specialists) and the formation of team approaches.

THE DEVELOPMENT OF THE TEAM APPROACH

However, the singular specialist, well trained within the limits of a discipline, may have difficulty in asking fundamental questions or providing answers for complex problems. Therefore the professional forms linkages with other professionals in order to share expertise, to deal with concerns which cross boundaries of disciplines.

This interdependency has been a powerful force in promoting team activity, and opens up to the members of the team the interdisciplinary exchange of the most recent knowledge and experience of each involved discipline.

This interdependency between health care specialists trained in different professions makes new demands but offers unique opportunities to the team members. The team approach requires communication skills, supported by a framework consisting of the ability to work comfortably with others, and an appreciation of one's own personal limits, and the desire to collaborate. Such professional relationships result in beneficial rewards such as personal and intellectual interactions, mutual support, and professional growth.

Additionally, new directions toward team approaches in special education and rehabilitative services are being mandated by federal laws, for instance, Public Law 99-457, the Education of the Handicapped Act, amended in 1986. This new legislation stresses the importance of the collaboration of professionals in assessing and developing initial treatment plans and caring for at-risk and handicapped infants and children. Therefore, federal law is now an additional driving force for team formation and collaboration in certain areas of health care.

CHANGING HEALTH CARE MODELS

The "traditional" medical model involved a biomedical approach limited to the identification of disease processes, in particular etiology, pathology, and signs and symptoms [11]. The dilemma with the traditional medical model is that

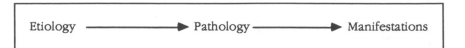

the "state-of-the-art" medical practice for chronic conditions is often limited in respect to an immediate or total cure. These long-term conditions involve both caring and curing, but caring involves a different problem solving approach to clinical practice than the traditional medical model. Chronic or long-term conditions such as cleft lip and palate involve curing, that is, the removal of a congenital defect, and also caring, that is, the long-term, often difficult person-oriented type of support and management of patients and their families. As in any rehabilitative approach the major goals are restoring and maintaining function which leads to independence. The traditional medical model may be conceptualized and is illustrated in Figure 4-1. This model is not satisfactory for those with chronic conditions or developmental disabilities. A more appropriate conceptualized model appears to be the World Health Organization health care model as illustrated in Figure 4-2.

Disease or disorder means a pathological process (the underlying etiology). *Impairment* is the consequent physiological, anatomical, or psychological loss, abnormality, or injury. *Disability* refers to the restriction or lack of ability to perform human activities. *Handicap* brings in societal attitudes and means the inability or lack of opportunity to perform socially expected roles [4].

In chronic or long-term conditions such as cleft lip and palate, the rehabilitative process is inclusive of medical, social, psychological, and vocational factors, after the characteristics of the etiology, pathology, and manifestation have been ascertained. Therefore, a "clinical team" is required in order to provide the "holistic" approach to the patient or client. This is because no single discipline can provide all the needed curing and caring.

THE CLINICAL TEAM

The definition of *team* in *Webster's Ninth New Collegiate Dictionary* [10] is "a group of specialists or scientists functioning as a collaborative unit" [the diagnostic team of psychiatrist, clinician, and social worker in a child guidance clinic]. This source defines teamwork as "work done by a

Figure 4-1. Traditional medical model. Determination of the etiology of the disease or disorder is the major driving force for the traditional model. (From Duckworth [2].)

number of associates with usually each doing a clearly defined portion but all subordinating personal prominence to the efficiency of the whole." Bringing together a group of professionals does not of itself create a team. Collaboration by the professionals is an absolute requirement, and such an interaction is based, at least partly, on the need to provide and care for the whole person.

Nine characteristics have been identified which are common to teams, and these suggested characteristics have been further divided into three main categories as follows: (1) composition, (2) functions, and (3) task [3].

COMPOSITION

Composition refers to the overall makeup of the team and has three characteristics:

1. *A team consists of two or more individuals.* Nonprofessionals, including the client and family, may be team members, but at least one professional must be on the team.
2. *There may be face-to-face or non-face-to-face configurations.* The team concept does not exclude individuals who communicate by the exchange of written reports or materials by phone. In special cases, such as emergency teams, communication may be by radio.
3. *There is an identifiable leader.* A singular individual must be identifiable who leads the team. This leadership role may change in regard to function and specific individual, as needed. This characteristic refers primarily to the need for an identifiable leader and does not specify the form the leadership should take.

FUNCTION

Teams are characterized by their several functions or methods of operation.

4. *Teams function both within and between organizational settings.* Teams are usually formed to

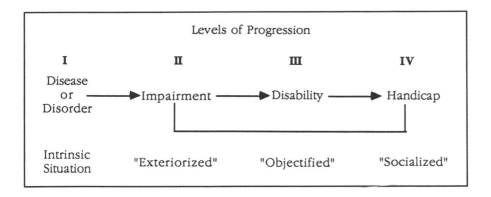

Figure 4-2. The World Health Organization (WHO) conceptualized health care model reveals the levels of progression starting from disease or disorder and leading sequentially to impairment, disability, and handicap. Disease or disorder (I) is the underlying problem (intrinsic situation). Impairment (II) is any abnormality or psychological, physiological, or anatomical structure of function ("exteriorized"). Disability (III) is any restriction or lack of ability to perform an activity in a manner considered to be normal ("objectified"). Handicap (IV) brings into account societal attitudes and is a disadvantage for a given individual, due to an impairment or disability, that limits or prevents the fulfillment of a role that is normal ("socialized"). (From World Health Organization [12].)

perform functions such as assessment fund raising, parent organizations to support schools, etc. Also teams can operate between organizations with members of the team representing different agencies or organizations.

5. *Roles of participants are defined.* The role of the team participants is generally defined by the disciplines and competency of the team members. Individual teams may determine the function of each participant and degree of overlap by the team members.
6. *Teams collaborate.* The team approach is a collaborative effort, combining the diverse expertise of the team members, to provide solutions to specific and often complicated problems. This collaboration is a key feature characterizing the team approach.
7. *There are specific protocols of operation.* Each team develops specific rules of operating specific methodologies to accomplish the defined goals or tasks. These may be unwritten and informal to formal and written procedural manuals. Of importance is that the protocol of operations be identifiable.

TASK

There are certain characteristics associated with the unique task of an interdisciplinary human service or health care team.

8. *The health care team is patient/client–centered.* The team is focused to serve the patient/client and exists primarily to fulfill this role.
9. *The team is task-oriented.* The team is task-oriented and exists to improve the conditions of the patient/client by dealing with the problems that have impacted on the patient/client's life requiring assistance by the team.

Other characteristics may be suggested such as the team is *family-centered,* which is being mandated by new federal legislation involving at-risk and handicapped infants and toddlers. Unique characteristics may evolve for an individual team depending on goals, roles of the members, and the team's stability over time.

Several types of team approaches have evolved over several decades to better meet the needs of children with chronic or handicapping conditions [1]. These children usually have multiple problems and needs that require assessment and intervention services from a number of professionals representing various disciplines. The team models that have been developed have been described as multi-, inter-, and transdisciplinary according to the amount and types of interactions and communication among members.

The *multidisciplinary team* approach, in wide use in health care settings, involves well-established, defined roles for the various professionals, with limited communication occurring among professionals on the team. In this model, each team member works independently of the others.

In the *interdisciplinary team,* the team members meet often to plan assessment, but then each professional performs an assessment independent of those done by team colleagues. This is followed by a sharing of findings, recommendations for intervention, and the preparation of a single report incorporating all recommendations. As in the multidisciplinary team approach, the assessments are done independently, but a greater degree of interaction occurs among team members.

In the *transdisciplinary team,* each discipline is responsible for an initial independent assessment, but then information is shared and members are permitted to cross over one another's previously traditional rule boundaries. Role release occurs in this approach — that is, the roles of most disciplines are released to one or two team members who are called "facilitators" and are responsible for delivering services to the child and family. The degree and type of release is governed by the particular needs of the child, the experience and competency of the facilitators, and common sense and legal concerns. Figure 4-3 outlines the interactive activities of a family-focused, collaborative team.

An extension of the transdisciplinary approach is an arena-style approach [11]. This involves not only participants, but active spectators. A primary

Figure 4-3. Team functioning in a family-focused model involves a series of activities with major objectives such as the assessment process leading to a diagnosis and the treatment plan dictating the intervention. The family is an integral part of all the activities. (Modified from Ducanis [3].)

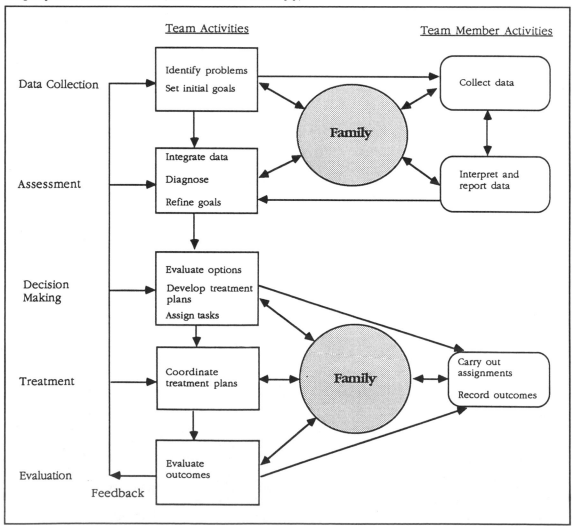

facilitator assesses the child in the presence of the team, and varying degrees of interaction occur on the part of team members. This approach has the advantage of reducing the handling of the child and prevents redundant questioning. In the arena approach, each team member is able to develop a more complete view of the child, while concomitantly increasing the knowledge of the other disciplines involved.

As professionals collaborate more closely, the evaluation, management, and services to children with chronic or handicapping conditions improve. In the past, the disciplines of medicine, education, and the health-related professions (e.g., physical therapy, occupational therapy, speech and language pathology and audiology, clinical psychology, social work, and nutrition) shared only one common bond — the child. Because these professionals approached the child from different frames of reference, they were generally unable to identify common areas of need for the child. Specifically, the professionals' lack of knowledge of the roles of the other professionals of the other disciplines created an obstacle to comprehensive care of the patient/client. The child and family were often left waiting for some kind of integrated assistance, guidance, and support due to the lack of collaboration. Therefore the team approach not only improved the evaluation and management of the patient/client by combining the diverse skills of the team, but the actual team interaction increased the database of team members. The ideal team interaction results in team members who not only learn about the other involved disciplines, but who can communicate comfortably in terms allowing for a unified frame of reference in regard to the patient/client.

THE CLEFT LIP-PALATE TEAM

The successful management of the child born with a cleft lip with or without a cleft palate requires improvement or restoration of the initial defect and preservation of all other anatomical, psychological, and social attributes of the child. The initial defect which occurs in utero results in a cascade of events after birth impacting on the child's growth and physical and psychosocial development. Problems are compounded by possible facial growth aberrations, communication abnormalities involving speech and hearing, disturbance of dental development, as well as psy-chosocial developmental problems. From the moment of birth, the family is challenged by a series of concerns about their child's ongoing needs beyond those encountered by the normal child.

The cleft lip and palate team has both a curing and caring role which helps minimize the impact of the initial defect. A major goal is to prevent the cleft lip or palate from becoming or causing a disability and handicap. This goal requires the expertise and cooperation of the various professionals representing the appropriate disciplines in a collaborative fashion — the interdisciplinary or transdisciplinary team.

More than 150 symptom complexes occur with clefts that involve one or more of the oral structures [7]. Cleft lip with or without cleft palate may exist without other clinically identifiable significant deformities in the body. However, it is not uncommon for other associated defects of structure or function to be found in the child with a cleft of the facial structures. Associated or accompanying defects may involve the skeletal, cardiovascular, and genitourinary systems.

The team function will be dictated by the population served, and this identified function will determine the number and types of specialists needed. Two general team types have evolved for the care of this population. Larger teams incorporating more disciplines have been developed to care for the child with multiple congenital abnormalities, while smaller teams with fewer specialists have cared for the child without other accompanying complications.

A team to serve a population with multiple deformities, in which cleft lip with or without cleft palate is represented, may include professionals from the following disciplines [17]:

Audiology
Clinical psychology
Genetic counseling
Neurosurgery
Nursing
Ophthalmology
Oral and maxillofacial surgery
Orthodontics
Otolaryngology
Pediatrics
Pedodontics
Plastic surgery
Prosthodontics
Social services
Special education
Speech pathology

The setting for the team may vary from private practice to a medical school academic center. A core group may be formed representing the "permanent staff," with other specialists being involved with children with multiple congenital anomalies. For the teams to function well professionally, the patient's scheduling needs to be carefully coordinated to take advantage of the available and appropriate expertise of the team members. Also, a driving force to maintain participation by team members is appropriate scheduling for the professionals themselves, allowing for the effective use of their time. A physician knowledgeable about child health care, such as a pediatrician with a special interest in cleft lip-palate patients, is important to oversee the total care of the child. Since the child with a cleft lip-palate may have associated malformations, multiple congenital anomalies, or an identifiable syndrome, a thorough history and physical examination is essential. Also, a monitoring of growth and development over time is critical with a special emphasis on speech and hearing. The pediatrician has a role to support and guide the family, and in concert with the team to develop treatment plans taking into account the total needs of the child and family. Therefore the pediatrician serves as an advocate for the child by taking a leadership role on the team.

THE TEAM IN FUNCTION

The population served, the clinical setting, the number of available different types of specialists, and their individual expertise will determine the function of the team. In contrast to the traditional medical model of determining the characteristics of etiology, pathology, and manifestations, the habilitation of the whole person should be the goal. By identifying such a goal, the team will maintain its appreciation of the need for an interdisciplinary team approach.

CLINICAL COORDINATOR

Various leadership roles are necessary for a well-functioning team to care for the scheduling and clinic operations and clinical needs of the patients. A cleft lip-palate or craniofacial team "coordinator" is essential for maintaining the clinical operations such as scheduling new and old patients, deciding which specialists need to attend the individual clinics, making sure that the

reports are sent out to the appropriate individuals or agencies, and serving as a single contact person for the patients to facilitate communication with the family. For large programs the coordinator may be involved in community education, fund raising, and home visits. In small programs an official coordinator may not be necessary, but some member of the team will need to take the responsibility for scheduling, completion of reports, and follow-up care.

TEAM DYNAMICS

Team dynamics refers to how the team conducts itself in regard to its determined activities, especially how it makes decisions and carries out the developed treatment plans. Research studies have concentrated primarily on small group dynamics, and these data may be used to infer the dynamics of interdisciplinary teams.

Interdisciplinary teams are usually part of a larger institutional setting such as a university, hospital, or similar organization. Also, the roles of the team members are usually assigned by professional expertise rather than by group consensus. Teams are formed usually as a part of a specific job responsibility, and the performance of a team member may be dependent on that individual's true interests.

The behavior of the members of the team are reflected by developed norms [6], which provide guidelines for expected behaviors. These norms are often unspoken and mandate appropriate behavior, regular attendance at team meetings and functions, contributions to the team, and use of team discussions for relevant material in a non-monopolizing manner. In some cases insensitive team members may not be aware of these unspoken guidelines and the result is team interaction difficulties. Some norms demand rigid adherence, while others are readily bypassed; some norms may be accepted by all members, while others may be opposed by a significant member of the team [9].

Norms impact on the team functioning and "the cost of failing to develop norms of flexibility, support and openness of communications is high indeed" since the team will fail to adequately examine the various alternatives in decision making and will be unable to become self-correcting [5].

Personalities of the team members may determine their roles on the team such as mediator, critic, "opinion-giver" and "energizer" [3]. In small groups, research reveals that an individual's profession will influence the status of team members. For example, psychiatrists may be more influenced by other psychiatrists than by psychologists, whereas psychologists appear to be equally influenced by both [8]. As team approaches become more widely accepted and professionals spend more time working with individuals outside of their own discipline, it is advantageous that all team members who offer appropriate expertise have an equal status on the team.

A team leader is important and this role is assigned or emerges spontaneously. Five aspects of "team leadership" of the primary health care team have been identified: (1) patient coordination and management, (2) team managment, (3) charismatic or spiritual leadershp, (4) primary patient relationship, and (5) medical decision making [3].

Since the team leader may not have all of these characteristics, other team members may fill some of these leadership roles. Research into group behavior in problem solving and action reveal that the leader's skill and employed methods directly determine the outcome. Exclusive authoritarianism by the clinical leader is usually unacceptable, and the team decisions must be a product of group interaction.

THE FUTURE OF
THE TEAM APPROACH

The interdisciplinary team approach involved in the care of individuals with cleft lip-palate is accepted as the standard of care. As the knowledge base for specialists continues to expand, the need for coordination of the professionals on the team will be critical to guarantee high-quality care for the client. Driving forces for increased collaboration between disciplines in a teamlike fashion will be the introduction of the team approach to preservice professionals and the new federal mandates for interdisciplinary approaches for at-risk and handicapped infants and children.

COORDINATION OF
CLEFT PALATE
TEAM PROGRAMS

Various leadership roles are necessary for a well-functioning team to care for the scheduling, clinic operations, and clinical needs of the patient. One of the most important is the role of a coordinator. According to *Webster's*, to coordinate implies bringing "into a common action, movement or condition," to harmonize or "to act together in a smooth concerted way" [10]. This can be quite a task for the coordinator who must work with several professionals, all of whom have different schedules and often work in different areas. This role is compounded by patients who may have limited access to services.

The role of the coordinator may vary greatly from team to team. In addition to coordinating clinical services, responsibilities or interests may include family counseling, patient advocacy, developing outreach or educational programs, clinical research, and practicing their own profession. While the other team members may be involved on a part-time basis, it is often the coordinator who is the full-time member. This allows time for dealing with some of the social and educational needs of the families along with programs for team development.

CLINICAL ORGANIZATION

The organization of the clinic depends on several factors, including individual team members' schedules and work settings, financial concerns, patient caseload, and availability of clinic space. University-based teams often have the luxury of seeing patients all at one time due to the team members' close proximity. In other situations in which private practitioners make up the team, patients may be seen in private offices and a discussion and treatment plan is developed at a later time.

Monetary reimbursement can also be an issue affecting clinical organization and the delivery of quality team care. Some practitioners may be forced into treating only patients with the ability to pay while others may volunteer their services for care of the indigent. Many states provide some reimbursement for indigent or low-income patients but it may not cover all the services (i.e., speech therapy and orthodontics) and may not be enough to cover basic overhead expenses. In some situations, teams and clinics are organized by how professionals are paid for their services. Entire teams may be funded by state dollars. However, this can limit families not funded by the state from benefiting from a coordinated team approach. The problem of funding for health care for children with clefts can have a major impact on the way teams are developed and organized.

Size of the patient caseload is another consideration when structuring a team clinic. Teams who see large numbers of children in each clinic may not be able to have every team member see each patient during each clinic visit. It is imperative in these cases, that team members discuss treatment planning among themselves to prevent confusion on the part of the team or family.

Reviewing the needs of the child prior to the clinic can often save time and expedite the evaluation process. This can be accomplished by studying the hospital records and department files. Interviewing the family either over the telephone or in person prior to beginning the evaluation can also be extremely helpful. The coordinator can then disseminate this information along with the medical history to the rest of the team members. The family may feel more positive about the evaluation if their concerns are addressed during the treatment planning process.

The coordinator must also be aware of the specific requirements of each of the active team members. How long does each member need to evaluate the patient or do certain team members evaluate the patient at the same time (i.e., pediatric dentist and orthodontist)? Can the team members' time commitments permit an organized schedule in the clinic setting (i.e., audiology and speech pathology at 1 p.m., pediatrics and clinical psychology at 2 p.m., dentistry and plastic surgery at 3 p.m.), or do other commitments require that team members come and go as their schedules permit?

The optimal treatment planning approach is a face-to-face discussion by all team members following the patients' evaluation. This is extremely helpful to the coordinator for several reasons. First, this process allows the team to develop a cohesive treatment plan with input from all team members. This eliminates confusion on the part of the team members, family, and others as to the priority and timing of treatment. The coordinator, who is involved in all discussions of treatment planning, should have a clear understanding of the team's plan for that particular child. The information can then be explained to the family without misunderstandings. This process is also advantageous because some appointments and procedures can be scheduled together if they are planned in advance. For example, the otolaryngologist may recommend PE tube insertion, which may be done at the time of other surgeries.

Also, genetic counseling sessions or other evaluations may be coordinated during a hospitalization. This is especially important for the families who must travel long distances or who have great difficulty scheduling hospital visits due to their jobs or the needs of their other children.

THE FAMILY AS A TEAM MEMBER

The coordinator should be in direct contact with the family and help them arrange follow-up appointments, and solve financial, insurance, and transportation problems. The needs and special circumstances of the family can effect treatment decisions. In large rural areas or when working with indigent patients, transportation problems can be the number one factor in the ability to provide any, much less optimal, patient care.

Often, the values and priorities of the patient are assumed to be the same as that of the team or professional. Understanding the social background of the family (socioeconomic status, religious beliefs, past experiences) can prevent many misunderstandings. The family's concerns and desires must be expressed when a treatment plan is being developed. It is helpful to ask the family at the onset of the clinic what their concerns are on that day and the specific questions they would like answered. The coordinator can also intervene if the family feels intimidated or reticent about asking specific questions. Often it is the responsibility of the coordinator to disseminate this information to other team members. Some families are hesitant to express these concerns to everyone who sees their child or to repeat it to every professional they see in one day. The coordinator can help the family become a part of the team and consequently involved in the decision making process for their child as mandated by federal law.

Counseling is an extremely important aspect of the coordinator's job. Because of this, it is imperative that he or she have basic knowledge of all areas of cleft lip-palate treatment. When visiting parents in the hospital or home after their child has been born, general questions regarding feeding, surgical repair, and speech development can be answered immediately. This seems to be more effective than having five or six different team members talk to the families individually. The family may still be dealing with the grief or shock of having a child with a cleft. Too much information too soon can be overwhelming and often ineffective. Unless another person from the team is designated, it is usually the coordinator who makes the initial contact with the family. That initial meeting is extremely important. The family's confidence must be secured by being knowledgeable about the treatment process and also sympathetic to their individual needs and circumstances. This is important if the team is going to be successful in treating their child for several years.

Having a good, overall knowledge of cleft lip-palate is also important when counseling the family during the clinic visit. The coordinator can summarize and discuss the team recommendations with the family and answer general questions. If treatment recommendations appear to be conflicting, the coordinator can recognize this and ask the individual team members making the recommendations to clarify and discuss them.

Providing families with information regarding funding and parent support groups available to them is always appreciated. Many teams have parents of older children with cleft lip-palate who are appointed to talk with families about their newborns. This can be a very successful program because it gives the family personal information that is sometimes absent in the clinical environment.

OUTREACH AND EDUCATION

One of the most important facets of the role of the coordinator is educating the parents, professionals, and the general public about cleft lip-palate. Many myths and misunderstandings still exist which can interfere with the child receiving optimal treatment. Inservices to rural hospitals, pediatricians, and nursery staff can be one way to achieve this goal. If these professionals do not see a large number of cleft lip-palate infants, they may not be aware of effective feeding methods and care of the newborn. A review of these is often helpful along with a discussion of current and long-term treatment approaches.

Home visits are quite important for a number of reasons. They can provide information about the family's social situation which lets the coordinator monitor the amount of education and assistance the family may need. Families often appreciate the fact that you have taken the time to visit them. They may ask more questions and be more receptive to counseling when they are in a home atmosphere. For infants, you can observe how they are feeding and the quality of the language stimulation they are receiving. Toddlers or older children

who may be reticent to talk in the clinic may be very communicative in their own environment.

Home visiting can also increase patient compliance. If families believe that you are genuinely interested in the care of their child they may be more willing to keep clinic appointments. It may also be reassuring to the family to have the name of one person whom they can contact with any question. This may eliminate confusion and frustration for the family. Even though the coordinator may not be able to answer every question, he or she should be able to find the answer or put the family in contact with a team member who can.

Education is also a major factor in patient compliance. If you can open lines of communication with parents who may be confused, they may be able to appreciate the importance of the clinic visits. For example, families may believe that once the initial lip-palate repair is done, no more treatment is necessary. Parents may become disillusioned when their child's treatment is going too slowly, without any immediate results (i.e., speech therapy or orthodontics). For these reasons, an ongoing counseling and educational process is necessary.

The establishment of parent support groups can also be an important outreach activity. When getting a support group started, it is often helpful to find one parent who seems to be interested and motivated in beginning a parent group. You can then provide him or her with the essentials to get started. These may include literature, meeting space, names of other interested families, and resource professionals. Initially, families may just want to get together and discuss their experiences rather than having any organized program. The support group is for the parents, so they should determine the goals and activities of their group. However, the coordinator can be a valuable resource to the parents (see available literature in Appendix).

CLEFT PALATE TEAM COMPOSITION: THE TRAINING AND GENERAL RESPONSIBILITIES OF TEAM SPECIALISTS

Health care delivery from a team is made much more efficient if general guidelines are established regarding clinical responsibilities of individual team members. These guidelines can help the coordinator in a number of ways. Clinics can be scheduled around the absences of certain members. If the needs of the patient are known, certain team members may not need to see the child. For example, a very young child may not need to see the orthodontist if it is the pediatric dentist who assesses early dentition and is responsible for maxillary orthopedics when and if necessary. The following is a description of the training requirements and general responsibilities for the individual team members; however, specific responsibilities may vary from team to team.

The *pediatrician* obtains an M.D. degree and then completes a 3-year pediatric residency. Board certification is obtained through the American Board of Pediatrics. The certification process involves successfully completing national medical examinations (boards) and the pediatric board examinations. The primary role of the pediatrician on the team is assessing and managing the overall medical care and treatment of the child.

The *plastic and reconstructive surgeon* receives an M.D. degree and continues training with a 5-year general surgery residency. After completion of the residency program, a 2-year plastic surgery fellowship is required. Accreditation is obtained through the American Board of Plastic Surgeons after completion of the fellowship. The plastic and reconstructive surgeon's role includes performing the primary surgical closures of the cleft lip and palate, secondary palatal procedures to correct velopharyngeal insufficiency, and later soft tissue reconstructions of the face.

An *oral-maxillofacial surgeon* begins training with a basic dental degree (D.M.D. or D.D.S.), followed by a 5-year residency involving 1 year of general surgery and 4 years of oral-maxillofacial surgery. Certification is obtained through the American Association of Oral-Maxillofacial Surgeons and requires both a written and oral examination. The role of the oral-maxillofacial surgeon as a member of the team involves predominately reconstructive surgery of the maxilla, mandible, and temporomandibular joints.

An *orthodontist* also begins training with a basic dental degree, either D.D.S. or D.M.D, then specializes in orthodontics during a 2-year residency. Board certification is obtained through the American Association of Orthodontics and requires both a written and oral examination. The orthodontist's primary role as a member of the team involves studying the alignment of the teeth and the jaw structure as influenced by facial growth. The orthodontist works closely with the pediatric dentist during the mixed dentition stage and also with

the oral-maxillofacial surgeon when orthognathic surgery is being planned.

The *pediatric dentist* receives a basic dental degree (D.M.D. or D.D.S.) and then spends 2 years as a resident in children's dentistry. Board certification is obtained through the American Board of Pediatric Dentistry and requires both a written and oral examination. Certification also requires a day office visit with three case histories presented. His or her primary role as a member of the team involves examining the dental health of the pediatric patient and assisting in recommendations based on that information. The pediatric dentist or orthodontist can fabricate feeding appliances for children with cleft palate who are having specific feeding problems. Also, palatal appliances may be made to cover oronasal fistulae.

An *otolaryngologist* begins training with an M.D. degree, then spends 1 year as a medical intern, 1 year as a general surgical resident, and 4 years doing a fellowship with otolaryngology and head-neck surgery. Board certification is obtained through the American Board of Otolaryngology/Head-Neck Surgery and requires a written examination. The otolaryngologist's role on the team includes examining the patient's ear and consulting with other surgeons regarding facial reconstruction. They will frequently be called on to insert PE tubes at the time of primary lip or palate surgery to manage the common problem of chronic otitis media.

The *medical geneticist* usually begins with an M.D. degree and then spends 2 years doing a clinical fellowship in genetics under the supervision of a certified geneticist. Certification is obtained through the American Board of Medical Genetics and requires a 2-day written examination. The geneticist's role as a member of the team involves analyzing specialized tests related to family history information and counseling the patient and family about recurrence risks as well as assisting in the diagnosis of syndromes.

The *clinical psychologist* completes 4 years of graduate training, a 1-year internship, and then receives a Ph.D. degree. After receiving the degree and participating in supervised clinical experience, he or she is eligible to take a national examination to obtain licensure. The licensing process varies from state to state and is monitored by the American Psychological Association. As a member of the cleft palate team, the psychologist helps families deal with the emotional and psychosocial problems of having a child with cleft lip and palate. The clinical psychologist may also counsel adolescents and adults who may have adjustment problems due to facial disfigurement or fear of hospitalization or surgery. Behavioral, developmental, and personality assessments are also part of the psychologist's role.

The *social worker* first receives a master's degree in social work. This is the terminal degree for all clinical practice. Board certification can be obtained from the National Association of Social Workers 5 years after the M.A. degree is obtained. The social worker can also become a member of the American Academy of Social Workers after successfully completing a national test. The social worker's role on the team consists of family and individual counseling, investigating local and state services available to the family, and helping them obtain these services.

The *nurse* involved with cleft palate teams usually receives either a 2- or 3-year A.S. or 4-year B.S.N. degree in prior training. Certification is obtained through the individual state nurses' association and requires a written examination. A nurse on the cleft palate team should have some background in craniofacial disorders. The role will vary depending on the needs of each clinic; however, it can include acting as a liaison between physicians and parents or assisting in obtaining referral and possibly financial aid for low-income families. The nurse is also an important support to the family since he or she helps prepare the patient and family for surgery with regard to preoperative and postoperative procedures and discharge teaching.

REFERENCES

1. Conor, F. P., Williamson, G. G., and Siepp, J. M. *Program Guide for Infants and Toddlers with Neuromotor and Other Developmental Disabilities*. New York: Teachers College Press, 1978.
2. Duckworth, D. The Need for a Standard Terminology and Classification of Disablement. In C. V. Granger and G. E. Gresham (Eds.), *Functional Assessment in Rehabilitative Medicine*. Baltimore: Williams & Wilkins.
3. Duncanis, A. J., and Golin, A. *The Interdisciplinary Health Care Team*. Germantown, Md: Aspen Systems, 1979.
4. Frey, W. D. Functional Assessment in the '80's. In A. S. Halpern and M. Fehrer (Eds.), *Functional Assessment in Rehabilitation*. Baltimore: Paul H. Brooks, 1984.
5. Fry, R. E., Lech, B. A., and Rubin, I. Working with the Primary Health Care Team. In H. Wire, R. Beckhand, I. Rubin, and A. L. Kyte (Eds.), *Making Health Teams Work*. Cambridge, Mass.: Ballinger, 1974.
6. Have, A. P. *Handbook of Small Group Research* (2nd ed.). New York: Free Press, 1976.
7. Koepp-Baker, H. The Craniofacial Team. In K. R. Bzoch (Ed.), *Communicative Disorders Related to Cleft Lip and Palate* (2nd ed.). Boston, Little, Brown, 1979. Pp. 52–61.
8. Left, W. F., Raven, B. N., and Gunn, R. L. A preliminary investigation of social influence in the mental health professions (abstract). *American Psychol.* 19:505, 1964.
9. Shaw, M. Communication Networks. In L. Berkowitz (Ed.), *Advances in Experimental Social Psychology*. New York: Academic Press, 1964. Vol. 1.
10. *Webster's Ninth New Collegiate Dictionary*. Springfield, Mass.: Merriam-Webster, 1988.
11. Wolery, M., and Dyke, L. Arena assessment: Description and preliminary social validity data. *J. Assoc. Persons Severe Handicaps* 9:231–235, 1984.
12. World Health Organization (WHO). *International Classification of Impairments, Disabilities, and Handicaps*. Geneva: World Health Organization, 1980.

APPENDIX

The following literature is available from The American Cleft Palate Foundation; 1218 Grandview Ave.; University of Pittsburgh; Pittsburgh, PA 15211; telephone (412) 481-1376.

For Parents of Newborn Babies with Cleft Lip/Palate
Cleft Lip and Cleft Palate — the Child from Birth to Three Years
Cleft Lip and Cleft Palate — the Child from Three Years to Twelve Years
Information for the Teenager Born with a Cleft Lip and/or Cleft Palate
Feeding the Infant with a Cleft
The Genetics of Cleft Lip and Palate: Information for Families
Organizing Support Groups for Patients and Parents of Children with Cleft Palate
Catalogue of Audiovisual Aids: Cleft Lip and Palate
Information About Financial Assistance
Information About Cleft Lip and Palate
Information About Choosing a Cleft Palate or Craniofacial Team
Information About the Dental Care of a Child with Cleft Lip/Palate
Information About Pierre Robin Malformation Sequence
Information About Crouzon Disease (Craniofacial Dysostosis)
Information About Treacher Collins Syndrome (Mandibulofacial Dysostosis)
Newsletter for Parents and Patients
Selected Bibliography for Parents of Children with Cleft Lip/Palate
Information about the National Cleft Palate Association

Other publications available for families:

The Child with Cleft Lip or Palate — A Guide for Parents, Nicholas G. Georgiade, M.D., D.D.S., and Edward Clifford, Ph.D., Facial Rehabilitation Center, Box 3098, Duke University Medical Center, Durham, NC 27710 (919) 684-2854
Your Cleft Lip and Palate Child — A Basic Guide for Parents, Gilbert Snyder, M.D., Samuel Berkowitz, D.D.S., Kenneth Bzoch, Ph.D., and Sylvan Stool, M.D., Mead-Johnson Nutritional Division, Evansville, IN 47721-0001

The Road to Normalcy for the Cleft Lip and Palate Child, Samuel Berkowitz, D.D.S., Mead-Johnson Nutritional Division, Evansville, IN 47721-0001

Bright Promise: For Your Child with Cleft Lip and Cleft Palate, Eugene T. McDonald, Ed.D. and Asa J. Berlin, Ph.D., National Easter Seal Society for Crippled Children and Adults.

Team Management for the Cleft Lip and Cleft Palate Patient, Lancaster Cleft Palate Clinic, 24 North Lime St., Lancaster, PA 17602

Team Approach to the Cleft Lip and Palate Child, Sidney K. Wynn, M.D., Milwaukee Children's Hospital Cleft Lip and Palate Center 1700 W. Wisconsin Ave., Milwaukee, WI 53222

Feeding An Infant with Cleft Palate: An Aid for Parents and Professionals, Diane Clapper, R.N. and Virginia Dixon-Wood, M.A., University of Florida Craniofacial Center, J-166, Gainesville, FL 32610 (Spanish edition in press)

Feeding Techniques for Children Who Have Cleft Lip and Palate, Marsha Dunn Klein, M.Ed., Therapy Skill Builders, 3830 East Bellevue, P.O. Box 42050, Tucson, AZ 85733

II.

DIAGNOSTIC ASPECTS

A. Evaluation of the Probable Causes of Related Communicative Disorders

CHAPTER 5

Etiological Factors Related to Managing Cleft Palate Speech

Kenneth R. Bzoch

Nature, as we often say, makes nothing in vain, and man is the only animal whom she has endowed with the gift of speech. And whereas mere voice is but an indication of pleasure or pain, and is therefore found in other animals (for their nature attains to the perception of pleasure and no further), the power of speech is intended to set forth the expedient and inexpedient, and therefore likewise the just and the unjust.

Aristotle [3]

Speech is a natural but also an extremely complex form of human auditory modality symbolic language behavior. However, it now appears that speech and language development in any human infant is dependent only in part on the physical integrity of the central nervous system and the many organs composing the hearing and speaking mechanisms of the body. Emergent language skills appear also to be only partially dependent on good environmental language stimulation and psychosocial developmental factors in the lives of infants. Speech and language skills in human infants are predisposed to develop. They do, even under some of the worst physical and environmental conditions present today.

Speech and language skills are clearly unique to mankind. What is particularly unique is that they depend primarily on auditory modality interactions from caretakers during infancy rather than visual or motor modality learning. All other animals seem to learn primarily through sight rather than sound. The uniqueness of speech and language behavior learning in mankind, within the animal kingdom, has long been a topic of philosophers and psychologists in the literature of Western civilization.

Through very earliest human evolution, the specialization of body parts composing the speaking mechanism and the auditory cortex, including a dominant hemisphere of the brain for language, either accompanied or preceded the devel-opment of symbolic speech and language behavior in *Homo sapiens sapiens*. This universally learned symbolic mediational behavior we call speech still seems to be our most unique and distinguishing characteristic as a species of animal today. The anthropologist Richard E. Leakey, considering our origins and survival as a single distinct species scattered across all continents of the earth, stated: "In the transition from *Homo erectus* to *Homo sapiens sapiens*, language was surely central in knitting together the social and cultural structures of the mingling populations" [43].

Language learning seems to have become possible in our earliest ancestors through biological changes in body structures leading to our evolutionary departure from having to depend on sight as the primary sense for individual learning. It seems clear that the primacy of visual memory learning has not changed for other intelligent living primates. This basic difference in our modes of learning now obviously limits the symboliclike learning potential of our most closely related living species, the great apes. They can learn well through visual symbolization conditioning learning as indicated by the recent primate language research literature. However, they do very poorly through auditory modality stimulus response learning.

In contrast, as Lennberg [44] pointed out, humans are born with a biological predisposition to learn speech and language skills through sound patterns, symbolically associated with visual motor experiences of the real world, in earliest life. Clinical experience with cerebral palsy, cleft palate, and other high-risk populations with primary language learning disabilities indicates that this is true, whether human infants are born with abnormalities of the speaking mechanism, such as cleft palate, or as healthy normal babies.

Cleft palate infants, then, also appear to be programmed through their prior evolutionary organic differences in brain and body from all other animal species to be ready to learn symbolic receptive and expressive language skills naturally through auditory modality interactive learning experiences with adults in the first 2 to 3 years of their development. This fact presents a particular need for very early intervention through language learning stimulation training by our profession for this population, whenever possible.

Symbolic learning through language, particularly early emergent language skills through speech and the understanding of language codes learned from the speech of caretakers, is what apparently introduced a new form of evolution to our species. This must have occurred many thousands and possibly millions of years ago [43]. Such universal early oral and auditory symbolic language skills enable human infants and preschool children today to quickly learn from the experiences of past generations. Our language cultures are passed on to all new members of human societies through emergent language skills.

Unfortunately, even at present, if cleft palate team management does not emphasize early treatment focused on preventing delayed language development, language development often remains markedly delayed for infants born with cleft palate [14]. This was a common finding in the past [7, 11, 23, 62, 90]. There is substantial evidence that delayed language development can and should be prevented for the majority of cleft palate infants born at this time [12, 13]. Early emergent speech and receptive language development of infants born with clefts or craniofacial disorders should be our first focus for preventing unnecessary communicative disorders in this population.

It is this earliest learning of oral language skills which generally frees most all human infants born in the world today from past animal forms of learning limited to spatial memory and personal visual motor experiences. It is only over the last 4,000 years that large segments of the human population have learned how to transfer speech back to a visual form for formal education through orthography (reading and writing). These latter visual forms of natural language through speech we call reading and writing are better able to hold learned information and thoughts over time. We can now all share the previous thoughts of past philosophers like Aristotle and the religious thinkers, psychologists, and political leaders who have shaped our different modern cultural societies through reading what they had written for more advance language-mediated learning.

Through language skills, then, over the past 4,000 years, mankind has learned how to anticipate and produce the many possible technical, environmental, and political changes in human life-styles which infants and children now experience early in our culture. The infants born today into our modern American culture apparently now improve these early speech and language potential skills more rapidly than in the past through existing technologies like television and the telephone and more recently through computer word processing.

The central importance of early speech and language to the individual and collective life of human infants is generally recognized in current learning and cognitive theories of human development. It is a major concern in the clinical management of infants born with cleft palate and related disorders. This is because it is also generally agreed that a somewhat characteristic and identifiable form of speech and early language learning defect, often termed *cleft palate speech*, is the frequently realized potential handicap of infants born with congenital clefts of the palate.

The remainder of this chapter is concerned with considering the several probable causes for the frequent and often severe early speech and language handicaps introduced by congenital cleft palate, the timing and methods of physical restoration evolved by modern cleft palate teams, and the several categorical aspects involved in such disorders. The following chapters will then cover current clinical and technical methods for studying the parameters of language development and presenting speech behavior abnormalities, and the basic theoretical and clinical methods that have been found to be useful in preventing, modifying, or correcting communicative disorders in the population with cleft palate or related craniofacial anomalies.

A speech-language pathologist or audiologist may engage in clinical practice with cleft palate and craniofacial clients as part of a functioning cleft palate team or in private practice, public school programs, or community or hospital clinics. For the purpose of this discussion, it is understood that only a limited number of speech-language pathologists and audiologists can actually specialize in the most effective means of managing the problems presented. Nonetheless, the same differential diagnostic questions must be investigated in each of these clinical settings. The unique opportunities and advantages as well as the limited disadvantages of working as part of a team approach for early management for prevention are emphasized in the following discussion of etiological factors.

The important role of the audiologist on a cleft palate team in identifying and referring for otological treatment or amplification and training the frequent developmental problems from hearing loss are detailed in Chapter 9. The more specific clinical screening tests required for evaluating possible causal factors through focusing on specific categorical aspects of cleft palate speech are covered in Chapter 8. The following discussion considers the several possible causes of communicative disorders frequently found in this population and the role of the speech pathologist on a cleft palate team in diagnosing and managing these factors.

BASIC CAUSAL FACTORS FOR EVALUATION

For an introductory consideration of speech and language learning problems related to cleft palate disorders, it seems necessary first to review the several physical and functional or developmental learning factors cited in the literature as the most usual causes of such findings in this population. This is done here in full recognition that some basic conceptual errors are introduced by any broad classification system of causal factors of communicative disorders. The population being considered is, in fact, a very heterogeneous group of human beings with often unique extents of clefting and associated physical and environmental conditions affecting their presenting conditions at initial evaluation.

It seems necessary, however, to first support the concept that several types of causal factors are related to defective speech in subjects born with clefts. This is done in order to counter the naive assumption that the cleft or craniofacial anomaly is necessarily *the* cause. Such an oversimplified hypothesis often leads to the fallacious inference that if the malformation is corrected surgically sometime in the life of the individual, the defective speech pattern should also be corrected.

ORGANIC AND FUNCTIONAL FACTORS

General semanticists have pointed out (with tongue in cheek) that there are really only two kinds of people in the world: those who divide everything into two kinds and those who do not. That is to say, there are people who usually see every problem as either due to A or to B, as either black or white. There are others who more correctly view everything rather as existing on a continuum with multiple possible causes. Communicative disorders in the cleft palate and related disorders population are due to multiple causes which exist on a continuum.

However, because of the limits and specialization of our profession to functional learning and behavioral problems in oral language communication, it seems useful and even important to me to divide the different possible etiologies of communicative disorders for cleft palate individuals into two broad categories as follows: (1) organic factors and (2) functional or learning factors. This is because the management of physical or organic problems usually requires treatment by other professionals, that is, from our colleagues in surgery, medicine, and dentistry. On the other hand, functional causes of communicative disorders can only be modified or corrected by clinical behavioral specialists such as speech and language pathologists, audiologists, and clinical psychologists.

The organic causes of communicative disorders are usually correctable today. They require referral to the specialized services of medical, surgical, and dental specialists. We should identify and refer such underlying problems to these specialists for treatment as early in our client's lives as possible to best support their learning of competent speech and language skills.

For our present purpose, organic factors can be defined as *diagnosable structural abnormalities that when corrected by physical management result in direct measurable improvement in speech behavior or hearing.* Examples of effective treatment for organic causal factors include palatoplasties for unoperated clefts to correct velopharyngeal insufficiency, orthodontic treatment to correct dental or occlusal hazards to clear speech, pressure equalization tubes (PE) inserted in the eardrums to correct recurring otitis media, etc. Functional factors may then be defined as *all other presumed learning, developmental, and psychosocial factors not treatable by physical management.*

Within this conceptual framework a speech disorder characterized by glottal stop substitutions for most pressure consonant sound elements in speech which does not change after effective secondary palatal reconstruction and maturation alone should be properly considered as being basically a functional or learned speech disorder. Such problems require speech therapy rather than further physical management for elimination in later speech behavior. However, the frequent distortion of pressure consonants in connected speech from nasal emission (which is most often eliminated by successful secondary surgical reconstruction of the velopharyngeal mechanism) should be properly related to its physical rather than functional etiology.

The basic differential diagnosis of functional versus organic causes of presenting speech disorders should be the major concern of the speech pathologist on a cleft palate team. Clearly, if speech deviations persist after demonstrable effective correction of suspected underlying physical defects, the persisting disorder should be established as being caused or maintained by functional learning factors in development. If, however, specific speech abnormalities are usually directly eliminated following physical management through surgery, prosthesis, or dental treatment, the organic etiology of these categories of disorder should be considered as being confirmed.

However, although some of the more unique and frequent errors in speech found by articulation testing of clients with cleft palate (such as the substitution pattern of glottal stops or pharyngeal fricatives for pressure consonants) are functional in nature, this is not to say that the physical correction of an underlying organic condition of demonstrated velopharyngeal insufficiency for speech is not first required to better achieve later functional changes through speech therapy. Pragmatically, both physical management and functional training steps are usually required under such circumstances in the case studies presented in Chapter 16.

Etiological factors that can be diagnostically identified from clinical tests, such as "velopharyngeal insufficiency for normal speech production" or "developmental dyslalia" (functional articulation disorders) or "delayed expressive language development," clearly indicate the need for either further physical management through surgery or prosthetic management or for behavioral changes through speech and language therapy. Speech therapy here refers to the processes of educating and directly training subjects or their parents to achieve such goals as (1) correction of sound substitutions such as p/f, w/r, s/t, etc. in the speech of a 5-year-old child with corrected cleft palate and demonstrable velopharyngeal adequacy, or (2) improvement in expressive language skills mea-

sured to be 1 year behind receptive language skills, by initiating a pragmatic home language stimulation program.

The several general factors selected from research and clinical experience for discussion in the following discussion are presented under these headings (i.e., organic or functional factors) to structure the information from more recent empirical and research information regarding the prevention, intervention, or correction of cleft palate speech and language development.

DIAGNOSTIC SPEECH EVALUATIONS

Clinical practice in speech and language pathology might best be likened to an exciting detective story. In the initial investigation of the problems of a new client, the speech clinician (detective) first needs to identify the possible criminal(s) responsible for defective oral communication in the life of the given human being. Within the area of children with cleft palate, the butler or most apparent suspect appears to be velopharyngeal insufficiency for normal speech and language learning caused by the congenital cleft palate. However, as in all detective stories, there should be other suspects. The challenge is to determine which of several, or what combination or gang of criminals are actually responsible for the crime. The butler (cleft palate) may turn out to be a rehabilitated citizen and the real criminals may be found to come from the neighborhood of functional factors.

ORGANIC FACTORS

What are the major physical or organic factors to be considered in the evaluation of a person with cleft palate or related disorders? A review of the literature and clinical experience indicate that there are three major problems which usually underlie defects of speech and oral language communication in this population. These are (1) velopharyngeal insufficiency to support clear voice and speech production, (2) dental or occlusal abnormalities contributing distorted articulation, and (3) acquired hearing loss from otitis media. Other physical or organic defects may also exist particularly for clients with chromosomal and syndromal abnormalities at birth.

VELOPHARYNGEAL INSUFFICIENCY

Velopharyngeal insufficiency* for clear speech and voice production is obviously present at birth for all infants born with clefts of the palate. For over two decades it has been known that the earlier this condition is corrected through surgical reconstruction, the better the speech and language development results of any protocol of team treatment. However, it is also know that if left untreated until early adult life, the position of the maxillary segments of the midface may be closer to normal than in unoperated adults.

There is considerable evidence to indicate that velopharyngeal insufficiency for normal speech production is often the direct cause of defective speech in the clinical cleft palate population. It is not the only cause [11]. Velopharyngeal insufficiency usually results from the interrelated functions of the velum with several skeletal and soft tissue structures surrounding the nasopharynx. Following primary reconstruction, the deficiency usually does not involve only one structural factor alone.

Rather, *velopharyngeal insufficiency* for speech is a condition which causes nasal emission distortion and hypernasal resonance distortion during acts of speech. It is due to interstructural inability for alternate sealing-off and opening of the nasopharynx in rapid coordinated physiological movements that are properly timed with the other articulators of the speaking mechanism.

RELATED STRUCTURAL FACTORS

Kingsley, as early as 1862 [39] and again in 1894 [40], recognized and emphasized the basic and critical importance of the velum as an organ of speech. He also properly criticized speech teachers of that era who ignored or did not understand its importance [39]:

I have known professors of elocution receive as pupils persons suffering from defective organs of speech, with the encouragement of perfect articulation held out as the result to follow under such circumstances. So far as I have read, it seems to me too little credit has been given to the velum, by physiologists, as an organ of speech. I would, therefore,

claim for it that it exercises a more important office in the modulation of sound than any other organ except the tongue.

Direct *cause-effect* relationships have been well demonstrated between the measurable presence of velopharyngeal insufficiency for speech and the distortion of speech attempts due to hypernasality or nasal emission or both [17, 56, 66, 89]. Clinical research studies of various age samples of the cleft palate population have most often demonstrated the presence of this one basic problem as related to nasalance distortions in cleft palate speech [7, 9, 16, 23, 80, 90]. Velopharyngeal insufficiency has even been found to correlate highly with measures of articulation skills [7–10, 50], although sound distortion, substitution or omission error patterns in speech are usually basically functional.

The sufficiency or insufficiency of velopharyngeal function for speech should be a determinable fact for each case in question through the application of clinical and instrumental tests and observations as described in the following chapters. If velopharyngeal insufficiency is evidenced on repeated testing after primary surgery, a second surgical reconstruction of the velopharyngeal mechanism is usually required. However, in inconsistent or phoneme-specific instances of nasalance distortions of connected speech, a period of diagnostic speech therapy, including indirect palatal training techniques and focusing on correct consonant productions, is often needed to decide if further physical management is really necessary.

The several structures that may contribute to the lack of achievement of this necessary physiological function have also been well identified and can now be specified through special instrumental studies and observations. Speech clinicians today may be involved in selecting and recommending specific surgical procedures which might best correct specific problems of structure or palatal function underlying a particular individual's velopharyngeal insufficiency for speech. A review of the literature indicates several possible contributing factors.

In the earliest literature on cleft palate speech, surgeons and speech clinicians alike tended to focus only on the single most obvious factor of diminished *length of the velum* as being directly related to good or defective speech. In 1927, for

---

* The term *velopharyngeal insufficiency* is used in this chapter as a synonym for palatopharyngeal inadequacy or incompetency.

instance, Kirkham wrote: "The reconstructed palate is usually too short to extend back to seal off the nasopharynx ... [and] the functional results as regards speech are far from good and in most instances bad."

However, even in the pre-1930 literature on the subject, two deficiency factors for postoperative velopharyngeal function were recognized: (1) velar length and (2) *velar mobility* [5, 34]. Hudson-McKuen [34] in particular emphasized the importance of somehow obtaining better velar mobility following surgery in a text describing operative procedures which made this impossible. He correctly stated: "It is this masterful inactivity of the palatal muscles seen following surgery that gives to the speech of cleft palate persons its characteristic quality, and it is the restoration of the function more than anything else which removes this disagreeable quality."

Unfortunately, it would be many decades before this insight would lead to effective techniques to free up and retropose the levator sling in particular (i.e., provide intervelar veloplasties) or retropose or lengthen the velum and provide nasal epithelial lining to achieve a mobile functioning velum following primary reconstruction of the palate. Early clinical research leading to today's more effective surgical techniques remained limited until the late 1950s. Ritchie [72] in 1937 reported a limited clinical investigation that compared estimates of velar length and velar mobility after surgery to subsequent nasal distortion of speech. He concluded that nasal emission was definitely related mainly to mobility of the postoperative velum and gave only seconday importance to velar length. The surgical reconstruction dilemma of somehow obtaining a mobile velum more frequently through primary palatal reconstruction continued to be emphasized in the literature until Graber [26] in 1949 challenged the efficacy of any surgical reconstruction of cleft palate before 4 years of age on the basis of probable exacerbation of midface growth arrest which was seen as a frequent sequelae at that time.

Most of the other structural aspects related to obtaining adequate physiological velopharyngeal function for speech were also anticipated, even before the advent of systematic x-ray cephalometry and later cine- or videofluroscopy and nasoendoscopy of normal and abnormal velopharyngeal function for speech production. In 1927 Wardill [87] determined from direct measurements of skulls that *the lateral dimensions of the nasopharynx* were often greater in persons with

cleft palate than in normal subjects, contributing to postoperative velopharyngeal insufficiency. This was probably more common in that distant past when surgery to correct wide clefts was deferred in favor of prosthetic speech appliances. This finding of posterior widening rather than collapse of the oropharynx was most probably due to the principle that abnormal muscle forces can affect the growth and position of bony structures of the head. Without early veloplasty or palatoplasty the posterior area of the oropharynx tends to widen rather than narrow on this basis (see Fig. 1-9 in Chap. 1). Be that as it may, Wardill first pointed out early that it was not enough to try to relate velar length and mobility of the velum to function for speech without also assessing differences in the skeletal and soft tissue framework within which the velum must function for speech [87].

A number of later investigators, using data obtained from more objective controlled cephalometric and laminographic studies, added to the list *the configuration of the soft structures in the roof of the nasopharynx and lateral walls* and confirmed frequent variations in the surrounding bony structures as factors often affecting the adequacy of velopharyngeal function for speech. Ricketts [69], for example listed *(1) the angulation of the cranial base, (2) the position of the nasal spine, (3) the length of the soft palate, (4) the range of function of the soft palate, and (5) the amount of forward bulging of the adenoid pad* as all being structural variations affecting the adequacy of function of the velum for speech.

Minor growth changes over time in the relative size of specific interrelated velopharyngeal structures have also been shown to be able to change early postoperative adequacy of the velopharyngeal mechanism to insufficiency at later ages, which finding gives credence to the importance of longitudinal reevaluations by cleft palate teams. Graber [27], for instance, determined that the loss of hyperplastic adenoid tissue and the decreased growth rate of the palate after surgery resulted in the loss of previously adequate velopharyngeal function and a return to nasal distortion of speech for some cleft palate subjects evaluated longitudinally. Pruzansky [65] in 1954 also related growth changes over time — specifically the degree of downward growth of the floor of the nose from the base of the skull between the ages of 6½ and 9½ years — to the loss of previous velopharyngeal adequacy for speech. The important fact for beginning clinicians established from longitudinal case studies dating back to the early literature is that several minor changes in the surrounding structures over time can affect velopharyngeal adequacy for speech. To best manage these clients, therefore, routine reevaluations testing the continued adequacy of the velopharyngeal support for normal speech production is necessary, particularly during the period of rapid growth of the midface up to 8 or 10 years of age.

PRIMARY CORRECTIVE SURGERY

Timing of Surgery

Primary reconstructive surgery is performed early in life in the United States today to restore normal form and function of cleft palatal structures. The timing of reconstructive surgery is considered an important factor for the effective habilitation of the infant's facial appearance, later growth of the midface, and early speech and language development. While there is little controversy over the early timing of cleft lip repair, there has been much controversy regarding the possible negative effects on maxillary growth of early palatal surgery since a seminal report on this factor by Graber in 1949 [26].

A 1986 survey by the American Cleft Palate Association (ACPA) reports that in patients with unilateral cleft lip and palate, lip repairs are now performed between 4 and 10 weeks of age in 42 percent of the teams reporting [47]. Forty-seven percent were performed after 10 weeks, with the remainder before 4 weeks. For the more complicated bilateral clefts of the primary palate (lip area), half of the patients received staged repairs (i.e., one side at a time). Lip adhesions followed by definitive reconstructons were used by 57 percent of the teams for wide unilateral or bilateral clefts. Some form of maxillary orthopedic appliance was used by 60 percent of the teams to help position and stabilize the cleft segment between the lip and palate surgeries.

The timing of complete palatal surgery is more controversial, although the latest survey of ACPA teams now shows that 73 percent of the teams repair the hard and soft palate clefts synchronously at between 6 and 18 months of age. This trend to earlier palatal surgery is based on the findings of two decades of cleft palate speech clinical research literature [7, 10, 12, 13, 19, 23, 56, 73, 79]. From numerous studies it became obvious that postponing correction of congenital velopharyngeal insufficiency over the earliest years of emergent speech and language development has an increasingly deleterious effect on developing habits of voice and articulation the longer it goes uncorrected. Postponing complete palatal closure out of fear of exacerbating midface growth potential also tends to delay emergent language skill development. It may not be necessary or advisable in the majority of cases.

Early attempts at clinical compromise by closing only the soft palate at about 18 months of age and obturating the hard palate area to provide for speech and language development were introduced by Slaughter and Pruzansky in 1954 [76] as a possible compromise for achieving both goals. However, the problems of effectively obturating the hard palate cleft over the critical speech developmental years while the maxilla is growing rapidly has led most centers over the past two decades to compromise by performing complete palatal reconstructions at between 18 to 24 months. This timing for primary palatoplasty remains the most common procedure in most communities today [51].

Unfortunately, the unsupported and misinterpreted impression against "early surgery" from the earlier clinical research reports of Graber [27] prevailed for over two decades and led to unsatisfactory compromises as regards speech and language development. Graber's report illustrated only that some of the repeated attempts at surgical reconstruction of combined clefts of the primary and secondary palates at that time (the 1950s) often contributed to additional lifelong stigma of grossly abnormal midface growth abnormalities (T. M. Graber, personal communication, June 1988) as evidence for the general condemnation of any "early surgery." Clinical researchers examining the adult status of unoperated subjects from Third World countries still show biased pictures of poorly managed operated cleft palate patients with gross facial deformities [33], contrasting these to the facies of unoperated subjects from these countries with more normal-appearing facies. However, these more normal-appearing facies also present with gross velopharyngeal insufficiency and the lifelong stigma of consequent cleft palate speech which are not demonstrable on facial slides.

Graber clearly considered early surgery to be attempts at reconstruction before 4 years of age [26].

We have seriously considered the propriety of early closure of cleft palates. It is becoming apparent that surgical correction will in some instances limit the growth potential of the maxillary denture (5/6th of which are accomplished laterally by the fourth year).

This preliminary report included only 45 cleft palate subjects widely ranging in age from 7 months to 58 years, reportedly selected at random. However, all but four were born with combined clefts of the primary and secondary palate structures, which is not typical of overall population samples. Three cases with very gross maxillary growth disturbances were emphasized in illustrations (case D.Q. had undergone 13 operations and case L.G., 15 operations) to point out the possible adverse effects of surgery and the timing of surgery as practiced at that time [26]. However, no data on the timing of these surgeries or methods used were presented.

On the positive side, Graber's criticism of the results of poor cleft palate surgery on midface development, as then evidenced, generated many relevant research questions for later animal and clinical research studies to test and qualify the effects of surgical techniques and the timing of operations. This research has slowly led to improved knowledge on the effects of specific surgical maneuvers on subsequent growth of the maxillary complex. Even today, however, many surgeons postpone early total reconstruction of clefts for speech development needs (i.e., by 12 months of age, whenever possible) on the basis of Graber's assertion, based on limited and selected data, that growth arrest results from early surgery.

The population sample in Graber's report is the same population whose speech and language development problems were studied by me up to 1960. The surgery of the older sample in this population often had both osteotomy procedures with wiring together of cleft segments in techniques described in Brophy [6] in 1915. Some of the younger cases had extensive push-back procedures [88] with much undermining of periosteum, no nasal epithelial covering of the retroposed palate, and, too frequently, repeated (10–20 operations) straight-line closure attempts. Younger cases had Langenbeck-type closures of palatal clefts with frequent attempts at later closure of the remaining fistula. However, none were operated on early by today's standards.

Some 75% of a total sample population of over 1,000 case studies presented with cleft palate speech characteristics. However, only 25 percent of the younger cases receiving two-stage closure procedures at 18 months and 4 years (with heroic efforts at prosthetically obturating the hard palate) developed cleft palate speech. It appears that the more recent approach of waiting at least until 18 to 24 months of age for complete primary sur-

gical reconstruction has also proved to be too late for about 25 to 30 percent of patients.

There has been a trend over the past 5 to 10 years toward more frequent earlier complete surgical repairs of cleft palates [12, 13, 35, 36, 63, 67, 68, 73]. However, only recently has there has been some objective research evidence indicating that such surgery before 1 year of age generally results in better midface growth than later or two-stage primary palatoplasties. It now appears that early complete closure may help to overcome midface tissue deficiencies present at birth [75].

Successful early palatal reconstruction providing velopharyngeal adequacy of speech and language development helps to prevent the development of cleft palate speech disorders, including delayed language development. The preliminary reports from programs documenting the results of complete palatoplasty in the first year of life indicate that early reconstruction can help in preventing both basic problems in this clinical population [2, 7, 10, 12, 35, 67, 73, 75].

Ross, in 1987 [75], analyzed and reported on the most extensive objective research on the question of the actual affect on midface growth of early palatoplasty (i.e., before 12 months of age). He conducted a detailed cephalometric analysis of the facial growth of a broad sample of 538 males, all born with complete unilateral clefts of both the primary and secondary palatal structures. He showed that the subgroup that was repaired prior to 12 months of age had better midface growth than those managed with delayed hard palate closures to enhance growth potential (hard palate closure delayed 4–9 years). Since early complete closure is one of the major factors recently documented as important for the prevention of cleft palate speech [12, 13], this is a long-awaited research verification of the clinical impression of a large number of speech pathologists working in this area over many years.

However, following palatal surgery at any age, it is the interrelationships of the several individual structures which change with growth of the head that determines adequate function to support clear speech production. In a sample of 60 cleft palate patients between 3 and 6 years of age, Bzoch [7] found that no single factor considered in the early literature as important to velopharyngeal adequacy for speech after surgery correlated well with measures of speech development. However, subjects with a combination of structural factors advantageous to velopharyngeal function were shown to have significantly better speech development than matched subjects without this combination of factors.

The developmental timing of when velopharyngeal adequacy for speech is obtained, rather than the age that primary surgery is performed, is the important factor in prevention of cleft palate speech. That is, 20 palatoplasties performed before 12 months of age with 50 percent failing to provide velopharyngeal adequacy are liable to show much poorer speech and language results than 20 palatoplasties performed at 18 to 24 months of age with all but one providing velopharyngeal adequacy.

Because of individual presenting differences in the structural deficiencies of tissue in the palatal shelves of the maxilla at birth, some early attempts at primary reconstruction will fail. Others will need to be postponed. However, our profession can probably contribute most to improved cleft palate care by advocating complete reconstruction as early as possible [51].

Also, speech pathologists can contribute to the prevention of cleft palate speech by objectively identifying those children shortly after primary surgery that have remaining problems of velopharyngeal insufficiency. These children should receive secondary palatoplasties as soon as possible. A more detailed discussion of both congenital and acquired forms of velopharyngeal insufficiency for speech, beyond the overt cleft palate population is presented in Chapter 6.

Figure 5-1. The basic V-to-Y technique of primary palatal reconstruction with goal of velar lengthening (used for over 3 decades). (From F. W. Pirruccello [63].)

Surgical Techniques

The complete history and step-by-step details of surgical techniques and procedures followed in modern cleft lip and palate repair may be found in the literature [14, 22, 23, 51, 52, 53, 54, 63, 91]. The student should examine this literature to acquire basic knowledge of what is possible, and of how abnormal structures presenting organic causes of speech and developmental disorders can now be corrected by cleft lip [52 53, 63], cleft palate [54, 63], orthognathic [51], and craniofacial [84] procedures. This literature and other basic texts [6, 37–39, 87, 88, 91] are available in most medical and university libraries.

Only the most basic techniques of palatal reconstruction are illustrated here. Over the past decade most early primary palatal reconstructions have been satisfactorily performed through modern refinements and modifications of two early techniques: Langenbeck's [46, 86], which is best suited for narrow palatal clefts, or the V-to-Y technique of palatal lengthening and closure developed by Kilner [37, 38] and Wardill [87, 88]. The latter approach to cleft palate repair attempted to provide for some primary soft palate lengthening to correct diminished palates cited in the early literature. The two basic techniques (see Figs. 5-1 and 5-2) appear to have been the most frequently performed operations, with refinements such as intervelar veloplasty, for primary palatal reconstructive surgery until the present time [45, 47, 50].

Lewin [45], in 1964, surveyed the basic procedures used by the membership of the American

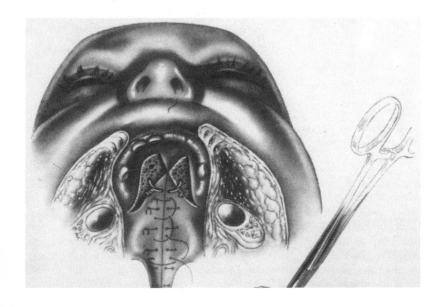

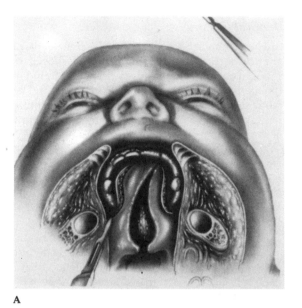

A

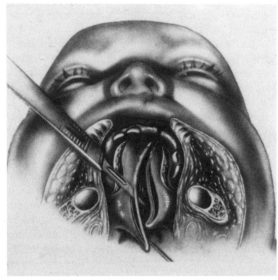

B

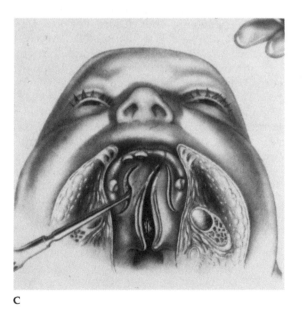

C

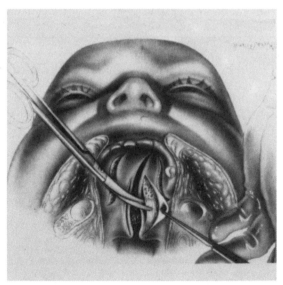

D

Figure 5-2. Basic step-by-step procedures for the more conservative Langenbeck primary reconstructive palatal operation; it has also been followed with intervelar palatoplasties as a frequently used procedure for primary palatal reconstruction. (From F. W. Pirruccello [63].)

Society of Plastic and Reconstructive Surgery in the United States and Canada. At that time, over half of the surgeons repaired cleft palates by sliding mucoperiosteal flaps with relaxing incisions, the classic Langenbeck procedure [86], as modified sometimes with retroposition of the levator sling. Unfortunately, most surgeons at the time repaired cleft palate without adding retroposition or suturing of the levator sling. However, many of the surgeons who did use retroposition in the primary repair also incorporated additional features to enhance success for velopharyngeal adequacy for speech following primary closure. Such additions included elongation of the neurovascular bundle, Z-plasty on the nasal surface, and narrowing of the nasopharynx [45].

This trend and a trend for even earlier complete attempts at primary repair of isolated cleft lip and cleft palate based on the demonstrated need for speech and language development continues up to the present time [2, 13, 21, 33, 34, 47–50, 57].

Primary reconstructions by using the modified basic Wardill [88] procedure involving a V-to-Y soft palate lengthening approach were then generally used by slightly less than half of those plastic surgeons reporting [45]. The technique of two-stage cleft palate repair with relatively early repair of the soft palate only, as advocated by Slaughter and Pruzansky [76] (I documented the speech results in about one fourth of the 1,000 cases preseneted in this book) were then adopted by only 12 percent of the surgeons reporting at that time. This conservative approach, which was developed to protect the growth potential of the maxilla by closing only the soft palate at about 18 months of age and attempting to obturate the hard palate with prostheses until 3 to 4 years of age, unfortunately resulted in the frequent occurrence of cleft palate speech. Ostiperiosteal flap closures were then used by only 6.7 percent of the surgeons reporting.

Current Trends in Timing and Techniques of Primary Palatoplasty

For a long time complete surgical reconstructions of cleft palate were generally postponed to an average age of 18 to 24 months [45, 51]. The most recent survey of practice in ACPA teams [47] indicates that clefts of the secondary palate are now repaired synchronously between 6 and 18 months of age in 73 percent of 186 teams reporting. This indicates a trend to earlier closures.

Two-stage procedures closing only the soft palate and attempting to obturate the hard palate until late adolescence are still followed in some European countries [57], reportedly with excellent midface growth but usually with a high incidence of cleft palate speech persisting into adult life. However, avoidance of a high frequency of cleft palate speech sequelae from a well-managed two-stage surgical approach appears to be possible, even if proved unnecessary. An intensive early treatment program in Zurich where hard palate closures are postponed to 5 years of age was recently reported to have avoided or corrected cleft palate speech in the majority of subjects undergoing this procedure [32].

The basic V-to-Y technique of palatal lengthening and closure is illustrated in Figure 5-1. This technique, along with modifications of the basic Langenbeck operation illustrated in Figure 5-2A, B, C, and D, has been 2 most frequently used techniques to correct palatal clefts over the last decade. A definite trend to incorporate intervelar veloplasty (i.e., specific retropositioning of the levator sling) with either of these basic operations has occurred since the 1970s [61].

More recently, a number of surgeons at large cleft palate treatment centers have adopted a newer timing protocol for complete cleft palate repair by 6 to 12 months of age. This protocol is based on newer proven techniques which should not exacerbate midface growth potential [2, 12, 13, 22, 47, 63, 67, 68]. Also, a new technique utilizing double-opposing Z-plasty elongation of the velum to improve velopharyngeal function for speech and closing hard palate clefts by simply dropping flaps of periosteum without cutting relaxing incisions near the alveolar ridges to close the hard palate early is presently under longitudinal study. This technique, conceived and introduced by Furlow [22], is illustrated in Figure 5-3. Furlow's technique, and other recent innovations designed to facilitate early complete velopharyngeal reconstruction [19] by utilizing microsurgical techniques and specific retroposition of the levator sling, offer hope for more frequent functional velopharyngeal reconstructions at an earlier age.

The fact that the early timing of surgery should not be considered an equal factor with the surgical technique followed or with the extent of the presenting deficiency of tissue for the potential growth of the midface is strongly suggested by the recent research report of Ross [75]. The techniques introduced in the last decade are available to help the next generation of infants born with cleft palate by providing for both lengthening of the soft palate and increased mobility by setting back the levator sling in early primary surgery. However, the long-term efficacy of these newer techniques requires that cases reconstructed earlier be followed into adult life [61]. Verification of long-term speech and maxillofacial growth results awaits further clinical research.

Further research is likewise needed to support the advocacy by speech pathologists for earliest possible complete reconstruction of speech mechanism defects in this population. In an excellent recent discussion of this topic, McWilliams, Morris, and Shelton [51] listed the major remaining unknown factors from clinical or basic research. These may be summarized as follows:

1. The variables used to decide the timing of surgery may also influence maxillofacial

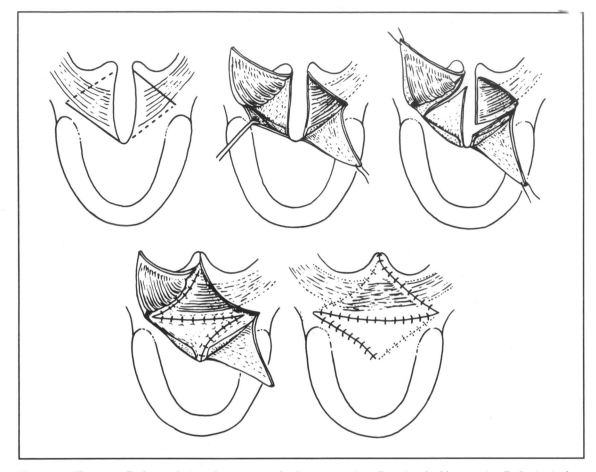

Figure 5-3. The newer Furlow technique for primary palatal reconstructions. By using double opposing Z-plasties in the velar area, this procedure attempts to accomplish both velar lengthening and intervelar veloplasty by retroposition of the levator sling in primary palatal reconstruction. (From L. T. Furlow [22].)

growth. That is, children receiving later primary surgery may also have larger deficits of palatal tissue.

2. There is no common agreement as to what constitutes a significant deficit. That is, is a minor difference of 1 to 3 mm of maxillary growth in cases long postponed for palatal surgery and correctable through orthodontic or later minor orthognathic procedures a difference of consequence in the lives of these patients?

3. We still do not know which recorded growth deficits arise from congenital deformities and which can be attributed to surgery.

4. Lip surgery, which is routinely carried out early, has been shown in animal research to affect maxillofacial growth adversely. Does this, rather than early palatal surgery, cause

the small differences measured and reported to date?

5. Techiques that might minimize the degree of midfacial deficiency with or without surgical intervention are not well-known.

6. There is a possibility that subsequent catch-up growth occurs after a lag following both lip and palatal surgery that is not recorded in the available research literature.

For these and other reasons, including parental and surgeons' preferences and individual differences in the presenting deficiency of the tissue available for reconstruction of the speech mechanism, I agree with McWilliams and colleagues. The preferred timing of complete cleft palate reconstructive surgery remains controversial and should not be determined a priori. However, on the basis

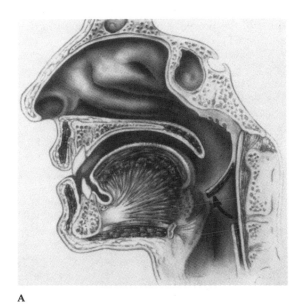

A

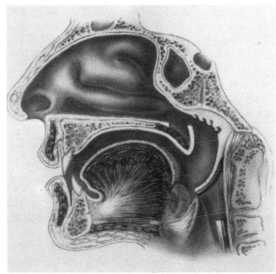

B

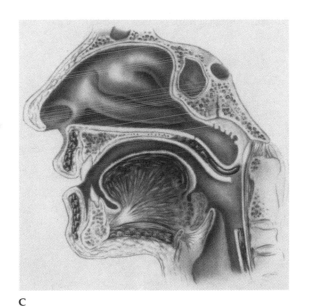

C

Figure 5-4. The basic reconstruction of the velopharyngeal mechanism involved in some primary, but more usually in secondary palatal reconstructions to correct velopharyngeal insufficiency for speech. A. Superior-based flap raised from posterior pharyngeal wall. B. Superior velar flap raised from velum to overlap and cover denuded area of pharyngeal flap, inserted into superior surface of velum. C. Completed pharyngeal flap reconstruction in midline attaching to velum to posterior pharyngeal wall. Lateral epithelialized openings must remain to allow for nasal breathing and nasal resonance during speech. (From F. W. Pirruccello [63].)

of clinical scientific reports in the literature as well as clinical experience, I join with McWilliams and colleagues [5] in advocating that, "The speech pathologist must be aggressive in informing other members of the management team that early surgery is more likely to give better speech results than late surgery." I would go one step further and define the ideal goal for timing of early surgery as complete reconstruction of all lip and palatal clefts before and including the 12th month of age.

Secondary Palatal Surgery

When velopharyngeal insufficiency for speech persists after primary reconstructive surgery, there is usually a need for referral for secondary operations to correct this condition. The most common basic secondary surgical procedure for correcting velopharyngeal insufficiency for speech now generally involves variations of the pharyngeal flap procedure. This procedure is illustrated in Figure 5-4.

In the early 1960s I compared the results of a large series of case studies treated for later velopharyngeal insufficiency by speech appliances with a large sample treated by this, then, newer approach [8]. I was impressed by the results of properly constructed obturating pharyngeal flaps. However, an obturating pharyngeal flap is an unphysiological substitute for the velopharyngeal mechanism. It can lead to mouth breathing or sleep apnea sequelae or both. Satisfactory opening and closing functions of the nasopharynx necessary for speech must be achieved by lateral wall movements in the nasopharynx. It should function successfully like a muscle tissue substitute for the speech bulb of a muscle-trimmed prosthetic speech appliance as described below.

Since then, more selective modifications of pharyngeal flap–type operative procedures have been developed. Selection of specific variations, based on objective presurgical analyses of individual deficiencies has been described by Sprintzen et al. [78] and the speech results of such procedures by Riski [70].

A pharyngeal flap can also be used in conjunction with a push-back operation to cover and epithelialize the nasal surface of the retroposed velum to maintain elongation for secondary palatoplasty [18]. In this case the velum rather than the pharyngeal flap must achieve adequate velopharyngeal function for speech.

Occasionally Teflon or other implants in the nasopharynx have been selected for correction of postprimary surgery velopharyngeal insufficiency problems with good results and avoidance of some of the problems of the obturating pharyngeal flap [21].

More recently, a modification of the Orticoachea operation [58–60, 71, 82] has been tried and initially evaluated. This operation was first developed as a standardized pragmatic approach to primary palatoplasty in a Third-World country to provide a higher frequency of velopharyngeal competency from a single operation. It involves insertion of the palatopharyngeus muscles, made surgically into a sphincter, into the nasopharynx behind the velum. In the United States this operation is performed as a later secondary veloplasty and the sphincter is inserted higher in the nasopharynx than originally described [58] in the area of closest approximation to velopharyngeal closure [71]. The sphincter thus created tends to close off the nasopharynx for oral syllable requirements and allows for nasal syllables due to its symmetry of innervation with the levator muscles. This basic technique, with recent modifications for use as a secondary corrective procedure, is well illustrated by Stratoudakis and Bambace [82].

CORRECTION THROUGH SPEECH APPLIANCES

In my earlier clinical experience, many problems of velopharyngeal insufficiency under conditions that did not allow for further or even for primary surgical reconstruction of wide clefts were corrected to eliminate nasalance through both temporary and permanent speech appliances constructed by a prosthodontist. Figure 5-5 illus-

Figure 5-5. Examples of prosthetic speech appliances with speech bulbs fitted to allow normal resonance characteristics during speech efforts. A. Temporary appliances constructed for young children to correct velopharyngeal insufficiencies when surgery for this purpose is not available. B. Large two-piece speech appliance with overlay denture and provision for hard-palate obturation and velopharyngeal function to support normal speech production.

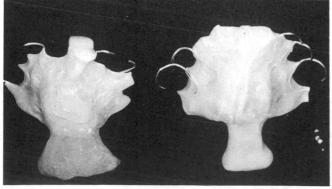

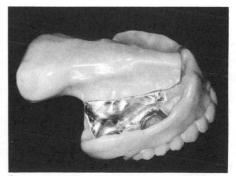

A   B

trates some of these primary and permanent dental appliances which can also accomplish satisfactory correction of this basic organic problem underlying speech production under special conditions today.

The art of constructing such speech appliances and details on their selective use can be reviewed in Adisman [1], Bzoch [8], Millard [55], and Rosen and Bzoch [74]. Although seldom required today because of the improved efficacy of complete early surgical reconstruction techniques, speech appliances, including the simpler lift appliance [24, 42] that is often useful for the neurogenic velopharyngeal acquired deficiencies discussed in Chapter 6, still need to be considered and made available to selected individuals today.

Prosthetic speech appliances or the temporary use of hard-palate obturators to cover palatal fistulae offer an important alternative to surgical physical management for correcting velopharyngeal insufficiency in cases where surgery is not advisable for special reasons.

DENTAL AND OCCULSAL HAZARDS

The second major organic factor to be considered in the evaluation of speech disorders of subjects with clift lip with or without cleft palate is the frequent presence of dental or occlusal abnormalities. These organic causal factors occur frequently, particularly in congenital unilateral or bilateral complete clefts of both primary and secondary palate structures.

Kingsley [40] conjectured, back in 1894, that a narrow and ill-formed jaw and an irregular dental arch were hindrances to speech. Since that time, research reports in the literature and discussions of the topic by clinical speech pathologists working at cleft palate centers have both confirmed and qualified Kingsley's early impression. The direct effect of improved articulation performance following correction of malocclusions of the dentition through orthognathic surgery in the absence of interventive speech therapy recently reported by Vallino et al. [85] seems to confirm

Figure 5-6. Some dental and occlusal hazard conditions which affected speech production for cleft palate subjects.

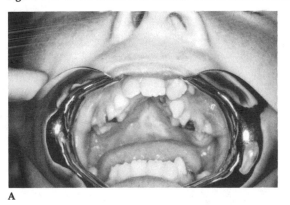

A

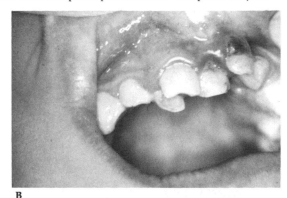

B

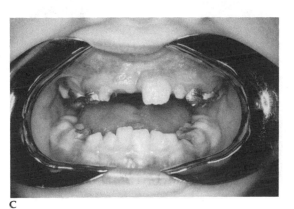

C

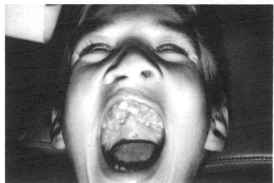

D

the suspected potential cause-effect relationship between dental malocclusions and speech.

The developmental nature of this organic cause of some cleft palate speech disorders was first suggested when Bzoch [7], Starr [79], and Counihan [16] carried out three interrelated studies in the mid-1950s. The studies examined in subjects with clefts in three different age groups. Bzoch [6] studied a group of 60 subjects aged 3 to 6 years and found no significant relationship between their dental and occlusal abnormalities and their poor performance on articulation tests. The sample population, however, was markedly delayed in articulation skills when compared to a matched group of 120 subjects without clefts. The 5- to 6-year old subjects with clefts actually scored below the 3- to 4-year-old normal subjects in producing correct articulation. Bzoch suggested that the failure to find articulation-dentition relationships might be due to the generally low level of articulation skills of the population studied [7].

Starr [79] studied a somewhat older group of cleft subjects (58 subjects aged 6–11 years). He found that the subgroup of subjects with malocclusions judged to be a hazard to speech made more articulation errors than the rest of the sample studied. These differences, in the expected direction, were found between subgroups with individual tooth variations as well as the subgroup whose maxillary arches were narrower than their mandibular arches.

Counihan [16] studied an older group of 55 subjects with clefts (aged 13–24). He found a similar high correlation between articulation skills and malocclusions limited to those subjects whose maxillary arches were narrowed.

The dental hazards to clear articulation of anterior consonant sounds in young children born with clefts can be very marked, as indicated by the examples in Figure 5-6. Remarkable changes in the architecture within the tongue must learn to articulate intelligible and normal-sounding speech sound elements developmentally are most often provided in cleft palate team management through early orthodontic treatment, as illustrated by the pre- and posttreatment cases shown in Figure 5-7A and B.

However, even some of the appliance procedures necessary for changing dental malocclusions (Fig. 5-8) can present hazards to clear speech. The close cooperation necessary between the dental pedodontist, orthodontist, or prosthodontist and the speech pathologist is facilitated by the cleft palate team approach and constitutes one of the most interesting interdisciplinary features of professional work in this area.

The usual interrelationships between dentition and speech behavior are difficult to verify objectively, although repeated clinical interrelationships are not uncommon in cleft palate team case studies. The difficulty in establishing objective research generalizations is due to the large number of uncontrolled variables affecting speech production in any sample of a population with specific dental abnormalities, but clinical experience clearly indicates that relationships do exist.

The urgings of speech pathologists for early correction of dental and occlusal abnormalities

Figure 5-7. Orthodontic casts illustrating the potential for clear speech production by removing dental and orthodontic hazards through effective dental specialty treatment.

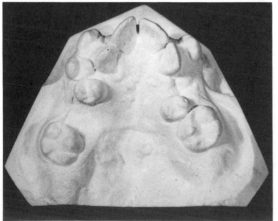

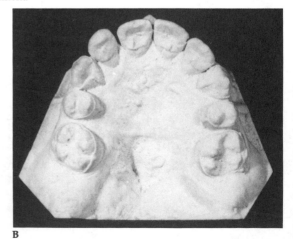

A

B

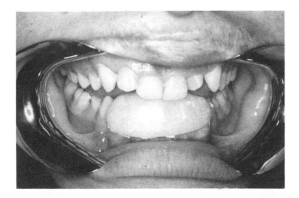
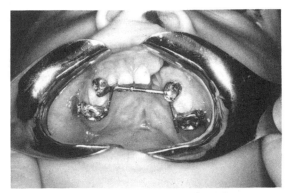
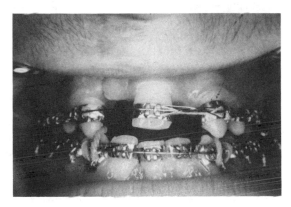
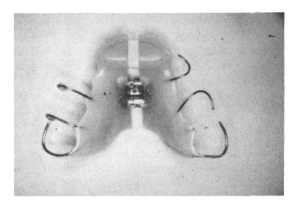

Figure 5-8. Dental appliances which, by themselves, created temporary and sometimes long-term hazards to clear speech production.

have provided the rationale for many early pedodontic, orthodontic, and dental prosthetic procedures for the cleft palate population. A narrow maxillary arch, in particular, or asymmetrical anterior malocclusions or missing lateral incisors often present a hazard to clear articulation, particularly for /s/ and /z/ articulation, into later childhood and early adult life.

Starr [80] later reviewed and evaluated the literature relating dental conditions to cleft palate speech disorders and to speech in otherwise normal subjects. He pointed out the difficulties of controlling for variables even in larger sample studies with data limited to clinical perceptual judgments of articulation. In his 1979 review of the literature [80], he summarized the trends that he found rather than any established cause-and-effect facts substantiated through research.

Several conclusions were drawn relating speech to dental hazards in subjects born with clefts. The early investigations by Bzoch [7], Starr [79], and Counihan [16], considered together, suggested that the possible negative effects of dental and occlusal abnormalities cannot be delineated until articulation skills are well advanced. The data reported by Counihan and Starr and those of Foster and Green [20] suggest that dental arch relationships may be the single most important dental factor affecting articulation.

A study by McDermott [49], along with the report of Foster and Green [20] and a study by Bankson and Byrne [4], indicated that missing teeth, but most often the number and combination of abnormal dental factors, often had a direct adverse effect on clear speech production. However, a study by Powers [64] as well as data in the literature indicate that good articulation skills can exist in the presence of even severe dental deviations.

From combined earlier literature on subjects with dental deviations without clefts as well as those specific cleft palate studies cited it may be concluded that:

(1) Under some conditions, dental deviations do affect articulation, (2) When dental variables are defined, it appears most probable that the number, severity, and combinations of dental deviations will be of primary importance, and (3) Single factors that will most likely be of importance are dental arch relationships, open bites, missing

incisors, and any other conditions that restrict relationships between the tongue and lower incisors.

The more recent research into dental arch and speech interrelations includes studies using experimental prosthetic alteration of the palatal contour of normal subjects to study their articulation compensations through palatographic methods [29–31]. These investigations have usually shown that compensations take place over a short period of time with some limitations in the first week of adjustment. However, McCutcheon et al. [48], using dynamic palatographic techniques related to dental models of normal speakers' hard palates, showed that palatal morphological differences as fine as variations in the rugae of the anterior maxillary alveolar ridge influence the /s/ and /z/ medial groove location and account for some laterality effects.

Compensation for the frequently more abnormal dental arch structures of cleft palate individuals probably requires learned compensatory effort for their usually greater deviations. This need for compensation may require *stressful effort* on the part of the speaker with cleft-related dental deviations as yet not well investigated through more sophisticated research.

However, because both clinical experience and research findings most often have demonstrated the capacity of individuals to compensate for even severe abnormalities of the dental or occlusal structures to produce intelligible speech, the presence of necessary cause-and-effect relations between dental hazards to clear speech and speech defects is *not* predictable. Such findings, for a given client, should be considered as possible or even as probable contributing hazards to clear speech production. They should not be presumed, a priori, to cause speech abnormalities.

The identification of dental abnormalities through interoral examinations by a speech pathologist thought to be related directly to specific articulation distortions (particularly lateral distortions of sibilant sounds on the side of missing teeth or alveolar clefts) is common in cleft palate team reports. Although training for compensation through speech therapy is possible, a better approach to avoid stressful speech effort is to have the dental abnormalities corrected as early as possible. The direct evaluation of individual cases, focused on recording observable relationships during speech production to dental abnormalities, should be a regular part of the cleft palate speech clinical evaluation.

HEARING LOSS

The third important major organic problem area to be investigated is the assessment of possible hearing impairment. Chapter 9 covers this subject in more detail.

While assessment of the contribution of hearing loss problems should be a necessary part of any speech and language evaluation, this topic is especially relevant here because of the almost universal finding of early and often chronic middle ear infection (otitis media) in newborns and infants presenting with congenital clefts of the palate [81]. Studies of hearing acuity in cleft palate subjects and otological examinations with discrete tests of middle ear and eustachian tube function have demonstrated the greater-than-average occurrence of hearing loss in this population [28]. More recent studies have implicated this frequent and difficult problem as most probably contributing to delayed language skill development in infants born with cleft palate.

Beyond the fact of the high frequency of repeated conductive hearing loss found in most infants born with congenital cleft palate [81, 83], there is an obvious need to manage complete conductive hearing loss with amplification and auditory training for congenital atresia of the external auditory canal. Atresia most frequently occurs bilaterally with *Treacher Collins syndrome* and unilaterally in many forms of *hemifacial microsomia,* as described in more detail by Smith [77] and in Chapter 2.

In addition to management of conductive hearing loss, there appears to be a possibility that infants born with clefts and related syndromal conditions might also have congenital or acquired sensory-neural hearing loss. This can be related to genetic syndromes with deafness or the use of ototoxic drugs in their early treatment. Deafness is listed as a frequent sequela of many of the chromosomal and syndromal craniofacial disorders presenting with or without cleft palate. The management of deafness and of significant hearing loss in this population is therefore a particularly important problem in the team management of children at high risk for communicative disorders. Effective management requires the services of a clinical audiologist, otologist, and speech and language pathologist for an effective team approach.

OTHER ORGANIC FACTORS

There are, of course, other possible organic or physical factors that need to be addressed and related to the clinical diagnostic speech evaluations for clients with clefts. On the modern craniofacial team, this is most often the responsibility of the team pediatrician who oversees the child's overall medical care.

While general mental retardation is not typically related to isolated cleft palate it occurs as a limiting factor to providing effective treatment for some children with syndromes including clefts and for most all infants born with chromosomal abnormalities. Also, false impressions of mental retardation due to facial disfigurement or cleft palate speech disorders of many intellectually normal children in this population needs to be corrected after objective developmental evaluation. This can usually best be provided by a team clinical psychology consultant working closely with other members of the team.

In the past, some forms of craniostenosis led to acquired brain damage with concomitant problems of motor retardation, general mental retardation, and blindness. These sequelae are today sometimes preventable with proper early diagnosis and treatment by a neurosurgeon and craniofacial surgeon working together on a specialized surgical team and through long-term craniofacial team management. Indeed, the different outcome of preventing retardation, motor, and sensory problems from developing in children born with many of the more common treatable craniofacial disorders, has become one of the most challenging and satisfying aspects of modern craniofacial center teamwork.

Many of the same types of children that were formerly committed to lifelong institutionalization with the severely mentally retarded today live productive lives within family units in communities that provide for their special early needs. The parents of these children also often need help in managing and guiding their children to their highest potential development, even those children who are severely retarded. This is an area of practice involving referral and coordination with developing community special education programs providing early intervention programs for high-risk infants and preschool children.

For the more typical infant with isolated clefting and a less significant congenital disorder that falls into one of the known syndromes, it is not known with what frequency teratogens causing multiple abnormalities of structures other than the head may also cause significant central nervous system abnormalities. Certainly, the *fetal alcohol syndrome* and other drug-related congenital disorders affect the potential development of many infants today beyond what might be accomplished for them through cleft palate team treatment.

Children with multiple congenital disorders were at one time categorized as part of the congenital cleft palate population. This contributed to the impression that children born with clefts were, in general, retarded. Syndromal subjects with clefts and other significant disorders constitute, rather, a limited subgroup of infants with clefts whom we need to study much further before knowing with confidence the limits of early intervention and stimulation programs. These experiments of nature and of detrimental environmental effects on their development therefore constitute the real challenge of the future.

Equally challenging today is the need for improving existing health care services by applying the treatment knowledge and the available information forged through decades of interdisciplinary clinical research. We need to more routinely *prevent* rather than try later to rehabilitate cleft palate speech.

INDIVIDUAL DIFFERENCES

It should also be remembered that in any sample population, whether classified in an organic area such as cleft palate or not, unique family and often significant individual differences and developmental learning experiences occur in the early life of each individual. A normal distribution curve, rather than either-or classifications, characterizes the early language learning environment of each child. Many children born with cleft palate, like many children essentially normal at birth, experience poor learning or traumatic environments as significant to their speech and language skill development as their presenting congenital abnormalities which label them clinically as "cleft palate children."

The developmental and medical case history information, therefore, is just as important as normative clinical speech and language tests for individual diagnostic evaluations. Always give equal importance to case history information in a differential diagnostic evaluation of presenting speech and language disorders, even though cleft palate is the obvious initial diagnosis.

In any definable human population, whether it be people with red hair or males in the New York City public school system, one should find a random distribution of human characteristics including intelligence and motor skills related to early speech and language development. Acquired diseases and accidents occur at predictable frequency for all children in a given environment, whether born with clefts or not. It follows, therefore, that the assessment of other possible significant physical factors should include a careful medical history, a family history, and an early developmental history of each patient. Factors such as illnesses, family traits, and accidents may have an important relationship to speech and language development which could be overlooked due to the diagnosis of cleft palate.

FUNCTIONAL FACTORS

We have discussed the literature that suggests that symbolic speech and language behavior is an innate biological predisposition in our species. This implies that human infants, whether born with clefts or not, are all predisposed to develop through predictable stages of prespeech, early speech, and mature speech behavior. However, biological predisposition and universal developmental patterns in no way negate the overwhelming evidence that for each human being, speech behavior must be *learned*. It is learned through interaction experiences with early caretakers in the home. It is this set of individual psychosocial, learning, and developmental experiences that the speech pathologist must assess and try to manage in order to prevent cleft palate speech, which is now considered broadly under the category of functional etiological factors.

There are several functional and learning factors which can negatively affect the speech and language development of children with clefts. These include (1) early bonding problems with parents and siblings after the shock of presentation at birth of a baby born with facial disfigurement; (2) the early feeding and breathing prob-

lems of Pierre Robin sequence and other multiply handicapped infants born with clefts; (3) the possible altered parenting and lowered expectation levels for early language skill on the part of parents of a child born with cleft palate; (4) the frequent lack of reinforcement of developing receptive language skills due to the substitution of gesture communication by an infant whose early expressive language efforts (speech) are difficult to understand by busy parents who anticipate needs and respond to and reinforce gesture communications; and (5) the habituation of modified speech patterns with effort through glottally initiated syllables in early speech (cleft palate speech habilitation in years 2 and 3 and beyond), leading to unintelligible speech, and other similar but not uncommon problems.

These developmental problems can usually be managed through counseling, by providing information on the stages and detailed patterns of normal language development, and by ascertaining with the child's parents the particular reasons for problems in achieving expected levels of speech and language competency. Information booklets from the ACPA and the American Cleft Palate Foundation and other sources as listed and discussed in Chapter 4 are helpful in reinforcing early interventive counseling. However, they do not take the place of face-to-face discussions between parents and the speech pathologist and other clinicians on a cleft palate team.

We have found that by monitoring each infant's month-by-month development, an individualized pragmatic home language stimulation program can be outlined and initiated during cleft palate clinic reevaluations. The Reel Scale or other developmental language scale or tests facilitate this service, which can usually be completed during routine team clinic recalls. By discussing the failure to achieve expressive language development skills at home when receptive skills have developed to higher levels, the therapist can help develop strategies for effective home language stimulation programs. This procedure has offset trends toward early delayed expressive language during our past decade of clinical experience.

A general consideration of the possible developmental learning and psychosocial factors needing review in discussions with parents and family members was presented in Chapter 3. A further discussion of the psychological aspects of competency in language skill acquisition follows in Chapter 7. The remainder of this chapter, therefore, is concerned primarily with a general explanation of the concept of learned functional speech disorders, which can become habituated in infancy and mantained indefinitely with maturation even after late physical restoration of congenital velopharyngeal insufficiency for normal voice and speech development. This concept is basic to the practice of speech and language pathology with this population. It is generally supported by current language and cognitive theories and by clinical research.

The empirical findings from clinical experience, that hundreds of subjects with cleft palate presenting with speech disorders have improved and achieved speech patterns comparable to their peers after limited periods of therapy, supports the concept that cleft palate speech is primarily a functional, learned disorder. Changes in speech disorders which did not improve with maturation alone before such training provides convincing evidence of the often functional nature of cleft palate speech. Also, the fact that in this age of accountability for our programs in schools, clinics, or private practice large numbers of individuals without any form of physical abnormality of the speech mechanism present with serious speech disorders that are modifiable through speech and language therapy programs, gives further credence to the reality of the concept of functional speech disorders.

MAINTENANCE OF LEARNED NEUROMOTOR PATTERNS IN SPEECH BEHAVIOR

The physical process of speech production by the human organism involves highly coordinated learned neuromotor patterns of behavior. Speech behavior, learned by most children during the first two years after birth, involves conditioning breathing, phonation, articulation, and resonance patterns of the movements of the speech mechanism. How these coordinated patterns are learned and stored is not completely understood. However, the essential requirements and typical developmental patterns of learning are known well enough to develop individual strategies for guiding children with cleft palate to essentially equal levels of speech and language achievement with their normal peers, particularly if their velopharyngeal insufficiency is corrected early.

Studies of language skill development in infants indicate that the basic motor speech patterns are usually laid down and reinforced during the first 2 to 3 years. These auditorially monitored encoding skills are preceded by the development of auditory decoding receptive language skills and usually develop to the level of the two- to three-word stage of expressive language by the child's second birthday. Infants born with cleft palate should develop similar levels of receptive and expressive language as noncleft infants.

These usual auditory decoding and neuromuscular encoding behaviors, however, need to be learned during a period of development when the majority of children born with cleft palate must try to produce speech intelligibly with velopharyngeal insufficiency. This condition, congenital velopharyngeal insufficiency, is unable to easily support an infant's unguided natural efforts at the early oral communication stages of speech development into the second and third years of development.

Infants born with velopharyngeal insufficiency are incapable of certain of the coordinated motor requirements to produce the usual sound patterns, even in early random vocalizations, and later in babbling, social babbling, jargon, and the first true word stages common to other infants during this period of development. They may struggle to produce understandable speech through compensatory neuromuscular patterns involving other organs of the speech mechanism. They can also habituate fairly normal articulation patterns distorted by nasalance but accepted and rewarded by the adults in their environment during their early development.

The physical condition most affecting early learning of compensatory motor patterns is velopharyngeal insufficiency. However, a management routine of fairly early reconstruction of the palate (i.e., reconstruction within the first year) does not of itself assure velopharyngeal adequacy for normal speech and language development. Some of the primary palatal reconstruction attempts, whether performed early or late, will fail to provide adequate function to support normal speech and language development. Through prior learning, although the palate is made potentially adequate, it may be some time before palatal function for speech is used after surgery, particularly for children with functionally delayed expressive language development. Clinical experience indicates that it may be a considerable period of time after either primary or later potentially adequate secondary palatal reconstruction before functional velopharyngeal adequacy for speech is both possible and used.

If abnormal neuromotor patterns were learned even through the limited social babbling, jargon, and first-word stages, they may be retained, without redirection through speech therapy, for an indefinite period of time. The fine coordination necessary among breathing, phonation, resonance, and articulation functions for even elementary speech production patterns involves specific and rapid muscular movements of the structures of the speech mechanisms. These underlying coordinated learned patterns are stored and automatically recalled and monitored by subconscious neurosensory systems in the brain. The control of speech production may be partly best understood as a cybernetic system monitored through proprioceptive as well as auditory feedback control. This concept is discussed and developed in finer detail in Chapter 18. The following is a simple overview of some of the basic facts involved in the sensorimotor learning of speech production.

NORMAL LEARNED FUNCTIONS OF THE SPEAKING MECHANISM

The speech mechanism of the body is energized by the outgoing breathstream. Speaking, therefore, first requires a learned preparatory major alteration in the pattern of breathing (inhalation-exhalation phase and mode). The inhalation phase of breathing is normally shortened, tidal air volume is increased, and the oral cavity is most often substituted for the nasal cavity to facilitate quick and easy inhalation in preparation for speech. The exhalation phase of breathing is prolonged for speech production due partly to the resistance of the vocal folds and partly to oral consonant restrictions on the outgoing breathstream from consonant articulations throughout utterances of several syllables for connected speech. Exhalation is also controlled subglottally to effect meaningful force and pitch changes of inflection used to communicate paralinguistic phonological differences in intended meaning.

The fundamental frequencies of the voice over speech utterances vary and are controlled at the level of the larynx by the coordinated adduction of the vocal folds under varying tensions. The vocal folds alternately close and open the glottis during speech. They close to vibrate at variable frequencies related to subtle changes in subglottic air pressure and internal muscle tone on different syllables. These fine, learned variations of intrinsic muscle tone and minor controlled vari-

ations in subglottic air flow and pressure must be learned to provide for rapid variations in both pitch and force of voice for introducing the paralinguistic features of our spoken language code. Even a 3-year-old child can usually utter even the single word "yes" and let you know that he or she really means "no" or "maybe" through these subtle connotative differences in meaning transmitted by oral language but not shared by orthography (the written form of language).

Spoken languages require that the vocal folds abduct and readduct within milliseconds in close coordination with the rapid co-articulation of lip, the front of the tongue, the back of the tongue, and the velar movement patterns underlying speech production. This is necessary to produce the unvoiced as contrasted to the voiced consonants in plosive and fricative manners of formation common to most languages. These contrasts in speech production are basic to the intelligible decoding of spoken English. The pharyngeal as well as the oral cavity resonating structures must also rapidly be altered in shape to produce the resonance changes required to distinguish the 17 vowel and dipththong elements used correctly by most 3-year-old children speaking a dialect of the English language.

Simultaneously with all these requirements, the velopharyngeal mechanism must be able to alternately close and open the nasopharynx in accordance with the alternate nasal and nonnasal syllable production of words in syntactical encoded utterances of the speaker. This articulation function of the palate must be coordinated perfectly with both lip and tongue valving in the oral cavity at the precise place of articulation required by the language system and anatomy of speech to produce intelligible sequences of syllables. This articulation function of the soft palate rather than only its resonance control functions is difficult to achieve early in the life of an infant born with congenital cleft palate. The fact that it can now be generally demonstrated to be an achievable goal under management of early team supervision of early development is the next topic of this discussion. However, since abnormal learned patterns of early motor speech behavior for infants born with cleft palate appear to often be learned before 2 years of age, it is important to recognize their early development. Some of the more typical learned functional patterns of cleft palate speech are described below.

SOME ABNORMAL EARLY LEARNED PATTERNS UNDERLYING CLEFT PALATE SPEECH HABITUATION

Infants born with cleft palate and related disorders present some unusual disorders and clinical symptoms to which the beginning clinician in communicative disorders needs to be alerted. Perhaps the most significant of these problems is in the area of delayed speech and language development. More unusual is their frequent development of atypical articulation patterns in speech production through early habituation of *gross sound substitution patterns* in early speech behavior. More subtle than these are their propensity for adjustments in both laryngeal and breath support functions affecting defects of phonation as a consequence of velopharyngeal insufficiency at birth. These differences in early speech and language development will be briefly discussed before proceeding to consideration of the categorical aspects of cleft palate speech.

Gross Sound Substitution Error Patterns of Articulation

The syllable, rather than the speech sound element (phoneme), should be considered as the basic unit of speech production for clinical purposes of evaluating expressive language skill development. Each syllable contains a perceivable vowel or vowellike sound element (syllabic element) which is voiced. Its distinguishing tone is dependent on the general shape of the resonating cavities from the larynx to the lips and particularly on the height of the tongue in the front or back of the oral cavity.

A syllabic element in speech may stand alone as a word symbol. More commonly, it will be initiated or closed off by one or more consonant (nonsyllabic) sound elements to form meaningful words in speech. The child with cleft palate may learn to form syllables for words in expressive language in a grossly abnormal manner in early infancy. The syllabic elements of words can usually be well approximated with some nasal distortion, even with an open cleft of the palate. However, the pressure consonant elements needed to produce intelligible first words are more difficult to approximate with velopharyngeal insufficiency. The cleft palate child is often more rewarded with understanding of his or her

early speech efforts by production of nonsyllabic speech sound elements initiated or closed off by glottal stop or by pharyngeal fricative substitutions for the oral consonants in words used to obtain wants and needs. A child developing this learned motor speech articulation error pattern is able to approximate many consonant sound elements by atypical movements of the vocal folds, the base of the tongue, and even the pharynx below the level of the velopharyngeal valve before he or she obtains velopharyngeal adequacy to support more typical infant speech patterns of articulation. Combining these learned laryngeal and pharyngeal noise elements with vowel sounds enables a child with velopharyngeal insufficiency to approximate more morphemic word symbols more intelligibly. They may thus learn to speak abnormally but understandably, even with an open cleft of the palate.

Such early speech experiences can initiate an abnormal pattern of movements of the articulators for speech production efforts over the early years of the child's life. The beginnings of development of these abnormal cleft palate speech patterns are diagnosable as early as 2 to 3 years of age through articulation tests which focus on error patterns in speech rather than on correct or incorrect judgments.

What we here refer to as gross sound substitution errors are errors characterized by a retracted place of articulation — sound elements produced at the glottis and laryngeal and oral pharynx and used as substitution sounds in words, particularly for plosives and fricatives. Such errors are not typical of the developmental articulation patterns of their peers at ages 2, 3, 4, or 5. Different efferent neuromotor pathways and specific muscles not normally conditioned in speech are being used when such errors are found in articulation testing. These patterns can be strongly reinforced and later continued even after complete and satisfactory reconstruction of the palatal structures. These abnormal neuromotor patterns underlying speech production may persist for a lifetime if not corrected through therapy. When identified, they require the intervention of direct articulation-focused speech therapy instituted at the earliest age possible to be effective.

WEAK AND ASPIRATE PHONATION

While there is often an opposite tendency toward hyperlaryngeal function related to gross sound substitution patterns of articulation, there is also a predisposition for weak and aspirate phonation. This appears to be related to its effect of masking nasalance distortions by minimizing the resonance distortion from velopharyngeal incompetency through weakening the fundamental frequency energy. This phonatory voicing pattern can limit the effective results of later correction of velopharyngeal insufficiency and articulation skill training.

Children with cleft palate may learn that they are better understood if they talk in this manner, that is, with breathy and weak phonation. This pattern later tends to be retained and becomes resistant to therapy after habituation. This is especially true for females since breathy voice characteristics are more common in the normal female voice and therefore not stigmatic or handicapping if continued.

DELAYED SPEECH AND LANGUAGE DEVELOPMENT

Studies of the receptive and expressive emergent language development of infants born with cleft palate [7, 15, 22, 56] indicate that these infants are often retarded in expressive language development. More recent clinical studies indicate that this delayed development can be effectively overcome through initiating routine early language stimulation programs in the home or through early direct language skill training when prevention is not possible [12, 57].

A child with cleft palate who obtains his or her wants and needs through gesture language along with very simple vocalizations from 2 to 3 or 4 years of age often develops unintelligible speech by early school age. This appears to be due to the development of higher levels of receptive and inner language skills without concomitant motor articulation skills through the pivot sentence and developmental grammar stages of emergent speech and language development. This propels such children to attempts at expressing themselves in long utterances with frequent omissions of sound elements and whole syllables that are difficult to understand, particularly for strangers unfamiliar with their speech patterns.

Delayed use of speech communication leading to delayed expressive language skills concomitant with good receptive and inner language often leads to functional speech articulation learning problems not directly caused by velopharyngeal insufficiency. This developmental learning problem also occurs in children with normal structures of the speech mechanism, particularly if they have been hospitalized or developmentally overprotected in the home. Faulty learning rather than organic factors such as velopharyngeal insufficiency may lead to articulation disorders with a pattern different from gross sound substitutions causing frequently unintelligible speech. These errors in speech will be perceived as a significant speech defect at school age. Such functional articulation disorders may occur concomitantly with a history of corrected velopharyngeal insufficiency due to congenital cleft palate and yet not be directly caused by this structural abnormality.

THE ROLE OF THE SPEECH PATHOLOGIST ON A CLEFT PALATE TEAM

The challenging role of the speech and language pathologist on a cleft palate team includes (1) primary responsibility for diagnosing developmental problems affecting normal patterns of emergent speech and language development, (2) repeated consultations with families and team members regarding the need and rationale for physical management procedures, including secondary palatoplasties necessary to normalize speech and emergent language development, (3) reevaluations to select cases needing early interventive speech and language therapy services for functional developmental problems, and (4) monitoring velopharyngeal functional support for maintaining normal levels of communication skills until early adult life.

For these purposes, it is recommended that routine speech and language evaluations should be a part of the cleft palate team evaluation for each patient starting before the early postnatal period of treatment. Periodic assessments should begin shortly after birth for each cleft palate child and the family. The evaluation period should allow time for face-to-face discussions of findings and recommendations with concerned family members and team colleagues.

During most longitudinal team evaluations, an objective clinical evaluation focusing on language skills and speech articulation error patterns should be accomplished. Such evaluations can be carried out during an approximately 20-minute evaluation period with a young patient and knowledgeable family members during team evaluations. The basic purpose should be to identify through case history information, observations, and objective screening tests, the presence or absence of possible organic or functional causes related to developmental speech and language disorders. These may include, but are not limited to, (1) velopharyngeal insufficiency to support normal speech and language development, (2) dental and occlusal hazards that directly affect speech articulation or communication behavior, (3) the presence of hearing loss problems that affect speech or language development or which need otological treatment or audiological amplification follow-up, or (4) specific functional learning problems such as delayed expressive language development or compensatory habits of speech sound production needing referral for therapy.

Chapter 6 considers other clinically similar problems presented by non–cleft palate subjects with congenital or acquired velopharyngeal insufficiency for speech. Chapter 7 considers the central problem of developmental competency in language skill acquisition for the cleft palate child and the wider high-risk population of clients.

REFERENCES

1. Adisman, I. K. Cleft Palate Prosthetics. In W. C. Grabb, S. W. Rosenstein, and K. R. Bzoch (Eds.), *Cleft Lip and Palate: Surgical, Dental, and Speech Aspects.* Boston: Little, Brown, 1971.
2. Aduss, H., Ziesemer, R., Dorf, D., Curtin, J., Schafer, M., and Cohen, M. Craniofacial growth following early complete closure of the palate (abstract 24). American Cleft Palate Association Annual Meeting, Williamsburg, Va., April, 1988.
3. Aristotle. *Politics,* Book I. In *Great Books,* Vol. 9. The Works of Aristotle, II. Chicago: Encyclopedia Britanica, Inc., 1952. P. 446.
4. Bankson, N. W., and Byrne, M. C. The relationship between missing teeth and selected consonant sounds. *J. Speech Hear. Disord.* 27:341, 1962.
5, Blair, V. P., and Toy, R. H. *Essentials of Oral Surgery.* St. Louis: Mosby, 1923.
6. Brophy, T. W. (Ed.). *Oral Surgery.* Philadelphia: Blakiston, 1915.
7. Bzoch, K. R. *An Investigation of the Speech of Pre-school Cleft Palate Children.* Thesis, Northwestern University, Evanston, Ill., 1956.
8. Bzoch, K. R. Clinical studies of the efficacy of speech appliances compared to pharyngeal flap surgery. *Cleft Palate J.* 1:275, 1964.
9. Bzoch, K. R. The effects of a specific pharyngeal flap operation upon the speech of 40 cleft palate persons. *J. Speech Hear. Disord.* 29:111, 1964.
10. Bzoch, K. R. Articulation proficiency and error patterns of pre-school cleft palate and normal children. *Cleft Palate J.* 2:340, 1965.
11. Bzoch, K. R. Measurement and Assessment of Categorical Aspects of Cleft Palate Speech. In K. R. Bzoch (Ed.), *Communicative Disorders Related to Cleft Lip and Palate* (2nd ed.). Boston, Little, Brown, 1979.
12. Bzoch, K. R. Clinical Evaluation and Management of Problems of Speech, Language, and Hearing. In F. W. Pirruccello (Ed.), *Cleft Lip and Palate: Plastic Surgery, Genetics and the Team Approach.* Springfield, Ill.: Thomas. Chap. 11.
13. Bzoch, K. R., Kemker, F. J., and Wood, V. D. The Prevention of Communicative Disorders in Cleft Palate Infants. In W. J. Lass (Ed.), *Speech and Language: Advances in Basic Research and Practice.* San Francisco: Academic Press, 1984. Vol. 10.
14. Calnan, J. S. V-Y Pushback Palatorrhaphy. In W. C. Grabb, S. W. Rosenstein, and K. R. Bzoch (Ed.), *Cleft Lip and Palate: Surgical, Dental, and Speech Aspects.* Boston: Little Brown, 1971. Vol. 1.
15. Costen, G., and Gould, E. Language development in the preschool cleft palate child (abstract). American Cleft Palate Association Annual Meeting, Williamsburg, Va., 1988.
16. Counihan, D.T. *A Clinical Study of the Speech Efficiency and Structural Adequacy of Operated Adolescent and Adult Cleft Palate Persons.* Thesis, Northwestern University, Evanston, Ill., 1956.
17. Curtis, J. F. Acoustics of Speech Production and Nasalization. In D. C. Spriesterbach and D. Sherman (Eds.), *Cleft Palate Communication.* New York: Academic Press, 1968.
18. Dixon, V., Bzoch, K., and Habal, M. Evaluation of speech after correction of rhinophonia with pushback palatoplasty combined with pharyngeal flap. *Plast. Reconstr. Surg.* 64:77, 1979.
19. Dorf, D. S., and Curtin, J. W. Early cleft palate repair and speech outcome. *Plast. Reconstr. Surg.* 70:74, 1982.
20. Foster, T. D., and Green, M. C. L. Lateral speech defects and dental irregularities in cleft palate. *Br. J. Plast. Surg.* 12:367, 1960.
21. Furlow, L. T., Williams, W. N., Eisenbach, C. R., and Bzoch, K. R. A long term study on treating velopharyngeal insufficiency by Teflon injection. *Cleft Palate J.* 19: 47, 1982.
22. Furlow, L. T. Cleft palate repair by double opposing Z-plasty. *Plast. Reconstr. Surg.* 78:724, 1986.
23. Fox, D., Lynch, J., and Brookshire, B. Selected developmental factors of cleft palate children between two and thirty-three months of age. *Cleft Palate J.* 15:239, 1978.
24. Gibbons, R., and Bloomer, H. H. The palatal lift. A supportive type speech aid. *J. Prosthet. Dent.* 8:362, 1958.
25. Grabb, W. C., Rosenstein, S. W., and Bzoch, K. R. (Eds.), *Cleft Lip and Palate: Surgical, Dental, and Speech Aspects.* Boston: Little, Brown, 1971.
26. Graber, T. M. Craniofacial morphology in cleft palate and cleft palate deformities. *Surg. Gynecol. Obstet.* 88:359, 1949.
27. Graber, T. M. The congenital cleft palate deformity. *J. Am. Dent. Assoc.* 48:375, 1954.
28. Halfond, M. M., and Ballenger, J. J. An audiologic and otorhinologic study of cleft lip and cleft palate cases. *Arch. Otolaryngol.* 64:58, 1956.

29. Hamlet, S. L., and Stone, M. Compensatory vowel characteristics resulting from the presence of different types of experimental prosthesis. *J. Phonetics* 4:199, 1976.

30. Hamlet, S. L. Aerodynamics and palatographic characteristics of early stages of speech adaptation to a dental appliance. *J. Phonetics* 12:157, 1984.

31. Hamlet, S. L. Speech compensation for prosthetically created palatal asymmetries. *J. Speech Hear. Res.* 31:48, 1988.

32. Holz, M., Perko, M., Nussbaumer, H., and Van Demark, D. Long term speech results of the Zurich two-stage palate repair evaluated by the Iowa Pressure Articulation Test (abstract). American Cleft Palate Association Annual Meeting, Williamsburg, Va., April, 1988.

33. Houston, W. The Sri Lankan cleft lip and palate project: Facial growth in the unoperated adult unilateral cleft lip and palate subjects compared with healthy non-cleft Sri Lankaan subjects (abstract). American Cleft Palate Association Annual Meeting, Williamsburg, Va., April, 1988.

34. Hudson-McKuen, T. In T. W. Brophy (Ed.), *Oral Surgery*. Philadelphia: Blakiston, 1915. P. 726.

35. Jackson, I. T., McLennan, G., and Scheker, L. R. Primary veloplasty or primary palatoplasty: Some preliminary findings. *Plast. Reconstr. Surg.* 72:153, 1983.

36. Kaplan, E. N. Early primary palate repair. Read before the American Cleft Palate Educational Foundation Symposium, Northwestern University, 1983.

37. Kilner, T. P. Cleft Lip and Palate Repair Technique. In R. Maigot (Ed.), *Postgraduate Surgery*. London: Medical Pub., 1931.

38. Kilner, T. P. Cleft lip and palate repair techniques. *St. Thomas Hosp. Rep.* 2:127, 1937.

39. Kingsley, N. W. *Congenital Cleft Palate*. New York: New York Printing Co., 1866. Reprinted from *Bull. N.Y. Acad. Med.* 6, 1862.

40. Kingsley, N. W. Treatment and education of cleft palate patients. *Dent. Cadmos.* 36:125, 1894.

41. Kirkham, H. S. Preliminary paper on the improvement in speech in cleft palate cases. *Surg. Gynecol. Obstet.* 44:244, 1927.

42. La Velle, W. E., and Hardy, J. C. Palatal lift prostheses for treatment of palatopharyngeal incompetence. *J. Prosthet. Dent.* 42:308, 1979.

43. Leakey, R. E. *Origins*. New York: Dutton, 1977, P. 124.

44. Lennberg, E. H. *Biological Foundations of Language*. New York: Wiley, 1967.

45. Lewin, M. L. Management of cleft lip and palate in the United States and Canada. *Plast. Reconstr. Surg.* 33:383, 1964.

46. Lindsay, W. Von Langenbeck Palatorrhapy. In W. Grabb, S. Rosenstein, and K. Bzoch (Eds.), *Cleft Lip and Palate: Surgical, Dental, and Speech Aspects*. Boston: Little, Brown, 1971. Chap. 26.

47. Marsh, J. L., and Lehman, J. A. Cleft care in 1986: An ACPA survey (abstract). American Cleft Palate Association Annual Meeting, Williamsburgh, Va., April, 1988.

48. McCutcheon, M. J., Hasegawa, A., and Fletcher, S. G. Effects of palatal morphology on /s/ and /z/ articulation. *J. Acoust. Soc. Am.* 67,s94. 1980.

49. McDermott, R. P. *A Study of /s/ Sound Production by Individuals with Cleft Palates*. Thesis, University of Iowa, Iowa City, 1962.

50. McWilliams, B. J. Articulation problems of a group of cleft palate adults. *J. Speech Hear. Res.* 1:68, 1958.

51. McWilliams, B. J., Morris, H. L., and Shelton, R. L. *Cleft Palate Speech*. Philadelphia: Decker, 1984.

52. Millard, D., Jr. *Cleft Craft: The Evolution of Its Surgery*, Vol. 1. The Unilateral Deformity. Boston: Little, Brown, 1976.

53. Millard, D., Jr. *Cleft Craft: The Evolution of Its Surgery*, Vol. 2. Bilateral and Rare Deformities. Boston: Little, Brown, 1977.

54. Millard, D., Jr. *Cleft Craft: The Evolution of Its Surgery*, Vol. 3. Alveolar and Palatal Deformities. Boston: Little, Brown, 1980.

55. Millard, R. Training for Optimal Use of the Prosthetic Speech Appliance. In K. Bzoch (Ed.), *Communicative Disorders Related to Cleft Lip and Palate* (2nd ed.). Boston: Little, Brown, 1979. Chap. 26.

56. Morris, H. Etiological Basis for Speech Problems. In D. C. Spriesterbach and D. Sherman (Eds.), *Cleft Palate and Communication*. New York: Academic Press, 1968.

57. Morris, H. L. (Ed.). *The Bratislava Project: Some Cleft Palate Surgical Results*. Iowa City: University of Iowa Press, 1978.

58. Orticochea, M. Construction of a dynamic muscle sphincter in cleft palates. *Plast. Reconstr. Surg.* 41:323, 1968.

59. Orticochea, M. Results of the dynamic muscle sphincter operation in cleft palates. *Br. J. Plast. Surg.* 23:108, 1970.

60. Orticochea, M. A review of 236 cleft palate patients treated with dynamic muscle sphincter. *Plast. Reconstr. Surg.* 71:180, 1983.

61. Pensler, J. Levator repositioning and palatal lengthening for submucous clefts (abstract). American Cleft Palate Association Annual Meeting, Williamsburg, Va., April, 1988.

62. Phillips, B. J., and Harrison, R. Language skills of pre-school cleft palate children. *Cleft Palate J.* 6:108, 1969.

63. Pirruccello, F. W. *Cleft Lip and Palate: Plastic Surgery, Genetics and the Team Approach*. Springfield, Ill.: Thomas, 1987.

64. Powers, G. R. Cineradiographic investigation of the articulatory movements of selected individuals with cleft palates. *J. Speech Hear. Res.* 5:59, 1962.

65. Pruzansky, S. The role of the orthodontist in a cleft palate team. *Plast. Reconstr. Surg.* 14:27, 1954.

66. Quigley, Y. F., Shiere, F. R., Webster, R. C., and Cobb, C. M. Measuring palatopharyngeal competence with nasal anemometer. *Cleft Palate J.* 1:304, 1964.

67. Randall, P., La Rossa, D. D., Fakhraee, S. M., and Cohen, M. A. Cleft palate closure at 3 to 7 months of age: a preliminary report. *Plast. Reconstr. Surg.* 71:624, 1983.

68. Randall, P., La Rossa, D., Solomon, M., and Cohen, M. Experience with the Furlow double-reversing Z-plasty for cleft palate repair. *Plast. Reconstr. Surg.* 77:569, 1986.

69. Ricketts, R. M. The cranial base and soft structures in cleft palate speech and breathing. *Plast. Reconstr. Surg.* 14:47, 1954.

70. Riski, J. E. Articulation skills and oral-nasal resonance in children with pharyngeal flaps. *Cleft Palate J.* 16:421, 1979.

71. Riski, J., Serafin, D., and Riefhohl, R. A rationale for modifying the site of insertion of the Orticochea pharyngoplasty. *Plast. Reconstr. Surg.* 73:882, 1984.

72. Ritchie, H. P. Cleft palate: a comparison of anatomic and functional results following operation. *Arch. Surg.* 35:548, 1937.

73. Robertson, N. R. E., and Jolleys, A. The timing of hard palate repair. *Scand. J. Plast. Surg.* 8:49, 1974.

74. Rosen, M., and Bzoch, K. R. The prosthetic speech appliance in rehabilitation of patients with cleft palate. *J. Am. Dent. Assoc.* 57:203, 1958.

75. Ross, R. B. Treatment variables affecting facial growth in complete unilateral cleft lip and palate. *Cleft Palate J.* 24:3, 1987.

76. Slaughter, W. B., and Pruzansky, S. The rationale for velar closure as a primary procedure in repair of cleft palate defects. *Plast. Reconstr. Surg.* 14:1, 1954.

77. Smith, D. *Recognizable Patterns of Human Malformation* (3rd ed.). Philadelphia: Saunders Co., 1982.

78. Sprintzen, R. J., Lewin, M. L., Croft, C. B., Daniller, A. I., Argamaso, R. V., Ship, A. C., and Strauch, B. Comprehensive study of pharyngeal flap surgery: tailor made flaps. *Cleft Palate J.* 16:46, 1979.

79. Starr, C. *A Study of Some Characteristics of the Speech Mechanism of a Group of Cleft Palate Children.* Thesis, Northwestern University, Evanston, Ill., 1956.

80. Starr, C. Dental and Occlusal Hazards to Normal Speech Production. In K. Bzoch, *Communicative Disorders Related to Cleft Lip and Palate* (2nd ed.). Boston: Little, Brown, 1979. Chap. 7.

81. Stool, S. E., and Randall, P. Unexpected ear disease in infants with cleft palate. *Cleft Palate J.* 4:99, 1967.

82. Stratoudakis, A. C., and Bambace, C. Sphincter pharyn-goplasty for correction of velopharyngeal incompetence. *Ann. Plast. Surg.* 12:243, 1984.

83. Sweitzer, R. S., Melrose, J., and Morris, H. The air-bone gap as a criterion for identification of hearing losses. *Cleft Palate J.* 5:141, 1968.

84. Tessier, P. The definitive surgical treatment of the severe facial deformities of craniofacial dysostosis, Crozon's and Aperts's diseases. *Plast. Reconstr. Surg.* 48:419, 1971.

85. Vallino, L., McWilliams, B. J., Pierce, J., and Andrews, J. Speech and hearing before and after orthognathic surgery (abstract). American Cleft Palate Association Annual Meeting, Williamsburgh, Va., April, 1980.

86. von Langenbeck, B. Die Uranoplastik mittels ablösung des mukös-periostalen Gaumenüberzuges. *Arch. Clin. Chir.* 2:205, 1861.

87. Wardill, W. F. M. Cleft palate. *Br. J. Surg.* 16:127, 1927.

88. Wardill, W. F. M. The technique of operation for cleft palate. *Br. J. Surg.* 25:117, 1937.

89. Warren, D. W. Nasal emission of air and velopharyngeal function. *Cleft Palate J.* 4:148, 1967.

90. Westlake, H., and Rutherford, D. *Cleft Palate.* Englewood Cliffs, N.J.: Prentice-Hall, 1966.

91. Yules, R. B. *Atlas for Surgical Repair of Cleft Lip, Cleft Palate, and Noncleft Velopharyngeal Incompetence.* Springfield, Ill.: Thomas, 1971.

CHAPTER 6

Congenital and Acquired Velopharyngeal Inadequacy

Doris P. Bradley

Velopharyngeal inadequacy can be a major diagnosable organic cause of communicative disorders in many conditions, in addition to cleft palate. Failure to achieve velopharyngeal closure during speech production is recognized as a major cause of faulty articulation (weak or distorted consonants, compensatory articulation productions), reduced oral breath pressure, improper oral and nasal air flow, and hypernasal resonance. In individuals with repaired cleft palate, it is estimated that 10 to 25 percent have residual velopharyngeal inadequacy. However, *the other conditions resulting in inadequate velopharyngeal closure are numerous.* These conditions include: (1) submucous cleft palate, which is identified by intraorally visible stigmata; (2) anatomical defects of the levator veli palatini muscles, the musculus uvulae, and the tonsillar pillars; (3) abnormalities in regional growth disturbances causing disproportionate size of nasopharynx or hard and soft palate; (4) mechanical interference with motion of the velopharyngeal system through restriction or incoordination; (5) injury to palatopharyngeal structures; (6) a wide variety of neuromotor deficits; and (7) faulty learning of unknown origin which results in palatopharyngeal inadequacy during production of one or two phonemes while all other pressure consonants are emitted orally.

Individuals with cleft palate and repaired clefts have received the most attention and study related to inadequate velopharyngeal closure. However, since cleft palate is discussed in detail elsewhere in this book, it is the many other conditions associated with velopharyngeal inadequacy which will be emphasized here. Reports of prevalence of velopharyngeal inadequacy are summarized, and its effect on articulation, resonance, and voice quality are described. Treatments for modification of velopharyngeal closure

are reviewed, and speech therapy procedures appropriate for individuals with inadequate velopharyngeal closure are discussed.

Trost [101] suggested that "velopharyngeal inadequacy" should be used as a generic term, reserving "velopharyngeal insufficiency" for cases in which there is an insufficiency of tissue, and "velopharyngeal incompetency" for cases in which movement patterns are inadequate. This suggested terminology is followed in this chapter except for quotations, even though it is not in agreement with the recommendations of Loney and Bloem [52]. The reader should remember that, generally, the literature uses the terms "palatopharyngeal" and "velopharyngeal" as synonymous terms. Also, "velopharyngeal inadequacy," "velopharyngeal insufficiency," and "velopharyngeal incompetency" often have been used synonymously by many authors.

PREVALENCE

The term *prevalence* is used in preference to incidence, since in epidemological terms it represents a measure or rate of existing cases in a population. Data regarding some of the many conditions associated with velopharyngeal inadequacy are still very limited. Clearly, the prevalence of velopharyngeal inadequacy is greater than the incidence of cleft palate. The various conditions in which velopharyngeal closure is inadequate are presented next with the prevalence figures that were located.

SUBMUCOUS CLEFT PALATE

One of the more frequent conditions with visible stigmata which you should learn to recognize is submucous cleft palate [10]. This condition consists of one to three of these observable symptoms: bifid uvula, midline diastasis of palatal muscles, and indentation at the posterior nasal spine.

Several attempts have been made to identify the prevalence of individuals with submucous cleft palate but sometimes results have been reported in terms of only one of the visual stigmata. In the United States, for instance, Gorlin, Čerrenka, and Pruzansky [32] reported that 1 in 80 whites have a bifid uvula. However, this report did not indicate how many of these bifid uvulae were accompanied by submucous cleft palate. Weatherly–White et al. [110] required the presence of bifid uvula, muscular diastasis of the soft palate, and bony defect of the hard palate. This more complete evidence resulted in identification of 1 in every 1,200 Colorado school children (10,386 sample size) with submucous cleft palate. Stewart, Ott, and Legace [96] reported that 28 percent of the individuals with submucous cleft in this Colorado sample had speech problems related to it. Bagatin [3] studied 9,720 Zagreb (Yugoslavia) children, 6 to 13 years of age, and reported 1 in 1,944 with submucous cleft and 1 in 44 with cleft uvula. B. L. Shapiro et al. [84] compared the occurrence of bifid uvula in four races with these results: Chippewa Indians, 10.25 percent of 605 individuals, Japanese, 9.95 percent of 4,726 individuals, whites 1.44 percent of 9,701 individuals, and blacks, 0.27 percent of 2,968 individuals.

In population studies such as the ones reported here, the symptoms of articulation errors of the type associated with velopharyngeal inadequacy and hypernasal resonance are sometimes present. Two of nine cases (22.2%) reported by Weatherly–White et al. [110] had the speech characteristics typical of velopharyngeal inadequacy and one of the five (25%) identified by Bagatin [3] demonstrated hypernasal resonance. These figures should not be construed to mean that submucous cleft palate is inconsequential with regard to speech. Weatherly–White [111] reported that 11 (25%) of 44 patients referred with submucous cleft palate had speech symptoms. Kona, Young, and Holtmann [45] reported velopharyngeal incompetency in 44 percent of the patients who had submucous cleft palate and cleft lip while 88 percent of the patients with only submucous cleft palate had velopharyngeal incompetency. Pruzansky et al. [77] stated that velopharyngeal incompetency cases accounted for 20 percent of all new referrals to their cleft palate center, but not all of these were submucous clefts.

While the prevalence figures continue to be somewhat confusing, it remains obvious that bifid uvula, midline diastasis of the palatal muscles, and a bony defect of the hard palate without overt cleft are observations that require further investigation if they exist in the presence of articulatory errors or hypernasal resonance.

ANATOMICAL DEFECTS

Minor anatomical defects have been described with regard to the levator muscles, the musculus uvulae, and the tonsillar pillars. In particular, variations in sites of muscle insertion can affect velopharyngeal adequacy for speech. Hoopes et al. [40] described two cases with velopharyngeal inadequacy due to anterior levator palatini insertions. Minami et al. [63] used the term "occult cleft palate" to describe the palate that looks normal but on operative dissection is found to have abnormal anterior insertion of the levator palatini muscles. Kaplan [43] described 23 cases without visible evidence of submucous cleft palate with abnormal insertions of levator palatini. Likewise, Trier [99] described 52 consecutive cases of velopharyngeal incompetency in the absence of clefts of the secondary palate. Forty-six (88%) of these patients had levator muscles with abnormal insertions. Twenty-nine (56%) of the 52 had no visible evidence of submucous cleft palate, but in all 29 patients, the levator muscles inserted into the

Figure 6-1. Appearance of submucous cleft palate with partial bifid uvula and midline diastasis of palatal muscles, leading to velopharyngeal incompetence.

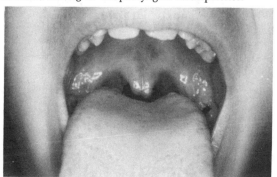

hard rather than the soft palate. Further support of this possible condition was supplied by Pruzansky et al. [77] who found that 40 percent of their total cases of congenital palatal incompetency without visual or palapable stigmata of submucous cleft palate had abnormal insertion of the levator muscles.

A significant role for the musculus uvulae in velopharyngeal incompetency was suggested when Maue–Dickson [59] stated that the central velar gap reported by Shprintzen et al. [89] would be consistent with hypoplasia or absence of the uvular muscle. Croft et al. [13] studied 20 patients with central velar gaps and found that all exhibited an absence of the musculus uvulae. Identification of the central velar gaps required frontal and base view cineradiography. Today, nasoendoscopy is effective in the identification of such causal anatomical defects. In the view of these authors, as well as Kuehn [46], the musculus uvulae contributes to the nasal bulk of the levator eminence. Undoubtedly, more evidence regarding the small abnormal anatomical variations of the musculus uvulae will continue to stimulate research. Meanwhile, it is important to investigate the presence of a possible central velar gap prior to assuming a functional etiology for hypernasal resonance or articulatory errors consistent with velopharyngeal inadequacy. More prevalence estimates must await such future research.

Abnormalities of the tonsillar pillars have been described in the early literature by Newcomb [69], and by Fridenburg [28], as being related to velopharyngeal incompetency. The anterior tonsillar pillars contain the palatoglossus muscle which according to Kuehn [46] is attached to the tongue inferiorly with variable insertions along the length of the velum. The possible role of the palatoglossus is the lowering of the velum or elevation of the tongue during speech, but its function varies in different individuals. Crikelair et al. [12] described two patients with "cleft palate speech" in whom the velum was anchored inferiorly by abnormalities of these pillars. Warren, Bevin, and Winslow [107] described two cases of posterior pillar webbing behind the uvula as well as one case of webbing that also caused palatopharyngeal displacement. Bradley [4] described the three cases reported by Warren et al. and an additional two cases both of whom had insertion of the posterior tonsillar pillars near the tip of the uvula resulting in restricted movement of the uvula and the appearance of the uvula tipping forward during the production of the vowel "ah."

Peterson–Falzone [74], however, reported two cases similar to those of Warren et al. [107] and Bradley [4] in whom the speech was normal. The Peterson–Falzone observation indicates that posterior tonsillar webbing, like bifid uvula, may be present without causing resonance problems in given individuals. It might seem that these few cases are insignificant in the large population with velopharyngeal incompetency. However, further observations and study may reveal that these differences often provide an explanation for many cases of hypernasality in the absence of clefts or other etiologies as was suggested by Warren et al. [107].

REGIONAL GROWTH DISTURBANCES

Many of the conditions associated with velopharyngeal inadequacy might be described under the general heading of regional growth disturbances which disrupt function. They affect various parts of the oral, pharyngeal, and nasal cavities. They may result in a soft palate that is too short to effect closure in a normal-sized pharynx or a normal soft palate that cannot effect closure in an abnormally deep pharynx. Growth disturbances are discussed in several sections.

PALATOPHARYNGEAL DISPROPORTION

Fletcher [23] reported on 10 patients with hypernasal resonance in whom he identified various regional growth disturbances. These included (1) abnormally obtuse basicranial angle, (2) large anterior-posterior dimensions of the pharynx at the level of the hard palate, and (3) reduced linear and vertical dimensions of the soft palate. Kaplan [43] described the combination of deep pharynx, short hard palate, and short soft palate as causes for velopharyngeal incompetency. Kaplan concluded that most cases he observed with congenitally short soft palate actually had occult submucous cleft palate. Previously, Dorrance [21] described the general condition of "congenital palatal insufficiency." Calnan [9] reported that a congenital large pharynx was present in 41 cases of hypernasal resonance without cleft palate. Saad [82] found 24 of 1,500 consecutive children admitted for tonsil and adenoid surgery to have had

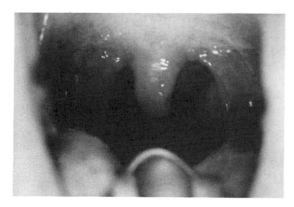

Figure 6-2. Appearance of palatal webbing in 7-year-old male, when palate was relaxed.

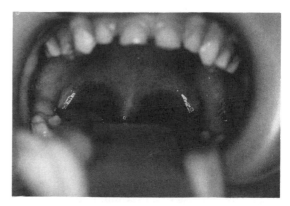

Figure 6-5. Appearance of extensive palatal web that limited palatal elevation of 4-year-old female patient.

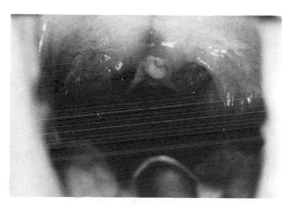

Figure 6-3. Appearance of palatal webbing and its apparent tethering effect in same patient as in Fig. 6-2, palate was elevated during phonation.

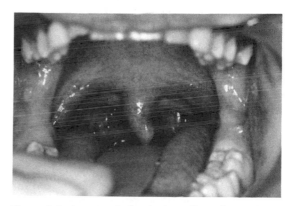

Figure 6-6. Asymmetrical tethering effect of palatal webbing upon velar elevation during phonation in teenage male with congenital velopharyngeal incompetence.

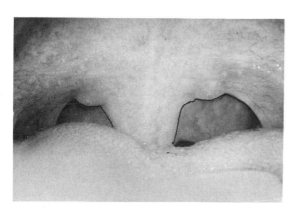

Figure 6-4. Appearance of palatal webbing in an 11-year-old male with an extensive web of tissue behind the posterior tonsillar pillars. Surgical removal of the web alone improved voice quality.

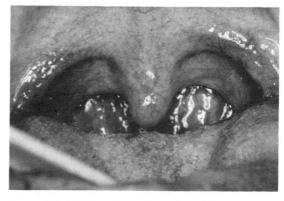

Figure 6-7. Weblike effect of insertion of the palatopharyngeus muscles into tip of uvula in a 54-year-old male with lifelong velopharyngeal incompetency requiring correction through utilization of a speech appliance.

an underdeveloped soft palate which resulted in velopharyngeal inadequacy postsurgically.

Another type of regional growth disturbance that affects velopharyngeal closure is the change in size of the tonsils and adenoids over time. Some authors [11, 23, 56, 65, 78] have indicated that adenoids generally assist in closure at young age levels and their surgical removal may stress the soft palate in attempts to reach the pharyngeal wall. Others, including Mason and Warren [58], state that even with gradual involution of adenoid tissue, velopharyngeal inadequacy may develop. Since this increase to a maximum point and then gradual decrease in size of adenoids and tonsils is considered normal growth and development, it may be inaccurate to suggest it is a regional growth disturbance. Nevertheless, in some individuals, it causes speakers who appeared to achieve closure early to lose the ability and thus it must be considered a possible cause of late acquired velopharyngeal inadequacy. Roberts [80] suggested that the soft palate might not develop adequately from disuse in the presence of large adenoids. A report by Greene [34] indicated a 6.6 percent occurrence of hypernasal speech following adenoidectomy, and Gibb [29] estimated hypernasality in 5 percent of cases after adenoidectomy. Various reports [33, 60, 87] have indicated that if structures are borderline inadequate, the normal involution of adenoids may result in the later development of inadequate velopharyngeal closure, causing faulty articulation and hypernasal resonance after earlier evidence of normal voice and speech characteristics. Witzel et al. [118] identified 137 patients in 8 years who had persistent hypernasality after adenoidectomy. They projected that 1 in 1,500 children undergoing adenoidectomy have persistent postsurgical hypernasality.

Peterson–Falzone [74] stated that other significant changes occur simultaneously with an increase or decrease of adenoid size: "The primary change is the descent of the hard palate away from the base of the skull, carrying the soft palate with it." According to Subtelney and Koepp–Baker [97], this hard palate descent regularly causes an increase in vertical size of the nasopharynx and an increased distance between the velum and the posterior pharyngeal wall. The distance may be increased more by the reduction of the adenoids.

While additional research is being conducted, it is important to carefully examine each patient for evidence of potential velopharyngeal incompetency prior to adenoidectomy. Morris et al. [65]

provided a list of symptoms present before adenoidectomy based on responses to parent questionnaires. It included evidence of neurological abnormality of velopharyngeal structures, family history of cleft lip or cleft palate and related disorders, early speech disorders, and nasal regurgitation during feeding in infancy.

INTERFERENCE WITH MOTION OF VELOPHARYNGEAL STRUCTURES

Mention has been made of abnormal anterior and posterior tonsillar pillars in the section on possible abnormal structures related to velopharyngeal incompetency. The reports of Warren et al. [107] and Bradley [4] indicated that in addition to such abnormal structures, there may be interference with movement of the soft palate. The insertion of the palatoglossus too far distally on the soft palate may actually pull the posterior third of the palate anteriorly instead of posteriorly during phonation. Although Peterson–Falzone [74] reported cases of abnormal posterior tonsillar pillars without problems of articulation or resonance, this condition should be considered as a possible cause for speech problems consistent with velopharyngeal inadequacy in the absence of cleft palate or submucous cleft palate.

Neiman and Simpson [70] documented increased velar mobility, increased height of velopharyngeal closure, and increased velar stretch after adenoidectomy, thus implying that movement was restricted by the adenoid mass. Previously, Subtelney and Koepp–Baker [97] had reported changes in activity of the soft palate following adenoidectomy, which consisted of less soft palate-to-pharyngeal wall contact in some patients but increased soft palate activity in those who maintained normal speech.

Still another modification of the structures which interferes with velopharyngeal closure can be maxillary advancement surgery. Witzel and Munro [117] and Witzel [119] found hypernasality in patients who had maxillary advancement and later demonstrated increased nasal resonance, increased nasal air emission, and inadequate velopharyngeal closure. The advancement of the maxillae in maxillofacial surgery resulted in a greater distance for the soft palate to move in order to make contact with the pharyngeal wall. Mason, Turvey, and Warren [57] reported on three cases of maxillary advancement in which two had speech deterioration after the surgery. In both cases such speech results could be anticipated from preoperative examination. It appears that velopharyngeal inadequacy may be created in 16 to 66 percent of this surgical population operated on with maxillary advancement procedures. Those patients with previously repaired cleft palate, who undergo maxillary advancement, are a greater risk for speech deterioration than are noncleft patients.

All patients being considered for maxillary advancement surgery should, therefore, receive careful evaluation of their velopharyngeal adequacy for speech to determine the possible effects of such surgery. Evaluations that include analysis of vocal resonance, endoscopic, or fluoroscopic visualization of velopharyngeal function, articulation analysis for weak consonant productions, or compensatory articulation errors should permit basic identification of such factors for use in preoperative counseling of these patients. Follow-up of many patients having maxillary advancement is needed to establish more adequate information regarding the frequency with which speech is made worse. Another structural modification is the pharyngeal flap which requires adjustments of muscle activity for achieving adequate velopharyngeal closure [33].

INJURY TO VELOPHARYNGEAL STRUCTURES

Trost [101] included traumatic injury to the palate and ablative palatal lesions related to cancer surgery as acquired structural impairments causing velopharyngeal inadequacy. No data on frequency of occurrence were provided and none have been located in the literature. Kuehn [47] listed trauma from accidents or surgery as major causes of acquired anatomical defects. Peterson–Falzone [74] also recognized ablative surgery defects as leading to a growing population in need of rehabilitation. Lotz and Netsell [53] reported that half of 415 cases fitted with a palatal lift prosthesis had experienced dysarthria of the velopharyngeal mechanism secondary to head injury. Aronson [2] included traumatic injury in the possible etiologies of hypernasality. Surgical removal of portions of the soft and hard palate because of tumors or damage to velopharyngeal musculature during tonsillectomy and adenoidectomy with scarring and stiffness as a residual or accidents re-

sulting in penetrating wounds of the palate are among the possible types of trauma. Gupta [35] reported the removal of foreign bodies from the nasopharynx of two infants and suggested that the lodging of foreign bodies in the nasopharynx may occur "particularly in patients suffering from incompetence or paralysis of the soft palate." More specific prevalence data for these types of acquired defect have not been located to date.

NEUROMOTOR DEFICITS

The broad category neuromotor disorders may be congenital or acquired and represents increasing numbers of individuals who now look to cleft palate teams for management of velopharyngeal incompetency affecting speech production. Virtually any disease process that affects innervation of the muscles active in velopharyngeal closure may be responsible for impairment of normal positioning of the speech structures and thus result in velopharyngeal incompetency. Peterson Falzone [74] cites approximately 23 different disease processes that may affect velopharyngeal function. Kuehn [47] proposed a classification of physiological disorders he considered in three categories: (1) "dysarthria and apraxia of speech, (2) speech of the deaf, and (3) nonorganic disorders." Netsell [68] distinguished two types of velopharyngeal dysfunction in the dysarthrias: (1) constant velopharyngeal opening and (2) intermittent and inappropriate velopharyngeal action. Aronson [2] stated that neurological disease may cause hypernasality by producing weakness (paresis or paralysis) or incoordination of the velopharyngeal muscles. He also cautioned that hypernasality and nasal emission may be early speech production symptoms of neurological disease. Hypernasality was a salient feature in flaccid, spastic, mixed, and hyperkinetic dysarthrias.

Prevalence data for each disease process are available but evidence regarding the prevalence of velopharyngeal inadequacy for speech in each disease process is unclear. Wilson [116] listed myasthenia gravis, multiple sclerosis, scoliosis, and mental retardation among the conditions in which hypernasality is most common. The population is large enough to include information on the characteristics present in speech of individuals with dysarthria or apraxia and the presentation of required treatment procedures in later sections of this chapter.

The presence of velopharyngeal inadequacy in many individuals who have mental retardation was reported by Bradley [4] who suggested that the prevalence of 40 percent was actually higher than in the repaired cleft palate population (about 20%). Others [15, 37, 40] have supported the presence of velopharyngeal inadequacy as a basic causative factor of speech problems in many speakers who are retarded. In addition to the lack of velopharyngeal closure, erratic and inconsistent movements of the articulators were reported.

FAULTY LEARNING

Faulty timing of velopharyngeal movements is now receiving increased attention. Stevens et al. [94] found timing to be a special problem in the intelligible oral speech production learning of deaf individuals because they substitute /m/, /n/, /ng/, for /b/, /d/, /g/, and vice versa. It is not known if timing of velopharyngeal movements is the basis for the hypernasality that is frequent among speakers who have severe hearing loss. Williams, Bzoch, and Agee [115] reported that many intelligent, young, adult, deaf speakers did not use velopharyngeal closure for sounds that required it and yet they obtained such closure often on sounds not requiring closure. Both Kuehn [47] and McWilliams, Morris, and Shelton [61] recognized the importance of timing in movements of the velopharyngeal mechanism. These movements must be coordinated with movements of other articulators in co-articulation if accurate speech is to be produced by any speaker.

Hardy [36] suggested that rate of speech production and timing of the velopharyngeal closure influenced each other. This idea was supported by Warren et al. [109] who proposed that timing errors compounded other problems associated with velopharyngeal closure. They found that duration of the pressure curve was shorter in the normals and cleft palate–inadequate speakers than in borderline and cleft palate–adequate velopharyngeal closure speakers. They hypothesized that the cleft palate–adequate speakers needed to impound air for a longer time to generate adequate speech. Fletcher's research [26] called attention to incoordination of the articulators with velopharyngeal closure by reporting that diadochokinetic performance accounted for 36 percent of the variance in his subjects. Karnell, Folkins, and Morris [44] combined spectrographic and cinefluorographic records to evaluate voice onset and voice offset with movements of the tongue, jaw, soft palate, and posterior pharyngeal wall. These authors speculated that timing adjustments might be made by the speakers with repaired cleft palate in an attempt to achieve velopharyngeal closure. Peterson–Falzone [75] concluded that timing differences exist, but the particular deviations, their magnitude, and the effects on perception of nasal resonance remain subjects for research.

An unusual type of velopharyngeal inadequacy is represented by the "phoneme-specific" cases of velopharyngeal incompetency. Lawson, et al. [49] recognized that some children had nasal emission on specific sounds and not on other sounds that require oral breath pressure and velopharyngeal closure. Peterson–Falzone [72] refined the description to include co-articulation sounds, nasal emission, or audible posterior frication on certain pressure consonants. Trost [100, 101] described the occurrence of nasal emission without hypernasal resonance on specific pressure consonants in noncleft velopharyngeal disorders and attributed its occurrence to articulatory mislearning. While productions of posterior nasal fricatives are common among this subgroup of velopharyngeal inadequacies, the posterior posturing of the tongue and lingual assistance to velopharyngeal closure are observable features too, but only on specific sounds. All cases of phoneme-specific velopharyngeal incompetency demonstrate adequate closure on most pressure consonants. Few cases of such phoneme-specific velopharyngeal inadequacy have been reported in the literature, so prevalence data were not projected.

STRESS VELOPHARYNGEAL INADEQUACY

Since 1970 when Weber and Chase [112] described an oboe player who demonstrated "nasal snorting" after 10 minutes of playing, several other reports [1, 19, 55, 74] of musicians experiencing velopharyngeal inadequacy for music but not for speech have appeared. These musicians have played various instruments such as clarinet, oboe, trumpet, and saxophone. This author adds two cases to the growing numbers in this category. One was a young college trombone player who did not demonstrate lack of closure on lateral view cineradiography either in speaking or blowing into the mouthpiece of the trombone.

However, his skill on the trombone deteriorated after 10 to 15 minutes of playing. He had no speech symptoms and chose to find another career and not pursue treatment. The second was a mature French horn player whose career was being threatened by his inability to "hit the high notes" after playing for some time or at the end of a day of teaching. He was referred to D. Dibbel and S. Ewanowski and elected to undergo pharyngeal flap surgery. Ewanowski (personal communication, November 1987) reported that they have now treated 14 musicians for velopharyngeal inadequacy associated only with instrument playing that requires unusual amounts of oral breath pressure. As with many conditions reported here, more research is needed to determine the prevalance of the problem.

This limited discussion reveals that speech in a wide range of speakers without cleft palate is influenced by inadequate velopharyngeal closure which is sometimes congenital and sometimes acquired. Suggestive prevalence figures are available for various conditions associated with velopharyngeal inadequacies and not available for others. Most of the affected individuals require the services of the professionals usually present on a cleft palate team and should be encouraged to seek treatment from such teams. Speech-language pathologists working in the area of cleft palate have a professional responsibility to become familiar with these other conditions that cause velopharyngeal inadequacy and affect communication skills.

EFFECTS OF VELOPHARYNGEAL INADEQUACY ON SPEECH PRODUCTION

Hardy [36] considered the speech-producing system to be an aerodynamic mechanical sound generator. Within this context, the velopharyngeal port functions to emphasize the dichotomy between the aerodynamic-mechanical and the acoustic aspects of speech production. If the velopharyngeal port is closed, the oral cavity is an efficient generator capable of producing sounds within the oral cavity without nasal leak. If the velopharyn-

geal port is open, sounds and air are directed through the nasal cavity. The opening of the velopharyngeal port also changes the acoustic characteristics of the the vocal tract and creates two air-filled resonating cavities that are acoustically coupled. The resonating characteristics of these cavities are modified by various positions of the articulators which are assumed for the production of vowels and consonants. Further, according to Hardy:

When the aperture of the velopharyngeal port is larger than the articulatory aperture in the oral cavity, a relatively large volume of air will leak through the nasal cavity. It may, therefore, be impossible to generate sufficient intraoral air pressure to force air at the needed particle velocity through the oral aperture for continuant consonants or to create the needed potential aerodynamic energy for plosion of stop consonants.

According to Netsell [68], this velopharyngeal system consists of the muscles of the soft palate, the muscles and structures of the upper pharynx, and the sensory receptors and peripheral neural innervations. The velopharyngeal structures function in various ways in different individuals to achieve velopharyngeal closure. Croft, Shprintzen, and Rakoff [14] described four patterns of velopharyngeal closure in which the structures were used in various combinations. Since various patterns of closure exist, it is crucial that evaluation of velopharyngeal closure include instrumental observations to support the information inferred from the analysis of speech production.

The precision of coupling and separating the oral and nasal cavities required for production of "normal" speech varies among individuals. Requirements regarding the firmness of velopharyngeal closure and timing of movements appear to be related to phonetic context of speech being produced. However, there are limits to the degree of variability that may be present without distorting speech productions. Warren [105] reported that velopharyngeal openings greater than 20 sq mm during speech permit enough nasal emission to interfere with oral air pressure necessary for production of plosives, fricatives, and affricatives. Openings less than 20 sq mm interfered with speech production for some individuals and not for others. If the velopharyngeal opening is less than 10 sq mm, Warren suggested therapy prior to surgery or other modifications of the speech mechanism [105].

The effects of inadequate velopharyngeal closure on speech [78] consist of five separate characteristics: (1) hypernasal resonance, (2) nasal emission of air, (3) weak (imprecise) production of consonants, (4) compensatory articulations and voice disorders of quality, and (5) loudness. These effects are complicated by the ability of the individual to compensate for the velopharyngeal inadequacy. McWilliams et al. [61] stated that a nasal obstruction might assist individuals with a large velopharyngeal opening in impounding oral air pressure. Increased rate and volume of air flow during speech was suggested as another compensation for velopharyngeal inadequacy. Such compensations may work at the syllable or word level and not be applied in conversational speech. Persons who have had normal speech may tolerate more velopharyngeal opening without effects on speech than speakers who are learning speech with inadequate velopharyngeal closure [96]. Likewise, persons with normally mobile articulators and normal respiratory systems may speak better in the presence of minimal velopharyngeal inadequacy than speakers with additional impairments [36].

HYPERNASALITY

Hypernasality is considered a "clinically significant manifestation of velopharyngeal incompetence" according to Hardy [36]. It is defined by Aronson [2] as excess resonance of vowels and voiced consonants within the nasal cavity. The sonorants and glides or liquids are the consonants affected the most [101]. Bzoch [8] preferred a more strict definition: Hypernasality is "the detectable distortion of syllabic elements in speech due to the effects of atypical coupling of the nasal resonating cavities produced under conditions of clear phonation and normal articulation." Support for the relationship between velopharyngeal inadequacy and hypernasality has been provided by Warren [104] who reported a clear tendency for orifice area and hypernasality to be covariant. Other variables influencing the relationship were amount of oral airway opening, airway resistance of nasal cavity, and oral cavity volume. Speakers with borderline velopharyngeal closure did not show clear relationships, but those with adequate and inadequate velopharyngeal closure showed normal resonance or hypernasal resonance.

The presence of hypernasal resonance may be evaluated by listener judgments [62, 113, 116]. It

can now also be evaluated by several instrumental methods such as TONAR [18] (see also Fletcher [25] on nasalance versus listener judgments of nasality and Chapter 15 on newer computer-augmented measurements of nasalance available today).

Other instrumental means of measuring or verifying clinical judgments of hypernasality include use of accelerometers [41, 93], sound spectrography [20, 22, 27, 83], sound pressure [86, 87], and spectral comparison [50, 104, 106]. Part II, Section C details the most frequently used instrumental means now available for objectified diagnostic evaluations of hypernasality.

The audiotape recordings that accompany the McWilliams and Phillips [62] scale represent attempts to decrease the influence of training and experience on listeners judgments of hypernasality. Aronson [2] suggested a speech sample to be used in making listener judgments of hypernasality. The existence of nasal resonance on a continuum makes the task of determining when there is excessive nasal resonance a very difficult one for the speech pathologist.

Careful descriptions of the method of assessing resonance and the speech samples used can increase the usefulness of assessments and provide the database for comparing information. Such a database for the neurogenic population was provided through the work of Darley, Aronson, and Brown [16] and by Johns [42]. No such database was located for other populations with velopharyngeal insufficiency.

NASAL EMISSION

Nasal emission is the nasal air flow which accompanies production of pressure consonants (stops, affricates, and fricatives). It can be audible or inaudible [71]. Like hypernasality, nasal emission of air except on the phonemes /m/, /n/, or /ng/ is characteristic of inadequate velopharyngeal closure. The inaudible nasal emission does not interfere with the speech signal so its significance is as an indicator of inadequate velopharyngeal closure. It may cause nasal grimacing or odd posturing of the lips and thus become a visual distraction during speech. Audible nasal emission may vary from awareness of the nasal air flow during speech to the substitution of "nasal snorts" or nasal fricatives for fricatives or affricatives. Nasal turbulence may be created by obstructions to the nasal air flow and may accompany any or all speech sounds.

WEAK PRESSURE CONSONANTS

The lack of velopharyngeal closure results in inadequate oral air pressure for the production of all pressure consonants. The /s/, /z/, and the other fricatives appear to be most sensitive, followed by affricatives, then plosives. The affected sounds fit the descriptive category Aronson [2] calls imprecise consonants. The degree to which consonants are affected seems to be related to respiratory volume available to the speaker, tongue postures used, and the degree of velopharyngeal inadequacy. Weakness (paresis or paralysis) of muscles used in articulation will increase the effects of weak oral air pressure. Also, control of the voicing features may be related to inadequate oral air pressure. As Trost [101] so succinctly stated, "reduced intraoral pressure diminishes plosive power and often renders even a correct labial or lingual articulatory gesture ineffective."

COMPENSATORY ARTICULATIONS

The use of nonstandard English sounds as compensatory articulation has been reported in the literature for many years [5–7, 38, 48, 61, 64, 76]. As a rule, the manner of articulation is maintained but the place of articulation is altered. Generally, the place of articulation is shifted posteriorly. Thus, glottal stops are frequently substituted for other stops (/p/, /b/, /t/, /d/, /k/, and /g/). Glottal stops may be co-articulated with the stops they replace. Glottal stops may be used for other purposes such as juncture markers, substitutions for words, or indicators of intonation [114]. In these capacities, glottal stops may distract the listener and reduce the intelligibility of the speech.

Peterson–Falzone [75] summarized the use of glottal stops and "backed" articulations as the speaker's attempt to "make some effective use of the airstream before it escapes into the nose." Trost [102] explained the speaker's use of compensatory articulations as efforts to approximate as perceptual-acoustic target, while Warren and Hinton [108] suggested that they served to maintain constant subglottic pressure. Trost–Cardamone [100] emphasized the importance of using the /ʔ/ phonetic symbol to indicate the occur-

rence of glottal stops in speech and indicating the co-articulation of glottal stops and regular stops as /$\frac{?}{p}$/.

Trost–Cardamone [100] described various compensatory articulations based on x-ray studies and therapy results. Her proposed phonetic symbols are useful for transcribing articulation errors. In addition to the glottal stop, the following six compensatory articulations were described. (1) The pharyngeal stops /$\frac{\overline{\underline{\varsigma}}}{}$/ and /ɬ/ are produced by contact of the lingual base to the pharyngeal wall. While the exact point of contact varies, the sound is perceptually distinct from /k/ and /g/. (2) The pharyngeal fricatives /ʕ̥/ and /ʕ/ are produced with lingual pharyngeal contact but the configuration of the tongue is different. They are substituted for fricatives and affricates or they are co-articulated with the fricatives and affricates. (3) The pharyngeal affricates /ʔʕ̥/ and /ʔʕ/ combine the glottal stop and the pharyngeal fricative productions. (4) The velar fricatives /x/ and /ɤ/ are made in the back velar place of articulation and appear perceptually as distortions of /k/ or /g/. They may be used as substitutions for sibilants. (5) The mid-dorsum palatal stops /ɛ/ and /ʒ/ are made at the same point of articulation as the glide /j/. These mid-dorsum palatal stops are used as substitutions for the /t/, /d/, or /k/, /g/. (6) The posterior nasal fricative /Δ/ shows variability in its production but is perceptually distinguishable from nasal air emission and the velar or pharyngeal fricatives. It is frequently heard in speakers with phoneme-specific nasal emission. This nasal fricative may be used as a co-articulation with all of the pressure consonants or it may replace the fricatives and affricates. Examples of compensatory errors are available on the tape recording in the Trost [101] audio journal presentation. McWilliams and Phillips [62] presented examples of compensatory articulation. Both of these recordings are useful in teaching students to recognize these sound productions that are considered to be compensatory.

VOICE DISORDERS

McWilliams et al. [61] reported that inadequate volume (soft voice syndrome), hoarseness, harshness, monotone, and aspirate voice may be the result of inadequate velopharyngeal closure. These authors stated that speech therapy which stresses the speech mechanism may result in hyperfunction of the vocal folds, the development of vocal nodules, and increased hoarseness.

TREATMENT OF VELOPHARYNGEAL INADEQUACY

The treatment of velopharyngeal inadequacy usually takes the form of surgery or a speech prosthesis. Direct and indirect muscle training and speech therapy continue to be viewed as possible alternatives in selected cases. The speech-language pathologist has a responsibility to contribute to the decisions about velopharyngeal inadequacy treatment by providing information about velopharyngeal function based on speech productions.

The speech pathologist should be alert to symptoms of inadequate velopharyngeal closure as reflected in the case history and the speech productions of speakers. Careful analysis of articulation, resonance, and voice characteristics of the speaker are the beginnings of diagnosing velopharyngeal inadequacy. If indications are present, further verification of velopharyngeal closure through instrumental assessment is necessary. The types of instruments available and the information available through their use are presented in Section C below. The most effective management decisions are usually made by teams with complete participation from various disciplines.

Classification of velopharyngeal function as adequate, inadequate, or borderline is essential. In patients with clearly inadequate velopharyngeal closure, physical modification has been considered necessary prior to speech therapy [5, 61]. If conditions delay physical restoration, speech therapy can be undertaken to achieve correct articulator placement for accurate sound production.

Golding–Kushner [30], Shprintzen [88], Warren et al. [109], and Henningsson and Isberg [38] have provided evidence that articulatory movements influence the movement of the velopharyngeal sphincter. In the Golding–Kushner study [30], 14 (93%) of the 15 subjects showed improved velopharyngeal closure after articulation therapy and this altered the surgical planning. Shprintzen [88] reported 70 percent correction of

compensatory errors with improved lateral pharyngeal wall motion in a group of 72 patients (50/72) with grossly inadequate velopharyngeal closure. No reports were located that indicate that control of the nasal airstream or reduction of hypernasal resonance have been achieved with therapy alone in the presence of grossly inadequate velopharyngeal closure.

Speech therapy is the clear treatment of choice when velopharyngeal closure can be demonstrated to be adequate and errors of articulation, resonance disorders, or voice disorders are present. Until recently, speech therapy was not recommended until after surgery or a speech prosthesis had provided adequate velopharyngeal closure. It now appears that achieving correct placement for articulatory productions may change velopharyngeal function. Currently, speech therapy is probably justified when velopharyngeal closure is borderline or inconsistent. Enough changes in velopharyngeal function have been documented [39, 88] to demonstrate that changes brought about with therapy determine differences in surgery and thus support decisions to conduct therapy preoperatively. Careful documentation of change and a 3- to 6-month time limit for achieving change seem prudent until more is know about the effects of articulatory change on velopharyngeal closure.

THERAPY FOR VELOPHARYNGEAL CLOSURE

As stated earlier, speech therapy for changing the function of the velopharyngeal structures generally has been considered unsuccessful. Surgical or prosthetic procedures were considered necessary to provide an adequate mechanism. However, concerns about providing overtreatment and being sure speakers use the mechanism to its full potential have prompted continued interest in therapy that might improve velopharyngeal function during speech. The conclusion reached by Spriestersbach et al. [92] was that velopharyngeal incompetency is not solved by speech therapy procedures. Ruscello [81] generally supported the conclusion reached by Spriestersbach et al., but reported that many speech pathologists continued to use velopharyngeal therapy techniques (blowing, sucking, swallowing, or direct palatal stimulation) despite the reports that such procedures are ineffective and obsolete. He conceded that palatal training might be a treatment for a very limited number of individuals with velopharyngeal inadequacy for speech. Warren [105] noted that approximately 90 percent of patients with borderline closure required surgery for hypernasal voice quality and nasal emission of air during speech. Support for the use of such procedures as blowing and sucking as effective means for modifying velopharyngeal function was not located in the literature.

Hoch et al. [39] reported that changes in velopharyngeal function through modification of articulation or biofeedback are possible in some types of velopharyngeal insufficiency. They stated that failure to show change was accounted for by lack of specificity regarding the cause of velopharyngeal insufficiency associated with hypernasality. They suggested the following types of velopharyngeal insufficiency: (1) consistently inadequate due to structural etiology; (2) consistently inadequate because of neurological problems; (3) inconsistent, of structural origin; (4) inconsistent, of neurological origin; (5) inconsistent, in otherwise normal speakers; and (6) arrhythmic valving. Hoch et al. [39] concluded that speakers with type (5) have the best chance of successfully changing closure with nasopharyngoscopic biofeedback. Speakers with types (3) and (6) also have shown improvement of velopharyngeal function with therapy. Speakers with types (1) and (2) were considered very poor candidates for biofeedback therapy because the structural problems were consistent and too great to overcome with biofeedback.

The "hard line" position continues to be that the mechanism should be adequate prior to speech therapy which cannot be expected to change velopharyngeal function. However, the research of Henningsson and Isberg [38] and the experimental therapy of Hoch et al. [39] suggest that therapy prior to modification of the speech mechanism should be considered for carefully selected individuals. As Ruscello [81] noted, results are too inconsistent to advocate speech therapy or nonspeech activities such as blowing as a means of changing velopharyngeal closure. See Chapter 20 for a more detailed discussion of this topic.

THERAPY FOR HYPERNASAL RESONANCE

Various biofeedback procedures have been used to monitor parameters that correlate with hypernasal resonance. These include: PERCI, developed by Warren [105] for nasal air flow; TONAR, developed by Fletcher [24] for an oral-nasal acoustic ratio; photodetection, reported by Dalston [17] for palate-to-pharynx contact; nasopharyngoscopy, reported by Siegel–Sadewitz and Shprintzen [91] for visualization of palatal-pharyngeal wall movements; and accelerometry, (utilized by Lippmann [51]) for tactile feedback of nasal vibrations. All of these feedback devices have been reported to be effective in the modification of hypernasal voice quality, but *all need further research support before being recommended as a general clinical procedure.*

According to Hoch et al. [39] improvement in articulation and hypernasal resonance was demonstrated with traditional articulation therapy in individuals with their type (5) velopharyngeal insufficiency by Tantillo [98] who used a combination of visual, auditory, and kinesthetic feedback. A program for modification of hypernasality generally consists of awareness and discrimination training of resonance patterns, production of utterances containing only oral sounds, production of oral and nasal sound sequences in structured speech, production of oral and nasal sounds in self-generated sentences, and gradual elaboration of the essential concepts during therapy.

Nasopharyngoscopic biofeedback was reported by Hoch et al. [39] to be effective for modification of articulation, hypernasal resonance, and movement of the velopharyngeal structures. In just four to nine sessions, six of nine speakers with types (3), (5), and (6) velopharyngeal insufficiency resolved the problem of inadequate velopharyngeal closure, hypernasal resonance, and articulatory errors with this combination of biofeedback and therapy. Rampp, Pannbacker, and Kinnebrew [79] advocated teaching soft contacts and shortened durations of sounds to reduce the perception of hypernasality and nasal emission of air. Shprintzen, McCall, and Skolnick [90] advocated a "whistling-blowing" technique which consisted of the following eight steps: (1) Teach simultaneous blowing or whistling phonation. (2) Keep repeating step (1) until phonation accompanied by whistling or blowing is consistently free of nasal escape. (3) Produce phonation without blowing or whistling until it is free of nasal escape. (4) Obtain vowel /i/ or /U/ with blowing, then nasal-free until consistent. (5) Eliminate whistling or blowing and produce vowel at 95 percent success. (6) Add nonnasal consonants to vowel. (7) Develop self-monitoring and self-operants. (8) Move from monosyllables to short sentences, longer sentences, and conversation while avoiding nasal emission.

Mysak [67] stated that an exaggerated and slowed articulation pattern with light articulatory contacts reduced perceived hypernasality. Darley et al. [16] acknowledged that speech therapy techniques for reducing hypernasality are limited, then suggested that increasing oral activity in speech and perceptual training that would enable the speaker to adjust his own mechanism were sometimes helpful. Moncur and Brackett [66] offered some suggestions for therapy that seem appropriate for speakers with borderline closure: (1) Develop appropriate timing of the velopharyngeal closure on nonnasal sounds preceding nasals, then on nonnasal sounds between consonants. (2) Lengthen vowel durations, if short, to permit better timing and articulation in the coupling-uncoupling function. (3) Use diagrams and other visual aids to explain and eliminate assimilated hypernasality. (4) Provide a complete program of sensory awareness and discrimination for auditory, visual, and kinesthetic systems. (5) Initiate vowels with a yawn to establish a nonnasal production, then initiate nasals and alternate. (6) Stabilize control for nasal and nonnasal productions in words, phrases, and sentences. (7) Stabilize new behaviors in all speaking situations.

These suggestions from the literature on hypernasality with various etiologies are offered for consideration. At present therapy for reduction of hypernasality should be used only on carefully selected speakers who show adequate velopharyngeal closure on some speech or speech-related task. The procedures and techniques used should be described in enough detail that replication studies can be conducted. Clinicians should not hesitate to terminate therapy if no progress is made and refer for surgery, palatal lift appliance, speech appliance, or one of the effective biofeedback procedures.

ARTICULATION THERAPY

Weak pressure consonant production with some hypernasal resonance is indicative of mild-to-moderate velopharyngeal inadequacy. Correct placement of the articulators may be used but the oral breath pressure cannot be impounded in the oral cavity or oral air flow cannot be controlled adequately to produce accurate stops and fricatives. Articulatory therapy techniques to modify this type of articulation include increasing the volume of air used in the speech process, exaggerated articulatory movements, and increased precision of articulator placement. No research or clinical studies of speech therapy specifically directed at weak pressure consonant production were located.

Compensatory articulations have generally signaled inadequate velopharyngeal closure or behaviors learned prior to surgery or placement of a speech appliance. Hoch et al. [39] observed that mid-dorsal sibilants and stops were used by speakers who had anterior palatal fistulae and suggested that closing the fistula should precede therapy. Routine placement techniques should correct these mid-dorsal productions after repair of the fistula.

The compensatory articulations labeled glottal stops, pharyngeal stops, pharyngeal fricatives, and pharyngeal affricatives, velar fricatives, palatal fricatives, or posterior nasal fricatives have been closely associated with inadequate velopharyngeal closure. The general consensus reflected in the literature has been that these articulation patterns are most often developed because velopharyngeal closure is inadequate. In most instances these articulatory productions occur inferior or posterior to the normal palatopharyngeal contacts and thus seem to represent attempts to valve the airstream at some point in the vocal tract at which the structures are adequate. Hoch et al. [39] proposed that productions inferior to the velopharyngeal port deprived the velopharyngeal valve of an opportunity to modify the airstream and might cause it to cease functioning to its capability. This hypothesis has been supported by the studies of Golding–Kushner [30] and Shprintzen [88] in which increased oral articulation was accompanied by increased motion of the soft palate and pharyngeal walls. Henningsson and Isberg [38] reported velopharyngeal movement or oral productions and lack of velopharyngeal movement on glottal articulations in the same speaker, which also supports the Hoch proposal.

Hoch et al. [39] provided an outline of therapy techniques used in the studies of Golding–Kusher [30] and Shprintzen [88]. The therapy goals were to move appropriate productions superior and anterior to the velopharyngeal port (bilabial, labiodental, lingua-alveolar) and to use the correct placement regardless of nasal air flow. Speech therapy was initiated after the speakers learned through five or six sessions of nasopharyngo-scopic feedback to move the palate and pharyngeal walls.

The salient known features about the therapy of Hoch et al. [39] are described here. The selection of sounds for therapy was made based on stimulability, place of production, visibility, appropriate maturational level, and the voicing feature. Facilitators were used to get the sounds selected into production. These included whispering the sound; using an aspirate /h/ between consonants and vowels; proceeding from simple to complex syllable and word structures; using visual, tactile, and auditory cues; and using co-articulation contexts for the targets phoneme. The speech pathologist attempted to obtain 70 to 100 accurate responses during each session. Results reported by Hoch et al. [39] indicated that over half of the speakers improved their velopharyngeal function and corrected 70 percent of their articulatory errors. This has provided encouragement that changes in articulation and velopharyngeal closure may be made through a combination of biofeedback and articulation therapy.

Trost–Cardamone [100] presented general principles of articulatory therapy that included "place mapping" for consonants; teaching place and durational contrasts; using maximal visual input and self-monitoring to complement auditory modeling; contrasting oral-nasal air flow; and teaching tactile-kinesthetic tracking for tongue placements. These general principles should be applied to any standard articulatory program. Specific goals for articulatory therapy with speakers who use compensatory articulations were eliminating glottal stops; modifying compensatory co-articulations; establishing fricative manner; moving backed articulations forward; and eliminating phoneme-specific nasal emission.

Lotz and Netsell [54] provided therapy suggestions for phoneme-specific cases of velopharyngeal closure in which they paired facilitative sounds with the error sound such as /t/ . . . /s/ or /f/ . . . /s/. The use of nose plugs to establish oral pressure and exaggeration of speech movements, increased mouth opening, increased loudness, projection of voice, and a bite-block to establish accurate sound productions were suggested. Further suggestions included structuring the speech stimuli from those requiring least to greatest demands on the velopharynx: oral-only consonants, nasal consonants, and oral and nasal mixed consonants produced in syllables, words, phrases, sentences, and conversation. Abutting oral-nasal

consonants in words like jump, bumper, hamper, and lumber were considered very difficult.

McCabe and Bradley [60] and VanDemark and Hardin [103] reported the use of the multiple-phoneme approach to articulation therapy with individuals who had repaired cleft palate and some of whom had questionable velopharyngeal closure. Both studies demonstrated much improvement with intensive (every day) therapy. The multiple-phoneme approach is too complex to present in detail here. Suffice it to say that it relies on stimulability through the use of auditory, visual, and tactile cues. Sound production is established in isolation, words, sentences, reading, and conversation. Subjects were seen 5 days a week for at least 1 hour of therapy. Behavior modification principles of establishment, stabilization, and generalization were used with external reinforcements being transferred to self-monitoring and self-reinforcement.

In this section an attempt was made to focus attention on (1) the effects of velopharyngeal inadequacy on speech regardless of its etiology and (2) to summarize the therapy techniques located in the literature that show effectiveness or promise of effectiveness in modifying the speech effects. Most aspects of the therapy process require more research and more precise descriptions of procedures so that replication studies can be conducted.

SUMMARY

Velopharyngeal incompetency may be congenital or acquired. It may be present at birth, as in all cases of cleft palate, or may occur at any time during the life span related to growth factors, accidents, diseases, or neurological deficits. The effects of velopharyngeal incompetency on speech are variable and appear to be influenced by the presence or absence of other defective structures or functions. Treatment includes all the surgical and prosthetic procedures now available to create an adequate velopharyngeal mechanism. In addition, various biofeedback procedures and numerous therapy techniques have been used to modify, improve, or correct function. Limitations of therapy techniques are major but enough success is reported to encourage continued limited therapy planned and reported with more precision. Coordination of the speech therapy with other rehabilitation procedures is essential and the team approach to management is the preferred delivery system.

REFERENCES

1. Argamaso, R., and Shprintsen R. Fanfare for a pharyngeal flap. A videotape presented at the American Cleft Palate Association, Denver, 1983, cited in Peterson–Falzone, S. Velopharyngeal inadequay in the absence of overt cleft palate. *J. Craniofac. Genet. Dev. Biol.* 1(Supp.):97, 1985.

2. Aronson, A. E. Nasal Resonatory Disorders. In A. E. Aronson (Ed.), *Clinical Voice Disorders.* New York: Thieme, 1985. Pp. 199–247.

3. Bagatin, J. Submucous cleft palate. *Maxillofac. Surg.* 13:37, 1985.

4. Bradley, D. P. Congenital and Acquired Palatopharyngeal Insufficiency. In K. R. Bzoch (Ed.), *Communicative Disorders Related to Cleft Lip and Palate* (2nd ed.). Boston: Little, Brown, 1979. Pp. 77–89.

5. Brooks, A. A., Shelton, R. L., and Youngstrom, K. A. Compensatory tongue-palate-posterior pharyngeal wall relationships in cleft palate. *J. Speech Hear. Disord.* 30:166, 1965.

6. Bzoch, K. R. A study of the speech of a group of preschool cleft palate children. *Cleft Palate Bull.* 9:2, 1959.

7. Bzoch, K. R. An investigation of the speech of preschool cleft palate and normal children. *Cleft Palate J.* 2:211, 1965.

8. Bzoch, K. R. Measurement and Assessment of Categorical Aspects of Cleft Palate Speech. In K. R. Bzoch (Ed.), *Communication Disorders Related to Cleft Lip and Palate* (2nd ed.). Boston: Little, Brown, 1979. Pp. 161–191.

9. Calnan, J. Congenital large pharynx: A new syndrome with a report of 41 personal cases. *Br. J. Plast. Surg.* 24:263, 1951.

10. Calnan, J. Submucous cleft palate. *Br. J. Plast. Surg.* 6:264, 1954.

11. Calnan, J. The investigation of nasality (nasal escape) in speech. *Speech* 1:59, 1957.

12. Crikelair, G., Kastein, S., Fowler, E., and Cosman, B. Velar dysfunction in the absence of cleft palate. *N. Y. State J. Med.* 15:263, 1964.

13. Croft, C. B., Shprintzen, R. J., Daniller, A., and Lewin, M. I. The occult submucous cleft palate and musculus uvulae. *Cleft Palate J.* 15:150, 1978.

14. Croft, C. B., Shrintzen, R. J., and Rakoff, S. J. Patterns of velopharyngeal valving in normal and cleft palate subjects: A multi-view videofluoroscopic and nasendoscopic study. *Laryngoscopy* 91:265, 1981.

15. Daly, D., and Johnson, H. Instrumental modification of hypernasal voice quality in retarded children: Case reports. *J. Speech Hear. Disord.* 39:550, 1974.

16. Darley, F. L., Aronson, A. E., and Brown, J. E. *Motor Speech Disorders.* Philadelphia: Saunders, 1975.

17. Dalston, R. M. Photodetector assessment of velopharyngeal activity. *Cleft Palate J.* 19:1, 1982.

18. Dalston, R., and Warren, D. W. Comparison of Tonar II, pressure-flow and listener judgments of hypernasality in the assessment of velopharyngeal function. *Cleft Palate J.* 23:108, 1986.

19. Dibble, D., Ewanski, S., and Carter, W. Successful correction of velopharyngeal stress incompetence in musicians playing wind instruments. *Plast. Reconstr. Surg.* 64:662, 1979.

20. Dickson, D. R. An acoustic study of nasality. *J. Speech Hear. Res.* 5:103, 1962.

21. Dorrance, G. Congenital insufficiency of the palate. *Arch. Surg.* 21:185, 1930.

22. Fant, G. Analysis and Synthesis of Speech Processes. In B. Malmberg (Ed.), *Manual of Phonetics.* Amsterdam: North Holland, 1968.

23. Fletcher, S. G. Hypernasal voice as an indication of regional growth and developmental disturbances. *Logos* 3:1, 1960.

24. Fletcher, S. G. Contingencies for bioelectric modification of nasality. *J. Speech Hear. Disord.* 37:329, 1972.

25. Fletcher, S. G. "Nasalance" vs listener judgments of nasality. *Cleft Palate J.* 13:31, 1976.

26. Fletcher, S. G. *Diagnosis and Speech Disorders from Cleft Palate.* New York: Grune & Stratton, 1978.

27. Forner, L. L. Speech segment durations produced by five and six year old speakers with and without cleft palates. *Cleft Palate J.* 20:185, 1983.

28. Fridenburg, P. Congenital detachment of faucial pillars and isolation of palato-glossus muscle. *Laryngoscope* 18:567, 1908.

29. Gibb, A. G. Hypernasality (rhinolalia aperta) following tonsil and adenoid removal. *J. Laryngol. Otol.* 72:433, 1958.

30. Golding–Kushner, K. The effect of articulation therapy on velopharyngeal closure. Paper presented at the Fourth International Congress on Cleft Palate and Related Craniofacial Anomalies, Acapulco, Mexico, 1981.

31. Goode, R., and Ross, J. Velopharyngeal insufficiency after adenoidectomy. *Arch. Otolaryngol.* 96:223, 1972.

32. Gorlin, R. J., Čerrenka, J., and Pruzansky, S. Facial Clefting and Its Syndromes. In D. Bergsma (Ed.), *Birth Defects: Original Article Series 6. Part II, Orofacial Structures.* Baltimore: Williams & Wilkins, 1971. Pp. 3–49.

33. Graham, W., Hamilton, R., Randal, P., Winchester, R., and Stool, S. Complications following pharyngeal flap surgery. *Cleft Palate J.* 10:176, 1973.

34. Greene, M. C. L. Speech of children before and after removal of adenoids. *J. Speech Hear. Disord.* 22:361, 1957.

35. Gupta, S. C. Nasopharyngeal foreign bodies in infants. *Ear Nose Throat J.* 61:72, 1982.

36. Hardy, J. C. *Cerebral Palsy.* Englewood Cliffs, N.J.: Prentice-Hall, 1983.

37. Heller, J., Gens, G., Moe, D., and Lewin, M. Velopharyngeal insufficiency in patients with neurologic, emotional and mental disorders. *J. Speech Hear. Disord.* 39:350, 1974.

38. Henningsson, G. E., and Isberg, A. M. Velopharyngeal movement patterns in patients alternating between oral and glottal articulation: A clinical and cineradiographical study. *Cleft Palate J.* 23:1, 1986.

39. Hoch, L., Golding–Kushner, K., Siegel–Sadewitz, V. L., and Shprintzen, R. J. Speech therapy. *Semin. Speech Lang.* 7:313, 1986.

40. Hoopes, J., Dellon, A., Fabrikant, J., and Soliman, A. Idiopathic hypernasality: Cineradiographic evaluation and etiologic considerations. *J. Speech Hear. Disord.* 35:44, 1970.

41. Horri, Y., and Lang, J. Distribution and analyses of an index of nasal coupling (HONC) in similated hypernasal speech. *Cleft Palate J.* 17:279, 1981.

42. Johns, D. F. *Clinical Management of Neurogenic Communicative Disorders* (2nd ed.). Boston: Little, Brown, 1985. Pp. 156–162.
43. Kaplan, E. N. The occult submucous cleft palate. *Cleft Palate J.* 12:356, 1975.
44. Karnell, M. P., Folkins, J. W., and Morris, H. L. Relationships between the perception of nasalization and speech movements in speakers with cleft palate. *J. Speech Hear. Res.* 28:63, 1985.
45. Kona, D., Young, L., and Holtmann, B. The association of submucous cleft palate and clefting of the primary palate. *Cleft Palate J.* 18:207, 1981.
46. Kuehn, D. P. Velopharyngeal anatomy and physiology. *Ear Nose Throat J.* 58:59, 1979.
47. Kuehn, D. P. Assessment of Resonance Disorders. In N. J. Lass et al. (Eds.), *Speech, Language, and Hearing.* Philadelphia: Saunders, 1982. Vol. 2, pp. 499–525.
48. Lawrence, C., and Phillips, B. J. A tethat fluoroscopic study of lingual contacts made by persons with palatal defects. *Cleft Palate J.* 12:85, 1975.
49. Lawson, L., Chierici, G., Castro, S., Harvold, E., Miller, E., and Owsley, J. Management of a patient with velopharyngeal incompetency of undetermined origin: A clinical report. *J. Speech Hear. Disord.* 37:390, 1972.
50. Lindbloom, B., Lubker, J. F., and Pauli, S. An acoustic perceptual method for the quantitative evaluation of hypernasality. *J. Speech Hear. Res.* 20:485, 1977.
51. Lippmann, R. Detecting nasalization using low cost accelerometer. *J. Speech Hear. Res.* 14:314, 1981.
52. Loney, R. W., and Bloem, T. J. Velopharyngeal dysfunction: Recommendations for use of nomenclature. *Cleft Palate J.* 24:334, 1987.
53. Lotz, W., and Netsell, R. Effects of velopharyngeal treatment for individuals with dysarthria: Follow-up and research needs. Paper presented at the Clinical Dysarthria Conference, Tucson, Ariz., 1984, as quoted in Netsell, R. *A Neurobiologic View of Speech Production and the Dysarthrias.* San Diego: College-Hill Press, 1986. P. 140.
54. Lotz, W., and Netsell, R. Treatment of Velopharyngeal Dysfunction. A miniseminar presented at the American Speech-Language-Hearing Association Annual Convention, New Orleans, 1987.
55. Massengill, R., and Quinn, G. Adenoid atrophy, velopharyngeal incompetence and sucking exercises: A two year follow up case report. *Cleft Palate J.* 11:196, 1974.
56. Mason, R. Preventing speech disorders following adenoidectomy by preoperative examination. *Clin. Pediatr.* 12:405, 1973.
57. Mason, R., Turvey, T. A., and Warren, D. W. Speech considerations with maxillary advancement procedures. *J. Oral Surg.* 38:752, 1980.
58. Mason, R., and Warren, D. W. Adenoid involution and developing hypernasality in cleft palate. *J. Speech Hear. Disord.* 45:469, 1980.
59. Maue–Dickson, W. The craniofacial complex in cleft lip and palate: An updated review of anatomy and function. *Cleft Palate J.* 16:291, 1979.
60. McCabe, R. B., and Bradley, D. P. Systematic multiple phoneme approach to articulation therapy. *Acta Symbolocia* 6:57, 1975.
61. McWilliams, B. J., Morris, H. L., and Shelton, R. L. *Cleft Palate Speech.* Philadelphia: Decker, 1984.
62. McWilliams, B. J., and Phillips, B. J. *Audio Seminars in Speech Pathology: Velopharyngeal Incompetence.* Philadelphia: Saunders, 1979.
63. Minami, R., Kaplan, E., Wu, G., and Jobe, R. Velopharyngeal incompetence without overt cleft palate. *Plast. Reconstr. Surg.* 55:573, 1975.
64. Morris, H. L. Etiological Bases for Speech Problems. In D. C. Spriestersbach and D. Sherman (Eds.), *Cleft Palate and Communication.* New York: Academic Press, 1968.
65. Morris, H., Krueger, L., and Bumsted, R. Indications of congenital palatal incompetence before diagnosis. *Ann. Oto. Rhinol. Laryngol.* 91:115, 1982.
66. Moncur, J. P., and Brackett, I. P. *Modifying Vocal Behavior.* New York: Harper & Row, 1974. P. 56–60.
67. Mysak, E. D. *Pathologies of Speech Systems.* Baltimore: Williams & Wilkins, 1976.
68. Netsell, R. *A Neurobiologic View of Speech Production and the Dysarthrias.* San Diego: College-Hill Press, 1986. Pp. 137–142.
69. Newcomb, J. Anatomical defects in the faucial pillars. *Laryngoscopy* 2:220, 1897.
70. Neiman, G. S., and Simpson, R. K. A roentgencephalometric investigation of the effect of adenoid removal upon selected measures of velopharyngeal function. *Cleft Palate J.* 12:377, 1975.
71. Peterson–Falzone, S. Nasal emission as a component of misarticulation of sibilants and affricates. *J. Speech Hear Disord.* 40:106, 1975.
72. Peterson–Falzone, S. Nasal distortions and compensatory articulations in velopharyngeal competent speakers. Paper presented at the Fourth International Congress on Cleft Palate and Related Craniofacial Anomalies, Acapulco, Mexico, 1981.
73. Peterson–Falzone, S. Resonance Disorders in Structural Defects. In N. L. Lass, L. V. McReynolds, J. L. Northern, and D. E. Yoder (Eds.), *Speech, Language, and Hearings.* Philadelphia: Saunders, 1982. Vol. 2, pp. 526–555.
74. Peterson–Falzone, S. Velopharyngeal inadequacy in the absence of overt cleft palate. *J. Craniofac. Genet. Dev. Biol.* 1(Suppl.):97, 1985.
75. Peterson–Falzone, S. Speech characteristics: Updating clinical decisions. *Semin. Speech Lang.* 7:269, 1986.
76. Powers, G. *Cleft Palate.* Indianapolis: Bobbs Merrill, 1973.
77. Pruzansky, S., Peterson–Falzone, S., Laffer, J., and Parris, P. Hypernasality in the absence of overt cleft: Commentary on nomenclature, diagnosis, classification and research design. Paper presented before the Third International Congress on Cleft Palate and Related Craniofacial Anomalies, Toronto, June 5–10, 1977.
78. Pruzansky, S. Roentgencephalometric studies of tonsils and adenoids in normal and pathologies states. *Ann. Otol. Rhinol. Laryngol.* 19(Suppl.):55, 1975.
79. Rampp, D. L., Pannbacker, M., and Kinnebrew, M. C. *VPI: Velopharyngeal Incompetency.* Tulsa: Modern Education Corp., 1984.
80. Roberts, W. J. Speech defects following adenoidectomy. *Rocky Mt. Med. J.* 56:67, 1959.
81. Ruscello, D. M. A selected review of palatal training procedures. *Cleft Palate J.* 19:181, 1982.
82. Saad, E. F. The underdeveloped palate in ear, nose and throat practice. *Laryngoscopy* 90:1371, 1980.
83. Schwartz, M. F. Acoustic Measure of Nasalization and Nasality. In K. R. Bzoch (Ed.), *Communicative Disorders Related to Cleft Lip and Cleft Palate.* Boston: Little, Brown, 1979. Pp. 263–268.
84. Shapiro, B. L., Meskin, L. H., Cervenka, J., and Pruzansky, S. Cleft Uvula: A Microform of Facial Clefts and Its Genetic Basis. In D. Bergsma (Ed.), *Birth Defects: Origi-*

nal Article Series, Part II, Orofacial Structures. Baltimore: Williams & Wilkins, 1971. Pp. 80–83.

85. Shapiro, R. S. Velopharyngeal insufficiency starting at puberty without adenoidectomy, *Int. J. Pediatr. Otorhinolaryngol.* 2:255, 1980.

86. Shelton, R. L., Knox, A. W., Arndt, W. B., Jr., and Elbert, M. The relationship between nasality score values and oral and nasal sound pressure level. *J. Speech Hear. Res.* 10:549, 1967.

87. Shelton, R. L., Arndt, W. B., Jr., Knox, A. W., Elbert, M., Chisum, L., and Youngstrom, K. A. The relationship between nasal sound pressure level and palatopharyngeal closure. *J. Speech Hear. Res.* 12:193, 1969.

88. Shprintzen, R. J. Surgery for speech: The planning of operations for velopharyngeal insufficiency with emphasis on the preoperative assessment of both pharyngeal physiology and articulation; cited in Hoch, L., Golding–Kushner, K., and Siegel–Sadewitz, V. L., Speech therapy. *Semin. Speech Lang.* 7:313, 1986.

89. Shprintzen, R. J., Lewin, M. L., Rakoff, S. J., Sidoti, E. J., and Croft, C. Diagnosis of small central gaps in the velopharyngeal sphincter. Paper presented at the annual meeting of the ACPA, San Francisco, May, 1976; abstract in *Cleft Palate J.* 13:415, 1976.

90. Shprintzen, R. J., McCall, G. N., and Skolnick, M. L. A new therapeutic technique for the treatment of velopharyngeal incompetence. *J. Speech Hear Disord.* 40:69, 1975.

91. Siegel–Sadewitz, V. L., and Sphrintzen, R. J. Nasopharyngoscopy of the normal velopharyngeal sphincter: An experiment in biofeedback. *Cleft Palate J.* 19:194, 1982.

92. Spiestersbach, D. C., Dickson, D. R., Fraser, F. C., Horowitz, S. L., McWilliams, B. J., Paradise, J. L., and Randall, P. Clinical research in cleft lip and cleft palate: The state of the art. *Cleft Palate J.* 10:113, 1973.

93. Stevens, K. N., Kalikow, D. N., and Willemain, T. R. A miniature accelerometer for detecting glottal waveforms and nasalization. *J. Speech Hear. Res.* 18:594, 1975.

94. Stevens, K. N., Nickerson, R. S., Boothroyd, A., and Rollins, A. M. Assessment of nasality in the speech of deaf children. *J. Speech Hear. Res.* 19:393, 1976.

95. Stewart, J. M., Ott, J. E., and Legace, R. Submucous Cleft Palate. In D. Bergsma (Ed.), *Birth Defects: Original Article Series, Part 11, Orofacial Structures.* Baltimore: Williams & Wilkins, 1971. Pp. 64–66.

96. Subtelny, J. Evaluations of Palatopharyngeal Valving: Clinical Research Procedures. In R. Lencione (Ed.), *Cleft Palate Habilitation.* Syracuse, NY: Syracuse University Press, 1968.

97. Subtelny, J., and Koepp–Baker, H. The significance of adenoid tissue in velopharyngeal function. *Plast. Reconstr. Surg.* 17:235, 1956.

98. Tantillo, M. W. Feedback articulation approach in the treatment of velopharyngeal insufficiency. Paper presented at the New York State Speech-Language-Hearing Association Convention, New York, 1984; cited in Hoch, L., et al., Speech therapy. *Semin. Speech Lang.* 7:313, 1986.

99. Trier, W. C. Velopharyngeal incompetency in the absence of overt cleft palate: Anatomic and surgical considerations. *Cleft Palate J.* 20:209, 1983.

100. Trost–Cardamone, J. From diagnosis to treatment: Speech remediation for persons with cleft palates and related disorders. Short Course Presentation, American Speech and Hearing Association Convention, Washington, D.C., 1985.

101. Trost, J. Differential diagnosis of velopharyngeal disorders. *Communication Disorders: An Audio Journal of Continuing Education* 6(7), July, 1981.

102. Trost, J. Articulatory additions to the classical description of the speech of persons with cleft palate. *Cleft Palate J.* 18:1933, 1981.

103. VanDemark, D. L., and Hardin, M. A. Effectiveness of intensive articulation therapy for children with cleft palate. *Cleft Palate J.* 23:215, 1986.

104. Warren, D. W. The determination of velopharyngeal incompetency by aerodynamic and acoustic techniques. *Clin. Plast. Surg.* 2:304, 1975.

105. Warren, D. W. PERCI: A method for rating palatal efficiency. *Cleft Palate J.* 16:279, 1979.

106. Warren, D. W. Aerodynamics of Speech. In N. J. Lass, L. V. McReynolds, J. L. Northern, and D. E. Yoder (Eds.), *Speech, Language, and Hearing.* Philadelphia: Saunders, 1982. Pp. 219–245.

107. Warren, D. W., Bevin, A. G., and Winslow, R. B. Posterior pillar webbing and palatopharyngeus displacement: Possible causes of congenital palatal incompetence. *Cleft Palate J.* 15:68, 1978.

108. Warren, D. W., and Hinton, V. A. Compensatory speech behaviors in cleft palate: A regulation/control phenomenon? *ASHA Rep.* 25:107, 1983.

109. Warren, D. W., Dalston, R. M., Trier, W. C., and Holder, M. B. A pressure flow technique for quantifying temporal patterns of palatal pharyngeal closure. *Cleft Palate J.* 22:11, 1985.

110. Weatherly–White, R. C. A., Sakura, C. Y., Jr., Brenner, L. D., Stewart, J. M., and Ott, J. E. Submucous cleft palate incidence, natural history and implications for treatment. *Plast. Reconstr. Surg.* 49:249, 1972.

111. Weatherly–White, R. C. A. Submucous Cleft Palate. In J. Calnan (Ed.), *Recent Advances in Plastic Surgery* Edinburgh: Churchill Livingstone, 1976. Vol. 1, pp. 58–67.

112. Weber, J., and Chase, R. Stress velopharyngeal incompetence in an oboe player. *Cleft Palate J.* 7:858, 1970.

113. Weinberg, B., and Shanks, J. C. The relationship between three oral breath pressure ratios and ratings of severity of hypernasality for talkers with cleft palate. *Cleft Palate J.* 8:251, 1971.

114. Wilbert, K., and Bradley, D. P. Relationship between perception of error type and spectrographic analysis of cleft palate and developmental speech. Paper presented at Florida Cleft Palate Association, Tampa, Fla., 1986.

115. Williams, W., Bzoch, K. R., and Agee, F. Functional versus organic patterns of velopharyngeal insufficiency for speech. Paper presented at the American Cleft Palate Association Meeting, Chicago, Ill., 1967.

116. Wilson, K. D. *Voice Problems of Children.* Baltimore: Williams & Wilkins, 1979. Pp. 78–82.

117. Witzel, M., and Munro, I. R. Velopharyngeal insufficiency after maxillary advancement. *Cleft Palate J.* 14:176, 1977.

118. Witzel, M., Rich, R. H., Margar–Bacal, F., and Cox, C. Velopharyngeal insufficiency after adenoidectomy: An 8 year review. *Int. J. Pediatr. Otorhinolaryngol.* 11:15, 1986.

119. Witzel, M. Speech problems in craniofacial anomalies. *Communication Disorders: An Audio Journal of Continuing Education* 8(4), April, 1983.

CHAPTER 7

Psychological Aspects of Competency and Language Development

Edward Clifford • Miriam Clifford

Communications research into problems associated with cleft palate have, until recently, focused primarily on a single aspect of language — speech production. A shift in focus has been taking place, resulting in greater emphasis on linguistics as well as on psychological aspects of communication. The earlier research, however, remains pertinent to the development of competent, fully functioning individuals born with palatal defects.

Speech deficits have been associated with language deficits because of the intimate association between speech and language. Morris [39] stressed the relationship between poor speech and an equivalent lack of language mastery. He found the verbal output of poor articulators deficient, both in terms of loquacity and vocabulary, and related this deficiency to velopharyngeal incompetency.

A point-for-point correspondence between speech deficits and language development does not seem to exist, however. Psychological factors have been perceived as intervening between the physical defect (velopharyngeal incompetency), the speech defect, and language competency. Linguistic skills were viewed as having a psychosocial basis in the affected child's experience in the home and in the attitudinal framework existing there [39]. Psychological factors were seen as either inhibiting or facilitating language competency, overlying or exacerbating structural deficiencies. In a similar vein Smith and McWilliams [61], finding children with clefts to be less creative on the language components of their measures than children without clefts stressed that the poorer performance of children with clefts could not be attributed to the physical defect itself. These authors emphasized the role of psychosocial variables intervening between the physical defect and the expression of the child's behavior.

An earlier review of language in children with clefts devoted only a total of 7.5 lines to language. Within this fourth of a page, four references were cited to support the general finding that while language problems associated with cleft palate were mild, children with clefts had reduced language skills. It was noted that average sentence length was shorter for children with clefts than for their unaffected peers. The expressive language of children with cleft palate was also found to be inferior to their receptive language [64]. A later review [5] suggested that the differences in language skills between children with clefts and normal children appeared to be decreasing. The decrease was attributed to greater emphasis on early treatment and increased language stimulation in the home.

This chapter examines relationships among psychosocial factors, competency, and language development. It examines the role of competency in development, cleft palate and issues of competency, intelligence and competence, developmental considerations of language, and maternal-child aspects of language development.

COMPETENCY AND DEVELOPMENT

We assume that children who exhibit age-appropriate competencies react and are reacted to differently from those who do not. During the course of development the acquisition of appropriate skills frees the child to progress to more advanced developmental tasks. Those who are not competent may have to devote much of their available energy to (1) becoming more competent, (2) defending themselves against their incompetencies, (3) defending themselves against a loss of esteem.

Lack of competencies affects the behaviors and attitudes of significant persons around the child exhibiting the lack. Attitudes, feelings, and behaviors of parents are modified in the presence of the child's abilities. The situation is exacerbated when a child with a birth defect exhibits incompetency. Differentiating issues of competency from the direct effects of the birth defect itself becomes a problem. For example, competent children with a birth defect may be praised for overcoming their handicap, while the incompetency of children with defects may be attributed to the defect itself.

The feedback provided to children about their performances have significant effects on their behaviors. When others, particularly those who are of importance to them, attribute characteristics to the children, they are likely to accept these for themselves. Negative attributions have the effect of impoverishing self-concepts, while positive attributions enhance them. Children are affected also by their own demonstrated abilities. They become aware of an inability to perform, which may lead in turn to depreciated feelings of self-worth. Conversely, feelings of self-enhancement or pleasure occur in the presence of the ability to perform well.

Early in life, competency is displayed by the child's attainment of the usual developmental milestones at appropriate age levels, for example, the development of locomotion and the utterance of the first word. However, infants do not await the unfolding of development passively; drives toward mastery are evident in their attempts to understand and manage their environments through the self-seeking of stimulation and of tasks [15]. Fogel and Thelen [19] point out that competency, including language and communication skills, evolves in an asynchronous, uneven sequence. A dynamic, systems theory model is posited in which the child's maturational status interacts with his or her experiences and takes place within a current context.

During the preschool period competency is manifested in more complex forms of behavior, so that by the time the child is of school age, relevant competencies are apparent in social, perceptual, cognitive, and language areas — skills needed for adaptation to school and prerequisite to adequate academic functioning. Levels of performance are changing and interacting during this period of development. As children increase their functioning levels, feelings of others about them may change as well.

In the case of the child with a cleft, the expression of competency occurs within the special context of a reparable birth defect that requires a succession of accommodations. More specifically, the fact that the child has a birth defect influences the mother. What continues to influence maternal attitudes and behaviors is not the existence of a cleft, but the series of experiences encountered in individual and team treatment processes. Shortly after infancy, parents may experience a growing awareness that other problems exist for the child and for themselves as well.

Accommodations may be made also in the light of accumulating evidence that their child with a cleft is demonstrating greater competency as he or she grows older. During the preschool and school-age periods, the parents are affected by the child's characteristics and continue to be affected by treatment events. The effects of having a child with a cleft in the family are variable and are dependent on the following:

1. The presence and nature of the sequelae associated with the original cleft condition
2. The intrusiveness of the child in terms of the amount of time, energy, and the perceived self-sacrifice involved in child care
3. The increasing ability of the child to demonstrate mastery, so that increasing independence can be perceived
4. The amount and kind of support available from the treatment efforts of cleft palate team members

In summary, competencies of all children have wide-ranging effects. They directly influence parental perceptions of the child, as well as directly affecting the perceptions of significant others, for example, teachers and peers. Children react to their own masteries, or lack of them, developing feelings of self-enhancement at one extreme or self-depreciation at the other. When achievements are low, poor performances may be rationalized and attributed to personal characteristics not involved in the task, that is, the presence of a birth defect like cleft palate. Unfortunately, in some cases, through generalization, other behaviors of the person become contaminated (a contagion effect) and a reputation for incompetency is obtained [13].

CLEFT PALATE AND ISSUES OF COMPETENCY

Cleft palate research has chiefly studied the effect of functional limitations on competency achievement. More specifically, the literature has emphasized predominantly two problematical functioning areas for children with cleft palate — poor speech and poor hearing. It is assumed that these are causative factors in an eventual lack of competency in children with cleft palate. We have mentioned previously that a relationship between poor speech and an equivalent lack of language mastery was stressed [39]. Similarly, Spriestersbach et al. [64], in a comprehensive review, concluded that children with cleft palate had lower achievement levels in language skills than children without clefts. The implication is clear; general language incompetency is a correlate of cleft palate.

Seeking etiological factors related to poor language mastery in preschool children with cleft palate, Nation [41] found that hearing loss and the amount of time the child was hospitalized played significant roles. Because variables other than functional ones were involved, Nation postulated a "cleftness syndrome" to account for poor language mastery.

Hearing impairment was one of the factors included in the syndrome. Psychological factors, reflected in the duration of hospitalization and the age at surgical procedures, were included as well. In effect, Nation [14] and Morris [39] agree in believing functional limitations (e.g., poor speech, poor hearing) interact with psychosocial components to induce a general lack of language mastery.

There is some evidence that the vocabulary development of children with clefts is below the level of their normal peers. Phillips and Harrison [47], using four different measures of language ability, found that preschool children with cleft palate performed below their chronological age levels in both receptive and expressive language. Nation [40] found that children with cleft palate, compared to both siblings and normal controls, developed vocabularies of use and of comprehension at a much slower rate. Smith and McWilliams [62], using the Illinoise Test of Psycholinguistic Abilities, found the performance of chil-

dren with cleft palate to show a general depression in language areas sampled by the test. Unfortunately, however, no control groups were used in these studies.

When written language was investigated, using the Myklebust Picture Story Language Test [16], no significant differences were obtained in a sample of children with clefts and a control group. Using the same test measure, a later study of slightly older children found they performed more poorly than the norm, scoring below the 50th percentile in the use of total words and the words used per sentence [24].

Several more recent studies question the generalizability of language retardation. Preschool children with clefts and intelligible speech compared favorably to normal controls on the Northwestern Syntax Screening Test [5]. J. J. Frick (unpublished data, 1973) compared language abilities of children with cleft palate between the ages of 7 and 14 to matched sibling controls. All children were asked to respond to five of the cards of the Thematic Appreception Test. Verbatim transcripts were analyzed for number of sentences, number of words per sentence, number of words, and grammatical usage of words. A large number of comparisons were made between the experimental and control groups; the number of significant differences did not exceed a chance level. Frick concluded that linguistic abilities of children with cleft palate and their siblings at this age level were equivalent.

Saxman and Bless [58] examined patterns of language development in children with cleft palate aged 3 to 8 years. Their carefully controlled study matched children with repaired palatal clefts and children without clefts for age. All had normal hearing. There was equal representation at each yearly age level between the ages of 3 and 8. Of particular interest was the use in this study of the following measures: the Belugi–Kilma Test of Grammatical Comprehension, the Northwestern Syntax Screening Test, The Osser Sentence Imitation Test, and the Utah Test of Language Development. Saxman and Bless concluded that the linguistic performance of children with cleft palate did not differ appreciably from that of their noncleft counterparts. Finally, adults with repaired cleft palates and normal adults were described as being similar in the use of syntax and vocabulary [46].

Recently, emphasis has been placed on the use of language, or communicative intent, by those with clefts. An observational study of gestural communication compared 10 normal children and 10 children with cleft lip and palate in play inter-actions with their mothers. Finding no significant differences between the groups, the investigators concluded that communicative intent and aware-ness was well established before the appearance of later language deficiencies in children with clefts [30].

The use of shorter sentences, of reduced vocab-ularies, and of inhibited verbal expressions in children with clefts may be associated with a re-luctance to talk any more than is absolutely neces-sary, even when they can [36]. Communicative intent is perceived as involving a combination of speech, language, and psychosocial, personality, and physical characteristics of children. Commu-nicative intent is also dependent on the relations between linguistic expressions and their users, that is, the linguistic behavior of the person in a social situation, known as pragmatics [55].

Warr–Leeper and her colleagues [67] examined communicative intent in a group of children with clefts in order to determine whether they differed from a normative population and to detect influ-ences on pragmatic test scores. The study in-volved two groups of children: 13 preschool chil-dren, age 3 to 5 and 14 school-age children, age 6 to 9. All had surgically repaired congenital facial clefts, no hearing deficits, normal IQs, and nor-mal receptive and expressive language. Speech intelligibility and acceptability of facial appear-ance were rated. The Test of Pragmatic Skills was used to evaluate communicative intent in four controlled play interactions where the child had to initiate or respond with language stimulated by the examiner's provocations. The linguistic ap-propriateness and the sophistication of each child's verbal responses were rated.

Neither IQ nor linguistic skills accounted for the level of performance on the Test of Pragmatic Skills; nor were appearance or intelligibility strong-ly related to pragmatic skills. There was an age factor, however. Preschool children with re-paired clefts did as well or better than the norms, while school-age children performed at or below the norms. In addition, the younger group com-municated more elaborately and appropriately than school-age children with clefts. The differ-ences are provocative and induce speculation. Perhaps the younger children, because of their in-teractions with cleft palate team members, were more comfortable in interactions with strangers. Perhaps their parents provided more stimulating linguistic environments. Factors such as negative

teacher or peer responses and increasing peer influence influenced self-perceptions which, in turn, may have induced poorer performances of the school-age children [67].

In a somewhat different approach to language evaluation, reading disabilities were contrasted for children with cleft lip and palate and for chil-dren with cleft palate only [52]. The investigators suggested that children with cleft palate only con-stitute a language disorder group while those with cleft lip and palate were more likely to have expressive verbal deficits. In a subsequent study, approximately one third of a group of 132 ele-mentary school children who had either clefts of the palate only or clefts of the lip and palate exhib-ited a moderate degree of reading disability; of these 17 percent demonstrated a severe reading disability. The finding that the incidence of read-ing disability in children with cleft lip and palate approximated the normal population (9%), while those with cleft palate only exhibited a much higher rate (33%), is provocative. The authors suggest that reading disabilities are related to ear-lier general language disorders for those with cleft palate only [53].

INTELLIGENCE AND COMPETENCY

In the search for the effects of a cleft and its se-quelae on functioning, considerable attention has been paid to the measured intelligence of chil-dren with clefts. Specific attention has been paid to the Wechsler Intelligence Scale for Children (WISC), because the division of scores into Ver-bal and Performance IQs has a parallel in the di-vision of language into expressive and recep-tive performance.

Children with clefts obtain IQ scores within the range of normal intelligence, although specific comparisons with other groups seems to demon-strate a slightly lower operational range for them. In addition, Verbal IQ scores on the average tend to be below Performance IQs [20, 26, 56, 57, 68]. The combined findings of lower WISC Verbal IQs for subjects with clefts compared to control sub-jects and the tendency for children with clefts to have lower Verbal IQs in contrast to their Perform-ance IQs are frequently cited to bolster the position that poor speech has resulted in poor verbal performance.

Using factor analysis, WISC verbal and performance scores were used to discriminate three groups of children based on low verbal–high performance profiles. One group contained children having a specific language disability; they also had good reasoning abilities. These children had adequate reading skills. The second group, also with a specific language disability, had good sequencing-motor skills; these children demonstrated somewhat poorer reading skills. The third group had a general language disability with associated poor performances in abstract reasoning and sequencing memory; these children read very poorly [54]. There were indications that a significant number of children with cleft palate only could be included in the last group [51–53].

In almost all of the studies IQ is seen as a dependent variable and depressed scores are seen as correlates of the cleft palate condition. IQ is rarely considered as an identifying characteristic separately from cleft palate. Its role as an independent variable is largely ignored. Intelligence may be related to a greater extent to genetic and environmental factors than to the existence of a cleft. In one study, when the correlation between parent-child IQ was taken into account, no significant differences among children with cleft palate, their siblings, and their nonaffected peers were in evidence [57].

The impact of hearing loss on the expression of IQ is not quite clear. Lamb, Wilson, and Leeper [25] examined the effects of hearing acuity on WISC Verbal, Performance, and Full Scale IQ scores. Significantly depressed Verbal IQ scores were obtained for children with cleft palate, even when hearing acuity was within normal limits. In a subsequent study these investigators examined 73 children with cleft palate using the WISC to ascertain the effects of cleft type and sex on IQ. No significant differences were found when subjects with cleft palate only were compared to those having cleft lip and palate. Again, IQ has been viewed as a dependent variable subject to influence by a functional limitation or by a specific birth defect.

In an extensive study of 166 children with clefts, 191 of whom were followed longitudinally from birth to 15 years of age, Estes and Morris [18] found that the depressed Verbal IQs could not be attributed to the fact that the children had communication problems, nor could the depressed scores be related to decreases in hearing

sensitivity. IQ scores were not related to the severity of problems with verbal communication effectiveness as reflected in speech scores. These investigators concluded that depressed scores were probably related to some other factor or combination of factors.

DEVELOPMENTAL CONSIDERATIONS OF LANGUAGE

Considerable attention has been paid to language acquisition in the developmental literature. Early developmental studies, for example, McCarthy's [32], emphasized the acquisition of words, sentences, and grammatical structure. The assumption that child language is an approximation or an imperfect version of adult language is implicit in this approach.

Historically, the early acquisition of speech and the association of meaning to sound used reinforcement theory as an explanatory principle. The child's production of sound was differentially reinforced. The sounds, retained within a specific culture in which children are reared, are positively reinforced, while those that are not part of a common linguistic code are either negatively reinforced or nonreinforced. Utilizing this model, it would seem that if the child is incapable of producing appropriate sounds, because of velopharyngeal competency, for example, it would be impossible for the child to be reinforced for producing the correct sound. It would be possible, however, to reinforce the meaning of words, despite the child's inability to produce appropriate sounds.

Some explanations of language acquisition use a combined imitative-reinforcement model. The expansion of the child's linguistic repertory is seen as being a result of the child's imitative efforts and these efforts in turn are differentially reinforced. Adults serve as the primary models as well as the primary reinforcers.

In the 1960s interest shifted to models of language acquisition that were more cognitive in their conception. McNeill [33] added the idea that processes within the child (e.g., cognitive noise) and the child's own rudimentary vocabulary filters the adult language. The development of language was recognized as an independent process following its own rules.

In order to understand language acquistion and how it proceeds, it is necessary to know what is being acquired [60]. This idea resulted in an emphasis on linguistics and the development of psycholinguistics as a field of interest. Early stages of language acquisition were considered to involve processes not directly related to adult language. Child language was perceived as a language in its own right that gradually conformed to adult language. In an excellent review of theories of language acquisition, Edmonds [17] explored three grammatical models:

1. *Finite-state grammars:* Grammar was analyzed by the sequence of words (left-to-right) in a sentence. It was assumed that in this sequence, each word as it occurs determines the following word or class of words. This analysis is akin to the chaining phenomenon described in learning theory, in which responses are added to responses in a stimulus-response chain. Chaining, however, proved to be an inadequate explanation for the generation of sentences or their understanding [37].

2. *Phase-structure grammars:* Grammar in this model was analyzed by the rules governing the usage of syntactic classes. Words in a sentence were no longer seen as dependent on their association with the immediately preceding word, but were perceived as dependent on grammatical rules. Analysis of linguistic production focused on the use of different syntactic classes. Developmental research, for example, might emphasize the frequency with which various syntactic classes were used by children at differing age levels.

3. *Transformational grammars:* Chomsky [9–11] proposed that sentence structure could be represented on two levels — surface structure and deep structure. The surface structure expresses meaning in the sound patterns, the sentence as spoken. Deep structure contains the semantic meaning; this structure is generated by grammatical rules (e.g., phrase structure may be altered by transformational rules). Different parts of the deep structure may be altered by transformational rules, producing or modifying the surface structure. Thus, only a finite set of rules is required to generate all sentences. Analysis, particularly with children, is based on recording spontaneous speech and writing a grammar that could account for the child's productions.

Since it is difficult for this approach to explain why the child is prepared to imitate at one level of development, and not at an earlier and perhaps less mature stage, McNeill [34, 35], Lenneberg [27, 28], and others claimed that humans innately possess the fundamental concepts of language. As soon as the ability to produce speech is found, the child's communications are grammatical and understandable to adults. According to McNeill the child has a language acquisition device (LAD) that is activated when the child is first exposed to language. Unfortunately, as Edmonds [17] asserts, the LAD concept sheds no further light on how language is acquired but merely shifts the explanatory burden to some other discipline, for example, developmental neurology.

An alternative explanation of language acquisition utilizes a cognitive hypothesis, assuming that children comprehend and productively use language if their cognitive abilities are sufficiently developed to enable them to do so [14, 48–50]. Language itself is perceived as a system of relations, classifications, and referents that are all in the service of thought [44, 60]. The development of thought is based on the child's progression through developmental stages during which, through gradual internal organization, the child is released from a dependence on the concrete here-and-now, and becomes able to use symbols that are independent of the specific referent. Through the processes of assimilation and accommodation the language structure is capable of modification.

Current views stress language acquisition and mastery within the context of a developing social and communicative system, rather than being understood only within a linguistic, genetic, rule-testing framework, that is, witness the growth of interest in pragmatics. As noted, previously individual differences were ignored. The basic assumption that grammar was innately given, operating under universal principles, was derived from the theories of Chomsky and others [10, 11, 33, 34]. This formulation resulted in expectations of finding a similar course of acquisition for all children; thus variation among individuals, cultures, and language communities could only be minor and irrelevant. Individual differences rather than similarities have been emphasized in this complex language system. In contrast to stage theories that focus on common points of similarity among children, the study of transitions is likely to uncover rampant dissimilarity [43].

MOTHER-CHILD ASPECTS OF CHILD DEVELOPMENT

Psychologists have long been interested in the effects of the caretaker on the developing child and, more recently, in the effects of the child on those who care for him or her. In an insightful and concise review of the effects of maternal behaviors on child development, Clarke–Stewart [12] summarized the effects of several relevant variables as follows:

1. The absence of the caretaker or the presence of an inadequate caretaker can lead to developmental retardation, especially in social, language, and cognitive areas. Provision of warmth, food, and hygienic conditions alone is insufficient for adequate development.

2. Not all maternal care variables are related to child development. Variations in feeding procedures and other superficial variables of caretaking demonstrate neither consistent nor significant relationships to infant development. In addition, maternal availability alone, that is, the total amount of maternal contact with the child, does not influence development.

3. Subtle rather than gross aspects of maternal behavior, for example, personality characteristics, feelings, and attitudes, influence the way the child develops. Maternal coldness and rejection have been shown to be related to be related to poor development; maternal anxiety and negative attitudes toward the child have been related to retarded intellectual development; and maternal attitudes indicative of eagerness for close interaction and an accepting attitude toward the child have been positively related to infant development.

4. The quality of maternal stimulation is related to the child's cognitive development. Distinctive and frequent verbal stimulation by the mother has been related to the child's frequent vocalization and his adequate development of language ability. In addition to serving as direct sources of stimulation, mothers serve as mediators of stimulation from the environment. Mothers who choose a great number and variety of play materials and activities and who choose materials for children commensurate with their skills with the objects have children who tend to be cognitively advanced. Mere exposure to a haphazardly stimulating physical environment has little or no effect on the child's cognitive development.

5. Responsiveness of mothers to infant behavior affects the infant. Mothers who are responsive to their child's behavior increase the likelihood of interactive responsiveness with the child. The mother's prompt, contingent responses to the child's signals enable the child to learn that his or her behavior has consequences — a necessary basis for further learning. Deliberate and playful maternal stimulation is a potent dimension of maternal influence.

6. Several related components of maternal behavior, rather than simple elements, may constitute a "syndrome of optimal care" related to maximal development of the child.

7. The child does influence mother-child interactions, a fact which has been neglected in studies of mother-child relationships. The child's reaction patterns, biological predispositions, immediate physical status, and acquired characteristics can influence parental behavior, facilitating or inhibiting the responses of caretakers. The child's ability to make his or her needs known clearly can affect communication between parent and child; determining the child's needs and wishes are not solely dependent on the parent's ability to read the appropriate cues. Finally, the effect of the child on parental behavior is sustained. Over time, the child has long-term effects on parental attitudes and behaviors.

MOTHER-CHILD ASPECTS OF LANGUAGE DEVELOPMENT

The language environment of young children has been the focus of many developmental studies [1, 6, 42, 63]. Seitz and Marcus [59] point out that the complexity of maternal linguistic behavior is commonly found to be related to the complexity of the young child's speech; both the child's and the mother's mean length of utterance increases systematically. Mothers seem to respond more readily to imitations of their speech or in response to their questions.

Nelson [42] stresses the importance of parental feedback and particularly emphasizes the relationship between positive feedback and the rapidity with which word acquisition is achieved. This feedback is crucial to the child's attempt at communication and may begin before the actual use of language. Lewis and Freedle [29], for example, refer to the early mother-child communication network as the "cradle of meaning."

Osofsky [45], in a study of 134 mothers and their newborn infants, found that infants who were alert and responsive had mothers who were alert and responsive. The finding is impressive, particularly as the mothers were all nonwhite and from lower socioeconomic status levels. Moerk [38] also examined the mother-child dyad and obtained recordings of verbal behavior in the homes of 20 mother-child pairs. He found that mothers from middle-class homes actively taught all aspects of language to their children. Moerk suggested the mother-child dyad is self-regulating and hence a relatively closed system.

Studies of parent-child behavior typically assume the child's behavior is the consequence of antecedent parental input [31]. This is the historical model of the socialization process. Seitz and Marcus [59] suggest that for language development, the quality of mother-child interactions needs to be examined in terms of maternal responsiveness to the child and, in turn, the child's responsiveness to the mother. In this system, not only is the mother the socializing agent, she is dependent on her child's characteristics and the cues the child brings to the interaction. If, as may be true in the case of the child with cleft lip and

palate, the child presents confusing or unclear cues or is not responsive to the mother, the early communication system can be affected. Seitz and Marcus would assert that in the presence of reduced child responsiveness, parents experience difficulty in knowing how to respond to the child and may misjudge whether the content or complexity of the child's language is appropriate.

The role of mother-as-teacher, particularly of language, has been emphasized as a way of directly assessing characteristic inputs of the mother. Studies used structured observational approaches to observe and assess maternal teaching behavior, employing a paradigm in which mothers have to instruct their children; the nature of the interaction is determined by the investigator [2, 7, 22, 23, 65]. Hess and Shipman [22] defined teaching styles in terms of the mother's characteristic verbal behaviors in interaction with the child. Verbal behaviors were recorded and analyzed according to whether restricted or elaborated verbal codes were used in instructing the children. The type of verbal strategy employed affected the child's learning. Similarly, teaching styles involving strategies of enrichment or stimulation were more effective than strategies of correction [7].

The direction that studies of maternal teaching strategies has taken is congruent with the familiar socialization paradigm. It has been suggested, however, that the influence of the child has been neglected and that examining the effects of the child on the caretaker can expand the socialization model [3, 31]. That characteristics of the child do influence parental behaviors has been reported by Terdal, Jackson, and Garner [66], who concluded that the nature of the feedback and its impoverishment on the part of retarded children had the effect of producing parental uncertainty, parental intrusiveness, and inefficient parental commanding. Kaplan and Kaplan [23] used an observation-teaching strategy approach in which mothers had to (1) encourage the child to play with a "curiosity" box for which there were no criteria for use and no goals to achieve, and (2) instruct the child on a specific task.

Mothers and two of their children were involved: one child had a functional speech impairment, the other, a like-sex sibling, did not. The verbal behavior of the mothers was recorded and coded. With the unstructured task, mothers demonstrated more negative verbalizations toward the child with a speech problem. In the direct instruction task mothers were more directive, expended more verbal effort, and were more verbally rejecting toward their children with speech problems. Because of the presence of interactive effects with age, Kaplan and Kaplan concluded that these mothers treated their children with speech problems as less mature or younger than their like-sex siblings [23].

Clarke–Stewart [12] examined interactions between mothers and their 9- to 18-month-old children over a 9-month period. She found a specific linear relationship between the mother's verbal stimulation and the child's language development. Her analysis of relationships over time is of particular interest; the mother's stimulating and responsive behavior affected the intellectual development of the child and the child's behavior influenced the mother in the area of social relationships with the child.

One examination of mother-infant interactions found that the mother and infant took turns. For example, they did not vocalize at the same time. This turn-taking interaction was characterized as an adultlike conversation. At times, infants vocalized in bursts of sound, just as babies suck in bursts. When this occurred, mothers filled in the pauses between bursts. Additionally, mothers adapted their responses to follow the baby's initiatory behavior. This interchange of responses formed communication patterns that were uniquely specific to the particular baby and mother by the time the infant was 7 months old [21].

Complexities in infant as well as maternal behaviors associated with language acquisition continue to receive increasing emphasis. A recent study investigated relationships between infants' emotional expressions and the emergence of their language. Neutral affect was found to support the early transition from prespeech vocalizations to language by allowing the reflective stance required for language learning. Antecedents for neutral affect could be found in the quiet alert states which support the cognitive activity of early infancy, necessary for the learning of words. The frequency with which infants expressed nonneutral emotions was related to a later onset of language achievements [4].

Currently, functional analyses involving the child in a linguistic-social context are being stressed. For children language is important because it becomes a way for them to get things done with words, that is, intentions are realized by the appropriate use of language [8]. Given the capacity to acquire language, the child also needs a support system which fosters communication. The interactions between the child's capacity to acquire language and a language support system facilitate the child's entry into the broader culture, the social linguistic community. This dynamic viewpoint stresses the importance of the dialogue pair, in most cases mother and child. Parents do more than provide linguistic modeling behavior; they negotiate communications with children and help them reach the objectives by enabling them to make their intentions clear. Parents can

1. Emphasize salient features of the child's language using simple words and syntax
2. Encourage new knowledge and the child's intentions by using lexical and phrasal extensions for known verbal and gestural communications
3. Use formal play situations, that is pretend, make-believe, and story-telling, which ritualize language usage
4. Routinize and generalize from one format to another, that is, the use of naming first to indicate, then to request

Not only does the child need to acquire a language system that can function in his environment — that is, has utility in that unique setting — but the persons in that environment must interpret the communication and understand its intent. Thus language learning, in addition to requiring knowledge of vocabulary and syntax, involves learning to master conventions for making intentions clear through the appropriate use of language [8].

It is clear that current concepts of language acquisition and development are becoming more dynamic and that rapid changes are taking place. In terms of taking the sequelae of clefting into account, the literature remains impoverished. We still do not know how the presence of a cleft affects lingusitic-interactional behaviors, nor do we know much about the effects of a cleft and its sequelae on mother-child interactions.

CONCLUSION

This chapter has focused on the psychological aspects of competency and language development. While some progress has taken place, much more needs to be done. A primary area for future research is the conceptualization and assessment of competency in children born with clefts and exposed to a lengthy treatment process. We strongly urge that considerations of language and communication take advantage of the sophisticated, dynamic methodologies and theories of language development and acquisition, going beyond the rudimentary aspects so frequently emphasized in cleft palate literature.

REFERENCES

1. Baldwin, A. L., and Baldwin, C. P. The study of mother-child interaction. *Am. Sci.* 64:711, 1973.
2. Bee, H. I., Van Egeren, I. R., Streisgath, A. P., Nyman, B. A., and Leckie, M. S. Social class differences in maternal teaching strategies and speech patterns. *Dev. Psychol.* 1:726, 1969.
3. Bell, R. O. A reinterpretation of the directions of effects in studies of socialization. *Psychol. Rev.* 75:81, 1968.
4. Bloom, L., and Capatides, J. B. Expression of affect and the emergence of language. *Child Dev.* 58:1513, 1987.
5. Bradley, D. P. Section VI. Speech and language aspects. *Cleft Palate J.* 14:321, 1977.
6. Broen, P. A. The verbal environment of the language learning child. *Am. Speech Hear. Assoc. Monogr.* No. 17, 1972.
7. Brophy, J. E. Mothers as teachers of their own preschool children: The influence of socioeconomic status and task structure on teachings specificity. *Child Dev.* 41:79, 1970.
8. Bruner, J. S. *Child's Talk: Learning to Use Language.* New York: Norton, 1983.
9. Chomsky, N. *Syntactic Structures.* The Hague: Mouton, 1957.
10. Chomsky, N. *Aspects of the Therory of Syntax.* Cambridge, Mass: MIT Press, 1965.
11. Chomsky, N. Deep Structure, Surface Structure, and Semantic Interpretation. In D. Steinberg and I. Jakobovits (Eds.), *Semantics.* London: Cambridge University Press, 1971.
12. Clarke–Stewart, K. A. Interactions between mothers and their young children: Characteristics and consequences. *Monogr. Soc. Res. Child Dev.* 38, 1973.
13. Clifford, E. *The Cleft Palate Experience: New Perspectives on Management.* Springfield, Ill.: Thomas, 1987.
14. Cromer, R. F. The Development of Language and Cognition: The Cognition Hypothesis. In B. Foss (Ed.), *New Perspectives in Child Development.* London: Penguin Education Series, 1974.
15. Dweck, C. S., and Elliott, E. S. Achievement Motivation. In E. M. Heatherington (Ed.), *Handbook of Child Psychology: Vol. 4 Socialization, Personality, and Social Development.* New York: Wiley, 1983. Pp. 643–691.
16. Ebert, P. R., McWilliams, B. J., and Woolf, G. A comparison of the written language ability of cleft palate and normal children. *Cleft Palate J.* 44:17, 1974.
17. Edmonds, M. H. New directions in theories of language acquisition. *Harvard Educ. Rev.* 46:175, 1976.
18. Estes, R. F., and Morris, H. L. Relationships among intelligence, speech proficiency, and hearing sensitivity in children with cleft palate. *Cleft Palate J.* 7:703, 1970.
19. Fogel, A., and Thelen, E. Development of early expressive and communicative action: Reinterpreting the evidence from a dynamic systems approach. *Dev. Psychol.* 23:747, 1987.
20. Goodstein, L. D. Intellectual impairment in children with cleft palate. *J. Speech Hear. Disord.* 4:287, 1961.
21. Harris, M., and Coltheart, M. *Language Processing in Children and Adults: An Introduction.* Boston: Routledge & Kegan Paul, 1986.
22. Hess, R. D., and Shipman, V. C. Early experience and the socialization of cognitive modes in children. *Child. Dev.* 36:869, 1965.
23. Kaplan, N. R., and Kaplan, V. C. Differential patterns of maternal behavior toward speech-defective and non-speech-defective children. In *Proceedings of the 76th Annual Convention of the American Psychological Association,* 353, 1968.
24. Kommers, M. S., and Sullivan, M. D. Written language skills of children with cleft palate, *Cleft Palate J.* 16:81-85, 1979.
25. Lamb, M. M., Wilson, F. B., and Leeper, H. A. A comparison of selected cleft palate children and their siblings on the variables of intelligence, hearing loss, and visual-perceptual-motor abilities. *Cleft Palate J.* 9:218, 1972.
26. Lamb, M. D., Wilson, F. B., and Leeper, H. A. The intellectual function of cleft palate children compared on the basis of cleft type and sex. *Cleft Palate J.* 10:367, 1973.
27. Lenneberg, E. H. Language, Evolution, and Purposive Behavior. In S. Diamond (Ed.), *Essays in Honor of Paul Radon.* New York: Columbia University Press, 1960.
28. Lenneberg, E. H. *The Biological Foundations of Language.* New York: Wiley, 1967.
29. Lewis, M., and Freedle, R. *Mother-Infant Dyad: The Cradle of Meaning.* Princeton, N.J.: Educational Testing Service, 1972.
30. Long, N. V., and Dalston, R. M. Gestural communication in twelve-month-old cleft lip and palate children. *Cleft Palate J.* 19:57, 1982.
31. Lytton, H. Observation studies of parent child interaction: A methodological review. *Child Dev.* 42:65, 1971.
32. McCarthy, D. Language Development in Children, In I. Carmichael (Ed.), *Manual of Child Psychology* (2nd ed.). New York: Wiley, 1954.
33. McNeill, D. Developmental Psycholinguistics. In F. Smith and G. A. Miller (Eds.), *The Genesis of Language.* Cambridge, Mass: MIT Press, 1966.
34. McNeill, D. *The Acquisition of Language.* New York: Harper & Row, 1970.
35. McNeill, D. The Development of Language. In P. H. Mussen (Ed.), *Carmichael's Manual of Child Psychology* (3rd ed.). New York: Wiley, 1970. Vol. 1.
36. McWilliams, B. J. Morris, H. L., and Shelton, R. L. *Cleft Palate Speech.* St. Louis: Mosby, 1984.
37. Miller, G. Some psychological studies of grammar. *Am. Psychol.* 17:748, 1962.
38. Moerk, F. I. Processes of language teaching and training in the interactions of mother-child dyads. *Child Dev.* 17:1064, 1976.
39. Morris, H. I. Communication skills of children with cleft lip and palate. *J. Speech Hear. Res.* 5:79, 1962.
40. Nation, J. E. Vocabulary comprehension and usage of preschool cleft palate and normal children. *Cleft Palate J.* 7:639, 1970.
41. Nation, J. E. Determinants of vocabulary development of preschool cleft palate children. *Cleft Palate J.* 7:645, 1970.

42. Nelson, K. Structure and strategy in learning to talk. *Monogr. Soc. Res. Child Dev.* 38, 1973.
43. Nelson, K. Individual differences in language development: Implications for development and language. *Annu. Prog. Child Psychiatry Child Dev.* 249–276, 1982.
44. Olson, D. R. Language and thought: Aspects of a cognitive theory of semantics. *Psychol. Rev.* 77:257, 1970.
45. Osofsky, J. D. Neonatal characteristics of mother-infant interaction in two observational situations. *Child Dev.* 17:1138, 1976.
46. Pannbacker, M. Oral language skills of adult cleft palate speakers. *Cleft Palate J.* 12:95, 1975.
47. Phillips, B. J., and Harrison, R. J. Language skills of preschool cleft palate children. *Cleft Palate J.* 6:108, 1969.
48. Piaget, J. *The Origins of Intelligence.* New York: Norton, 1952.
49. Piaget, J. *The Construction of Reality in the Child.* New York: Norton, 1954.
50. Piaget, J. *Play, Dreams, and Imitation in Childhood.* New York: Norton, 1962.
51. Richman, L. C. Cognitive patterns and learning disabilities in cleft palate children with verbal deficits. *J. Speech Hear. Res.* 23:447, 1980.
52. Richman, L. C., and Eliason, M. J. Type of reading disability related to cleft type and neuropsychological patterns. *Cleft Palate J.* 21:1, 1984.
53. Richman, L. C., Eliason, M. J., and Lindgren, S. C. Reading disability in children with clefts. *Cleft Palate J.* 25:21, 1988.
54. Richman, L. C., and Lindgren, S. D. Patterns of intellectual ability in children with verbal deficits. *J. Abnorm. Child Psychol.* 8:65, 1980.
55. Roth, F. P., and Spekman, N. J. Assessing the pragmatic abilities of children: Part I. Organizational framework and assessment parameters. *J. Speech Hear. Disord.* 49:2, 1984.
56. Ruess, A. A comparative study of the cleft palate children and their siblings. *J. Clin. Psychol.* 21:354, 1965.
57. Ruess, A., and Lis, F. F. *A Multidimensional Study of Handicapped Children.* Final report to Maternal and Child Health Services, Health Services and Mental Health Administration, U.S. Dept. of Health Education, and Welfare. Grant No. MC-R-170007-04-0, 1973.
58. Saxman, J. H., and Bless, D. M. Patterns of language development in cleft palate children aged 3 to 8 years. Paper presented at American Cleft Palate Association. Oklahoma City, May 1973.
59. Seitz, S., and Marcus, S. Mother-child interactions: A foundation for language development. *Except. Child.* 43:445, 1976.
60. Sinclair-de-Zwart, H. Developmental Psycholinguistics. In D. Elkind and J. H. Flavell (Eds.), *Studies in Cognitive Development.* New York: Oxford University Press, 1969.
61. Smith, R. M., and McWilliams, B. J. Creative thinking abilities of cleft palate children. *Cleft Palate J.* 3:275, 1966.
62. Smith, R. M., and McWilliams, B. J. Psycholinguistic abilities of children with clefts. *Cleft Palate J.* 5:238, 1968.
63. Snow, C. Mother's speech to children learning language. *Child Dev.* 43:549, 1972.
64. Spriesterbach, D. C., et. al. Clinical research in cleft lip and palate: The state of the art. *Cleft Palate J.* 10:113, 1973.
65. Steward, M., and Steward, D. The observation of Anglo-Mexican, and Chinese-American mothers teaching their young sons. *Child Dev.* 11:329, 1973.
66. Terdal, L., Jackson, R., and Garner, A. M. Mother-child interactions: A comparison between normal and developmentally delayed groups. Paper presented to the Banff International Conference on Behavior Modification. Alberta, Canada, March 1974.
67. Warr-Leeper, G., et al. A comparison of the performance of preschool children with cleft lip and/or palate on the *Test of Pragmatic Skills.* Presented at the Annual Convention of the American Cleft Palate Association. Williamsburg, Va., April 1988.
68. Wirle, C. J. Psycho-Social Aspects of Cleft Lip and Palate. In W. C. Grabb, S. W. Rosenstein, and K. B. Bzoch (Eds.), *Cleft Lip and Palate: Surgical, Dental, and Speech Aspects.* Boston: Little, Brown, 1971.

B. Evaluation of Basic Causes of Related Communicative Disorders

CHAPTER 8

Measurement and Assessment of Categorical Aspects of Cleft Palate Language, Voice, and Speech Disorders

Kenneth R. Bzoch

The acoustic image of cleft palate speech is distinctive and unmistakable. Once they have heard it, few students have difficulty distinguishing it.
Charles Van Riper [3]

An objective measurement of speech is required for both research and clinical diagnostic evaluations carried out by speech pathologists on, or receiving referrals from, cleft palate teams. Obtaining, recording, and evaluating objective measurements of speech and behavior and assessing developmental levels of language skills within the short periods of time available during team clinics is the major responsibility of a team speech and language pathologist. This and the following chapters in Part II give the reader a brief but overall review of the state of the art of current clinical and instrumental techniques being used in diagnosing the basic causes of cleft palate communicative disorders and in clinical research in this area.

Before considering clinical tests or instrumental measurements that might objectively record some of the components of speech behavior, it seems advisable to first review for beginning professional students the nature of the energy systems we are referring to as "speech." Before turning to and interpreting instrumental measurements of speech, it is necessary to first use a number of clinical tests whose results are based on the perceptual judgments of a speech pathologist. This can best be accomplished if you first identify, separate, and test for several definable categorical aspects of possible speech deviations often found in speakers born with cleft palate. The need for

this becomes clearer when one first considers the limitations of specific instrumental measures.

In general, scientific instruments are designed to pick up and display or to give the examiner a new or enlarged direct view of only certain parts of the energy forms or physical movement patterns of articulators or of acoustic or air flow outputs involved in the oral language communication process we call speech.

ENERGY FORMS INVOLVED IN SPEECH PRODUCTION AND RECEPTION

Communication through speech is a distinctively human process that involves energy transduction in the body through several different measurable forms. Figure 8-1 suggests the four major forms of energy transmission involved. Note that the same forms are present in reverse order for receptive language functions as those found in expressive language (speech) behavior. Each distinctive form of energy in expressive oral language behavior may be measured in a different way by different instruments. Perceptual judgmental techniques can be best used first to infer probable underlying physical or functional abnormalities of the total process when evaluating abnormal speech behavior. These inferences can then be best verified by specific instrumental tests when possible.

The letter A in Figure 8-1 in the head of the speaker on the left represents the first form of energy in oral language communication. Cognitive functioning is intimately related to what one might here call the potential language encoded thought or idea in the head of the potential speaker. One can start with a scientific description of this aspect of speech behavior as chemical-electrical activity in the central nervous system of the speaker. It exists first as changing waves of chemical-electrical energy generated by inner language, whose patterns of discharge can be partly measured from the skull of the speaker as changing electrical potentials from the cortex of the human brain. These energy forms are measurable by electroencephalography (EEG) and by newer techniques such as positron emission tomography (PET), and variations of magnetic resonance imaging (MRI).

As the thoughts and feelings existing in the conscious mind of a speaker and mediated by language begin to be expressed in speech, they are next channeled as multiple-patterned chemical-electrical discharges in the efferent neural pathways leading to the many muscles controlling the breathing, phonatory, resonance, and articulatory organs of speech. In the muscles of these organs this neural energy is again transduced into neuro-motor discharges (B). These next result in the co-ordinated contraction and relaxation of the many muscles in the breathing, phonatory, and articulatory organs of speech. This second form of energy involved in the speech process might be recorded and measured and has often been studied, in part, by electromyography (EMG).

The contraction and relaxation of muscles throughout the speech mechanism next create actual movements of the supralaryngeal organs of resonance and articulation and of the adduction and abduction of the vocal folds. Such movements of organs of the speech mechanism are represented by the letter C in the oral cavity of Figure 8-1. Visualization and measurements of these movements of organs can be made through cine- or videoflurographic techniques (which limit x-ray exposure through electronic intensification) as reviewed in Chapter 11. Chapter 12 reviews the clinical techniques needed to view and study or evaluate velopharyngeal function during speech more directly through another important technique, nasopharyngoscopic examinations recorded on videotapes. Movements of the velum

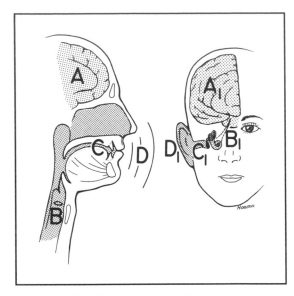

Figure 8-1. The four major types of energy transduction in speech expression and reception.

and surrounding tissues can be viewed directly and can also be recorded on videotapes for later more detailed analysis, as discussed in Chapter 12. Also, more recently, measurements of electrical capacitance change of transducers placed on the palate, which indicate the approach or contact of the dorsum of the tongue, and visual images of tongue movement patterns in speech or swallowing activities recorded by ultrasonography, have been employed to study or infer movement patterns of the tongue or other portions of the organs of articulation during speech.

Multiple-view speech videofluoroscopy with a synchronized sound track appears to be the best technique for visualization and measurement of the several interrelations of phonation and coarticulation involved in the supralaryngeal speech process during this speech organ movement–energy transduction stage of speech production. Nasopharyngoscopy has proved to be the most useful for detailing the several possible structural factors which might contribute to a condition of velopharyngeal insufficiency to support normal speech production.

These physical movements modify the resonance characteristics over the fundamental acoustic waves from the vibration of the vocal folds, affecting resonance quality of voice while shaping the vowel tones and syllabic elements during speech. Also, the physical movements of articulators impinge on the egressive airstream creating the turbulence, stops, and bursts of acoustic energy we call phonemes or distinctive consonant speech sound elements through precise co-articulatory movement patterns. Through these processes, the speech effort is transduced into a final form of energy (D). This form is acoustic energy or sound waves capable of traveling through space at 332 meters per second at sea level at 0°C. The acoustic energy of speech combines (1) the modulated phonatory acoustic waves produced by the vocal folds at the glottis, interrupted by (2) frequent noise elements introduced by turbulence or bursts of sound from the articulated egressive airstream in the oral cavity, and (3) dampening and shifting of resonance formats related to the opening and closing of the velopharyngeal mechanism and also modifications of the resonance chambers in the pharynx and oral cavities from movements of the tongue.

Prior to or just after its emission from the body, instruments sensitive to varying acoustic, air flow, air pressure, or sound pressure energy levels can be used inside or just outside the oral or nasal cavities to measure a transition stage between C and D (see Fig. 8-1) in a speech process. The aerodynamic and computer-augmented oral-nasal acoustic instruments capable of measurements of this final energy tranduction stage are reviewed in Chapters 13 and 14.

The final encoded speech message exists as acoustic energy in the air with embedded meaning from morphemic, syntactic, and semantic speech sound patterns. Acoustic energy can be picked up (transduced) by several types of microphones, recorded and stored for later analysis on tape and several newer recording devices, and displayed on monitors or hard-copy printouts as spectrograms (computer-analyzed voiceprints). Objective acoustic analysis as related to velopharyngeal dysfunction is discussed and illustrated in Chapter 15.

None of the instrumental measures mentioned above really evaluates the totality of speech intelligibility or the correctness of the linguistic message encoded in the acoustic speech energy. This can only be evaluated in total by perceptual judgments of a trained speech and language pathologist. A speech pathologist should develop the skills necessary to further analyze and classify the syllables heard into definable phonetic units; record judgments of omissions, substitutions, and distortions of speech sound elements, relating these to patterns of their several distinctive features; judge phonatory and resonance aspects of

voice quality; and evaluate the correctness of the phonemic, morphemic, syntactic, semantic, and pragmatic aspects of an oral language sample through systematic perceptual judgments of direct or recorded speech utterance samples on standardized tests.

Communication through speech also requires a listener to decode and respond to the expressive speech behavior energy just described. On the right of Figure 8-1, D_1, C_1, B_1, and A_1 represent the necessary transduction process through these same four major energy forms in inverse order, as happens in speech reception. The patterned acoustic energy transmitted by sound waves (D_1) is first changed back into physical movement patterns of body parts by the tympanic membranes of the ears of the listener (C_1). The membrane movements also move the ossicles that transmit the waveform energy next through perilymph and endolymph to transduce physical movements (C_1) back into chemical-electrical energy (B_1) at the hair cells of the cochlea. This chemical-electrical energy is then carried through afferent neural pathways (the eighth cranial nerve) to the central nervous system. In its final form, the energy winds up again as A_1 in the brain of a listener — an auditorially transmitted symbolic communication of meaning between two or more human beings. The audiometric instrumental tests available to record aspects of speech and language reception are covered in Chapter 9.

Through this energy transduction process, A_1 should almost equal A; the psychological phenomenon of conscious awareness of symbolic meaning in the mind of the speaker is transferred to the mind of the listener. The systematic judgments of a trained speech pathologist or of a speech and language scientist regarding aspects of the total process of speech behavior can be recorded through articulation tests, language scales and tests, intelligibility or voice-quality rating scales, or phonetic transcription of connected speech behavior. Such data better measure the end product of the total encoding processes. These data are, however, somewhat subjective judgments, dependent on the skills of the decoder or listener. Only under controlled conditions can these data be shown to be as reliable as most automatic instrumented data.

However, instrumental data can describe only part of the underlying functions leading to speech perception. The ear and auditory cortex of most human beings is an extremely sensitive and reliable extensor sense when properly trained in a speech pathology curriculum of studies. It is as discriminating in certain types of fine auditory perceptions as the eye is in the visual modality. Discriminations for both modalities require the use of the investigator's judgment based on prior knowledge of developmental differences in the modal average of speech and language skills in a cultural language population. In the final analysis, measurements provided by "objective" instruments still also depend on the "subjective" discrimination and interpretations of the visual data produced. They are limited to a part rather than to the total process of speech communication.

Considered in this frame of reference, it seems clear that none of the possible scientific instrumental measures alone can really measure what is called "speech." Each possible instrument responds to and records only limited energy patterns of a portion of one of the transduced forms of energy involved in the process we call human speech communication. Each of the instruments discussed in the following chapters, however, does present a valuable, reliable, and objective means of recording data confirming the speech pathologist's inferences regarding the possible causes of cleft palate speech disorders. However, such data can also be misinterpreted unless logical and operationally defined categories of aspects of the total speech behavior are clearly understood and better illustrated by the instrumental data obtained.

CATEGORICAL ASPECTS OF CLEFT PALATE SPEECH

To say that speech is defective or disordered usually means that a sample of someone's speech behavior has been judged by a given listener to be noticeably unlike the speech of others. The biases of the judge of speech behavior, and the particular conditions under which the speech sample was judged, are therefore significant variables in studies of defective speech for subjects with cleft palate.

Certainly, such undefined terms as *good speech results, normal speech, fair speech,* or *bad speech,* which have been used commonly in the medical and dental literature to support specific medical or surgical procedures or the timing of treatment

are no longer appropriate judgments for future clinical research. Reports based on the general impressions of clinicians in medical or dental specialties or from our own, hopefully, more objective clinical and research profession can still lead both to contradictory and to questionable findings regarding the efficacy of new methods of treatment.

Early examples in the literature which illustrate the probable effects of specialty bias in reported observations include Kingsley's [19] advocacy of dental prostheses to correct velopharyngeal incompetency ("I suppose that there are surgical operations which have enabled the beneficiary to speak correctly — but in all my 40 years of experience I have never seen one") and Oldfield's [24] assessment of 183 of his own cleft palate surgical cases, in which he reported that 90.7 percent of the patients had "normal or good speech." Turner's [39] early assessment of 44 of his surgical cases, in which he indicated that 7 (16%) had "normal speech," 20 (45%) had "good speech," 14 (32% had "fair speech," and only 3 (7%) had "bad speech," shows an effort at more detailed reporting of clinical impressions but is equally questionable on scientific grounds. Objective perceptual judgment tests that are standardized and confirming instrumental indices of abnormal speech behavior should be required in speech and language pathology today.

The need, therefore, for categorizing definable aspects of speech behavior in such a way that they can be more reliably rated or scored or instrumentally measured for verification to yield more objective indices and more detailed data for comparative or controlled clinical research on current treatment methods is indicated by a review of the literature. The need for objective clinical tests as well as instrumental measurements of speech behavior has been recognized for many years.

However, several problems in the former broad classification of speech disorders appear to have imposed limits on past efforts of clinical research in the cleft palate area. These problems include (1) the usual form of basic classification (categorization) of speech disorders by speech pathologists, (2) terminology — the use of different terms by different speech researchers to describe the same problems or phenomena of abnormal speech behavior common in cleft palate speech disorders, and (3) the limitations of instrumental measurements that measure only one part of the speech production process and yet are often used as the only data in reports on the clinical aspects of managing cleft palate speech disorders.

TERMINOLOGY AND CLASSIFICATION PROBLEMS

The concept of defective speech, as used in clinical speech pathology today, includes (1) speech behavior that is a source of embarrassment to a speaker or his listener; (2) speech patterns that generally distract a listener from attending to what is being said, even though it may be completely intelligible; and (3) speech that can be intelligible or not distracting only under conditions of unusual or extreme effort by the speaker. Defective speech is universally understood to refer to any speech behavior that is completely or partially unintelligible.

The term *speech defect* connotes some inadequacy of the physical mechanism for producing speech or an inadequacy of prior learning affecting function. The term is usually not applied to problems such as foreign or regional or even black English dialectical differences as the language is spoken today in the United States. However, these are also problem areas needing our attention and understanding. Such differences do not fit, although they may overlap, the more basic speech problems of cleft palate individuals. Nor should mispronunciation of single, unfamiliar words generally be considered as part of a speech disorder.

Clearly, the speech defects defined above may not be considered defects by some medical or dental clinical investigators on cleft palate teams. Similarly, minor occlusal deviations or cosmetic imperfections considered as defects requiring orthodontic or surgical treatment might be considered as essentially normal conditions by clinical investigators in speech pathology.

For purposes of basic classification, speech disorders are usually classified by speech pathologists as disorders of either (1) articulation, (2) voice, (3) rhythm, and (4) symbolization. However, specific symptoms of defective speech of cleft palate individuals may be very difficult to discuss under these broad terms, particularly for subjects with more complex craniofacial disorders.

Two Special Problems

It appears that two forms of frequent abnormal speech behavior in subjects with clefts, namely, (1) the distortion of consonant sound elements due only to nasal emission, and (2) the substitution of laryngeal or pharyngeal articulations for consonants, are intimately related to judgments of disorders of voice (e.g., they affect voice quality judgments and even some instrumental measurements of hypernasality). They are also related to judgments of disorders of articulation. Speech phenomena related to these two aspects of deviant speech behavior have been, unfortunately, considered with varying terminology as types of either voice or articulation disorders (or both). Their relation to velopharyngeal insufficiency was left uncertain due to this ambivalent categorization.

Nasal Emission: A Voice or Articulation Disorder?

The problem of distortion from nasal emission during the articulation of pressure consonant sounds may be a major reason for the distinctive or identifiable character of cleft palate speech. Nasal emission during the articulation of consonant sounds was considered by Berry and Legg [3] as early as 1912 as an aspect of defective articulation, rather than as a disorder of voice quality. McMahon, however, in 1916, described nasal emission distortions as "an undue amount of nasal resonance and of air passing over the soft palate into the nasal cavities during the production of many of the consonant sounds" [20].

The considerable problem presented to the speech diagnostician of trying to fit the phenomenon of nasal emission into the conceptual framework of voice-versus-articulation disorders of speech led to the use of varying descriptive terminology. Masland [21], for example, referred to consonant distortion from nasal emission as a "nasal aspirate." Brown and Oliver [4] appear to have previously described this same phenomenon as "snorting." Backus [1] used the term *nasal snort* to mean a form of subsitute sound in cleft palate articulation errors. Van Riper and Irwin [43] later distinguished between the hissing nasal escape of air (nasal emission distortion) and a nasopharyngeal snort (apparently a phoneme-specific nasal substitution) as two types of articulation errors in speech.

The problem of recognizing the differences in distortions of consonant sounds due to phoneme-specific or general nasal emission distortions on most pressure consonants, in addition to the accompanying problem of distortion of voice quality on the vowel sounds or syllabic elements, as a resonance voice disorder is critical in the differential diagnosis of underlying velopharyngeal insufficiency, which usually requires secondary surgical reconstruction of the palate. General distortions of speech samples from both nasal emission on most pressure consonants and hypernasal resonance distortion of vowels both appear to be features of cleft palate speech related directly to continued velpharyngeal incompetency and occasionally to nasal habituation after correction of velopharyngeal insufficiency. These subjectively evaluated speech symptoms have been variously considered as either articulation or voice disorders in the past literature.

West, Kennedy, and Car [44] more correctly discussed nasalization distortions of speech from velopharyngeal insufficiency as affecting both of these aspects in subjects with cleft palate:

The nasalization of uranoschillia has two aspects that are mechanically separate: (1) The distortion of the vowels and semivowels by improper resonance of the vocal tone in, and its emission through the nasal chambers; and (2) the distortion of the "pressure" consonants by escape, through the nares, of air that should be impounded in, and directed through, the oral passages.

The overlap of the problem of nasal emission and hypernasal distortion of syllabic elements related to velopharyngeal insufficiency for speech into the former broad categories of *articulation* and *voice disorders* has presented a semantic barrier to uniform testing, measurement, and discussion of cleft palate speech disorders. Nasal emission is a definable and easily measured aspect of deviant speech behavior. There is evidence that its frequency of occurrence under given conditions can be reliably recorded clinically by trained speech pathologists.

The occurrence of nasal emission distortion can also be directly recorded on several objective instruments. However, an equally reliable clinical count of the frequency of abnormal nasal emission occurrence can also be obtained from direct clinical test observations. The employment of any one of several simple devices that produce a visible movement of a paddle, or condensation on a mirror, or enhanced sound signals indicating nasal emission to the tester, improve the reliability and validity of such tests.

Several such early used clinical devices for detecting the occurrence of nasal emission were described insightfully by Morley [22] as early as 1958. The simple *air paddle nasal emission test* first described by Bzoch in 1979 [8] is a current and convenient clinical means of objectively identifying abnormal nasal air flow during pressure consonant articulation without dependence on expensive instruments.

Since nasal emission distortion of consonant sounds is a definable and recordable entity, I suggest that it be regularly considered as *a separate categorical aspect* of articulation in cleft palate speech disorders. It should be distinguished from hypernasal distortion of syllabic elements, which is a resonance voice disorder symptom. It is a second indicator of velopharyngeal insufficiency along with objective indices of hypernasality. This symptom, however, should be distinguished from phoneme-specific nasal emission on only one or a few consistent consonant articulations and from functional types of articulation errors including gross sound substitutions in speech.

Laryngeal and Pharyngeal Gross Substitutions of Consonant Sound Elements

The second special problem frequently found in cleft palate subjects with speech disorders, namely, laryngeal and pharyngeal articulation substitutions for oral consonants, also appears to need a separate classification. Such error patterns usually originate in early infancy due to speech efforts learned during periods of velopharyngeal insufficiency. They should be considered only as evidence of a functional (learned) articulation disorder. This is in contrast to distortions from nasal emission which indicate the continued presence of velopharyngeal incompetency as evidenced during the production of the speech sample. Nasal emission distortions evidence a probable organic speech disorder, namely, a concurrent problem of velopharyngeal insufficiency; gross sound substitutions do not necessarily evidence the same etiology.

However, because gross sound substitution error patterns are associated initially with velopharyngeal insufficiency, and the pattern affects both perceptual judgments and acoustic measures related to hypernasality, it affects clinical judgments of velopharyngeal insufficiency and of voice resonance characteristics as well as articulation. The speech abnormality of a client with frequent gross substitution errors should therefore be classified as a separate functional learning problem in phonology (a functional articulation habit pattern) which is separate from hypernasality. It should be understood that it can be present with or without an underlying problem of velopharyngeal insufficiency for normal speech production.

LIST OF CATEGORICAL ASPECTS

The limited usefulness for clinical or research purposes of simple counts of correct or erroneous sounds on articulation tests, of scaled judgments of nasality or intelligibility, or of phonatory voice disorders required the development of defined *categorical aspects of cleft palate deviant speech*, which could be perceptually measured during a short clinical testing period and which could be obtained from very young as well as older cleft palate subjects. The number of such categories for routine screening testing was expanded from the six discussed by Bzoch [7] in 1961 to the following more complete list of 11 categories. The following list appears in order of their frequency of occurrence in 1,000 consecutive longitudinal case studies evaluated between 1956 and 1970 [8]. Each of these 11 aspects of abnormal speech behavior can be reliably identified and rated or measured under specific, controlled clinical test conditions. The categorical aspects of deviant speech are as follows:

1. Habituation of gross sound substitution error patterns in which laryngeal, pharyngeal or palatal substitution errors of consonant sound elements occur in single words or in connected speech
2. Delayed expressive or receptive language development not accounted for by concurrent problems of deafness, hearing loss, or mental retardation factors alone
3. Hypernasal resonance distortion of vocal quality perceived as distortions of vowels and other syllabic sound elements due directly to atypical nasal resonance
4. Distortion of consonant sounds due to abnormal nasal emission of air flow from velopharyngeal insufficiency or palatal fistulae
5. Developmental dyslalia (e.g., occurrence of an excessive number of functional articulation errors more typical of younger subjects than of cleft palate speech)
6. Dysphonia characterized by weak and aspirate (breathy) voice
7. Lisping and other articulation distortions which can be directly related to specific dental or occlusal abnormalities (e.g., dental-related articulation distortions which appear to require dental or occlusal treatment before speech therapy can be most effective)
8. Hyponasal (denasal) resonance distortions of voice quality (e.g., perceived and measurable atypical denasality affecting the quality of vowels, syllabic, and particularly nasal consonants)
9. Hoarse voice quality (e.g., dysphonia characterized by a rough or uneven fundamental laryngeal vibration suggesting hyperlaryngeal function or a possible laryngeal pathological condition)
10. Speech disorders or delayed receptive-expressive language skills related to hearing loss or deafness (e.g., an early history of chronic or recurrent otitis media, congenital atresia in craniofacial syndromes such as Treacher Collins syndrome and hemifacial microsomia, or occasional sensorineural deafness.
11. Communication problems from visual distraction of the listener due to habituated nasal or facial grimacing during speech related to excessive nasal emission from velopharyngeal insufficiency

The speech pathologist on a cleft palate team needs to be able to identify, distinguish, and measure all of these possible forms of common articulation, voice, and language problems. This is especially important during the early preschool years when normal peers also present with developmental differences in speech, voice characteristics, and in emergent language skills. Language, voice, and articulation skills are immature and rapidly changing developmentally during this period of development between 1 and 4 years of age.

The speech clinician will usually have only limited time to gain sufficient rapport with clients aged 2 to 4 years to conduct direct test-response measure of articulation and voice quality characteristics (both phonatory and resonance-related) or to conduct a complete assessment of the phonemic, morphemic, syntactic, semantic, and pragmatic levels of oral language skill development. Therefore, a test battery including direct standardized tests of nasal emission, hypernasality, hyponasality, phonation, and a broad-ranging screening speech articulation error pattern test, along with a parent interview language development scale measure, have proved useful for this purpose. A further discussion on interpreting developmental and error pattern articulation test data and of language development evaluations under these conditions therefore precedes specific discussion of management of each of the 11 categorical aspects listed above.

RECOMMENDED CLINICAL TEST BATTERY

Figure 8-2 illustrates the form used to record a set of five basic short clinical test procedures which have been studied and shown to yield sufficient reliable test data to infer judgments regarding the adequacy or inadequacy of velopharyngeal function for speech and the presence of functional abnormal articulatory or phonatory speech patterns in cleft palate clinics. This short battery, along with normative language scale measures and audiometric tests, has proved useful for standardized routine evaluations of communicative disorders in infants and children in cleft palate team clinics. It is equally applicable for adult patients. Data from such tests can be used in clinical research regarding the comparative efficacy of differing treatment procedures within and between team centers [9, 12]. The following is a brief discussion of the rationale and procedures to be followed in administering and interpreting the test battery illustrated in Figure 8-2.

The Nasal Emission Test

The nasal emission test has proved to be the single most valuable speech evaluation procedure for drawing an inference regarding the adequacy or inadequacy of velopharyngeal function to support normal voice and articulation development following primary surgical reconstruction of cleft palate. It is particularly useful for testing 2- to 4-year-old cleft palate subjects.

A difficult but important responsibility of the speech pathologist on a cleft palate team is the decision as to the adequacy or inadequacy of velopharyngeal function following primary surgery during a period of development of rapid changes in developmental speech and language skills for all children. At this most critical period of development, objective instrumental studies are often difficult to obtain because of the inability to cooperate of very young subjects and the cost and availability of instruments for use in small clinical settings. The nasal emission test can be completed by an experienced speech pathologist in 2 to 3 minutes of direct testing. The procedure for the initial short nasal emission test is described below. We first review its rationale and validity.

The rationale for the nasal emission test seems evident from basic principles of speech physiology and phonetic sciences. If there is any leak in a pneumatic system, air under pressure should

flow (be emitted) through that opening. If the hard palate is intact and the velopharyngeal mechanism is able to seal completely for pressure consonant sounds, air should not flow through the nose under the conditions of this test procedure.

The validity of this rationale was tested in the pediatric screening clinic at our institution when the test was adopted as a standard procedure for all longitudinal speech evaluations in our craniofacial center weekly clinics. A rural normal population of 100 children, 50 males and 50 females, aged 2 years, 6 months to 5 years, 7 months were tested. All tests (100% of bisyllable word utterances) yielded an index of 0/10 (no clinical evidence of nasal emission) for each subject tested. Further, a retrospective study of the level of agreement of independent judgments of the adequacy or inadequacy of velopharyngeal function for 40 clinical case studies, based on this test alone and separately from speech cinefluorographic studies alone, yielded a 96 percent agreement.

Finally, studies of nasal emission in the literature using more refined instrumental measures have reported similar findings. A study reported by Thompson and Hixon in 1979 [37] was in total agreement with our studies. They used an individually custom-formed mask that was placed over the nose of the subject to detect air flow with a pneumotachometer coupled to a differential air pressure transducer. Each subject spoke the nonsense syllables /iti/, /idi/, /isi/, and /izi/, embedded in a carrier phrase. Their normal sample included 112 subjects, 59 females and 53 males, ranging in age from 3 year to 37 years, 6 months. They found zero nasal flow for 3,996 individual utterances of these syllables. It appears from the above that an index of 1/10 to 10/10 indicates some level of velopharyngeal inadequacy, particularly for simple two-syllable utterances repeated after oral stimulation.

The nasal emission test was standardized on a set of 10 two-syllable words, each containing either two unvoiced or two voiced bilabial plosives, /p/ or /b/. The words are generally easily repeated by subjects 2 years of age or older. A simple air flow paddle held under the nose, as described by Bzoch [8], or a small mirrored surface, or a headset listening device suffice to enhance the visual or auditory perceptions of the tester to detect occurrences of nasal air flow timed with visible bilabial articulations. The procedure to be followed is simply to observe and record evidence of atypical nasal emission occurring during the impounding and explosive phases of

CRANIOFACIAL CENTER COMMUNICATIVE DISORDERS CLINICAL TESTS - 1982-A
K. BZOCH, Ph.D.

Name _____ Birth _____ Age ____ Sex ____ No. _____

Examiner _____ Date _____ Stimulus Oral/Reading/Pix

I. Nasal Emission Test:

Circle words or syllables uttered that evidenced nasal air flow (i.e., indicated Velopharyngeal insufficiency); air flow checked by FLA II ☐ , Paddle ☐ , Bubble ☐ , other _____ .

a. people   paper   puppy   pepper   piper

   baby   Bobby   bubble   B.B.   bye-bye

b. For infants test (pi) syllable ten times:

   P   P   P   P   P   P   P   P   P   P

Nasal Emission Score _____/_____

II. Hypernasality Test:

Circle words or vowels on which a shift in tone quality occurred when nares were closed (i.e., indicated Velpharyngeal insufficiency); ask patient first to repeat word loudly then to say again while nares are pinched.

a. Beat   bit   bait   bet   bat

   bought   boat   boot   but   Bert

For infants or speechless try simpler test of alternately pinching and opening nares as patient utters prolonged vowels /i/ as in see and /u/ as in new; circle those that shift.

b. /i/ /u/ /i/ /u/ /i/ /u/ /i/ /u/ /i/ /u/

Hypernasality Score _____/_____

III. Hyponasality Test:

Circle words or nasal sounds which sound the same (i.e., indicated block nasal passages) when nares are pinched closed as when open; otherwise proceed as above.

a. meat   mit   mate   met   mat

   moat   moot   mut   Mert   might

For infants or speechless, have patient hum (i.e., prolong /m/ then /n/ as tested).

/m/ /n/ /m/ /n/ /m/ /n/ /m/ /n/ /m/ /n/

Hyponasality Score _____/_____

IV. Phonation Test

	Duration	Aspirate	Hoarse
/i/	Sec. _____	Yes/No	Yes/No
/a/	Sec. _____	Yes/No	Yes/No
/u/	Sec. _____	Yes/No	Yes/No

©

V. Error Pattern Screening Articulation Test

C = Correct $\tilde{I}$ = indistinct from nasal emission alone
D = distortion (.5 error) SS = simple substitution (1.0 error)
GS = gross substitution (1.5 error)   O = (2.0 error)

PLOSIVES		C	$\tilde{I}$	D	SS	GS	O
/p/	aPPle						
/b/	baBy						
/t/	mounTain						
/d/	canDy						
/k/	chiCKen						
/g/	waGon						

FRICATIVES							
/f/	elePHant						
/v/	shoVel						
/ө/	tooTHbrush						
/ᵭ/	feaTHer						
/s/	bicyCLe						
/z/	sciSSors						
/ʃ/	diSHes						
/ʒ/	televiSion						

AFFRICATES							
/tʃ/	maTCHes						
/dʒ/	briDGes						

GLIDES							
/w/	sandWich						
/l/	baLLons						
/y/	onIOns						
/r/	aRRow						

NASALS							
/m/	haMMer						
/n/	baNana						
/ŋ/	haNGer						

BLENDS							
/sp/	SPider						
/str/	STRawberries						
/st/	STar						
/SK/	SKirt						
/sm/	SMoke						
/bl/	BLock						
/kl/	Clown						
/br/	BRoom						

ARTICULTATION SCORE $C + \tilde{I}$ = _____

.5x___ 1x___ 1.5x___ 2x___

ERROR SCORE = _____

Figure 8-2. Standard battery of craniofacial clinical tests for use during cleft palate team evaluations.

bilabial articulation of the set of words on the form as repeated by the subject after the tester.

Experience indicates that most 2- and 3-year-old subjects can be tested completely to determine a base 10 index of nasal emission. However, the test is invalid if glottal co-articulation occurs with the bilabial articulations. This can be determined by first holding the air flow paddle or positioning the end of the headset listening device at the lips. If glottal co-articulation is occurring habitually there will be little or no release of impounded air pressure for the explosive phase of the plosive productions on /p/ and /b/ syllables. A training session (a period of diagnostic therapy) will be necessary before a valid nasal emission test can be given under these conditions.

The Hypernasality Test

The hypernasality test was standardized on a set of 10 one-syllable words, each beginning with a /b/ and ending with a /t/. The syllabic elements in the words selected sample the vowel triangle from high-front to low-back to high-back tongue positions for vowels. The purpose of the test is to yield a base 10 count of the frequency of occurrence of hypernasal resonance on single words with vowels in a plosive environment. These should always have no nasal resonance under conditions of normal velopharyngeal valving. The syllabic elements are initiated and closed off by pressure consonant sounds, a condition which predisposes to complete velopharyngeal seal and no nasal resonance in normal speech production.

The tester simply asks the subject to repeat each word 2 times. On the second utterance, the subject or tester pinches the nares closed, changing the open nasal resonator into a cul-de-sac or closed resonator. A perceptual judgment is made by the tester comparing the quality of the first and second utterances. Words that shift in quality under the second cul-de-sac resonance conditions are circled on the recording form. The total number of words with apparent hypernasal resonance on the vowel elements yields a base 10 index of hypernasality.

The validity of this test was demonstrated by O'Shea [25]. She demonstrated a 91+ percent exact agreement between data from this procedure alone and vocalic peak amplitude measures of 10 subjects producing oral and nasal syllables measured by a piezoelectric microphone transducer attached to the bridge of the nose. She also determined that the variable of fundamental frequency

of male or female subjects had no significant effect on the validity of this test or the similar test for hyponasality described below. Since the clinical hypernasality test enhances the tester's perception of the presence of hypernasal resonance by shifting formats and creating a greater distinction between oral and nasal syllables, it is particularly useful for use in the often noisy environments prevalent during cleft palate team clinical speech evaluations.

The Hyponasality Test

The hyponasality test is conducted similarly to the hypernasality test. However, the rules for recording judgments of abnormal productions are reversed, as the stimulus words selected should be produced with perceivable nasal resonance since they are all initiated by the bilabial nasal consonant /m/. The same alternate open-and-closed cul-de-sac resonance test procedure should be followed. However, a perceivable shift in resonance should occur under the conditions of this test. Therefore, if a difference is not perceived when the nares are closed, an abnormal denasal syllable production occurred indicating the presence of hyponasality from some blockage of the nasal resonating chambers or at the velopharyngeal mechanism. This test is particularly useful following an obturating pharyngeal flap procedure or the placement of a muscle-trimmed speech appliance.

A shift in resonance quality between the conditions of open and closed nares is to be expected. If not perceived, the test words should be circled. The number of words initiated by nasal consonants produced without nasal resonance provides a clinical index of hyponasality.

The Phonation Test

A routine phonation test is also called for during cleft palate team speech evaluations. Both hoarseness and weak aspirate voice production occurred frequently in past samples of this population of clients. Pragmatically, a short isolated vowel phonation test appears to be adequate for identifying such phonatory voicing problems along with impressions from conversational speech. Since vowels and syllabic elements are only rarely misarticulated in developmental phonology in this population, but hyper- and hyponasal resonance characteristics may be common, the cleft palate team speech pathologists need to look specifically for phonatory compensations which may have been learned and habituated in compensaton for velopharyngeal insufficiency in early life. Specifically, the presence or absence of habituated hoarseness or aspirate voice quality should be identified during routine team speech reevaluations. Also, since phonatory judgments have been shown to be influenced by the consonant environment of the words evaluated, this test should be limited to judgments of phonatory quality during sustained vowel phonation.

The standardized test procedure is simply to ask the subject to repeat the sounds /i/, /a/, and /u/, first with the tester and then in isolation, as long as possible on one inhalation. Unless aspirate phonation is strongly habituated, subjects should be able to sustain isolated vowel phonation for 10 or more seconds with motivation on two or three trials. If phonation cannot be sustained and the quality of the voice sounds aspirate and weak, it is an indication of habituated breathy voice. This judgment can be confirmed by close observations of interruptions of connected speech for frequent inhalation that disturb thought group phrasing during propositional speech.

Any perceived roughness of the fundamental laryngeal vibrations during isolated prolonged vowel phonation should be interpreted as hoarseness. If confirmed by impressions of hoarse voice in connected conversational speech, this clinical impression should lead to further investigation through indirect or direct laryngeal examinations to determine the possible presence of vocal nodules or other pathological conditions.

The Error Pattern
Screening Articulation Test

The Error Pattern Screening Articulation Test has been described in some detail [8, 9]. The test words selected and the order of testing are indicated by the recording form in Figure 8-2. Further clinical experience has verified that this short 31-word oral stimulus testing procedure yields very valuable information and usually provides a sufficient test sample to aid in several judgments regarding the functional or organic basis of speech deviations for early preschool children as well as adult subjects born with clefts and evaluated for rehabilitation of related cleft palate speech disorders.

This test or some alternate form of single-word articulation testing is usually required to make several judgments regarding the nature and level of phonological skills. However, client's responses must be related to developmental age and the apparent presence or absence of underlying organic problems needing surgical or dental correction. Articulation error pattern test data are also especially needed to develop the focus of needed speech therapy service programs.

The screening test procedure consists simply of the speech pathologist making several judgments of the correctness or of the type of articulation errors which occur on 31 speech sound consonantal elements (first for medial–word position consonants and then in consonant clusters). The words are repeated after the tester by the subject. Elementary words known by most young subjects constitute the stimulus word set. All single-consonant sound test elements are embedded in medial word positions predisposing to the types of errors which occur in connected speech. The speech sound elements tested sample the skills required for plosive, fricative, affricate, glide, and nasal consonants followed by a sampling of the most common two- and three-consonant clusters occurring in kindergarten word lists.

Figure 8-2 also indicates the types of judgments required of the tester for error pattern analysis to aid in management decisions. Error pattern judgments require that correct productions of the target sound be simply checked in the C (for correct) column. Perceived distortions which are judged correct in motor speech articulation for both place and manner of formation but which are distorted by nasal emission are checked in the I (for indistinct due to nasal emission distortion alone) column. The nasal air flow paddle, or a similar device, should be used to confirm such judgments whenever the tester is uncertain. Enhancement through visual or auditory cues from simple clinical instruments such as an air flow paddle or a listening device held under the nares helps in the judgments of frequency of occurrence of errors related to nasal emission alone.

Articulation errors that are judged to be allophones of the target sound, but to be somewhat distorted due to imprecise articulation, should be recorded by a check in the D (for distortion error) column. Perceived lateral distortions related directly to malocclusions or missing teeth can be verified by holding an air flow paddle to the middle or lateral portions of the lips during the production of test words with the target sounds /s/, etc. Dentally related lateral lisping distortions should also be checked in the D column with a note as to their apparent dental-related etiology.

Whenever an error on a target sound is perceived as more like an allophone of other American English phoneme (e.g., more like an indistinct

/t/ than a /k/, or more like an indistinct /p/ than an /f/), that specific sound substitution error should be recorded in the SS (simple substitution) error column rather than in the D column. Record as It/k or as Ip/f to enable a better kinetic analysis of existing error patterns in the subject's speech habits.

Any occurrence of gross sound substitution errors for single-consonant elements or in consonant clusters should be recorded in the GS (gross substitution) column with the appropriate phonetic symbols for glottal stops, pharyngeal and velar fricatives, and related sound substitutions as reviewed in Chapter 6.

The reliability of clinical judgments of omission errors is simplified on this test since the omission of medial-position consonant sounds has to be uttered as a single syllable rather than as a two-syllable word utterance. Errors of omission of a target sound or complete cluster are simply checked in the O (omission) column.

DEVELOPMENTAL EVALUATIONS OF PHONOLOGICAL SKILLS OF PRESCHOOL CHILDREN

When conducting direct articulation test evaluations with young children, it is necessary to pay close attention to the types of errors made rather than the number of sound elements correctly or incorrectly produced. Since articulation errors in general have been shown to be inconsistent, it is recommended that the examiner record only the most severe type of error on any repeated testing of a test element. It is also recommended that auditory stimulus-response testing rather than picture stimuli be used. This saves time for other testing and yields more relevant data for error pattern analysis of young preschool children. This is because when an examiner first clearly pronounces a test word and the child responds by repeating that word with an error in production of a test sound element, that specific error type is strongly habituated in the speech behavior of the child. If the child had self-corrected on some of the sound elements because he heard the word first, those errors he might have additionally made by naming pictures are probably of little

diagnostic value during this period of rapid maturation, learning, and improvement in articulation skills by all children.

Arranging the set of articulation test words by manner of formation of test sound elements, limiting the test sound elements to nonsyllabics (i.e., consonants and their blends), and using the medial position for screening tests of single consonants further facilitates error pattern analysis, although any standardized articulation test procedure can be similarly interpreted.

The usual developmental articulation mastery patterns of children without clefts before the age of mastery were indicated long ago by the Templin [35] or Poole [27] norms. The more characteristic developmental substitution errors on unmastered sound elements were described by Bzoch [6, 8] and compared with errors of a matched cleft palate sample. These comparative data are shown in Table 8-1. Recent studies in developmental phonology before and after 2 years of age support these earlier findings in regard to sounds usually mastered in speech and developmental errors which often occur in normal maturation, and present greater detail for the interpretation of developmental error pattern test findings. It appears from recent reports that most developmental phonological systems develop rapidly during the months prior to the second birthday [16, 17, 28].

The literature on developmental phonology now provides beginning clinicians with the data needed to identify the usual developmental error patterns which should change with maturation alone through infancy and early childhood and to distinguish these from the usual error patterns that develop in cleft palate infants and young children [16, 17].

Preisser, Hodson, and Paden [28] reported in 1988 in some detail on the usual developmental error patterns found for 60 normally developing children aged 18 through 29 months. Their findings, which are particularly pertinent to this discussion, are paraphrased below:

1. Consonant cluster reductions such as /pun/ for /spun/ were the most common form of omissions.
2. The frequency of occurrence of such error patterns diminished rapidly for subjects who were 2 years, 2 months or older.
3. The most liquid were most often omitted in clusters that consisted of an obstruent and a liquid.

TABLE 8-1. A COMPARISON OF THE MOST FREQUENT TYPES OF ARTICULATION SUBSTITUTION ERRORS MADE BY PRESCHOOL CHILDREN BORN WITH CLEFTS AND A MATCHED GROUP OF NORMAL CHILDREN

Speech Sound Element Tested	Templin Norm [34]	Poole Norm [27]	Errors of Control Subjects (N = 120, 3–6 yr.)	Errors of Cleft Palate Subjects in Order of Frequency of Occurrence (N = 60, 3–6 yr.)
/p/	3	3.5	None	?/p, PF*
/b/	4	3.5	p/b	m/b, ?/b
/t/	6	4.5	d/t	?/t, PF, k/t
/d/	4	4.5	t/d	?/d, PF, n/d
/k/	4	4.5	t/k	?/k, PF, t/k
/g/	4	4.5	k/g, d/g	?/g, d/g, PF
/f/	3	5.5	p/f, b/f, s/f	?/f, PF, p/f
/v/	6	6.5	b/v, f/v	b/v, ?/v, m/v
θ	6	7.5	t/θ, s/θ, f/θ	?/θ, PF, t/θ
/ð/	7	6.5	d/ð	d/ð, ?/ð, PF
/s/	4.5	7.5	θ/s, t/s	PF, ?/s, t/s
/z/	7	7.5	s/z, θ/z, d/z	PF, ?/z, s/z
/ʃ/	4.5	6.5	s/ʃ, tʃ/ʃ	PF, ?/ʃ
/tʃ/	4.5	—	ʃ/tʃ, s/tʃ, t/tʃ	PF, ?/tʃ, ʃ/tʃ
/dʒ/	7	—	tʃ/dʒ, d/dʒ, ʒ/dʒ	PF, ?/dʒ, ʒ/dʒ
/l/	6	6.5	w/l	w/l, ?/l
/j/	3.5	4.5	?/j	?/j, w/j, l/j
/r/	4	7.5	w/r	w/r, j/r, PF
/w/	3	3.5	j/w	?/w, l/w
/m/	3	3.5	b/m	PF, ?/m
/n/	3	4.5	m/n	?/n, j/n
/ŋ/	3	4.5	n/ŋ	n/ŋ

* PF = either pharyngeal or velar fricative substitution.

4. In consonant clusters of two obstruents, the strident segment was deleted most often.
5. Deletion of postvocalic singleton obstruents (omission of the final consonant sound elements in words) was the second most frequent omission pattern with a mean occurrence of 21 percent overall.
6. Syllable reductions (omission of the final whole syllables in two- and three-syllable words) had a 19 percent occurrence overall.
7. Omission of final consonants or syllables occurred frequently for children aged 1 year, 6 months to 1 year, 9 months (45% and 43%, respectively), while children 1 year, 10 months to 2 years, 1 month of age had such error patterns only 13 and 10 percent of the time, respectively, and most children over 2 years old had learned to close syllables and sequence syllables in words.
8. Prevocalic singleton obstruent deletions were infrequent (e.g., initial consonants were seldom omitted although substitutions of sounds occurred in initial word positions), even for the youngest children.
9. Regressive velar assimilation (e.g., /k/ for /t/ substitutions) were the most frequent assimilation process.
10. Depalatization and deaffrication substitu-

tions (e.g., /wats/ for /watʃ/ or /zus/ for the word juice (/dʒus/) were fairly common.
11. One third of the subjects evidenced palatization errors (e.g., /ʃup/ for /sup) and affrication errors (e.g., /tsup/ for /sup/).
12. The only other phonological processes, used mainly by the youngest subjects, were metatheses (e.g., /p/ for /k/ or /k/ for /p/) and/or prevocalic voicing.

From a more pragmatic articulation error pattern frame of reference, these more linguistically labeled findings mean simply that developmentally one may find frequent omissions of single-consonant sound elements in the final position of test words in the usual phonological patterns of 1- and 2-year-old children. These same sound elements, however, may be correctly produced in the initial position but substituted for or distorted in medial positions in words uttered at this age.

Omissions of final consonants at 3 years of age or older should signal a developing problem of developmental dyslalia or functional articulation skill disorder.

The correct production of clearly articulated initial oral pressure consonants (plosives or fricatives) should indicate to the tester a potential velopharyngeal adequacy to support normal speech production with maturation and learning. Errors in the production of initial bilabial consonants /p/ and /b/ should be very infrequent at 1 and 2 years of age.

Substitution errors of medial-position test sound elements in words are common at age 2 and are still frequent at 3 years of age, as compared to correct production of initial consonants in single-word utterances. However, the substitution of /p/for /f/ by a 2- or 3-year-old client with corrected cleft palate is not uncommon in any word position. It also reveals the ability to produce stop consonants without nasal distortion, indicating potential velopharyngeal adequacy to support normal speech production.

The substitution of plosives for fricatives at 2 up to 3 years of age, or of cognate substitution errors such as /t/ for /d/, or the use of /w/ for /r/ or /l/, are frequent at age 2 and occasionally at 3 years of age in normal development. These substitutions should change to distortions and then to correct productions for most fricative sounds by 4 years of age with maturation alone. Similar types of substitutions may often occur in initial–word position test elements, but these are usually correctly produced before the established norms for the fricative phonemic elements in overall developmental speech mastery.

The two- and three-consonant clusters are usually produced as single-sound elements developmentally (e.g., /p/ for /sp/, /t/ for /st/ or /str/, /m/ for /sm/, /b/ for /bl/, /p/ for /pl/, etc.) up to 2½ years of age. However, before 3 years of age they are usually developmentally mastered by maturation alone.

Table 8-1 presents an earlier recorded listing of the most common types of articulation sound substitution errors found for 120 children without clefts aged 3 to 6 years who were considered to be "normal" compared to those found for 60 matched children with cleft palate. The table clearly shows that basically different articulation error patterns may occur between these two population samples. The subjects evaluated were closely matched in age, race, sex, and family socioeconomic levels [5]. The tendency early to develop atypical articulation skills as well as voicing disorders in cleft palate speech, speech production errors that are basically functional in nature, supports the need for early articulation-based testing and intervention therapy in this population.

ON ARTICULATION TESTS (PHONOLOGICAL EVALUATIONS) IN GENERAL

It appears from past clinical research experience that the assessment or measurement of articulation skills of any infant or preschool-age cleft palate client should include tests which sample a subject's ability to produce sets of particular speech sound elements (phonemes) in single words organized in a particular pattern. A panel of seven speech pathologists experienced in the cleft palate area recently recommended that some form of error pattern articulation test be included in any method of assessing speech in relation to velopharyngeal function [14].

Diagnostic single-word articulation tests are best for both clinical assessments and for planning therapy or as a means of obtaining reliable scores describing speech behavior for clinical management and research. Such tests usually attempt to evaluate the correctness and level of precision of the majority of the basic motor articulations of the organs of speech required by the phoneme units of our language system.

However, a single-word diagnostic articulation test should only be a major part of any complete developmental phonological assessment of speech articulation skills. The articulation errors in a sample of connected speech need to be identified and compared with the errors on single-word utterances. The subject's ability to correctly imitate sounds in isolation after stimulation for the sound elements misarticulated in words should also be evaluated. If time does not allow this further evaluation during the cleft palate clinic, a referral for more in-depth testing should be recommended.

Published standardized articulation tests often used in cleft palate studies include the Templin-Darley Screening and Diagnostic Tests of Articulation [36]; the Iowa Pressure Articulation Test, evaluated by Morris, Spriesterbach, and Darley [23], for assessing competency of velopharyngeal closure; and the Bzoch Error Pattern Diagnostic Screening Articulation tests [8].

An experienced speech pathologist can also conduct reliable articulation evaluations using other types of materials, including recording for later analysis of oral readings of phonetically selected sentences or paragraphs by older patients. Analyzing free conversational speech samples directly or as recorded on a tape recorder and played back for phonetic analysis is another useful method of evaluting phonological speech articulation developmental status.

However, most experienced speech pathologists use some form of systematic single-word diagnostic articulation test to gather descriptive data about patients with a congenital cleft palate condition. This is because articulation test data in particular can be used to make inferences regarding several underlying variables of learned abnormal articulation patterns as contrasted to errors caused directly by velopharyngeal insuffiency of the test subjects. Articulation test data should be used to better determine the need for and to interpret instrumental data to form a judgment regarding abnormal physical mechanisms or the more probable functional causes of abnormal speech behavior in cleft palate individuals.

DIAGNOSTIC ERROR PATTERN ARTICULATION TEST

The more detailed diagnostic articulation test described here was designed to facilitate identification of error patterns related more to velopharyngeal insufficiencies than to functional learning problems. It is described below, in part, along with its rationale and the rules for error pattern–type classifications of speech articulation behavior that are important for developing early preventive and interventive cleft palate speech disorder therapy management programs.

Specific types of articulation error patterns are more easily identified on the recording form illustrated in Figure 8-3. The target sound elements are in the initial, medial, and final morphemic word utterance positions in which they occur in connected speech utterances. A kinetic phonemic analysis of errors is facilitated by grouping test sound elements by manner of formation, place of articulation, and voicing differences. The recording form indicates the order of testing from top to

bottom and from left to right. The symbols above the columns indicate the six types of judgments to be made, as in the screening test, for each test sound element or cluster.

The rationale of the error pattern diagnostic articulation test is based on research findings by Bzoch [5] of the most frequent characteristics of articulation errors in developmental cleft palate and matched normal control subject speech behavior differences between 3 and 6 years of age. It appeared from the data that the vowel sounds and the majority of the syllabic consonant sound elements and glides (with the exception of /w/) were usually mastered early in the speech of both groups of normal and cleft palate preschool children.

These syllabic speech sound elements, which constitute a large part of other articulation test items, were therefore not considered to be generally of sufficient import for inclusion in diagnostic articulation error pattern articulation testing for cleft palate subjects. In general, the testing of vowels or repeated word sets of syllabic consonants failed to distinguish or to add much information needed to distinguish or delineate the several abnormal speech articulation patterns most characteristic of cleft palate speech development.

The term *speech articulation* is here considered to refer to the perceived effects of underlying movement patterns of the organs of speech including the velopharyngeal mechanism (i.e., the co-articulation of lips, front of the tongue, and back of the tongue with velopharyngeal valving), which relate directly to the acoustic output of speech. Syllables, that is, the basic physiological units of speech encoding, as contrasted to nonsyllabic speech sound elements, are generally formed by moving from a greater constriction in the speaking mechanism through a vowel or semiconsonantal shaping of the oral and pharyngeal cavities to the next nonsyllabic articulation constriction. The focus of articulation competency testing in this test, therefore, is on the more specific areas of constriction which produce the nonsyllabic or consonant sound and cluster elements in connected speech. These speech sound elements are more directly affected by velopharyngeal incompetency than are syllables.

Errors of habitual consonant sound misarticulation present information bearing directly on underlying possible abnormal motor speech habit patterns or on the presence of evidence of velopharyngeal insuffiency. This is particularly true in

BZOCH ERROR PATTERN DIAGNOSTIC ARTICULATION TEST #1   1982-A

K. R. BZOCH, Ph.d.

	PLOSIVES	C	T̂	D	SS	GS	O		C	Ĩ	D	SS	GS	O		C	T̂	D	SS	GS	O
/p/	Pencil							aPPle							cuP						
/b/	Ball							baBy							tuB						
/t/	Table							mounTain							boaT						
/d/	Dog							canDy							beD						
/k/	Cat							chiCKen							booK						
/g/	Gun							waGon							piG						

FRICATIVES
		C		D	SS	GS	O				D	SS	GS	O				D	SS	GS	O
/f/	Fork							elePHant							kniFE						
/v/	Vase							shoVel							stoVE						
/ǝ/	THumb							tooTHbrush							mouTH						
/ʒ/	THis							feaTHer							baTHE						
/s/	Sun							bicyCLe							houSE						
/z/	Zipper							sciSSors							noSE						
/ʃ/	SHoe							diSHes							fiSH						
/ʒ/	XXXXX							televiSion							garaGE						

AFFRICATIVES
| /tʃ/ | CHair | | | | | | | maTCHes | | | | | | | waTCH | | | | | | |
| /dʒ/ | Juice | | | | | | | briDGes | | | | | | | oranGE | | | | | | |

ASPIRATES
| /h/ | Horse | | | | | | | grassHopper | | | | | | | XXXXXX | | | | | | |

GLIDES
/w/	Window							sandWich							XXXXXX						
/l/	Lion							baLLoons							doLL						
/y/	Yarn							onIOns							XXXXXX						
/r/	Rabbit							aRRow							caR						

NASALS
/m/	Man							haMMer							druM						
/n/	Nail							baNana							traiN						
/ŋ/	XXXXXX							haNGer							swiNG						

BLENDS
	SPider							STar							neST						
	STRawberries							SKirt							boX						
	SLide							SMoke							SNake						
	PLiers							BLock							beLT						
	worLD							CLown							FLag						
	PResent							BRoom							TRuck						
	DRess							heaRT							swoRD						
	CRy							GRapes							coRK						
	FRog							THRead							aRM						
	dropPED							inseCT							siFT						
	WHeel							teNT							haND						

COLUMN TOTALS = _____ _____ _____ _____ _____ _____   _____ _____ _____ _____ _____ _____   _____ _____ _____ _____ _____ _____
C T̂ D SS GS O   C T̂ D SS GS O   C T̂ D SS GS O

ARTICULATION SCORE   =   TOTAL CORRECT _____   +   TOTAL INDISTINCT FROM NASAL EMISSION ALONE _____ = _____

ERROR SCORE = .5 X D ERRORS _____   +   1 X SS ERRORS _____   +   1.5 X GS ERRORS _____   +   2 X 0 ERRORS _____ = _____

Figure 8-3. Bzoch Error Pattern Diagnostic Articulation Test recording form indicating order of testing and types of clinical judgments based on target sounds to be made.

errors judged to occur from distortion due to nasal emission alone.

The sound elements produced by consonant constrictions in this test are organized in the order following their manner of formation of sounds as classified by Thomas [38]. The evaluation begins with the truest nonsyllabic category, the *plosives*. Within each grouping the most peripheral articulations, moving to the most posterior place of articulation, are tested first. Cognate pairs (sounds articulated alike except for laryngeal voicing) are listed in sequence through the *plosive, fricative,* and *affricate* categories. The unvoiced precedes the voiced cognate sound.

The basic diagnostic test has four alternate forms for research purposes, each with a different word set. Each set of test words permits the evaluation of articulation precision on a total of 100 nonsyllabic elements. The majority are single-consonant elements, which are tested in the initial, medial, and final word positions. In addition, there are 33 two- or three-consonant cluster elements which occur frequently in early speech and language behavior. These are the blends that occur most frequently in common English words.

A total of 100 test elements was chosen to facilitate percentage and decimal calculations, because a base of 100 forms the basis of many standardized tests in psychology and education, and because the length of the test was deemed adequate for clinical and research purposes without being unduly lengthy or time-consuming.

The following rules and operational definitions were developed to enable each tester to make similar judgments and to help establish a high level of reliability of the error judgment data.

Rules for judging and recording articulation errors on single-consonant elements: Record all judgments regarding the subject's correct or incorrect responses to test words, testing each phoneme first in the initial, then in the medial, and then in the final position. If the test sound is produced correctly by the subject on the first attempt (regardless of other errors in the word), record the judgment of the correct response by placing a check in the C (correct) column. If the test sound is articulated correctly but perceived as indistinct due to concomitant nasal emission alone, place a check in the I (indistinct) column. Tabulate such errors separately but add their number to the correct number for determining the total correct motor articulation score. When a test sound element is produced in error on the first attempt, have the subject repeat the same word again, 2

more times. Record on the test form only the most severe error perceived in accordance with the following order of error-type severity: (1) *distortion,* (2) *simple substitution,* (3) *gross substitution,* and (4) *omission* as defined below:

1. *Distortion* (D). A distortion error is defined as a phonemic sound element of a syllable judged by the tester to be somewhat distorted by imprecise articulation production but nevertheless a close approximation of the sound attempted. If the distortion is great enough to approximate an allophone of another phoneme, that error should be recorded as a simple substitution (SS). For example, if the production of a medial /k/ sound approximated a /t/ but would be judged distorted as a /t/, record D^t/k in the SS column after the test word *chicken* on the recording form. This indicates front in place of back lingual gesture and thus facilitates kinetic error pattern analysis.

2. *Simple substitution* (SS). A simple substitution is the use of another phoneme in place of the phoneme being tested, whether or not the sound substituted is clearly produced. The error should be recorded by placing the phonetic symbol of the sound substituted in the SS column.

3. *Gross substitution* (GS). Gross substitution is defined as the use of glottal catch, pharyngeal fricative, or velar fricative in place of the phoneme being tested. Close attention should be paid to the use of the glottal catch as the substitute sound in the medial and final word positions. These errors should be recorded as gross substitutions and not as omissions of the sound tested. Record the errors in the GS column as follows: for glottal stop substitutions, the phonetic symbol for the glottal stop /ʔ/; for pharyngeal or velar fricative, PF.

4. *Omission* (O). Omission errors are characterized by the absence of any phonemic element in place of the sound being tested. They should be recorded with the symbol O in the omission column.

Rules for judging consonant blends (consonant clusters): For the purpose of this test the two- and three-consonant blend elements are considered as a single nonsyllabic speech sound element. Therefore deletion on part of the cluster is to be recorded as a substitution error on the cluster (e.g., as t/st or k/kl rather than as an omission.

5. If the entire blend is produced correctly, place a check mark in the correct column.
6. If an error occurs, have the subject repeat the word 2 more times, and record only one judgment of the error, as on a single-consonant sound test.
7. If all elements of the blend are present, but one or more of the elements are distorted due to misarticulation, record the error by placing a check mark in the D (distortion) column.
8. If any part of the blend is missing, or if other sounds are used in the cluster tested, record the error as a simple substitution rather than as an omission (e.g., record as simple substitutions, /pr/ for /spr/, /st/ for /sk/, /p/ or /pl/, etc.).
9. Any substitution errors that include a gross substitution element should be recorded in the GS (gross substitution) column. Record the gross substitution as accurately as possible, including the phonetic symbols and the special symbols for glottals, velar fricatives, pharyngeal fricatives, etc.
10. Record an O in the omission column only if all elements of the blend listed are missing in the subject's response.

RELIABILITY OF ERROR PATTERN TESTING

The identification of each of the several possible forms of articulation disorders, categorical aspects 1, 4, 5, 7, and 10, depends in large part on analysis of error types and patterns of errors found on single-word articulation tests. These errors must be related to the age of the subject and the treatment received to date as well as to the developmental norms by manner of formation and the place of articulation of the target sounds. The reliable and uniform classification and identification of consonant articulation errors appears to require the acceptance of a uniform rationale and operational definitions for classifications of error types.

Philips and Bzoch [26] demonstrated that experienced speech pathologists judging only tape-recorded samples of defective cleft palate speech showed good agreement on the classification of error types such as *omissions, gross substitutions,* or *simple substitutions.* However, comparison of the data from 10 experienced judges indicated that interjudge agreement on classification of error types from tape-recorded samples of speech alone was not sufficiently reliable for collaborative research purposes. This is not to say that sufficient reliability of articulation test data was not demonstrated for clinical research by a single investigator or group with established high interjudge reliability.

However, under conditions of direct simultaneous testing with supplemental visual checks of articulation movements and air flow patterns using an air flow paddle, Schendel and Bzoch [29] demonstrated high interjudge agreement on specific error types for reliable identification of such categorical forms of disordered speech. They reported 95.3 percent exact agreement among three judges simultaneously recording the specific errors of 10 cleft palate speakers on all 100 elements of the Bzoch Error Pattern Diagnostic Articulation Test. Exact agreement ranged from a low of 90 percent to a high of 100 percent, as contrasted to the wide discrepancies found in the broader study of tape-recorded speech samples.

Articulation testing with systematic error pattern analysis followed by the selective instrumental measurement of underlying parameters of speech energy can lead to reliable quantified measurements of speech behavior needed for clinical studies of preschool age as well as of older cleft palate individuals.

EVALUATION OF EMERGENT LANGUAGE SKILLS

Language skill development through speech in human infants is the only natural and universal form of symbolic language development known today. With very few exceptions the human infant essentially learns to master the complex, four-level symbolic code system of one or more languages used in his or her linguistic environment by 3 years of age. From this time on, symbolic language behavior almost completely interpenetrates most of our later human perceptions, thoughts, learning, and consciously remembered experiences throughout life.

During the process of learning language behavior, *receptive language* skills always precede in timing and complexity those similar linguistic skills evidenced in *expressive language*. For example, by 6 months of age, an infant usually recognizes his or her own name and evidences specific meaningful responses to words such as "no," "bye-bye," or names used to refer to family members or loved objects or pets. This early linguistic decoding skill is evident long before such words are spoken (encoded) for the first time.

The first use of true words generally occurs 2 months before or after an infant's first birthday. By this time the infant is already regularly decoding the meaning of most commands or statements of his parents as encoded in simple sentence (semantic) structures. This is a full year before use of basic sentence (syntactic) sequences in speech. These language learning accomplishments are no mean task, for the skills required for understanding and communicating through speech involve learning the codes and rules of the (1) phonemic, (2) morphemic, (3) syntactic, and (4) semantic levels of a specific language system.

Early language development studies of cleft palate subjects, by Bzoch [5] and Starr [33] in 1966, and by Spriesterbach, Darley, and Morris [30], and Smith and McWilliams [32] in 1968, all reported that samples of the cleft palate population appeared to be retarded in expressive language skills. However, these early investigations were based on rough and limited language data such as sentence length, articulation skills, measures of receptive vocabularies, and performance on the Illinois Test of Psycholinguistic Abilities. Since that time many specific and sophisticated tests and scales of language skills have been developed and published and much has been learned in detail about the nature and norms of emergent and early childhood language development. Clinical research experience to date with several language development test procedures, however, indicates that much time and excellent rapport are required to obtain valid direct test-response measures of language skills of young children, particularly before 3 years of age. A 3-year-old child who is able to talk her parents into a new tricycle for Christmas may respond to an initial attempt at direct language assessment only sufficiently to indicate the 12- to 14-month level of language development in an unfamiliar multidisciplinary clinical setting. Several language development scales that depend more on systematic parent interview scaling measures of both receptive and expressive language behavior skills as evidenced in the home are therefore recommended for initial and routine longitudinal language measures for children less than 3 years of age.

INFANT LANGUAGE ASSESSMENT TESTS

Table 8-2 presents some of the specific language item–develomental norms found for the receptive as compared to the expressive language behavior skills typically achieved by well infants in stimulating linguistic environments. The table is taken from the REEL Scale [10] and presents only those language skills achieved regularly between 6 and 12 months, 18 and 24 months, and 30 and 36 months of age for normal developing children in a stimulating environment without congenital abnormalities of the speech or hearing structures.

Bzoch and League early developed the REEL scale [10] for the specific purpose of providing a quick and valid receptive and expressive language development screening measure for children up to 3 years of age in clinical test settings with limited time available. Similar scales are now available including the *Preschool Language Scale* of Zimmerman, Steiner, and Evatt [45], the recently revised *Birth to Three Scales* of Bangs and Garrett [2], and the *Early Language Milestone Scale* of Coplan [13].

Since the REEL Scale [10] was used in the several past studies reported here, its rationale and procedures will be described. It is particularly useful for managing delayed language development in cleft palate subjects since REEL Scale evaluations require only a short parent interview format applicable to the usual time limits available during most cleft palate team evaluations.

The greatest number of receptive and expressive language learned new behaviors occur in the first year of life. There are six specific items on the REEL Scale for each month of development after birth: three receptive and three expressive over the first 12 months of development. The second year of development is assessed in 2-month intervals, with six items in each interval. The third year is assessed in 3-month intervals, with six items in each interval. Technical vocabulary is avoided and a glossary of terms is provided in the handbook *Assessing Language Skills in Infancy* [10], which provides directions for the current use of this language scale.

TABLE 8-2. RECEPTIVE AND EXPRESSIVE LANGUAGE DEVELOPMENT ITEMS (TAKEN FROM THE REEL SCALE [10])

SIX TO SEVEN MONTHS

____ R19. Appears to recognize names of family members in connected speech, even when the person named is not in sight

____ R20. Responds with appropriate gestures to such words as "come," "up," "high," "bye-bye," etc.

____ R21. Gives some attention to music or singing

____ E19. Begins some two-syllable babbling (repeats combinations of 2 or more different sounds)

____ E20. At least half of the time responds with vocalizations when called by name

____ E21. Uses some wordlike vocal expressions (appears to be naming some things in his own "language")

SEVEN TO EIGHT MONTHS

____ R22. Frequently appears to listen to whole conversations between others

____ R23. Regularly stops activity when his (her) name is called

____R24. Appears to recognize the names of some common objects when their names are spoken

____ E22. Occasionally vocalizes in sentencelike utterances without using true words

____ E23. Plays speech-gestures games like "pat-a-cake" or "peek-a-boo"

____ E24. Occasionally "sings along" with some familiar song or music without using true words

EIGHT TO NINE MONTHS

____ R25. Appears to understand some simple verbal requests

____ R26. Regularly stops activity in response to "no"

____ R27. Will sustain interest for up to a full minute in looking at pictures if they are named

____ E25. Uses some gesture language (such as shaking head appropriately for "no," etc.)

____ E26. Often mimics the sounds and number of syllables used in vocal stimulation by others

____ E27. Utterances now contain more consonants than at the 6-month stage

NINE TO TEN MONTHS

____ R28. Appears to enjoy listening to new words

____ R29. Generally able to listen to speech without being distracted by other sounds

____ R30. Often gives toys or other objects to a parent on verbal request

____ E28. Speaks first words often ("da-da," "ma-ma," "bye-bye," or the name of a pet or a toy)

____ E29. Uses some exclamations like "oh-oh"

____ E30. Often uses jargon (short sentencelike utterances of four or more syllables without true words)

TEN TO ELEVEN MONTHS

____ R31. Occasionally follows simple commands like "Put that down"

____ R32. Appears to understand simple questions like "Where is the ball?"

____ R33. Responds to rhythmic music by bodily or hand movements in approximate time to the music

____ E31. Usually vocalizes in varied jargon patterns while playing alone

____ E32. Initiates speech-gesture games like "pat-a-cake" or "peek-a-boo"

____ E33. Occasionally tries to imitate new words

ELEVEN TO TWELVE MONTHS

____ R34. Demonstrates understanding by responding with appropriate gestures to several kinds of verbal requests

____ R35. Generally shows intense attention and response to speech over prolonged periods of time

____ R36. Demonstrates understanding by making appropriate verbal responses to some requests ("Say bye-bye")

____ E34. Uses three or more words with some consistency

____ E35. "Talks" to toys and people throughout the day using long verbal patterns

____ E36. Frequently responds to songs or rhymes by vocalizing

EIGHTEEN TO TWENTY MONTHS

____ R46. Upon verbal request points to several parts of the body and various items of clothing shown in large pictures

____ R47. Demonstrates understanding by appropriate responses to such action words (verb forms) as "sit down," "come here," "stop that," etc.

____ R48. Demonstrates understanding of distinctions in personal pronouns (such as "give it to her," "give it to me," etc.)

____ E46. Imitates some two-word and three-word sentences

____ E47. Imitates environmental sounds (such as motors, animals, etc.) during play

____ E48. Has a speaking vocabulary of at least 10 to 20 words

TWENTY TO TWENTY-TWO MONTHS

____ R49. Follows a series of two or three very simple but related commands

____ R50. Recognizes new words daily at an ever-increasing rate

____ R51. Recognizes and identifies almost all common objects and pictures of common objects when they are named

____ E49. Begins combining words into simple sentences (like "go bye-bye," "daddy come," etc.)

____ E50. Speaks more and more new words each week

____ E51. Attempts to tell about experiences using a combination of jargon and some true words

TWENTY-TWO TO TWENTY-FOUR MONTHS

____ R52. Upon verbal request selects an item from a group of five or more varied items (such as comb, spoon, etc.)

____ R53. Appears to listen to meaning and reason of language utterances, not just words or sounds

____ R54. Understands most complex sentences (e.g., "When we get to the store, I'll buy you an ice cream cone")

____ E52. Occasionally uses three-word sentences (such as "There it is," "Play with blocks," etc.)

____ E53. Refers to self by using his (her) own name

____ E54. Begins using some pronouns but makes errors in syntax

THIRTY TO THIRTY-THREE MONTHS

____ R61. Demonstrates an understanding of all common verbs

____ R62. Understands very long and complex sentences

____ R63. Demonstrates an understanding of most common adjectives

____ E61. Tells gender when asked, "Are you a boy or a girl?"

____ E62. Names and talks about what he (she) has scribbled or drawn when asked

____ E63. Gives both first and last name when asked

THIRTY-THREE TO THIRTY-SIX MONTHS

____ R64. Shows interest in explanations of "why" things are and "how" things function

____ R65. Carries out three simple verbal commands given in one long utterance

____ R66. Demonstrates an understanding of prepositions (such as on, under, front, behind, etc.)

____ E64. Regularly relates experiences from the recent past (what happened while he (she) was "out" or separated from parent)

____ E65. Uses several verb forms correctly in relating what is going on in action pictures.

____ E66. Uses some plural forms correctly in speech

From K. R. Bzoch and R. L. League, *Assessing Language Skills in Infancy: A Handbook for the Multidimensional Analysis of Emergent Language.* Austin, Tex.: Pro-Ed, 1971, With permission.

The regular achievement of essentially normal levels of emergent language developmental skills by subjects with isolated clefts involving the palate [12] was considered the main criterion for efficacy of cleft palate team management of the problems presented by the birth of infants with cleft palate. That this is an achievable goal has recently been demonstrated from clinical research reports [9, 12] using this scale.

MANAGEMENT OF THE CATEGORICAL ASPECTS OF CLEFT PALATE SPEECH

MANAGEMENT OF GROSS SUBSTITUTION ERRORS

The articulation error pattern briefly referred to as *gross substitution errors* is considered to be an early definable aspect of cleft palate deviant speech. It is often found in speakers born with cleft palate It can be reliably identified by the frequent occurrence of articulation errors of the form perceived of as produced by the vocal folds (glottal stops) or by articulated constrictions of the pharyngeal, velar, or palatal areas (pharyngeal or velar fricatives or related sounds) as detailed by Trost [39] in 1981.

When this type of articulation error pattern is present, the articulation test recording form shown in Figure 8-2 would reveal patterns of frequent errors in the gross substitution column. For initial identification of a gross substitution error pattern, the shorter *Error Pattern Screening Test* shown in Figure 8-2 is usually sufficient for identifying this problem. This is because the habitual use of glottal stops or velar or pharyngeal fricatives tends to persist in medial word positions even after they have been modified to correct productions in initial or final single-word utterances.

The commonest definable category of abnormal speech found for 1,000 consecutive cleft palate clinical case studies was this occurrence of gross sound substitution errors for normally orally articulated sounds. In effect, the subjects articulated noise elements judged and classified as glottal stop, pharyngeal fricative, or velar fricative substitutions in place of the consonant sounds being judged on the test words. This form of deviation occurred in 564 of the 1,000 (56.4%) cases studied. Errors of this type appeared in great frequency, particularly for the 3- to 4-year-old clinical population studied by Bzoch [5]. Those infants who acquired early error patterns of this type tended to maintain them through the preschool and school years, refining them in such a way that the glottal stop continued mainly as a substitute for the plosive sounds at later ages. The pharyngeal fricative errors continued longest for the lin-

gual oral fricative articulations. Generally, glottal stops persisted for the longest period, with therapy and maturation for the /k/ and /g/ sounds and particularly in medial word positions on single-word tests. Pharyngeal and velar fricatives tended to persist longest for /s/ and /z/ articulations, including consonant blends with these sounds.

The insidious nature of such learned compensatory patterns of misarticulation appears to lie in the fact that early habituation to extremely atypical neuromuscular-conditioned motor patterns used to form syllable pulses in speech is hard to extinguish. The patterns were almost always learned and reinforced in infancy and childhood (2–6 years of age). The maintenance of these articulation substitutions in the school-aged and even the adult population was frequent. The clinical problem of retraining was difficult and in general correlated with the age of the subject when therapy was started. Therapy during the earlier, more flexible periods of phonological development was always more efficacious.

There is good evidence that although this form of articulation error pattern developed mainly in the presence of congenital velopharyngeal incompetency, it is not necessarily continued by velopharyngeal incompetency. Isshiki, Honjow, and Monimoto [18] have demonstrated that artificial velopharyngeal incompetency created in mature subjects by polyvinyl tubes results in nasality and nasal emission but not in the development of glottal stop or pharyngeal fricative errors. Hundreds of case studies similarly demonstrate that some infants with obvious velopharyngeal incompetency (open clefts of the palate) for years of their early development did not learn to speak with gross substitution patterns.

The simple fact that this manner of early speech behavior involves efferent neuromuscular pathways completely different from those utilized in normal emerging speech patterns in early childhood is good reason for the relative difficulty of modifying such patterns after they have been reinforced over a considerable period of time. Clinical studies indicate that automatic central programming or habituation of general speech motor patterns takes place in infancy. By 2 years of age most children are using short sentences and many words to express their wants and needs.

Table 8-1 clearly reveals that there is often a considerable difference between the usual speech errors of 2- to 3-year-old or even 4- and 5-year-old children with cleft palate in demonstrations of this error pattern. The main past difference was in regard to the development of laryngeal, pharyngeal, and palatal place articulation gross substitution error patterns.

The usual errors of noncleft infants are characterized by simple articulation substitutions for more complex sounds and by frequent omissions of final consonants of words or elements of consonant clusters. Errors such as /t/ for /s/, /w/ for /r/, /p/ for /f/, or /b/ for /v/ are typical rather than abnormal in the speech of many children aged from 2 to 2½ years. However, the use of glottal stop substitutions or pharyngeal fricative substitutions for the majority of plosive or fricative sounds is infrequent and generally absent in the speech of preschool children without cleft palate [5].

There is evidence from cinefluorographic studies that grossly abnormal articulation movements involving constrictions of the entire laryngeal area and the epiglottis and base of the tongue underlie the errors perceived and recorded as pharyngeal fricatives and glottal stops. Figure 8-4 illustrates the abnormal laryngeal constriction of an 8-year-old subject with cleft palate who used glottal substitutions for all consonants. Significant increased use of glottal stops by infants with cleft palate can be found even in the first year of life. Glottal stop articulation usually involves much abnormal hyperconstriction of the larynx during speech.

The presence or absence, and a measure of the frequency of occurrence, of this categorical aspect of deviant speech in subjects with cleft palate can be reliably obtained from standardized diagnostic error pattern articulation tests. Areas of abnormal articulation and co-articulation can be identified from lateral cinefluorographic film studies with synchronized sound tracks, as illustrated in Figure 8-4. Acoustic displays of samples of speech involving misarticulations of glottal stops or pharyngeal fricatives can be distinguished from the normal acoustic displays on sonograph records.

DIAGNOSTIC PROBLEMS IN EVALUATING GROSS SOUND SUBSTITUTION ERROR PROBLEMS

The category of laryngeal and pharyngeal gross substitution errors presents several special problems, both for the clinical diagnostician on the cleft palate team and for the measurement of speech behavior for research studies. First, the need to identify the problem early due to its nature presents a need for reliable articulation testing in the early preschool years, including reliable identification of error types. The screening articulation test is usually sufficient to identify the problem early. Picture stimulation or word-repeating techniques in diagnostic tests are most often possible with children after the age of 2 years. Less formal impressions or more time-consuming methods of repeated short periods of testing over time, with analysis of recorded connected speech utterances, are sometimes required to identify the presence of strong glottal stop and

Figure 8-4. Line drawings of cinefluorographic study of the abnormal laryngeal area constrictions that accompanied speech efforts of a patient with glottal-stop error pattern. The central ellipse outlines the ventricle of Morgagni. The outline of the hyoid bone is found at the left of each drawing. The excessive constriction of the ventricle, laryngeal vestibule, and areyepiglottic fold in B accompanied all efforts at speech and was atypical of studies of normal speakers. A. Larynx outline at rest. B. Laryngeal constriction accompanying glottal stop articulation.

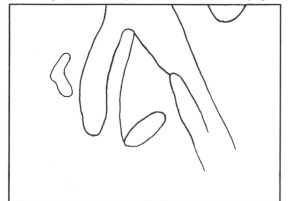

A

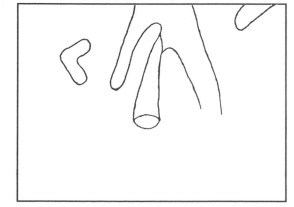

B

pharyngeal fricative articulation substitution patterns in very young children who are reticent in clinical diagnostic environments.

The need for early articulation testing during a time when normal children have many articulation differences that are not unusual for their age range requires a familiarity with the standard developmental misarticulations of this age range of normal phonological development. The problem of classification of errors on a uniform basis is partially solved only by an agreement on operational definitions and rules for classifying speech sound errors. For example, the articulation of the medial /p/ sound in a word such as "paper" may be produced in such a way that two syllables are perceived, but a glottal pulse initiates the second syllable. Under the rules of the screening test illustrated in Figure 8-2, such a difference would be uniformly classified as the substitution of a glottal stop (a gross substitution error) for a medial /p/ sound rather than as an omission of the /p/ sound. However, if a single syllabic utterance were made in the attempt to say the word, the rules of classifying errors would uniformly classify the error as an omission of the medial consonant element.

After a period of maturation, and particularly in the initial stages of articulation training, children who have previously become habituated to gross substitution patterns usually develop a *glottal co-articulation* period of speech production. During this period a glottal pulse is formed simultaneously with the usual lip or tongue articulations in the production of the /p/ in the word "paper," for example. The tester might see the normal bilabial articulation for initial or medial /p/ and yet perceive some distortion of the intelligibility or quality of the test sound in the word. If unsure as to whether this was due to the use of a glottal stop or to some other timing difference on the articulation of /p/, the examiner might classify the error as a distortion rather than a gross substitution.

The simple device of using an air paddle at the lips during the articulation test, as illustrated in Figure 8-5, can lead to more consistent and correct classification. Normally the impounded air pressure behind the lips on a voiceless plosive such as /p/ is sufficient to visibly move the air paddle placed in front of the lips. This is also true for the other plosive and fricative sound elements. There should be no nasal air flow during articulation of plosives or fricatives.

If, however, there is no nasal air flow and no oral air flow when such sounds are produced, there is a clear indication of co-articulation of a glottal stop, if speech was produced at the normal place and in the normal manner of formation. This leads us to another special problem related to this category of misarticulation.

When an overt glottal stop or glottal co-articulation error pattern occurs in speech, the difference directly affects the air pressure and air

Figure 8-5. Air paddle test gives visual evidence of presence or absence of air flow at lips and nares to help determine presence or absence of glottal co-articulation and to identify frequency of abnormal nasal emission on pressure consonants in standard base 10 test. Examiners observe patient's lips and paddle as he or she produces sets of words initiated by /p/ sound. The release of impounded oral air pressure results in a marked bending of the paddle, unless abnormal vocal fold (glottal stop) co-articulation occurs.

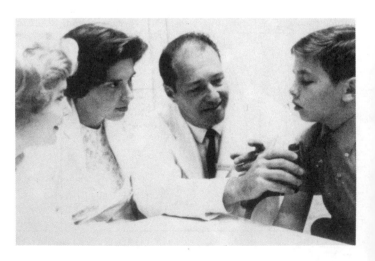

flow characteristics recorded by the instrumental method being conducted. Instruments designed to measure nasality by acoustic analysis may be generally affected by this abnormal form of articulation, yielding false-negative findings of hypernasality. Detailed articulation testing should therefore precede the use of instrumented research into voice characteristics or air flow or sound pressure–level studies. The error pattern data should be used to interpret the instrumented measure data obtained for research purposes.

A final, special problem is the fact that gross sound substitution error patterns also affect the usual clinical tets for velopharyngeal competency and related ratings of nasality. The latter may not be valid in speech samples in which gross substitutions predominate. A simple solution to this is to postpone final evaluations of velopharyngeal competency based on clinical tests of nasal emission, x ray, air flow, sound pressure, nasality scaling, or articulation data until after a period of diagnostic therapy. Train the child first in the simple production of a bilabial plosive such as /p/ to a level where it can be repeated in syllables such as (pi-pi-pi-) or (pa-pa-pa) at a normal rate with evidence of air pressure released at the lips. After this much has been learned, testing for nasality and nasal emission during such syllable utterances will yield a more valid inference as to whether or not the velopharyngeal mechanism can function adequately during speech.

MANAGING DELAYED LANGUAGE DEVELOPMENT

Delayed expressive language development, particularly after 1 year of age, along with some delay in receptive language development, was a frequent finding for the cleft palate sample of 1,000 consecutive cases referred to previously. Some 502 patients, or 50.2 percent of the population, were classified as having a problem of delayed language development. The diagnosis was based on the patient's having significant deviations from the established norms in such general factors as age at first word, expressive vocabulary, first use of sentence utterances, length of response, and general level of syntactic development.

Our focus on more detailed language development studies of cleft palate infants began in 1971 with the development of the Reel Scale [10] as a standard longitudinal early language test. Initial

data revealed an even more frequent occurrence of very early delay in emergent language development up to 3 years of age than had been previously estimated. Table 8-3 shows the average receptive and expressive language ages and the receptive-minus-expressive language difference for the first 25 consecutively born infants with cleft lip and palate studied with this tool, as reported by Bzoch et al. in 1973 [11]. It can be seen from Table 8-3 that there was an almost consistent and significant delay in expressive language skills. Such a delay was found in 23 (92%) of the 25 infants on initial testing at that time.

A broader cleft palate language development study was indicated from these early data and an investigation extended to four team centers was described by Swanson [34] in 1973. She included 37 infants with cleft lip or palate from four cleft palate team centers, and found similar findings for both frequency and type of delayed language development. Swanson's study included an initial factor analysis of the possible significant variables of age, sex, race, type of cleft, and order of birth in the family. Table 8-4 presents Swanson's findings in the form of language quotients for years 1, 2, and 3 and includes the combined language quotient scores. The pattern of delayed expressive language development with essentially normal receptive language development appears to be

TABLE 8-3. MEAN LANGUAGE AGE AND LANGUAGE QUOTIENT SCORES OF 25 CONSECUTIVE PATIENTS WITH CLEFTS (M = 14, F = 11, PREPALATE ONLY = 4, PALATE ONLY = 9, COMBINED = 12)

Mean Age	RLA	ELA	R-ELA Diff.	RLQ	ELQ
18 mo.	19.9	15.9	4 mo.	103	94

Key: RLA = receptive language age; ELA = expressive language age; R-ELA Diff. = receptive-minus-expressive language age difference; RLQ = receptive language quotient; ELQ = expressive language quotient.

TABLE 8-4. LANGUAGE DIFFERENCES RELATED TO AGE FOR 37 CHILDREN WITH CLEFT LIP AND/OR CLEFT PALATE

Language Quotient	Year 1 (N = 10)	Year 2 (N = 11)	Year 3 (N = 16)
RLQ	98.1	104.7	99.5
ELQ	93.1	94.1	91.2
R-ELQ	5.0	10.6	8.3
CLQ	95.6	99.5	95.4

Key: R-ELQ = receptive-minus-expressive language quotient; CLQ = combined language quotient; see also footnote, Table 8-3.

present throughout this period of time up to 2½ years of age and is especially marked in year 2.

A comparison of the average language differences found for female as compared to male cleft palate subjects is presented in Table 8-5. It can be seen from this table that although the female sample studied was generally higher in both receptive and expressive language scores than their male counterparts, they actually had greater receptive-minus-expressive language differences.

Thirty percent of the female sample, and 21 percent of the male subjects had a delay in their expressive language age of 3 months or more from their chronological ages. A receptive-minus-expressive age difference of 3 months or more was found for 49 percent of the female subjects as compared to 21 percent of the male subjects.

Although the language quotients of the white compared with the black and of the first-born compared with the non-first-born tended to be generally higher, the receptive-minus-expressive language quotient differences were essentially identical for both comparisons.

Perhaps the one factor compared in this study that bears most directly on a frequent common cause for the finding of delayed expressive language development in this population is suggested by the analysis of differences related to type of cleft.

Table 8-6 presents a breakdown of language quotient scores of the subgroups with clefts of the primary palate only, clefts of the secondary palate only, and with combined clefts. Although the sample is too small for generalizations to the population, the finding that some children with cleft lip only reveal as much or more delay in expressive language development as children with cleft palate suggests that the effect of a facial deformity stigma on speech and language development may be as great as congenital velopharyngeal insufficiency and its usual concomitant problem of conductive hearing loss.

Many special problems are involved in clinical management and research into delayed speech and language in this population. The determination of major factors (independent variables) other than cleft palate that influence speech development, and the difficulty of early differential diagnosis of possible general mental retardation or hearing impairment in syndromal cases with cleft palate, are basic problems needing collaborative research between large centers. Major functional factors, particularly those involving mother-child relationships and environmental in-

TABLE 8-5. LANGUAGE DIFFERENCES RELATED TO SEX

Language Quotient	F (N = 22)	M (N = 14)
RLQ	104	94
ELQ	95	88
R-ELQ	9.83	5.28
CLQ	100	91.5

Key: See footnotes, Tables 8-3 and 8-4.

TABLE 8-6. LANGUAGE DIFFERENCES RELATED TO TYPE OF CLEFT

Language Quotient	Primary (N = 5)	Secondary (N = 14)	Combined (N = 18)
RLQ	104.8	100.3	99.8
ELQ	94.6	92.3	92.2
R-ELQ	10.2	8.0	7.6
CLQ	99.6	96.3	96.2

Key: See footnotes, Tables 8-3 and 8-4.

fluences, require much further study. Despite this, the early identification of, and possible intervention in, problems of developing speech and language skills in infancy and early childhood promises to be a major area for advancement in overall cleft palate management and treatment in the near future. Future research in this area can add to the knowledge needed for effective parental counseling and the further development of direct and indirect language stimulation techniques as discussed in the following chapters.

Over the past decade, it has been demonstrated at our center [9, 12] that delayed speech and language development can also usually be prevented in a large sample of cleft lip and palate neonates. The early and repeated counseling of families regarding receptive and expressive language norms, measurement and treatment of ear disease, complete surgical reconstruction of palatal clefts in the first year of life, and institution of pragmatic home or direct language training programs are some of the major management factors instituted at our center that apparently led to almost routine elimination of delayed language development in the preschool years. Unfortunately, reports of serious delays in the language development of preschool children with cleft palate continues to be reported from current clinical research. Coston [14] in 1988 reported a comparative study of the language development of 20 children with cleft palate aged from 1 year, 4 months to 6 years 6 months with a group of noncleft children matched in age, race, sex, and socio-economic level. Using the Revised Preschool Language Scale he determined that the subjects with cleft palate were significantly ($P = .0001$) delayed in language development as compared to their matched peers. There was a 14.39-month mean difference in language age. The mean difference in language quotients was 30.22. Clearly, the regular prevention of delayed language development requires a team approach focused on the first 3 years of life with early correction of velopharyngeal insufficiency and management of hearing loss, and particularly a routine early language counseling and pragmatic home language stimulation program.

MANAGEMENT OF HYPERNASALITY

Although hypernasality was generally considered the major deviation in cleft palate speech disorders, the identification of that categorical aspect of speech defect for the clinical sample of 1,000 cases reported here totaled only 431 case studies, or 43.1 percent. However, in light of the advancement in earlier surgical treatment for the correction of velopharyngeal insufficiency and the relationship between hypernasality and velopharyngeal incompetency for speech, the current frequency of postsurgical reconstruction hypernasality is estimated to range at reporting clinical team centers from 25 percent to only 5 or 10 percent. This remains a significant area of deviant speech needing improved management. Management is through frequent monitoring of speech behavior over time looking for evidence of velopharyngeal insufficiency through developing and persisting symptoms of nasal emission distortions of pressure consonant sounds and hypernasal distortion of vowels.

A frequency of over 40 percent of postsurgical clinical case studies evidencing hypernasality, as in the 1950s and 1960s, is no longer typical of current practice. More recent studies, which indicate that only 5 percent to a later 10 percent of primary palatal reconstructions of palatal clefts should result in further evidence of velopharyngeal incompetency for speech production, means that these cases should be identified and treated as early as possible. Too many treatment programs identify the problem but fail to treat it until the child is 5 or 6 years of age when confirmation from instrumental measures is obtained. Such decisions are made by three years of age in an effective total management team program.

The direct cause-effect relationship between overt velopharyngeal incompetency and true hypernasality in the cleft palate population has already been discussed. As most commonly used, the term *nasality* (hypernasality) refers to an abnormal voice quality as judged subjectively by a listener who has learned to associate particular acoustic features with this term. However, an objective measure of hypernasality must be restricted by definition and conditions of identification to reliable clinical judgments supported by instrumental verification.

If velopharyngeal incompetency were the only factor related to the subjective perception of a voice quality generally identified as nasality, there would be no problem in scaling judgments or in obtaining instrumental measurements of this aspect of defective speech. However, certain phonatory variations, articulation errors, and distortions of voice quality from pharyngeal or oral cavity variations (all generally unrelated to either velopharyngeal insufficiency or to direct effects on speech by the nasal cavities or structures) influence perceptual judgments of broadly defined or undefined nasality. Similarly, acoustic and nasal instrumental indices used for the measurement of nasality may also indicate nasality when they respond to speech characteristics unrelated to the direct effects of coupling the nasal cavity with the oral and pharyngeal cavities.

The general impression of hypernasality in the speech of a patient is related to mode of phonation, precision of articulation of the consonant sounds, age and sex, the general fundamental frequency of voice, the speech sample studied, the rate of articulation of speech, the subject's level of fatigue or anxiety, and to velopharyngeal insufficiency.

Only if the term *hypernasality* is defined and strictly limited in use to refer to *the detectable distortion of syllabic elements in speech due to the effects of atypical coupling of the nasal resonating cavities produced under conditions of clear phonation and normal articulation* can hypernasality be reliably identified or logically discussed in clinical or speech science research.

Carefully identified and verified problems of hypernasal distortion of speech are treatable through physical management, either by surgical correction of inadequate velopharyngeal valving or by the utilization of a well-fitted prosthetic speech appliance. Yules [45] and others have proposed methods to reduce hypernasal speech distortions. Voice therapy and direct training of velopharyngeal function through speech therapy is adequate to remove the disorder only when it is maintained on a functional basis. Voice therapy and muscle training should generally be tried before resorting to physical management when the diagnosis is uncertain.

Studies by Schendel and Bzoch [30] of the results of intensive summer training programs which attempted to minimize hypernasal distortion in a group of subjects with velopharyngeal incompetency have demonstrated the fact that ratings of degrees of hypernasal distortion may falsely indicate that nasality can be modified or improved for such subjects, but such perceptual improvement changes do not remain over short periods of time. The changes recorded in the degree of perceived nasality were due to adjustments of the phonatory and articulatory aspects of speech learned by the subjects after training in a summer speech camp for cleft palate clients from rural Florida. The evidence of lasting improvement in severity of nasality *was never* complete and was only temporarily demonstrated for subjects with inadequate velopharyngeal mechanisms. These findings suggest that although several reliable methods for scaling or measuring degrees of perceived hypernasality have been developed, they are not necessarily valid indicators that speech therapy rather than physical management is needed to eliminate the stigma of hypernasal speech.

Hypernasality, as defined, can be reliably demonstrated to be either present or not present. Only a combination of evidence from pre- and posttreatment clinical nasal emission and hypernasality resonance test measures and from the instrumental tests described in this book should be considered as adequate verification that hypernasality has been actually managed satisfactorily. It now seems probable that only if degrees of hypernasality are based on inconsistent evidence from clinical or instrumental tests (i.e., an index of nasality of 2/10 or 7/10, etc., or phoneme-specific hypernasal distortions) are they valid indicators for trial speech therapy rather than physical management.

Techniques of indirect and sometimes direct palatal muscle training can occasionally successfully eliminate velopharyngeal incompetency for speech and result in the permanent elimination of the defect of hypernasality. Chapter 20 reviews the past and current literature on clinical palatal training procedures that have been used with limited success at cleft palate centers to manage

problems of hypernasal distortion of speech. The reader is cautioned strongly, however, not to consider palate and pharyngeal muscle training therapy techniques for the goal of only *reducing* nasality or of *improving* velopharyngeal valving. The only defensible goal for surgical, prosthetic, or speech therapy treatment should be to establish completely adequate velopharyngeal function to support clear speech production devoid of the stigma of hypernasal distortion.

The experience of long clinical practice with cleft palate subjects indicates that voice training techniques for increasing oral and pharyngeal resonance modify perceived hypernasal distortion. They do not correct an underlying problem of velopharyngeal insufficiency that needs correction. However, training for relaxed and balanced resonance rather than elimination of hypernasality is often helpful and meaningful, both before and after secondary palatal reconstruction.

Limited periods of diagnostic voice therapy and direct palatal muscle training should be given selectively before decisions for major secondary medical or prosthetic treatment procedures are recommended, unless physical evidence clearly reveals the impossibility of complete velopharyngeal closure. Indices of nasality from objective instrumental tests should be used whenever possible to confirm the presence or absence of hypernasality. The use and limitations of radiographic techniques are reviewed in Chapter 11, of nasopharyngoscopy in Chapter 12, of aerodynamic assessments of velopharyngeal function in Chapter 13, of TONAR and new computer-augmented measures of nasal and oral sound pressure levels in Chapter 14, and of acoustic analysis related to velopharyngeal dysfunction in Chapter 15.

The presence or absence of hypernasal distortions of voice can best be determined by direct clinical tests in which the abnormal effects of nasal resonance on syllabic elements are exaggerated by alternately closing and opening the nares. This changes the nasal cavity alternately from an open into a cul-de-sac resonator while the patient repeats vowel sounds or words. The hypernasality test in Figure 8-2 described above has proved to be a useful clinical procedure for identifying hypernasality during routine cleft palate team reevaluations. Under the conditions and simple procedures of this test, it does not take the trained ear of a voice specialist to determine and count the frequency of occurrence of abnormal nasal resonance. However, the same special problems and qualifications that are discussed in the following section on nasal emission errors with consonants must be considered in relating velopharyngeal function to clinical test evidence of hypernasality.

MANAGING DISTORTIONS OF PRESSURE CONSONANT SOUND ELEMENTS DUE TO NASAL EMISSION

Nasal emission on pressure consonant sounds occurred in the speech of 423 out of the 1,000 case studies, or 42.3 percent of the case studies, making it one of the more frequent symptoms of defective speech in subjects with cleft palate.

The distortion of consonant sounds due to audible or detectable nasal emission alone has already been defined and discussed. It is a symptom that is usually directly related to the presence of underlying velopharyngeal insufficiency for normal speech production. It is recommended that nasal emission of pressure consonant sounds be considered separately from nasality as an aspect of consonant sound distortions in articulation measurable by articulation test techniques and due directly to velopharyngeal insufficiency for normal speech production.

Counihan demonstrated that the presence or absence of this abnormality can be determined during administration of articulation tests [15]. The occurrence of nasal emission on pressure consonant sounds is direct evidence of velopharyngeal insufficiency for normal speech production. The short nasal emission test presently used for a standard clinical test of nasal emission is illustrated in Figure 8-2. The oral-nasal air paddle technique and the auditory tube listening device are the most convenient means for clinically detecting the presence or absence of abnormal nasal emission distortions in the speech utterances of patients with cleft palate. This abnormal finding from clinical or instrumental tests must be related to other aspects of articulation, phonation, voice, and language assessments. Consistent findings of nasal emission distortion of pressure consonant sounds indicates persistent velopharyngeal inadequacy for normal speech production.

The finding of audible or visible (or both) abnormal nasal air flow during articulation of pressure consonant sounds is a valuable speech measure directly related to velopharyngeal incompetency. Special caution should be taken, however, in interpreting the relationship between nasal emission and organic insufficiency. Special problems include the following:

1. It is not unusual for a deviated septum or enlarged concha (or both), or for a simple cold in the head at the time of testing, to be the cause of little or no visible or audible distortion from nasal emission on pressure consonant sounds in the presence of overt velopharyngeal incompetency. The patency of the nasal air passages should be checked first and the presence or absence of deviations of nasal structures studied and recorded.

2. If the subject being tested uses a gross substitution articulation error pattern, there will be little or no nasal air flow in the presence of velopharyngeal incompetency. The simultaneous checking of oral air flow with nasal air flow can be used to determine whether or not this is the case. If there is no oral or nasal air flow, the lack of nasal emission in that speech sample cannot be related to velopharyngeal function for that subject until speech training is given.

3. An anterior perforation in the hard or soft palate may also result in nasal air flow unrelated to the velopharyngeal mechanism. Close observation and recording of such perforations should precede testing to avoid misinterpretation of findings. If present, the fistula should be temporarily obturated with dental wax or gum or a dental appliance under supervision of the team dental or medical consultant, and the patient tested with and without perforation obturation.

4. Subjects who use extremely weak or aspirate voices may show minimal abnormal air flow, even with velopharyngeal incompetency. Voice therapy should precede nasal emission testing in such cases.

5. If velopharyngeal insufficiency is indicated by the finding of nasal emission, the possibility that this is a functional rather than an organically determined insufficiency should be evaluated. A period of diagnostic therapy, particularly one that uses articulation training with the oral air paddle for strong pressure consonant release and direct muscle training techniques, is usually advisable. Cinefluorographic film studies can be used to distinguish suspected timing abnormalities of palatal movements from true organic insufficiencies.

6. It is important to assume that if the findings indicate that some of the plosive and fricative sounds are produced with good oral air pressure and there is no indication from the air paddle or other clinical devices or instruments of simultaneous abnormal nasal air flow, a potential for adequate velopharyngeal function is present. This is true even if the general impression from connected speech is one of extreme hypernasality and nasal distortion.

Management of nasal emission distortions of speech as of hypernasal distortions of voice usually requires successful secondary palatal reconstructive surgery rather than speech therapy.

MANAGEMENT OF DEVELOPMENTAL DYSLALIA

Developmental dyslalia is here defined as *patterns of articulation errors in speech that are generally typical of the errors found in younger normal children* when such differences could not be due to a depressed level of intelligence (mental age). The category assumes a learning disability in speech skills related to factors such as overprotection in the home, poor learning models, or general social immaturity, and not one directly attributable to structural abnormalities or to general mental retardation.

The case studies of 340 out of the 1,000 children with cleft palate (34%) were interpreted as indicating the presence of this category of speech disorder in addition to or exclusive of the other 10 categories described in this chapter. Identification or measurement of the extent of differences attributable to developmental dyslalia depends primarily on articulation test analysis and identification of errors on sounds and error types similar to or typical of those usually found in much younger children.

There appears to be a relationship between the problem of delayed speech development already discussed and the later finding of articulation errors that fit the category of developmental dyslalia. The relationship is clearer in studies conducted on preschool children, since the developmental language data indicating delayed speech development were recorded in the cleft palate team records for infants and young preschool children and almost invariably were followed by a finding of developmental dyslalia for the same

children as they approached school age. Correlated case and family history studies generally present supportive evidence of environmental problems that can also affect speech for children without cleft palate. Particularly for the 5-, 6-, and 7-year-old samples studied, a low social quotient (SQ on the Vineland Social Maturity Scale, significantly below the IQ level) gave evidence of or support to the diagnosis of social immaturity with developmental dyslalia.

Studies of the articulation error characteristics of a group of 120 normal children between 3 and 6 years of age [4] indicated that they also made sound substitution errors on 16.54 percent of the sounds they attempted, that they distorted about 4 percent, and that they omitted about 2 percent of sounds. The 3-year-old children made simple substitution errors on about 27 percent of the sounds they attempted, but 5½-year-old children had such errors on only 8 percent of their attempts. By age 5½ years the relative frequency of distortions was only 3 percent of the sounds attempted in single words, and omission errors had dropped to less than 1 percent. At 3 years of age, however, omission errors occurred in 5 percent of the consonant sounds attempted and were found primarily in the final word positions on a single-word type of articulation test.

On the average, then, 3- to 5-year-old children may still present with simple substitution errors in 10 percent of their attempts on sounds on /s/, /t/, /d/, and /b/, etc., and still be within normal developmental measures for articulation skills. Noncleft subjects also presented with substitution errors on over 4 percent of attempts on /k/, /f/, /p/, /w/, and /y/. However, their most typical substitution errors were /p/ for /b/, /t/ for /d/, /t/ for /k/, /k/ for /g/, /b/ for /v/, /t/ for /θ/, /d/ for /q/, /θ/ for /s/, /s/ for /z/, /s/ for /f/, /f/ for /y/, /ga/ for /dʒ/, /w/ for /r/, and /l/ for /j/. When errors of this type are found in articulation testing in case studies of children with cleft palate, particularly before 5 years of age, there appears to be no reason to assume they are directly related to velopharyngeal insufficiency or to dental and occlusal abnormalities.

The elimination or modification of speech disorders in this category of children with a palatal defect apparently depends on factors other than surgical, medical, or dental treatment. Also needed are instruction by someone trained in techniques of parental counseling, indirect and direct articulation therapy, training through arrangement of frequent social interaction with peers to aid in development of social maturity and speech skills, and reinforcement of speech training in the home.

MANAGEMENT OF DYSPHONIA CHARACTERIZED BY ASPIRATE VOICE

The type of dysphonia discussed here is defined as a *habituated laryngeal voice abnormality caused by the adjustment of the intrinsic muscles of the larynx muscles of the larynx to produce a partial opening of the glottis during voice production.* Its habituated production may include, as well, a general lowering of the subglottic air pressure by exhalation adjustments during speech. It is considered as a laryngeal compensatory voice disorder separate from hoarseness or roughness of the fundamental frequency and may be confirmed as a functional voice disorder only when otolaryngological examination indicates clearly that there is no muscular weakness or lesion on the vocal folds or other structural abnormality limiting the abduction of the vocal folds.

The use of a weak and aspirate voice was identified as a categorical aspect of abnormal speech behavior in 313 of the 1,000 cleft palate case studies. Trained judges can agree on classifying a voice as aspirate by simply listening to samples of the patient's conversational speech. For the clinical identification of this category of disorder, the phonation test illustrated in Figure 8-2 was regularly used to confirm the impression from listening to connected speech samples. By paying careful attention to the breathing patterns during conversational speech and by timing the number of seconds a subject can sustain phonation of isolated vowels, subjects with habituated aspirate phonation characteristics can be identified. Subjects with habituated aspirate voice were most often unable to sustain vowels for 10 seconds or more on three trials for each vowel. A short period of diagnostic voice therapy indicating that the subject can produce clear and loud phonation of vowels with good quality gives further evidence of a functional aspirate voice adjustment pattern. It is possible to illustrate differences between normal phonation and aspirate or breathy phonation from sound spectrographic characteristics discussed in Chapter 16.

Aspirate phonatory voice quality appears often to be developed by these children early in order to improve the intelligibility of their speech when they must communicate while they have velopharyngeal insufficiency. The distortion from velopharyngeal insufficiency due to both nasal emission and hypernasal resonance characteristics is greatly increased perceptually when the patient speaks with clear phonation as contrasted to weak aspirate phonation. Speech therapists may inadvertently or consciously train patients with velopharyngeal insufficiency to adjust their phonation to aspirate production and to use minimal subglottic air pressure and minimal air flow during speech practice sessions in an effort to correct hypernasal distortion of speech. However, since aspirate phonation is itself a voice disorder that would limit the patient's ability to project the voice, this approach to modifying nasality should neither be encouraged nor recommended. Rather, the presence or absence of aspirate phonation should be determined in the initial speech evaluation study. If adequate velopharyngeal function for speech is confirmed, the subject who has previously become habituated to aspirate phonation should be trained in voice exercises to increase the volume of his or her voice and to use clear phonation characteristics.

A special problem is often presented in case studies of real concern to the plastic surgeon. Subjects using habituated aspirate phonation may speak fairly intelligibly, with little perceived nasal distortion, before surgical treatment to correct velopharyngeal insufficiency for speech, but their voice quality after successful physical management and correction of velar insufficiency may be perceived as about the same as before the treatment, or even worse.

The most difficult problem faced by clinical speech therapists at cleft palate centers is probably the correction of gross articulation error patterns such as the glottal stop. One may be quite successful at this with little acknowledged improvement by family or patient. If the therapist follows up articulation training with voice training to instill the habit of clear, relaxed phonation, the improvement is usually marked and noticed by all. If regular attention is paid to the correction of aspirate voice deviations, the speech therapist may find that he or she can receive reinforcement and support from the patients and their families and the professional staff to a degree far beyond the effort involved.

MANAGEMENT OF LISPING AND OTHER ARTICULATION DISTORTIONS RELATED DIRECTLY TO DENTAL OR OCCLUSAL ABNORMALITIES

The characteristics of articulation errors that might be directly related to dental or to occlusal hazards or both affecting normal speech articulation skills have been covered in some detail in Chapter 5. As considered here, it is recommended that the articulation test profile and direct oral examinations of each patient with cleft palate be used regularly to identify the presence of such dentally related distortions of articulation errors. One should observe closely and repeatedly the motor patterns of the lips and tongue in relation to the dental arches in the production of sounds in words in order to identify the presence or absence of articulation disorders in this category.

There were 128 subjects out of the 1,000 case studies (12.8%) who presented articulation distortion errors in this category in early studies. This percentage has not changed much in recent studies [9, 12]. A majority of the errors so identified involved articulation of /s/, /z/, /ʃ/, /tʃ/, and /dʒ/ sounds. Unilateral or bilateral lisping, particularly evident in the /s/ sound articulation, was the commonest single error related to dental abnormalities. Confirmation of lateral lisping was routinely accomplished by placing the air paddle in the middle and to the right and left of the center of the mouth during the patient's production of sustained sounds and of words containing these sounds for additional visual indication of the area of lateral air flow emission. By relating these findings directly to observations of tongue placement in preparation for and during the production of the consonant sounds distorted, it was possible for two or more judges independently evaluating the same subject to agree completely on the relationship of certain articulation disorders to the dental abnormalities.

In general, the correction of the occlusal and dental abnormalities should be undertaken and completed before such errors are modified. However, in cases of lisping characterized by unilateral or bilateral emission, when a patient is just beginning a long period of orthodontic treatment for the correction of malocclusions, it is often possible to correct the articulation errors on the sounds and, through training during the period of treatment and before final correction of the dental abnormality, to direct the airstream centrally.

MANAGEMENT OF HYPONASAL (DENASAL) RESONANCE DISTORTIONS OF VOICE QUALITY AFFECTING VOWELS OR NASAL CONSONANTS

Hyponasal distortion of speech may be identified as a separate categorical aspect by the careful assessment of correlated information from perceptual tests and physical measures. Hyponasal disorders are here defined as *defects of speech characterized by the abnormal absence of nasal resonance characteristics in vowel sounds, particularly those articulated in juxtaposition to nasal production of the consonants /m/, /n/, and /ŋ/.*

Problems of hyponasal distortion rather than hypernasal distortion of speech were found for some period of time in the case histories of 120 of the 1,000 case studies (12%) evaluated. The most common reason was obturation of the nasopharynx from a recent broad pharyngeal flap operation. The second most common reason was a speech bulb on a speech appliance that was not properly fitted or modified over time.

Figure 8-2 shows the short cul-de-sac test and the test procedure routinely used at cleft palate team clinics to identify and develop an index of the severity of this problem. The test procedure followed is generally the same as for the test of hypernasality except for the criterion for designating words that evidence the problem. In this test words should be circled that *do not represent a perceivable shift in vowel tone quality,* that is, that *sound the same* when the nares are pinched closed.

Clinically, this problem is manageable by the removal of obstructing tissue of the nasopharynx (modifications of pharyngeal flaps to open the lateral margins). The modification of speech bulbs on speech appliances is usually all that was needed in past cases treated by a speech appliance rather than a surgical procedure. Occasionally, hyponasal distortion of speech in postoperative pharyngeal flap cases appeared to be improved through speech therapy. Training was directed to the production of the nasal consonants as sounds, then in words, and then in connected speech.

Surgical procedures to widen the orifices lateral to a pharyngeal flap are not too complicated, and were successful in most cases of post–pharyngeal flap obstructions of nasal resonance, breathing, and of occasional sleep apnea.

MANAGEMENT OF DYSPHONIA CHARACTERIZED BY ROUGH OR UNEVEN FUNDAMENTAL LARYNGEAL VIBRATIONS (HOARSENESS)

As a categorical aspect of cleft palate speech, roughness or hoarseness is distinguished from aspirate or breathy voice. It may be identified reliably by ear by a trained speech pathologist who perceives roughness of the fundamental frequency on sustained vowels and samples of connected speech. For routine clinical purposes, hoarse voice judgments are made and recorded during the administration of the phonation test illustrated in Figure 8-2 and discussed above. Interjudge agreement on identification of hoarseness limited to this description is very high. Physical evidence of hoarseness can usually be confirmed by a sound spectrograph, which reveals an uneven vibration of the vocal fold energy.

Roughness of the fundamental frequency of voice can be caused by either weak subglottic air pressure driving tense vocal folds leading to vocal fry phonation or from vocal abuse that is usually related to effortful phonation associated with glottal stop substitutions in articulation of consonants (gross sound substitutions) and a general high level of laryngeal hypertonicity. Hoarseness related to vocal nodules or contact ulcers from long-term vocal abuse usually results in some aspirate as well as rough phonatory characteristics. There were 150 case studies out of 1,000 cleft palate case studies (15%) who were judged to have hoarseness characterized by roughness of the laryngeal vibration.

Hoarse or rough voice characteristics are speech deviations that are directly related to phonatory function of the larynx rather than to velopharyngeal valving. Voice abnormalities can also be caused by resonance balance changes between the oral, pharyngeal, and nasal resonating cavities. Hoarseness in cleft palate subjects appears to be a somewhat frequent deviation demanding separate identification and consideration for ther-

apy. About 50 percent (74 of the 150 hoarse subjects) had a habituated pattern of glottal stop articulation errors. The standard test for dysphonia characterized by rough laryngeal vibration was sustained phonation of the vowels /i/, /a/, and /u/ repeated 3 times by the patient. Two or more trained judges confirmed the abnormal voice judgment. All cases of confirmed or suspected hoarseness were routinely referred to an otolaryngologist for laryngoscopic examination. The possibility of lesions unrelated to vocal abuse demands immediate medical referral. However, all 150 patients cited in this report were found to have either normal larynges or small vocal nodules. Nodules were identified by otolaryngological examination in 36 cases.

Management through vocal re-education (voice therapy), rather than surgical excision of vocal nodules and voice rest, was considered the preferred approach to hoarseness related to vocal nodules in young cleft palate subjects presenting with this problem. Voice therapy is recommended for all subjects presenting with hoarseness. Surgical exision of vocal nodules should usually be postponed when voice therapy is available, even for the older subjects, because of the highly probable causal relation between habitual vocal abuse and the development of vocal nodules.

Voice therapy for hoarse voice usually includes management of stressful speaking situations in the home or school and direct training for relaxed clear phonation.

MANAGEMENT OF COMMUNICATIVE DISORDERS RELATED TO HEARING LOSS AND OCCASIONAL ESSENTIAL DEAFNESS DEVELOPMENTAL SYNDROMES

Moderate-to-severe levels of hearing loss may lead to distortions or omissions of the high-frequency, weak-energy consonant sounds and affect loudness and pitch monitoring of voice quality. An error pattern of distortions or omissions primarily for unvoiced fricative and plosive sounds and audiological evidence of frequent significant (moderate-to-severe) hearing loss indicates possible cause-effect relationships for both speech production monitoring and emergent language development communicative disorders. If supported by case history and other evidence, the characteristic speech production errors and language development delays should be considered as a separate category of cleft palate speech.

In 60 of the 1,000 case studies (6%) there was audiometric evidence of significant bilateral hearing loss, a case history that indicated chronic or repeated disease resulting in diminished hearing acuity, the evidence of auditory discrimination problems on words with elements such as /s/, /f/, and /t/ (particularly when the speaker was not visible to the patient), and the presence in articulation profiles of frequent distortions or omissions (or both) of the same sounds, which led to this classification. With only two exceptions the patients were under 25 years of age. Forty-two patients had a sensorineural component to their hearing losses as determined by audiometric testing.

Chapter 9 details the more recent experience in developmental audiological testing and otological management of the frequent problems of recurrent mild-to-moderate hearing loss secondary to otitis media. This early management protocol is necessary for the prevention of delayed language development as well as for the development of normal speech articulation skills. The problems in communication skills learning, related to a considerable air-bone gap or conductive component in the hearing loss, and occasional deafness can be treated effectively today by audiologists and otologists.

In the presence of significant bilateral sensorineural hearing impairments, which are found in some syndromes of craniofacial disorders, or of complete bilateral or unilateral conductive loss from congenital atresia as in the Treacher Collins and hemifacial microsomia syndromes, early amplification through hearing aids, auditory training and even speech-reading techniques, and early articulation therapy directed toward clear production of the distorted sounds can greatly assist the patient with these problems.

MANAGEMENT OF COMMUNICATION PROBLEMS CAUSED BY VISUAL DISTRACTION OF THE LISTENER FROM NASAL AND FACIAL GRIMACING

The early cleft palate literature described rabbiting movements of the nares and facial muscles as a symptom frequently observed during speech efforts. When this is a presenting symptom, close observation usually reveals that movements of the nasal alae or facial muscles are timed with the intervals of oral articulation on pressure consonant sounds. Further testing usually reveals that nasal grimacing is initiated by or accompanies nasal escape during connected speech.

Although it is generally reported that nasal grimacing ceases when velopharyngeal competency is established and nasal emission eliminated, the pattern is sometimes strongly habituated and persists. Of the case records of 1,000 consecutive cases, 42 (4.2%) were noted to have nasal or facial grimacing obvious enough to be considered a defect or problem in communication. When the problem failed to be eliminated by correction of velopharyngeal incompetency and elimination of nasal emission on pressure consonant sounds, direct conditioning training that employed mirrors for visual monitoring and feedback information for the patient was usually successful. In a few cases, however, the problem was strongly habituated and ingrained and presented a continuing problem to the patients due to their inability to come to the clinic for therapy.

RECORDING OF CLINICAL DIAGNOSTIC JUDGMENTS

The experience of over three decades of participation in cleft palate team evaluations has shown the value of consistently recording all diagnostic findings and interpretations possible at each clinic from a short and standard battery of tests and observations. The five short clinical direct stimulus–response tests illustrated in Figure 8-2 can usually be completed in 20 minutes by an experienced speech pathologist. When the data from these short tests and observations are supplemented with current information obtained from tympanometric and audiometric tests and case history information, informed clinical judgments as to the presence or absence of organic or functional problems needing further treatment can be made and should also be recorded. With the additional administration of the REEL Scale [10] or other language tests for older preschool children, *yes* or *no* judgments can and should be recorded for the 11 categorical aspects of cleft palate speech discussed in this chapter.

ORAL FACIAL COMMUNICATIVE DISORDERS CLINICAL EVALUATION FORM 1980 - A

K. R. BZOCH, Ph.D.

I. ORGANIC PROBLEMS NEEDING PHYSICAL MANAGEMENT:　　　　YES ☐　　NO ☐

　　1. Velopharyngeal insufficiency　　　　　　　　　　　　YES ☐　　NO ☐

　　2. Dental - occlusal hazard　　　　　　　　　　　　　　YES ☐　　NO ☐

　　3. Hearing loss: conductive _____ Sensori Neural _____　　YES ☐　　NO ☐

　　4. Other _____

II. FUNCTIONAL PROBLEMS NEEDING THERAPY　　　　　　　　YES ☐　　NO ☐

　　Rx _____

　　_____

　　_____

　　_____

III. CATAGORICAL ASPECTS CHECK:

　　1. Nasal emission distortion, ratio: : _____/10　　　　YES ☐　　NO ☐

　　2. Hypernasal, resonance distorton, ratio : _____/10　YES ☐　　NO ☐

　　3. Nasal and or facial grimace　　　　　　　　　　　　YES ☐　　NO ☐

　　4. Hyponasal distortion, ratio: : ___ ___/10　　　　　YES ☐　　NO ☐

　　5. Gross substitution error pattern, ratio: : _____/30　YES ☐　　NO ☐

　　6. Dysphonia; aspirate voice:　　　　　　　　　　　　YES ☐　　NO ☐

　　7. Dysphonia; hoarse voice:　　　　　　　　　　　　　YES ☐　　NO ☐

　　8. Dental related artic errors:　　　　　　　　　　　　YES ☐　　No ☐

　　9. Artic errors related to hearing loss:　　　　　　　　YES ☐　　NO ☐

　　10. Developmental dyslalia (functional artic):　　　　　YES ☐　　NO ☐

　　11. Delayed speech and language: Reel Scale　RLA _____　ELA _____　YES ☐　　NO ☐

　　　　(Language Test scores _____

　　_____

IV. FOLLOW-UP RECOMMENDATIONS:

　　_____

　　_____

　　_____

　　_____

　　_____

　　_____

Figure 8-6. Oral Facial Communicative Disorders Clinical Evaluation Form indicating the several types of clinical judgments based on tests, observations, and case history data recorded at cleft-palate team clinics. The form is intended to be a guide for beginning clinicians in the field of communicative disorders.

Figure 8-6 shows the single-page team clinic recording form that was developed to ensure that these important decisions are made and recorded as a guide for new clinicians. The decisions to be made at cleft palate team clinics include clinical judgments as to the presence or absence of velopharyngeal insufficiency. This important decision, to be made as early as possible after primary surgical reconstruction of the palate, depends primarily on the presence or absence of hypernasal distortion of vowels, distortion of pressure consonants from nasal emission, and general impressions of nasal distortion in conversational speech. Van Demark et al. [41] discuss current methods of assessing speech in relation to velopharyngeal function in more detail than is appropriate here. It seems particularly important for a clinical speech pathologist on a cleft palate team to always be willing to hazard a decision on this, even from limited clinical data on initial testing of a new client. A high index on both the nasal emission test and the hypernasality test shown in Figure 8-2 and discussed above is considered good clinical evidence of velopharyngeal incompetency for speech.

The judgment as to the presence or absence of dental and occlusal hazards affecting speech production requires relating careful observations of abnormalities of dental structure to articulation gestures that result in distorted production of speech sound elements during administration of the screening articulation test.

The presence or absence of hearing loss should be determined by standard audiometric and tympanometric tests, but the effect of diminished hearing levels on communication skills, language learning, and behavior is a judgment to be drawn as well from the case history, observations, and phonatory and articulation test findings.

Depending on these clinical diagnostic decisions regarding the causal relations of organic factors to observed speech behavior, the follow-up recommendations might be for referral for secondary palatal surgery, dental prosthesis, dental or orthodontic treatment, otological care, diagnostic or long-term speech or language therapy, or any one of a number of special instrumental tests such as cinefluorography of velopharyngeal functions for speech. The following chapters in Part II of this book consider in more depth the broad area of clinical and instrumental diagnostic evaluations of cleft palate communicative disorders.

REFERENCES

1. Backus, O. *The Child with a Cleft Palate.* Ann Arbor: University of Michigan Press, 1943
2. Bangs, T. E., and Garrett, S. D. *Birth to Three Assessment and Intervention System.* Helen, Tex.: DLM Teaching Resources, 1987
3. Berry, J., and Legg, T. P. *Harelip and Cleft Palate.* London, Churchill, 1912.
4. Brown, S. F., and Oliver, D. A qualitative study of the organic speech mechanism deformities associated with cleft palate. *J. Speech Hear. Disord.* 18:121, 1953.
5. Bzoch, K. R. *An Investigation of the Speech of Pre-School Cleft Palate Children.* Dissertation, Northwestern University, Evanston, Ill., 1956.
6. Bzoch, K. R. A study of the speech of a group of preschool cleft palate children. *Cleft Palate Bull.* 9:2, 1959.
7. Bzoch, K. R. Six mechanisms of disturbance in cleft palate speech. *Cleft Palate Bull.* 2:26, 1961.
8. Bzoch, K. R. Measurement and Assessment of Categorical Aspects of Cleft Palate Speech. In K. R. Bzoch (Ed.), *Communicative Disorders Related to Cleft Lip and Palate* (2nd ed.). Boston: Little, Brown, 1979. Pp. 161–191.
9. Bzoch, K. R. Clinical Evaluation and Management of Problems of Speech, Language, and Hearing. In F. Pirruccello (Ed.), *Cleft Lip and Palate: Plastic Surgery, Genetics and the Team Approach.* Springfield, Ill.: Thomas, 1987. Chap. 11.
10. Bzoch, K. R., and League, R. L. *Assessing Language Skills in Infancy: A Handbook for the Multidimensional Analysis of Emergent Language.* Austin, Tex.: Pro-Ed, 1971.
11. Bzoch, K. R., Morley, M., Fex, S., Laxman, J., and Heller, J. Development of speech and language in cleft palate children. In Proceedings of the Second International Congress on Cleft Palate, Copenhagen, 1973.
12. Bzoch, K. R., Kemker, F. J., and Wood, V. L. D. The Prevention of Communicative Disorders in Cleft Palate Infants. In W. Lass (Ed.), *Speech and Language: Advances in Basic Research and Practice.* Orlando, Fla.: Academic Press, 1984. Vol. 10, p. 59.
13. Coplan, J. *ELM Scale: The Early Language Milestone Scale.* Tulsa, Okla.: Modern Educational Corp., 1987.
14. Coston, G. W. Language development in the preschool cleft palate child. American Cleft Palate Association 45th Annual Meeting Program, Williamsburg, Va., April, 1988.
15. Counihan, D. T. *A Clinical Study of the Speech Efficiency and Structural Adequacy of Operated Adolescent and Adult Cleft Palate Persons.* Dissertation, Northwestern University, Evanston, Ill., 1956.
16. Ingram, D. Phonological rules in young children. *J. Child Lang.* 1:49, 1974.
17. Ingram, D. *Procedures for the Phonological Analysis of Children's Language.* Austin, Tex.: Pro-Ed., 1981.
18. Isshiki, N., Honjow, I., and Monimoto, M. Effects of velopharyngeal incompetence upon speech. *Cleft Palate Bull.* 5:297, 1968.
19. Kingsley, N. W. Treatment and education of cleft palate patients. *Dent. Cadmos.* 36:125, 1894.
20. MacMahan, C. In W. A. Lange, *Cleft Palate and Hare-Lip.* London: Medical Publishing Col, 1916. Pp. 62–73.
21. Masland, M. W. Testing and correcting cleft palate speech. *J. Speech Hear. Disord.* 11:309, 1946.
22. Morley, M. E. *Cleft Palate and Speech* (4th ed.). London:

Livingstone, 1958. P. 153.

23. Morris, H., Spriesterbach, D. C., and Darley, F. L. An articulation test for assessing competency of velopharyngeal closure. *J. Speech Hear. Res.* 4:48, 1961.

24. Oldfield, M. Modern trends in hare-lip and cleft palate surgery: With a review of 500 cases. *Br. J. Surg.* 37:178, 1949.

25. O'Shea, M. B. An analysis of two indexes of hypernasality. Thesis, University of Florida, Gainesville, Fla., 1982.

26. Philips, B. J. W., and Bzoch, K. R. Reliability of judgments of articulation of cleft palate speakers. *Cleft Palate J.* 6:24, 1969.

27. Poole, I. Genetic development in articulation of consonant sounds in speech. *Elementary English* 2:159, 1934.

28. Preisser, D. A., Hodson, B. W., and Paden, E. P. Developmental phonology: 18–29 months. *J. Speech Hear. Disord.* 53:125, 1988.

29. Schendel, L. L., and Bzoch, K. R. Tests and procedures for evaluation of young cleft palate children. ASHA Program of Annual Convention of the American Speech and Hearing Association, Chicago, November, 1967.

30. Schendel, L. L., and Bzoch, K. R. Advantages of Intensive Summer Training Programs. In K. R. Bzoch (Ed.), *Communicative Disorders Related to Cleft Lip and Palate* (2nd ed.). Boston, Little, Brown, 1979.

31. Spriesterbach, D. C., Darley, F. L., and Morris, H. L. Language skills in children with cleft palates. *J. Speech Hear. Disord.* 1:279, 1968.

32. Smith, R. M., and McWilliams, B. J. Psycholinguistic abilities of children with clefts. *Cleft Palate J.* 5:238, 1968.

33. Starr, C. D. *A Study of Some Characteristics of the Speech and Speech Mechanisms of a Group of Cleft Palate Children.* Dissertation, Northwestern University, Evanston, Ill.: 1956.

34. Swanson, J. F. *Language Development in Young Cleft Palate Children.* Thesis, University of Florida, Gainesville, Fla.: 1973.

35. Templin, M. C. Certain language skills in children, their development and interrelationships. *Inst. Child Welfare Mongr. Ser.* 26, Minneapolis: University of Minnesota Press, 1957.

36. Templin, M., and Darley, F. *Screening and Diagnostic Tests of Articulation.* Iowa City: Bureau of Educational Research and Service Extension Division, State University of Iowa, 1960.

37. Thompson, A. E., and Hixon, T. J. Nasal air flow during normal speech production. *Cleft Palate J.* 16:412, 1979.

38. Thomas, C. K. *An Introduction to the Phonetics of American English.* New York: Ronald, 1947.

39. Trost, J. E. Articulatory additions to the classical description of the speech of persons with cleft palate. *Cleft Palate J.* 18:193, 1981.

40. Turner, G. The treatment of cleft palate by operation. *Proc. R. Soc. Med.* 20:1891, 1927.

41. Van Demark, D., Bzoch, K., Daly, D., Fletcher, S., McWilliams, B. J., Pannbacker, M., and Weinberg, B. Methods of assessing speech in relation to velopharyngeal function. *Cleft Palate J.* 22:281, 1985.

42. Van Riper, C. *Speech Correction Principles and Methods* (3rd ed.). Englewood Cliffs, N.J.: Prentice-Hall, 1958. P. 464.

43. Van Riper, C., and Irwin, J. V. *Voice and Articulation.* Englewood Cliffs, N.J.: Prentice-Hall, 1958.

44. West, R. W., Kennedy, L., and Carr, A. *The Rehabilitation of Speech.* New York: Harper & Brothers, 1947.

45. Yules, R. B. The training method for reduction of hypernasality in speech. *Plast. Reconstr. Surg.* 43:180, 1969.

46. Zimmerman, I. L., Steiner, V. G., and Evatt, R. L. *Preschool Language Manual.* Columbus, Ohio: Merrill, 1969.

CHAPTER 9

Audiological Management in Patients with Cleft Palate

F. Joseph Kemker • Deborah R. Zarajczyk

Persons with cleft palates constitute a unique population that requires an interdisciplinary team approach for the treatment and management of their various associated problems. The team should consist of professionals representing many specialties including plastic surgeons, prosthodontists, otolaryngologists, oral surgeons, speech pathologists, audiologists, orthodontists, and other related professionals [56, 58]. Each professional is an integral part of the team and therefore must have consistent involvement in and understanding of the management and treatment objectives. The optimal treatment plan can only be achieved through the cooperative effort of these concerned professionals. For example, the coordination of the initial speech therapy with the surgeon, orthodontist, and other team members requires a very close working relationship to ensure appropriate and timely management. In addition to understanding the more obvious visible defects and speech problems related to cleft lip and palate, the interdisciplinary team cannot fail to recognize the high incidence of hearing loss and aural pathological disorders (otological abnormalities) in this population.

The purpose of this chapter is to describe the audiological tests, test results, and techniques to be used in managing the hearing problems of children born with cleft palates.

In order for the audiologist to provide adequate and timely management he or she should work closely with every member of the cleft palate team. There is an extensive body of research literature reporting a high incidence of hearing loss and aural pathological conditions in the cleft palate population as compared to the noncleft population [28, 36, 43, 53]. Broad generalizations are difficult to make when discussing the cleft palate population in relation to the degree of hearing loss observed. This fact is due to the number of variables involved and the different methodologies and definitions that have been employed in the literature. A few of these variables are (1) the definition of a hearing loss and aural pathological findings, (2) the age of the sample population studied, (3) pre- and postsurgical repair status, (4) the genetic defects of the sample population reported, and (5) the audiological standard used in obtaining the hearing loss data.

Despite these qualifications, it can be stated that the hearing problem in this population is generally bilateral, conductive, and in the mild-to-moderate severity range (see example in Fig. 9-1). As shown in Figure 9-1, bilateral air conduction thresholds are elevated and bone conduction thresholds are normal.

Aural pathology, as discussed in this chapter, refers to the study of medical problems (otologi-

Figure 9-1. Mean and range of conductive hearing loss of cleft palates seen at the University of Florida Craniofacial Center.

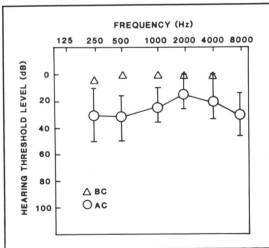

cal abnormalities) of the external auditory meatus and middle ear, including the eustachian tube.

Otitis media is an inflammation of the mucous membrane (mucoperiosteum) lining of the eustachian tube and middle ear [63], and the hearing loss will be within a range of almost no air-bone gap (5 dB or less) to as great as 50-dB air-bone gap. Possible causes of inflammation include bacterial infecton, respiratory viral infections, and allergies. Infant feeding practices such as bottle feeding and supine positioning are associated deleteriously with otitis media [37, 51, 56]. Northern and Downs [37] delineated three categories of otitis media: (1) serous, (2) acute, and (3) chronic otitis media. It is possible to find aural pathological conditions without a measurable hearing loss.

INCIDENCE OF HEARING LOSS AND AURAL PATHOLOGICAL FINDINGS

The high incidence of hearing loss and aural pathological findings in cleft palate patients has been examined and reported for over a century. Skolnik [50] and Bluestone [7] summarized earlier reports dealing with cleft palate and middle ear pathology. Alt [1], Gutzmann [20], Variot [59], and Brunck [11] found high incidence of middle ear problems in the cleft palate population. Pagnamenta [40] documented hearing sensitivity in 150 patients following surgical repair of palatal defects and found 30 percent continued to have hearing loss. A well-known study by Messiner [34] found hearing loss in 27 percent and pathological disorders in 83 percent of 213 cleft palate patients. These early reports were excellent documentations of the auditory problems associated with cleft palate.

When reviewing the more recent studies there are a number of important variables in the auditory data collected that must be distinguished in order to appreciate the effects of the different conditions on cleft palate management. These variables include the age of surgical repair and the age of the subject at the time of audiological testing. Even though there has been substantial improvement in surgical techniques and changes in audiometric standards which affect the collected data, the findings of the early studies cannot be ignored. They point out the importance of research in this area and the very high incidence of hearing loss and pathological problems associated with cleft palate.

EXTENT OF HEARING LOSS

The average incidence of hearing loss in the cleft palate population across studies is approximately 58 percent [3, 19, 25, 27, 32, 41, 48, 50, 52, 55, 61]. The age range for reporting hearing loss in the cleft palate subjects of the above studies ranged from 1 to 41 years with the majority of the studies reporting hearing loss from subjects in the age range from 2 to 18 years of age. In addition, the degree of hearing loss ranged from a 5 dB average hearing loss from 500 to 2000 Hz [19] to 30 dB average hearing loss from 125 to 2000 Hz [35]. It must be noted from these studies that the incidence of hearing loss was less than the incidence of aural pathological findings. If the criteria used for pathological disorder is the presence of a hearing loss, then a high percentage of middle ear problems will be overlooked. Therefore, the incidence of pathological problems in the cleft palate population may be higher than reported. For example, Bess, Lewis, and Cieliczka [6], using a 25-dB conductive hearing loss criterion at any one frequency between 250 and 4000 Hz found that 45 percent had a hearing loss and 60 percent had aural pathological findings, whereas if a 10-dB air-bone gap criterion was used, 79 percent of this group had a hearing loss [6, 25, 47]. The incidence of aural pathological problems in the noncleft palate, pre- and elementary school–aged group would be higher, approximately 20 percent, if a more stringent hearing loss criterion is used [6, 16, 43, 65, 66].

Aural pathological disorders during the first 2 years of life affect approximately 25 percent of the average population and do not show a decline until approximately age 7 [31]. Paradise [46] lists a number of factors which may contribute to the higher prevalence of otitis media in the first 2 years of life: greater susceptibility to infections; abundant quantity of nasopharyngeal lymphoid tissue; drinking of cow's milk as compared with human milk; susceptibility of invasion into the eustachian tube as a result of feeding in the supine position; *and decreased competency of eustachian tube functions.* The last factor — abnormal eustachian tube function — is particularly suspect as the main reason for increased hearing problems in the cleft palate populations. Otitis media is a common childhood disease, second to upper respiratory infections as a reason for a visit to a physician.

The Definition and Classification Panel of the Recent Advances in Otitis Media with Effusion Conference stated that "otitis media in its various forms is the single most common problem seen by pediatricians (9.1%) and otolaryngologists (16.7%), in percentages for their clinical caseloads documented as ascribable to these problems [43]. It was estimated that as many as 15 to 29 percent of all school-aged children have middle ear disease. In addition, the panel of physicians on the Epidemiology and Natural History of the Recent Advances in Otits Media with Effusion Conference summarized the current research findings as follows [49, 51]: More males than females are found with the disease but since males show a greater susceptibility to infection than females, this may be artificial. There is an increased incidence of otitis media during the cold winter months. Environmental factors such as crowded housing, social class, and care of children in day care centers are significant factors. In addition, it was reported that American Indians and Alaskan Eskimos show a high incidence of middle ear disease. White and hispanic children show a greater incidence than black children. The cleft palate group, in contrast to the general population, is highly affected by the same conditions and in addition to decreased competency of eustachian tube function. Falk and Magnuson [17], in 1984, suggested that a primary cause of diseased ears in the cleft palate population is eustachian tube closing failure.

As Paradise [46] stated, the universality of otitis media in patients with cleft palate during infancy could possibly be due to abnormalities of structure and function of the eustachian tube and inadequate velopharyngeal valving, with disturbed aerodynamic and hydrodynamic relationships in the nasopharynx and proximal portions of the eustachian tubes. The histological findings of inadequate development of the eustachian tubes of fetuses with cleft palate would support the higher incidence of otitis media in cleft palate infants [39].

In contrast to the observance of 100 percent aural pathological findings by some investigators, studies of the incidence of hearing loss in the 0- to 2-year-old cleft palate group are sparse because of the difficulty of assessing an infant's hearing. However, Harrison and Philips [23] and later Zarajczyk [67] found, with sound-field testing, a 100 percent reduced hearing sensitivity for this cleft palate age group. The hearing loss occurred along with aural pathological findings that were confirmed otoscopically in these studies.

NATURE OF HEARING LOSS

Age of the cleft palate patient plays an important role in the incidence of hearing loss and aural pathological findings. There is general agreement in the literature that the nature of the hearing loss is usually bilateral and conductive [6, 24, 33] but not necessarily symmetrical [67]. The frequency of pathological problems within this group varies considerably with age, with the most frequent occurence during infancy and early childhood.

Hearing sensitivity generally improves with age. Koch, Neveling, and Hartung [32] and Zarajczyk [67] demonstrated that there is not only a decrease in the incidence of hearing loss, but also in the degree of hearing loss as a function of the age of the child at testing. In Zarajczyk's study, the incidence of hearing loss decreased from 100 percent in the 0- to 2-year-old group to 63 percent in children aged 6 years and older. The mean air-bone gap also improved approximately 5 dB from the younger (2–5 years) to the older (6+ years) group. In 1970, Heller, Hochberg, and Milano [25] similarly reported mean pure-tone averages to be 5 dB better in 7- to 12-year-old children than in the 3- to 6-year-olds. Chaudhuri and Bowen-Jones [13] found the incidence of hearing loss dropped to 50 percent in children above 10 years of age as compared to younger children. Correspondingly, Aschan [2] reported that as high as 75 percent of all individuals with cleft palate have eardrum abnormalities, adhesions, perforations, and cholesteatoma. However, Webster [62] reported that although the majority of middle ear problems resolve, there is a significant percentage of permanent conductive hearing impairment in the adult cleft palate population.

There may be a continued decline in hearing loss and aural pathological problems in the adolescent and adult cleft palate population, but the condition, nevertheless, appears to remain for a lifetime for a large number of individuals with cleft palate. For example, Cole, Cole, and Intaraprason [14] reported a 40 percent incidence of pathological findings in cleft palate patients aged between 14 and 29 years. Bennett [4] found a 51 percent incidence of pathological conditions in subjects with cleft palate between the ages of 14 and 77 years, and emphasized the obvious need for long-term otological management for this population.

EUSTACHIAN TUBE FUNCTION AND AURAL PATHOLOGICAL DISORDERS

It is generally accepted that the etiological basis for this population's middle ear pathological problems and hearing loss is eustachian tube dysfunction. Eustachian tube dysfunction is thought, in general medical practice, to be caused by a functional obstruction from adenoid tissue. In cleft palate patients, however, more recent research indicates that impairment in infancy is more likely related to the lack of contraction of the tensor veli palatini muscle and to increased compliance of the tubal wall [7, 44]. Bluestone et al. [9] studied eustachian tube function in 25 infants with unrepaired cleft palates. Using roentgenographic evaluations, they observed normal prograde clearance radiopaque medium in 42 of 44 ears examined. Retrograde flow, however, was absent in all ears tested, indicating a block or nonfunctional eustachian tube orifice at the nasopharyngeal end of the tube. They concluded that this was a major factor in the pathogenesis of middle ear disease in infants with unrepaired cleft palate.

Maue-Dickson, Dickson, and Rood [39] studied histologically a number of fetuses with cleft palate. They found a decreased tubal width, decreased luminal surface area, increased tubal cartilage surface area, increased pharyngeal width, and decreased height. These findings might account for the higher frequency of poor eustachian tube function and related otitis media in cleft palate infants, separate from obstruction from adenoid hypertrophy.

Gereau and Shprintzen [18], utilizing direct observation of the eustachian tube nasopharyngeal orifice in 300 subjects with cleft palates, found that the eustachian tube orifice was displaced in a posterior-inferior direction compared to normal, and the levator muscle sling filled the orifice so that during swallowing and speech the orifice was seen to be occluded by the levator. This observation was found to correlate strongly with a history of chronic middle ear disease. Therefore, the incidence of aural pathological findings and hearing loss in cleft palate populations appears to range from approximately 100 percent of cleft palate infants [8, 67] to approximately 42 percent of cleft palate adults [14]. The frequent hearing loss and presence of aural pathological conditions in this population appears related to several congenital and developmental causes all adversely affecting eustachian tube function.

HEARING LOSS AS A FUNCTION OF TYPE OF CLEFT

There appears to be no clear relationship that can be found in the literature, at this time, between the incidence of hearing loss and aural pathological findings for the different types of clefts. Skolnik [50] reported that the maximum frequency of occurrence of aural pathological findings (73%) was in those with submucous clefts. The minimum incidence in their sample (31%) occurred in those with clefts of the hard and soft palate only. This difference, however, was significant only in the preschool group. He found no substantial difference across cleft types in the school-age group. Drettner [15], however, noted a higher incidence of tympanic membrane changes in a sample cleft lip and palate group (74%) than in a sample of cleft palate–only subjects (43%). Masters et al. [33] found a similar relationship. Other researchers have found other types of cleft relationships in limited sample populations. For example, Pannbacker [41] reported a higher incidence of hearing loss in those with cleft palate only (82.1%) than in those with cleft lip and plate (50.8%). In addition, she noted a 25 percent incidence rate in those with velopharyngeal insufficiency without overt clefts. Caldarelli [12] reported the incidence in cases of velopharyngeal insufficiency to be the same as in cases of overt clefts. Spriesterbach et al. [52] and Heller et al. [25] found a trend toward higher incidence in cleft palate–only groups. Sweitzer et al. [55] found no real difference between a cleft lip and palate group as compared to a cleft palate–only sample population. Zarajczyk [67] showed an incidence of hearing loss of 63.5 percent in the cleft lip and palate subjects and 71.4 percent in the cleft palate–only group. She also reported that there was close agreement in the occurrence of abnormal impedance findings in the cleft lip and palate group (55.3%) as compared to the cleft palate–only group (59.2%). It appears from these studies that findings vary according to population samples and that there is generally no consistent, significant difference in the high incidence of hearing loss and aural pathological findings across type of clefts.

PRE- AND POSTSURGICAL FINDINGS

Earlier studies found no improvement in auditory problems following surgical repair of the palatal defect. However, more recent investigations appear to agree, in general, that auditory function usually improves as a result of palatal repair. This is thought to be due, in part, to the use of newer surgical techniques which attempt to create a palate that is functional for speech and to enhance eustachian tube function. In 1960, Masters et al. [33] compared hearing test results from two different types of surgery. They found a 47 percent incidence of hearing loss in those whose palates had been repaired using the Langenbeck [60] procedure compared to a 29 percent incidence in those who had a combined closure and lengthening procedure (push-back and V–Y advancement). They felt that early restoration of tensor

palati and levator palati muscles was important in restoring eustachian tube function and thus in preventing hearing loss. Spriesterbach et al. [52] earlier had found a greater incidence of hearing loss only in those patients who had prosthetic rather than surgical management of their clefts.

Graham and Lierle [19], in an investigation into the efficacy of pharyngeal flap surgery, found no higher incidence of hearing loss or middle ear disease following such surgery. Zarajczyk [67] reported the incidence of hearing loss and aural pathological findings to be approximately 50 percent in subjects who underwent surgical repair using either the pharyngeal flap or push-back with pharyngeal flap procedures as compared to an incidence of approximately 83 percent in those whose palatal defects were repaired using either a push-back alone or a Langenbeck procedure. Yules [64] reported a decreased incidence of serous otitis media and improvement in hearing following a combined Dorrance push-back and superior high-base pharyngeal flap procedure. Prior to surgery, 40 (58%) of his 69 subjects, aged 5 to 48 years, had hearing loss. The postsurgical incidence was 46 percent. Bluestone et al. [8] found normal eustachian tube retrograde function in 12 (55%) of their 22 subjects following palatal repair, compared to impaired function in 100 percent prior to surgery. In addition, the incidence of serous otitis media had decreased from 100 percent prior to surgery to 52 percent in their 6- to 12-month-old group following surgery. Bluestone et al. [10] reported better equilibration of applied positive middle ear pressure in infants following palatal repair. Therefore, it appears that there is evidence that a positive relationship exists between palatal repair surgery and a decreased incidence of hearing loss, especially with some type of pharyngeal flap surgery. This apparently results from at least partially restoring eustachian tube function.

AGE AT SURGERY AND HEARING LOSS

An important issue at this time is whether or not early improvement in hearing loss and aural pathological conditions results from early palatal repair. Several studies have evaluated the relationship between auditory impairment and age at time of palatal surgery, with some investigators concluding that early closure did not result in improved hearing levels or a change in the aural pathological condition [21, 22, 27, 50]. In contrast, Masters et al. [33] noted that as age at surgery increased after 18 months, the percentage of subjects with hearing loss increased in nearly arithmetic progression.

Considered together with the findings of Bluestone et al. [10], and Too-Chung [57], who advocated palatal closure at about 4 months of age, the Masters et al. [33] study raises the logical inference that early surgical reconstruction does somewhat improve hearing function. However, as with other variables, there is at present an unclear relationship between the age of surgery and the frequency and severity of later hearing loss in the cleft palate population.

AUDIOLOGICAL TESTING PROCEDURES

It is recommended [67] that all children with cleft palate be seen for a complete audiological examination as soon as possible, regardless of their age. Each child should receive a test battery that includes either sound-field testing or pure-tone air and bone conduction thresholds under headphones, speech audiometry, and immittance measures. A follow-up otological examination should be performed as indicated from the hearing test battery.

A routine complete test battery should be repeated at the time of each cleft palate team reevaluation. Basic questions to the parents about their child's speech and language ability should be included during each audiological reevaluation. In addition, information from the family concerning the child's response to home environmental sounds and speech should be recorded. Any recent history of ear problems should also be noted. All case history information is considered as a valuable part of the audiological diagnostic evaluation.

In our experience, most parents are accurate in reporting how their child responds to sound. The reported responses were used, along with the formal audiological findings, in counseling the parents. The audiological test battery and case history record usually required 20 to 30 minutes

per patient during the cleft palate team's longitudinal clinic. The test results were used as a guide to future management of the child regarding further testing, home language stimulation, possible hearing aid use, and educational programming. Each consultant on the team could review the test findings during cleft palate team clinics. The audiological test findings, in conjunction with the findings of the other team members, were consolidated and used for specific treatment recommendations and consultation with each family.

METHOD OF AUDIOLOGICAL TEST PROCEDURE

Audiological tests provide information about the medical and rehabilitation needs of each patient. The type and extent of the hearing loss must always first be determined. In our team practice over the past 10 years we have attempted each audiological test with every child, regardless of age or cooperative state of the child at the time of testing. Although more difficult to obtain, useful information can be obtained even from a crying child.

It has been our experience with very young children that the first auditory test attempted should be a measurement of the speech awareness threshold in sound field. This test provides an estimate of hearing threshold for voice. For this test the mother generally holds the infant in her lap while positioned between two loud-speakers in a sound-treated room. An observer in the test room and the audiologist in the test suite monitor changes in the child's behavior. The observer looks for the reflexive (Moro's) response in the less-than-1-month-old infant, localization in the 4- to 12-month old child, and ability to point to familiar pictures and possible conditioned play audiometry at age 2 to 3 years. The practice of using an experienced observer in the same room with the child clearly increases the reliability of observations. Two excellent sources of developmental norms for observational audiometry in young children are Northern and Downs's [38] Auditory Behavior Index for Infants, and Hodgson's [26] Developmental Responses to Sound in Infants and Young Children.

Narrow-band noise or warble tones can next be used to measure sound-field auditory thresholds. When testing the very young child, sometimes only one response is obtained. Therefore, specific high-frequency information should be obtained first at 4000 Hz. If a sensorineural hearing loss exists, the loss will most often be in the high frequencies. These two measures (speech awareness and 4000-Hz thresholds) provide a sufficient baseline to assist the audiologist in counseling the parents with regard to language development and future management. The audiologist should obtain additional thresholds at frequencies of 2000, 1000, 500, and 250 Hz whenever possible.

Bone-conduction audiometry is next performed first at 250 to 4000 Hz to determine the integrity of the sensorineural system. We are looking here for the presence or absence of air-bone gap as shown in Figure 9-1. Sensorineural loss in the cleft palate population occurs [5] at least at the same prevalence as in the general population and probably greater. Therefore, sensorineural reserve should be obtained, if possible, for proper management of each child. Because many children can show 0 dB hearing levels by air conduction and yet have substantial middle ear problems, we next assess middle ear function using immittance audiometry. Every child seen by the team, regardless of his or her hearing threshold levels, was administered an immittance test battery. Our clinical battery usually includes complete measurements by tympanogram, acoustic stapedial reflex thresholds, and eustachian tube function. Acoustic stapedial reflexes cannot be obtained if there is excessive movement by the child. Acoustic reflexes are usually not attempted on children below 18 months of age.

Tympanometry is an objective measurement of the compliance of the middle ear system. It requires passive cooperation from the child but no active responses. In our craniofacial center routine, the infant or very young child sits in the parent's lap during assessment. The audiologist first examines the child's external canal otoscopically to determine if the canal is open or has excess cerumen, drainage, or gross abnormalities. The audiologist then inserts the impedance probe into the external canal. He or she obtains a middle ear volume measurement to assure that the end of the probe is not against the canal or plugged with cerumen, and then sweeps the external air pressure from +200 to −300 to 400 mm H_2O pressure and records the compliance of the system from the reflected sound pressure level. The tympano-

gram is derived from this measurement. Although the resulting tympanogram of an uncooperative child may not always be a textbook drawing of middle ear function, an audiologist often can determine the approximate function of the middle ear system of the child from irregular tympanometric patterns. Researchers have reported a variety of tympanometric patterns in infant testing. These range from normal tympanograms produced by all newborns [29, 30] to a statement that inaccurate and unreliable results may be obtained for infants under 7 months of age [45]. However, tympanometric findings in infants often reveal normal middle ear movement, whereas otoscopy may show middle ear effusion. The suggested cause is the highly distensible external auditory canal wall of infants.

Whenever possible, we also assessed *eustachian tube function*. The eustachian tube function test provides information on tubal opening, the presence of tympanic membrane perforation, and PE tube integrity. A PE tube is a pressure-equalizing tube surgically embedded in the typmanic membrane to ventilate and possibly drain the middle ear. The PE tube must be open (not plugged with wax, debris, etc.). Eustachian tube function is evaluated by monitoring a change in compliance or pressure on the tympanometer when the child swallows or performs the Valsalva maneuver.

Immittance audiometry has proved to be an extremely valuable tool to use with the cleft palate population because *bone-conduction audiometry* frequently is unsuccessful with the young child. However, the audiologist should also attempt bone-conduction audiometry on each child, even if unmasked, to determine the sensorineural reserve. If either the pure-tone or immittance results suggest aural pathological changes, a referral should be made for a complete otological evaluation. Following medical management of the ear condition, the cleft palate infant or older child should be seen for regular audiometric screening to determine the effect of either medication or the function of PE tubes, if present. Follow-up visits should be at 3- to 6-month intervals for the young child.

From a decade of experience, we cannot overemphasize the importance of maintenance of good auditory function during the critical language development period (ages 0–4½ years), when ear disorders also are most common in the general population. Although the conductive hearing loss found with the majority of the cleft palate population seems to decrease somewhat in frequency as age increases, it should not be allowed to be maintained during this critical period. Systematic audiological and otological care for the young cleft palate child is difficult, but we believe from our experience that it is a necessary and important part of all cleft palate or cranial facial team evaluations.

Since infants with cleft palate or craniofacial congenital disorders are an important part of the high-risk, hearing-impaired population, brainstem audiometric assessments of the population should be part of any state-wide screening programs being established for high-risk infants. Figure 9-2 is a typical example of a normal auditory brainstem response of an infant.

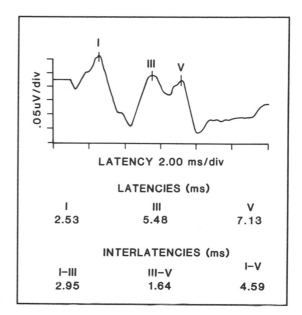

Figure 9-2. Typical example of a normal auditory brainstem response of a 1-day-old infant.

MANAGEMENT OF HEARING PROBLEMS

The degree of hearing loss and the frequency of aural pathological findings will be greatly influenced by the frequency of audiological and otological care provided in each health care system. Generally, such care appears to help prevent any long-standing conductive hearing loss that could interfere with speech and language development, based on our experience and that of others [28, 67].

CASE STUDY

A typical example of the management of hearing for cleft palate infants through the recommended standard audiological test procedure described is subject G.H.

G.H. was born with a unilateral complete cleft of both primary and secondary palates and was first seen by the team at 10 months of age. At that time, average sound-field thresholds were 500, 1000, and 4000 narrow-band noise at 40 dB hearing level (HL). The speech awareness threshold was 35 dB HL. Tympanometry indicated no middle ear movement, and acoustic stapedial reflexes were absent. The child was referred immediately for otological management and was placed on medication. The middle ear problem did not respond to medication, and therefore PE tubes were inserted in both ears.

At age 1 year, 5 months, he was again seen by the craniofacial team, and sound-field responses were obtained at a threshold average of 20 dB HL. Tympanometry then indicated that both PE tubes were open. The child was scheduled to be seen by the otologist again in 1 month. Recall for the team clinic was in 6 months.

On recall, the child was 1 year, 11 months old and was easily conditioned with play audiometry. The pure-tone

average under earphones at this time was 5 dB in both the right and left ears, with a speech reception threshold of 10 dB in the right ear and 15 dB in the left ear. Tympanometry indicated that both PE tubes were open.

He was seen by the team again at age 3½. The left ear had a pure-tone average of 5 dB and the right ear had a pure-tone average of 20 dB. The PE tubes had been removed prior to this appointment. The tympanogram indicated slight negative pressure in the left ear and no middle ear movement in the right ear. The child was again scheduled for otological evaluation and management.

This case illustrates the fact that continued and consistent otological and audiological management is usually necessary for this population. There were numerous children seen in this clinic who had hearing that fluctuated considerably due to middle ear involvement but, with immediate and frequent otological management when needed, hearing was returned to a normal range within a reasonable amount of time.

RECOMMENDATIONS REGARDING AUDIOLOGICAL TESTS

The use of the air-bone gap as a basis for the identification of hearing loss appears to be the most valid procedure required for the cleft palate population. The greater-than, or equal-to, 10-dB air-bone gap average criterion for either frequencies 500, 1000, and 2000 Hz or 500, 1000, and 4000 Hz was most effective in identifying medically significant losses when compared with otological findings [67]. This very strict criterion for the identification of medically significant hearing loss results in better agreement with otological findings and should result in a greater identification of pathological cases. However, this criterion should not be the sole basis for identification of medically significant hearing losses. For example, 12 percent of the cases in this study demonstrated less than a 10-dB air-bone gap average but had abnormal immittance results and verified otological problems.

For the children under the age of 18 to 24 months, the use of a 25-dB average sound-field pure-tone threshold at 500, 1000, and 2000, and 4000 Hz was an effective and valid criterion for identifying hearing loss, but was ineffective for identifying medically significant hearing problems. The 25-dB sound-field average was used as a basis for counseling regarding possible future problems in speech and language development due to reduced hearing sensitivity. In those children in whom pure-tone thresholds could not be identified for each ear separately, more reliance was placed on immittance audiometry for identification of a medical problem.

There was good agreement in this study between both audiometry and immittance measures with otoscopy, but neither was able to identify all cases completely. Normal pure-tone findings did not preclude abnormal immittance findings, and normal immittance findings did not preclude a significant hearing loss. It was therefore concluded that pure-tone audiometry and immittance audiometry should be used together in evaluation of cleft palate patients. They should definitely be used to supplement one another in the identification of medically significant problems within the auditory system, especially when the cleft palate team does not have the routine direct services of an otologist.

In the very young child, after obtaining a speech detection threshold, the threshold results should be obtained first for the high frequencies (e.g., 4000 Hz) to give an indication of any potential sensorineural hearing loss. The lower-frequency thresholds can give an indication of conductive pathological condition. If, therefore, the cooperativeness or attention span of the child allows time only for testing the high frequencies, then tympanometry can be used to confirm existing information about middle ear dysfunction. It has been our experience that tympanometry is a more valid tool for determining middle ear problems in the very young child.

It should be noted, however, that in our study there was good agreement between pure-tone findings and otoscopy (86.6%) in older children and adults, using the 10-dB or greater air-bone gap average as the criterion for medically significant hearing loss. Across all age groups in this study, there was very good agreement between tympanometry and otoscopy (90%).

TYMPANOMETRY AND OTOLOGICAL AGREEMENT

It seems apparent from our reported findings and previous studies in the literature that the cleft palate population will generally have significant recurrent hearing loss and aural pathological findings throughout most of their lifetimes due to their poor eustachian tube function. In conclusion, our most recent clinical studies are in agreement with those of most investigators in the literature and support the conclusion of Paradise [45], who stated that those cleft palate children who underwent aggressive early audiological testing and otological treatment evidenced the highest degree of language development and intelligence, making this a desirable management procedure.

REFERENCES

1. Alt, A. Heilungder Tabustummheit erzielte durch Beseitigung einer otorrhöe und einer angeborenen Gaumenspalte. *Arch. Augen Ohrenheilled.* 7:211, 1878. Cited in C. D. Bluestone, Eustachian tube obstruction in the infant with cleft palate. *Ann. Otol. Rhinol. Laryngol.* 189(Suppl. 2):1–7, 20–27, 1971.
2. Aschan, G. Hearing and nasal function correlated to postoperative speech in cleft palate patients with velopharyngoplasty. *Acta Otolaryngol.* 61:371, 1966.
3. Bennett, M., Ward, R. H., and Tait, C. A. Otologic audiologic study of cleft palate children. *Laryngoscope* 78:1011–1018, 1968.
4. Bennett, M. The older cleft palate patient. *Laryngoscope* 82:1217, 1972.
5. Bergstrum, L. V., and Hemmenway, W. G. Otologic problems in submucous cleft palate. *South. Med. J.* 64:64–71, 1971.

6. Bess, F. H., Lewis, H. D., and Cieliczka, D. J. Acoustic impedance measurements in cleft-palate children. *J. Speech Hear. Disord.* 40:13–24, 1975.
7. Bluestone, C. D. Eustachian tube obstruction in the infant with cleft palate. *Ann. Otol. Rhinol. Laryngol.* 189(Suppl. 2):1–7, 1971.
8. Bluestone, C. D., Paradise, J., Berry, Q. C., and Wittel, R. Certain effects of cleft palate repair of eustachian tube function. *Cleft Palate J.* 9:183–193, 1972.
9. Bluestone, C. D., Wittel, R. A., and Paradise, J. L. Roentgenographic evaluation of eustachian tube function in infants with cleft and normal palates. *Cleft Palate J.* 9:93–100, 1972.
10. Bluestone, C. D., Beery, Q. C., Cantekin, E. I., and Paradise, J. L. Eustachian tube ventilatory function in relation to cleft palate. *Ann. Otol. Rhinol. Laryngol.* 84:333–338, 1975.
11. Brunck, W. Die systematische Untersuchung des Sprachorgans bei angeborenen Gaumendefekte. Dissertation, Leipzig, 1906. Cited in C. D. Bluestone, Eustachian tube obstruction in the infant with cleft palate. *Ann. Otol. Rhinol. Laryngol.* 187(Suppl. 2):1–7, 20–27, 1971.
12. Caldarelli, D. D. Incidence and type of otopathology associated with congenital palatopharyngeal incompetence. *Laryngoscope* 88:1970–1984, 1978.
13. Chaudhuri, P. K., and Bowen-Jones. Otorhinological study of children with cleft palates. *J. Laryngol. Otol.* 92:29, 1978.
14. Cole, R. M., Cole, J. E., and Intaraprason, S. Eustachian tube function in cleft lip and palate patients. *Arch. Otolaryngol.* 99:337–341, 1974.
15. Drettner, B. The nasal airway and hearing in patients with cleft palate. *Acta Otolaryngol.* 52:131–142, 1960.
16. Eagles, E. D., Wishik, S. M., Doerfler, L. G., Melnick, W., and Levine, H. Hearing sensitivity and related factors in children (monograph). *Laryngoscope* 73, 1963.
17. Falk, B., and Magnuson, B. Eustachian tube closing failure. *Arch. Otolaryngol.* 10:10–14, 1984.
18. Gereau, S. A., and Sphrintzen, R. J. Structural and functional eustachian tube abnormalities in patients with palatal clefts. Program American Cleft Palate Association, Annual Meeting, Williamsburg, Va., 1988.
19. Graham, M. D., and Lierle, D. M. Posterior pharyngeal flap palatoplasty and its relationship to ear disease and hearing loss. *Laryngoscope* 72:1755–1760, 1962.
20. Gutzmann, H. Zur Prognose und Behandlung der angeborenen Gaumendefekte. *Mschr. Sprach Heilkd.* 1893. Cited in E. M. Skolnik, Otologic evaluation in cleft palate patients. *Laryngoscope* 68:1908–1949, 1958.
21. Halford, M. M., and Ballenger, J. J. An audiologic and otorhinologic study of cleft lip and cleft palate cases. I. Audiological evaluation. *Arch. Otolaryngol.* 64:58–62, 1956.
22. Halford, M. M., and Ballenger, J. J. An audiologic and otorhinologic study of cleft lip and cleft palate cases. II. Otorhinologic evaluation. *Arch. Otolaryngol.* 64:335–340, 1956.
23. Harrison, R. J., and Philips, B. J. Observation on hearing levels of preschool cleft palate children. *J. Speech Hear. Disord.* 36:252–257, 1971.
24. Hayes, C. S. Audiological Problems Associated with Cleft Palate. In *Proceedings of the Conference on Communicative Problems in Cleft Palate.* Washington, D.C.: American Speech and Hearing Association, 1965. Vol. 1, p. 83.
25. Heller, J. C., Hochberg, I., and Milano, G. Audiologic otologic evaluation of cleft palate children. *Cleft Palate J.* 7:774–783, 1970.
26. Hodgson, W. R. Testing Infants and Young Children. In J. Katz (Ed.), *Handbook of Clinical Audiology* (2nd ed.). Baltimore: Williams & Wilkins, 1978. Pp. 397–425.
27. Holmes, E. M., and Reed, G. F. Hearing and deafness in cleft palate patients. *Arch. Otolaryngol.* 62:620–624, 1955.
28. Hubbard, W., Paradise, J. L., McWilliams, B. J., Elster, B. A., and Taylor, F. H. Consequences of unremitting middle-ear disease in early life. Otologic, audiologic, and developmental findings in children with cleft palate. *N. Engl. J. Med.* 312:1529–1534, 1985.
29. Keith, R. W. Impedance audiometry with neonates. *Arch. Otolaryngol.* 97:465–467, 1973.
30. Keith, R. W. Middle ear function in neonates. *Arch. Otolaryngol.* 101:376–379, 1975.
31. Kessner, D. M., Snow, C. K., and Singer, J. *Assessment of Medical Care for Children: Contracts in Health Status.* Washington, D.C.: Institute of Medicine, National Academy of Science, 1974. Vol. 3, pp. 38–54.
32. Koch, J. G., Neveling, R., and Hartung, W. Studies concerning the problem of ear disease in cleft palate children. *Cleft Palate J.* 7:187–193, 1969.
33. Masters, F. W., Bingham, F. W., Bingham, H. G., and Robinson, D. W. The prevention and treatment of hearing loss in the cleft palate child. *Plast. Reconstr. Surg.* 25:503–509, 1960.
34. Meissner, K. *Ohrenerkrankungen bei Gaumenspalten. Der Huls Nasen Ohrenartz.* 30:6, 1939. Cited in E. M. Skolnik, Otologic evaluation in cleft palate patients. *Laryngoscope* 68:1980–1949, 1958.
35. Miller, M. H. Hearing losses in cleft palate cases: The incidence, type, and significance. *Laryngoscope* 66:1492–1496, 1956.
36. Miller, P. Otopathology and hearing loss in cleft palate patients during this 15 years of life. Presented at the Second International Conference on Cleft Palate, Copenhagen, Aug. 26–32, 1973.
37. Northern, J. L., and Downs, M. P. *Hearing in Children* (2nd ed.). Baltimore: Williams & Wilkins, 1984.
38. Northern, J. L., and Downs, M. P. *Hearing in Children* (1st ed.). Baltimore: Williams & Wilkins, 1979.
39. Maue-Dickson, W., Dickson, D., and Rood, S. Anatomy of the eustachian tube and related structures in age-matched human fetuses with and without cleft palate. *Trans. Am. Acad. Opthalmol. Otolaryngol.* 82:159–163, 1976.
40. Pagnamenta, E. Anatomische u. functionelle sprachresulate von 150 Gaumentspalten Separationen. Dissertation, Zurich, 1932. Cited in E. M. Skolnik, Otologic evaluation in cleft palate patients. *Laryngoscope* 68:1908–1949, 1958.
41. Pannbacker, M. Hearing loss and cleft palate. *Cleft Palate J.* 6:50–56, 1969.
42. Paparella, M. M., Sipi, P., Juhn, S. K., and Jung, T. T. Subepithelial space in otitis media. *Laryngoscope* 95:8, 1985.
43. Paradise, J. L., and Bluestone, C. D. Early treatment of the universal otitis media of infants with cleft palate. *Pediatrics* 44:35–42, 1969.
44. Paradise, J. L. Middle ear problems associated with cleft palate. *Cleft Palate J.* 12:42–47, 1975.
45. Paradise, J. L. Management of middle ear effusions in infants with cleft palate. *Ann. Otol. Rhinol. Laryngol.* 85(Suppl. 25):285–289, 1976.

46. Paradise, J. L. Otitis media in infants and children. *Pediatrics* 65:917–943, 1980.
47. Prather, W. F., and Kos, C. M. Audiological Otological Considerations. In D. C. Spriesterbach and D. Sherman (Eds.), *Cleft Palate and Communication.* New York: Academic Press, 1968. Pp. 169–200.
48. Sataloff, J., and Fraser, M. Hearing loss of children with cleft palate. *Arch. Otolaryngol.* 55:61–64, 1952.
49. Shwin, P. A., Giebink, G. S., Ingvarsson, L., Karma, P., Klein, J. O., Pestalozza, G., Roydhouse, N., Tos, M., Cauwenberge, P. V., and Wood, R. P. Epidemiology and Natural History. In D. J. Lim (Ed.), *Recent Advances in Otitis Media with Effusion. Ann. Otol. Rhinol. Laryngol* 94:10–11, 1985.
50. Skolnik, E. M. Otologic evaluation in cleft palate patients. *Laryngoscope* 58:1908–1949, 1958.
51. Steward, I. A., Kirkland, C., Simpson, A., Silva, P. A., and Williams, S. M. Some Factors of Possible Etiologic Significance Related to Otitis Media with Effusion. In D. J. Lim, C. D. Bluestone, J. O. Klein, and J. D. Nelson (Eds.), *Recent Advances in Otitis Media with Effusion.* Philadelphia: Decker, 1984. Pp. 25–27.
52. Spriesterbach, D. C., Lierle, D. M., Moll, K. L., and Prather, W. F. Hearing loss in children with cleft palate. *Plast. Reconstr. Surg.* 39:336–347, 1962.
53. Stool, S. E., and Randall, P. Unexpected ear disease in infants with cleft palate. *Cleft Palate J.* 4:99–103, 1967.
54. Strauss, R. P., and Broder, H. Interdisciplinary team care of cleft lip and palate: social and psychological aspects. *Clin. Plast. Surg.* 12:543–551, 1985.
55. Sweitzer, R. S., Melrose, J., and Morris, H. L. The air-bone gap as a criterion for identification of hearing loss. *Cleft Palate J.* 5:141–152, 1968.
56. Teele, D. W., Klein, J. O., and Rosner, B. Epidemiology of otitis media in children. *Ann. Otol. Rhinol. Laryngol.* 89(Suppl. 68):5–6, 1980.

57. Too-Chung, M. A. The assessment of middle ear function and hearing by tympanometry in children before and after early cleft palate repair. *J. Plast. Surg.* 36:295–299, 1983.
58. Trier, W. C., Evaluation and treatment planning for patients with cleft lip and cleft palate. *Clin. Plast. Surg.* 12:553–572, 1985.
59. Variot, G. Écoulement de lait pour l'oreille d'un nourrisson atteint de division congénitale du voile du palais. *Bull. Soc. Pediatr. Paris* 6:387, 1904. Cited in E. M. Skolnik, Otologic evaluation in cleft palate patients. *Laryngoscope* 68:1908–1949, 1958.
60. Von Langenbeck, B. Die Uranoplastik mittles Ablösung des mukös-periostalen gammenüberzuges. *Arch. Klin. Chir.* 2:205, 1861. Cited in W. C. Grabb, S. W. Rosenstein, and K. R. Bzoch, *Cleft Lip and Palate: Surgical, Dental, and Speech Aspects.* Boston, Little, Brown, 1971.
61. Walton, W. K. Audiometrically normal conductive hearing losses among the cleft palate. *Cleft Palate J.* 10:99–103, 1973.
62. Webster, J. C. Middle ear function in the cleft palate patient. *J. Laryngol. Otol.* 94:34–37, 1980.
63. Widerhold, M. L., Zajtchuk, J. T., Vap, D. G., et al. Hearing loss in relation to physical properties of middle ear effusions. *Ann. Otol. Rhinol. Laryngol.* 89 (Suppl. 68):185–189, 1980.
64. Yules, R. B. Hearing in cleft palate patients. *Arch. Otolaryngol.* 91:319–323, 1970.
65. Yules, R. B. *Atlas for Surgical Repair of Cleft Lip, Cleft Palate, and Noncleft Velopharyngeal Incompetence.* Springfield, Ill.: Thomas, 1975.
66. Yules, R. B. Current concepts of treatment of ear disease in cleft palate children and adults. *Cleft Palate J.* 12:315–322, 1975.;
67. Zarajczyk, D. L. R. Audiometry in cleft palate children. Thesis, University of Florida, Gainesville, 1979.

CHAPTER 10

Evaluation of Abnormal Articulation Patterns

Hughlett L. Morris

A few introductory remarks about speech sound articulation in general seem appropriate before considering articulation patterns of cleft palate speakers specifically. More detailed discussions are available elsewhere. An excellent one is provided by Bankson and Bernthal [1]; the same authors consider the topic in even more detail in their textbook [3]. In brief, speech sound articulation is regarded as the process of verbal production of the various speech sounds in the spoken language. Articulation refers usually to the physiological act, but in another sense it refers to the acoustic event perceived by the listener. A different way of describing articulation is to say that it has to do with the mechanics of speech rather than the linguistic content.

Within the confines of any language system, there is a range of acceptability of articulation of a speech sound which is defined as normal. In evaluating speech sound articulation, that range or perhaps some measure of central tendency taken from the distribution within that range is used as the standard for "correct articulation." In many discussions of speech sound articulation, and particularly in discussions relating to clinical problems of speech sound articulation, there is the implication that speech sounds can be viewed individually, or separately, or in isolation from other speech sounds. Hence speech pathologists talk about testing the adequacy of articulation /s/. There is general agreement that such a point of view may be a gross oversimplification. Rather one should consider the "articulations" of /s/, connoting that there may be variations in the articulation of /s/ depending on such factors as phonetic context [5]. In spite of these important theoretical implications, in view of our current level of knowledge it is still most convenient to consider the various speech sounds as entities, particularly for discussions such as the material presented here.

RELEVANCE TO COMMUNICATION PROBLEMS

There is clear justification for concern about the articulation problems of persons with cleft palate. Those persons with cleft palate and severely impaired speech sound articulation have speech that is not readily intelligible to listeners and so they are not able to communicate effectively with other people. Persons with cleft palate and moderately impaired speech sound articulation have speech that is intelligible in most situations, but their manner of speaking may be so distracting to the listener that their effectiveness as speakers is reduced.

Articulation proficiency may be particularly relevant to the development of communication skills [4, 10]. The young child with cleft palate frequently has speech that is only partially intelligible because of oral structural deficits. Since the development of language is in part contingent on its effectiveness as a social tool, the child whose speech is of limited intelligibility may not be rewarded sufficiently to achieve an appropriate level of development of language skills.

PURPOSE

Available research findings and clinical observations demonstrate clearly that there is tremendous range in the articulation skills of speakers with cleft palate [16]. So heterogeneous is the cleft palate population in variables relating to communication skills that it is difficult, if not downright impossible, to describe meaningfully "cleft palate speech." Many of these variables — for example, velopharyngeal function, age, adequacy of dentition, adequacy of hearing level, and intelligence — are discussed later in this chapter. Identification of variables of etiological significance indicates which diagnostic and management techniques are to be considered in the treatment of the communication problems demonstrated by individuals with cleft palate.

The purposes of this chapter are to describe the speech sound articulation problems demonstrated by cleft palate speakers, to enumerate and describe certain etiological bases for these problems, and to provide a general rationale for the selection of diagnostic and therapy techniques. (The discussion here considers principally the articulation of consonants rather than vowels. The primary difficulty that cleft palate speakers have with vowels is excessive nasal resonance and not misarticulation.)

DESCRIPTION OF THE PROBLEM

DISTORTION BY NASAL EMISSION

The type of error sometimes referred to as the distortion-nasal is typical of what most listeners regard as cleft palate speech and is demonstrated by many cleft palate speakers. It results from an inability to obtain velopharyngeal competency during the articulation of pressure consonants (plosives, fricatives, and affricates). Air pressure that would normally be directed through the mouth during the production of a plosive, fricative, or affricatives escapes from the oral cavity into the nasal cavity through the velopharyngeal port. The air pressure is emitted through the nostrils during the production of these speech sounds. If the escape is sufficient in quantity, the nasal emission of air pressure is audible and distorts the acoustic signal of the speech sound. (If the nasal emission of oral air pressure does not affect the way the sound is perceived, it does not create a problem in speech perception.)

There is great variability among speakers in the amount of nasal emission demonstrated during

speech. Factors such as rate of oral air flow or the presence of nasal obstructions (as from a deviated septum) may contribute to the amount of and perceptibility of nasal emission. The major determinant of the amount of nasal emission, however, appears to be the size of the velopharyngeal opening.

There is probably less variability in the amount of nasal emission in the speech within speakers than between speakers. The observed variance may well be related to phonetic context. Within-speaker variation is likely to be greater for the group of individuals with small velopharyngeal openings than for the group with large velopharyngeal openings.

Nares constriction is frequently observed in speakers who demonstrate nasal emission. Sometimes the constrictive movement is barely visible, but sometimes the movements are of such extent that the brow and upper lip are involved. Speakers who show nares constriction are apparently attempting to prevent, at the nostrils, the nasal emission of air pressure that they cannot prevent at the velopharyngeal port. Nares constriction is generally an indicator of velopharyngeal incompetency unless the patient has only recently had surgical or dental management affecting the velopharynx. However, not all patients with velopharyngeal dysfunction demonstrate nares constriction.

ORAL DISTORTIONS

In addition to distortion by nasal emission, the cleft palate speaker may also demonstrate speech sound distortions that are oral in nature. In other words, the issue here is not whether the air release during the speech task is properly oral or abnormally nasal. Rather the issue is whether the release, though properly oral, results in a "normal" acoustic event that will in turn be perceived as "normal." Such oral distortions are not unique to the group of persons with palatal problems and are demonstrated occasionally by the general population considered to be "normal" for most purposes.

Of the various types of speech sounds, fricatives are most likely to be orally distorted, probably because fricatives are continuants and are subject to more variation than other speech sounds, such as plosives. Any activity during the production of a fricative that changes the pattern of release of air pressure through the constrictions in the anterior portion of the oral cavity can result in the oral distortion of that speech sound. For example, missing teeth, a problem of many patients with cleft palate, may result in an inadequate dental cutting edge across which the airstream is often released in the production of /s/. The lack of an adequate cutting edge can change the acoustic event enough so that the /s/ is still recognized as an /s/ but is judged to be abnormal or defective. The same type of change can result from a tongue position during /s/ — for example, one that directs the airstream laterally rather than centrally. Missing teeth and faulty tongue position can affect the articulation of other fricatives, such as the /f/ or /v/ or either of the th sounds /θ/ or /ð/.

Structural problems in the lips can result in defective speech sounds, although they are not very likely to. For example, if the speaker can close his lips, lip structure and function are probably adequate for speech production.

Although the amount of research regarding the frequency of occurrence of such distortions is limited, indications are that such speech problems occur at least as often in the cleft palate population as they do in the normal population, and perhaps more often. Based on available information, the inference is that within-speaker variability in demonstrating such problems is comparable to that shown by noncleft palate speakers.

SUBSTITUTIONS

The substitution of one speech sound for another speech sound is not uncommon in several types of speech disorders. Generally such speech sound substitutions are seen in speech problems that are characteristic of young children who are still in the process of learning speech. In these instances, the substitution may be a /t/ for /k/ or a /θ/ for /s/, and the speech sound that is substituted is usually made in an appropriate manner (i.e., without nasal emission).

Speakers with cleft palate may demonstrate substitution errors, although this type of error is not generally as common as that of nasal distortion, for example. Some writers have referred to the fact that speakers with cleft palate substitute a nasal consonant for a consonant that requires intraoral pressure (e.g., substituting /m/ for /b/). It seems more meaningful in the majority of instances to regard this response as a nasally distorted /b/ rather than the substitution of /m/. Viewed in this context, the speech sound error clearly points to velopharyngeal incompetency rather than inappropriate learning.

The cleft palate speaker with velopharyngeal incompetency may substitute a nasally distorted speech sound for another speech sound. This speech behavior indicates either the inability to direct the airstream orally because of the structural inadequacy, or the possibility of confusion between the substituted and the appropriate speech sound, or both.

The speaker with velopharyngeal dysfunction or a history of dysfunction may also show two special substitutions in his or her speech: glottal stops and pharyngeal fricatives. The glottal stop is a coughlike sound, of a plosive nature, in which the air flow is restricted at the level of the larynx. Typically, the substitution is made for back plosives, and is observed most frequently in very young children or in older patients (children and adults) who have had velopharyngeal dysfunction for an extended period of time. The pharyngeal fricative is the result of restricting the airstream at some level of the pharynx, is most often substituted for some other fricative, and is also observed frequently in patients who have had velopharyngeal dysfunction for an extended period of time.

The incidence of these two special patterns does not appear to be high for cleft palate subjects who receive physical management resulting in normal or near-normal velopharyngeal function at a relatively early age. For example, Van Demark [14] found glottal stops and pharyngeal fricatives in 3 percent and 1 percent, respectively, of 108 Iowa subjects who had palatoplasty at 13 years and in 1 percent and 0.2 percent, in Danish subjects who had palatoplasty at 2 years. In contrast, Bardach, Morris, and Olin [2] found such patterns in 37 (86%) of 43 German subjects who had early primary veloplasty surgical repair of the soft palate cleft, but late surgical closure of the anterior, hard palate cleft not until the age of 13 years.

It seems likely that these two articulation patterns may be regarded as "compensatory," in the sense that the patient adopts them in an attempt to produce a satisfactory perceptual result. To the extent that such is the case, they should be considered as learned behavior that continues even after the physical deficit (lack of partition between the oral and nasal cavities) has been satisfactorily resolved.

Trost [13] has suggested the probability that there are still other, more subtle, abnormal articulatory patterns to be considered in this light. That likelihood merits further study.

OMISSIONS

A final type of error is that of omission in which a speech sound is simply left out of a word. Omission errors have been reported as being typical in the speech of very young children and in the speech of individuals with so-called functional articulation problems. Omission errors have also been described as part of the articulation problems demonstrated by persons with cleft palate.

Clinical observation indicates that omissions may not be as prevalent in various types of speech disorders as reported. If any attempt is made to produce the speech sound, the speech sound is not omitted. For example, a cleft palate speaker may use a relatively weak glottal stop for the /k/ in the word *look* so that the appropriate phonetic transcription is [l u ʔ]. If the glottal stop is not considered as an attempt to produce the /k/, then the speech sound is classified erroneously. Only by the critical use of the error type of omission can the observation be interpreted in a meaningful way.

CONCLUDING COMMENTS

Unfortunately the cleft palate patient does not always present misarticulations as easily categorized as the foregoing discussion implies. For example, frequently there is both substitution and nasal emission, such as the substitution of a nasally distorted /θ/ for /s/. Another example is a tongue-tip placement distortion of /s/ accompanied by nasal emission, or dentally related distortion of /s/ accompanied by nasal emission. These "combination" misarticulations are frequently difficult for the beginning clinician to recognize and properly diagnose, but with clinical experience, the task becomes easier.

ETIOLOGICAL FACTORS

From the above description of the types of articulation errors that cleft palate speakers may demonstrate, the following factors are identified as being of etiological significance. All are described in greater detail elsewhere in this book.

INABILITY TO PREVENT NASAL ESCAPE OF ORAL AIR PRESSURE

The deficiency of velopharyngeal incompetency is the major factor in a speaker's inability to direct the airstream orally in speech. This certainly is the case for the individual with an open cleft palate. In addition, it is the case in a large proportion, perhaps as large as a third, of persons who have had cleft palate repaired by a surgical procedure. It is also true for a portion of patients who have had secondary palatal surgery, such as pharyngoplasty or a pharyngeal flap, which was not successful. It may also be true for some persons who have obturators. Finally, it is true for some individuals who have had no overt cleft palate but who have palates that are too short or that are immobile for various reasons.

It follows then that persons with velopharyngeal incompetency demonstrate, at the very least, speech sounds which are distorted by nasal emission of oral air pressure. They also may demonstrate glottal stops and pharyngeal fricatives because they are not able to produce acceptable oral plosives and fricatives. They may or may not demonstrate nares constriction. They may or may not demonstrate oral distortions and substitutions. They may or may not demonstrate omissions.

INABILITY TO PROVIDE AN ADEQUATE DENTAL CUTTING EDGE

The individual with cleft palate may have a number of other structural anomalies. Of these, dental deficits are most likely to affect speech production, so that kind of deficit is singled out for discussion here. Other structural deficits are discussed later.

If the cleft palate extends through the alveolus, the patient is likely to have dentition problems, which at one time or other may result in distorted fricatives. The speech pathologist should be alert for such a problem, particularly in children who are younger than 10 years of age. Frequently a prosthesis is constructed to provide missing teeth, and orthodontic treatment is provided for the maintenance of a proper occlusion. It is important, however, to recognize that if articulation problems are related solely to dental inadequacies, those speech sound errors will be characterized by an oral, not nasal, direction of air flow.

INABILITY TO HEAR SPEECH MODELS

Much has been made of the fact that persons with cleft palate have a high frequency of middle ear disease and associated conductive hearing problems, particularly during the first 6 years of life. The possible effect of a hearing problem of this kind and extent on speech has been examined elsewhere. In summary, it seems rather unlikely that a conductive hearing loss which is of mild-to-moderate extent and which fluctuates greatly in severity could be a major etiological factor in causing the speech problems which cleft palate speakers demonstrate as a group, although it could be significant for certain individuals.

INABILITY TO LEARN

There is considerable evidence to suggest that the mean IQ of the cleft palate population is slightly lower than that of the normal population. It is important to realize, however, that most patients with cleft palate demonstrate levels of intellectual function higher than that which is relatively certain to adversely affect speech and language development. Clearly, then, the level of intelligence is not a major cause of articulation problems in the majority of cleft palate cases.

INABILITY TO ADOPT APPROPRIATE ARTICULATION MOVEMENTS

Many of the articulation problems demonstrated by speakers with cleft palate are not related to any structural defect but are apparently learned behavior. The mechanisms whereby this inappropriate learning takes place are not well understood, either for the subject with a so-called functional articulation problem or for the person with cleft palate.

Typically, the previously described articulation errors of (oral) distortion, substitution, and omission are considered to be problems of inappropriate learning. Glottal stops and pharyngeal fricatives may also be learned behavior, although, as pointed out previously, the adoption of the latter two speech sounds may be related to structural deficits. It is highly unlikely that a person would have learned to use nasal distortions, but the possibility exists, however remote.

The role of inappropriate learning is relatively clear in the case of substitution and distortion errors. Apparently the individual may learn the response [tʌm] for [kʌm] (*come*). Or, in the example used earlier, the individual uses [lʊʔ], instead of [lʊk] (*look*). In the instance of a distorted /s/, it may be that the speaker has learned inappropriate placement of the tongue so that the airstream is not directed centrally. Or it may be that the individual has not learned to "close his teeth" for the production of /s/, and so there is not sufficient constriction anteriorly of the oral cavity. Other examples can be cited. The role of inappropriate learning is less clear in the case of omission errors. Apparently the speaker is simply not sufficiently aware of the speech sound to make an attempt at it.

The major part of this discussion has been related to articulation errors on plosives, fricatives, and affricates, since these three classifications of speech sounds are most frequently in error in speakers with cleft palate. Articulation errors are made also on the glides /r/ and /l/. These speech sounds are most commonly distorted, although substitution errors may be made also. Since /r/ and /l/ do not require great amounts of intraoral pressure, nasal emission of oral air pressure does not result in perceptual distortion. Instead, the distortions on /r/ and /l/ made by speakers with cleft palate are essentially similar to those made by speakers with normal oral structures and are related to inappropriate articulation movements, which have been learned, probably movements of the tongue. These types of articulation errors are not uncommon in the cleft palate population [11].

In summary, velopharyngeal incompetency and inappropriate learning have been identified as the two major factors of etiological importance for the articulation problems demonstrated by speakers with cleft palate [15] There is the possibility that, for certain individuals, level of intellectual function and recurrent hearing loss may result in articulation errors, but it seems unlikely that, for the group, intelligence and hearing level are significant in this respect. In the same way, dental deficiencies may result in difficulties in articulating speech sounds. In addition, there may be deviations of other oral structures which may be significant for certain individuals. One such deviation is a low, narrow palatal vault, which may make normal tongue carriage and position difficult. Enlarged tonsils may have the same effect. A very large tongue may hamper articulation of speech sounds, but this is not frequently observed. A number of years ago there was concern about the adequacy of tongue flexibility in the cleft palate group. This contention has not been supported by research evidence, however, and the majority of speech pathologists who are knowledgeable in cleft palate speech problems discount the importance of this factor. Finally, the possibility of the effect of a number of the above factors in combination must be considered.

DIAGNOSIS AND TREATMENT

PROCEDURES FOR DESCRIBING THE ARTICULATION PROBLEM

Essentially the task is to provide for a method of determining what the errors are and when they occur. Learning when they occur is as important as learning what they are, since the context in which the errors occur frequently gives clues about appropriate treatment techniques.

At the beginning of this chapter, reference was made to the fact that the articulation of a speech sound may show considerable variation as a result of several factors — for example, phonetic context. Diagnostic articulation testing procedures must be designed in such a way that this kind of variance is examined as much as possible. Typically, then, an effort is made to sample the ability of the individual to make and to use the various speech sounds in single words, under some relatively well-controlled circumstances, and in connected speech. The choice of procedure used to elicit the speech sample depends on the age of the individual being tested and the purposes for which the material is to be used. Sometimes there is need to compare the articulation skills of a cleft palate patient with those of the normal population, and that is possible, to a limited degree, with one test: the Iowa Pressure Articulation Test (IPAT) [8]. The IPAT was derived from the Templin-Darley tests of articulation [12] and the norms for the IPAT have been taken from the original normative data for the Templin-Darley tests. Also, norms for the IPAT and the Templin-Darley Screening Test are available for Spanish-speaking Mexican-American children [9]. Generally, however, the size of the articulation test score is not as meaningful as the identification of the speech sounds which are made in error, the types of errors demonstrated, and the variance with which the errors occur.

Of special relevance in testing cleft palate patients is information about error type. A primary distinction to be made is whether the error is nasal or oral since, as indicated earlier in this discussion, the etiologies of the two types are likely to be different and may indicate need for different treatment procedures.

One of the important aspects of articulation testing, from the standpoint of providing a rationale for treatment, is to assess the results of auditory and visual stimulation of speech sounds that are consistently made in error. This information about stimulability is useful in the case of the person with a so-called functional articulation problem, because from it one can predict the degree to which articulation behavior can be changed, assuming the absence of a structural deficit [6]. The relevance of this procedure for patients with cleft palate has been described in some detail by McWilliams, Morris, and Shelton [7]. Essentially it is that inferences can be made from the results of the stimulation test, not only about the possibility of behavioral change, as with the so-called functional articulation problems, but also about the adequacy of the velopharyngeal mechanism as if functions during speech.

PROCEDURES FOR ASSESSING BASES FOR THE ARTICULATION PROBLEM

It is clear from the foregoing discussion that one of the bases for the articulation problems demonstrated by speakers with cleft palate is inappropriate learning. Speech is learned behavior, and patients with cleft palates are as likely as "normal" individuals, or even more so, to demonstrate certain articulation errors simply because they learned speech that way.

The objective of procedures to assess the role of inappropriate learning as a possible etiological factor is to determine whether the correct production of the speech sound in question is in the repertoire of articulation responses of the individual and, if it is not, to attempt to predict the relative difficulty to be encountered in teaching the appropriate production of the speech sound. If the individual can make the sound correctly some time during the articulation testing procedure, or if he or she can be stimulated by auditory and visual means to make it correctly, then it is to be inferred that the articulation of the speech sound is in the individual's repertoire. Sometimes, of course, trial speech therapy is necessary to determine whether the individual is capable of making the behavioral change.

It is always difficult to assess the relative importance of inappropriate learning in understanding the causes of articulation errors. Sometimes speech pathologists find it convenient to look for structural bases for articulation errors first, and if no such bases are discovered, they infer that the problem is learning and proceed on that assumption. Such a position seems acceptable from a theoretical point of view so long as the speech pathologist does not wholly discount the possibility that there may be structural deficiencies, such as minimal neurological deficits, that have not been diagnosed. Continued pressure for behavioral changes, which in reality are impossible or very difficult to effect, can be harmful to the individual. Additional discussion about this matter is presented in later chapters.

As indicated above, the major structural basis for articulation problems in the person with cleft palate is velopharyngeal incompetency. Several techniques have been devised to assess velopharyngeal function. They are described in critical detail elsewhere in this book. As indicated in these discussions also, all have limitations and give perspectives about function which are necessarily incomplete in the amount and kind of information provided. In light of these limitations, then, there is no technique that can be used as a single test or observation; the information obtained is most meaningful when interpreted together with other types of observations.

Two methods in current use, as indicated elsewhere in this book, are aerodynamic measures (air pressure and flow), which provide additional information about patterns of function of the velopharyngeal mechanism, and nasoendoscopy, which provides additional information about structural aspects of the velopharyngeal mechanism. Other methods, perhaps less often used, are various types of radiographic procedures and techniques such as accelerometry or sound spectrograph data analysis.

The question of what degree of velopharyngeal competency is required for *normal* speech sound articulation is not yet sufficiently answered. Although a number of attempts have been made to determine whether normal-sounding speech can be produced by speakers with incomplete closure

of the velopharyngeal space, none have yielded definitive findings. On the basis of present information, it seems likely that individuals with a normal mechanism do not always need to close the velopharyngeal space during speech. However, individuals with a physical deficit of the mechanism, such as cleft palate, must have physical management of the deficit such that she or he is capable of closing the space during connected speech. If that is not the case, the individual will show uncontrollable nasalization of speech.

An examination of the oral mechanism is necessary for assessing the role of the teeth, tongue, and lips as etiological factors. (The adequacy of the velopharyngeal port cannot be assessed by such an examination, since the area of contact between the palate and the pharyngeal wall is hidden from view.) There are no normative data for comparing observations regarding adequacy of dental cutting edge, tongue size, and so forth, and thus subjective clinical judgments must suffice.

Evaluation of hearing level and intelligence must be conducted by the appropriate professional personnel. The decision regarding the influence of any such problems on articulation skills must be made by the speech pathologist, taking into consideration all available information.

DECISIONS REGARDING TREATMENT

Decisions about management of articulation problems of a speaker with cleft palate are based on results of diagnostic tests and considerations of possible etiologies. If the speaker demonstrates misarticulations which are considered to be functional in nature (not related to a structural deficit), then speech therapy is indicated. If the speaker demonstrates misarticulations which are considered to be related to a structural problem or to some other behavioral problem, such as extreme personality maladjustment, then the speech pathologist should refer the patient to appropriate professional workers. For example, patients who do not demonstrate the ability to achieve velopharyngeal competency should be referred to a plastic surgeon for secondary surgery or to a prosthetic dentist for construction of an obturator.

Sometimes patients with cleft palate demonstrate articulation problems that warrant speech therapy and referral for other kinds of treatment at the same time. In that case, the speech pathologist should make clear to all concerned the goals of his therapy and the basis for his referrals.

The goals of clinical management vary with the individual and his needs. Some persons may choose to be content with speech which is understandable but not "normal," if taking steps to seek "normal" speech skills involves surgery. Others continue to seek help because their speech is distorted by a relatively minimal amount of nasal leakage of oral air pressure during speech. In the final analysis, the person with the "problem" should be the one to judge whether he or she wishes additional treatment of whatever kind indicated. Those involved in providing that treatment, however, have an obligation to be honest in their appraisals of his problems and candid in their predictions of the effectiveness of their treatment.

REFERENCES

1. Bankson, N. W., and Bernthal, J. E. Articulation Assessment. In N. J. Lass, L. V. McReynolds, J. L. Northern, and D. E. Yoder (Eds.), Speech, Language, and Hearing. Philadelphia: Saunders, 1982. Chap. 22.
2. Bardach, J., Morris, H. L., and Olin, W. H. Late results of primary veloplasty: The Marburg project. Ann. Plast. Surg. 12:235, 1984.
3. Bernthal, J. E., and Bankson, N. W. Articulation Disorder. Englewood Cliffs, N.J.: Prentice-Hall, 1981.
4. Bzoch, K. R. Articulation proficiency and preschool error patterns of cleft palate and normal children. Cleft Palate J. 2:340, 1965.
5. McDonald, E. T. Articulation Testing and Treatment: A Sensory-Motor Approach. Pittsburgh: Stanwix House, 1964.
6. McReynolds, L. V., and Elbert, M. F. Articulation Disorders of Unknown Etiology and Their Remediation. In N. J. Lass, L. V. McReynolds, J. L. Northern, and D. E. Yoder (Eds.), Speech, Language, and Hearing. Philadelphia: Saunders, 1982. Chap. 23.
7. McWilliams, B. J., Morris, H. L., and Shelton, R. L. Diagnosis of Articulation Disorders. In Cleft Palate Speech. Burlington, Ont.: Decker, 1984. Chap. 17.
8. Morris, H. L., Spriesterbach, D. C., and Darley, F. L. An articulation test for assessing competency of velopharyngeal closure. J. Speech Hear. Res. 4:48, 1961.
9. Paynter, E. T. Articulation skills of Spanish-speaking Mexican-American children: Normative data. Cleft Palate J. 21:313, 1984.
10. Philips, B. J., and Harrison, R. J. Articulatory patterns of preschool cleft palate children. Cleft Palate J. 6:245, 1969.
11. Pitzner, J. H., and Morris, H. L. Articulation skills and adequacy of breath pressure ratios of children with cleft palates. J. Speech Hear. Dis. 31:26, 1966.
12. Templin, M. C., and Darley, F. L. The Templin-Darley Tests of Articulation (2nd ed.). University of Iowa, Bureau of Educational Research and Service, Extension Division, 1969.
13. Trost, J. E. Articulatory additions to the classical description of the speech of persons with cleft palate. Cleft Palate J. 18:193, 1981.
14. Van Demark, D. R. A comparison of articulation abilities and velopharyngeal competency between Danish and Iowa children with cleft palate. Cleft Palate J. 11:463, 1974.
15. Van Demark, D. R. Misarticulations and listener judgments of the speech of individuals with cleft palates. Cleft Palate J. 1:232, 1966.
16. Van Demark, D. R., Morris, H. L., and VandeHaar, C. Patterns of articulation abilities in speakers with cleft palate. Cleft Palate J. 16:230, 1979.

C. Objectified Instrumental Diagnostic Evaluations

CHAPTER 11

Radiographic Assessment of Velopharyngeal Function for Speech

William N. Williams

Radiography is recognized as an indispensable aid to diagnosis throughout medical, dental, and speech pathology practice. Its power to differentiate the aberrant from the normal, however, presupposes that the range of normal structure and function is known. In the field of speech pathology, definition of the normal functioning of the speech mechanism and identification of what constitutes abnormalities by means of roentgenographic studies are still incompletely defined. There are two important purposes of the x-ray technique in the field of speech pathology: (1) research to further define the range and variation of normal function; and (2) examination of the functioning of the oral structures of those patients whose speech has been classified as abnormal. The data obtained from both normal speakers and individuals with speech disorders can provide a baseline to use in better understanding the operation of the speech structures.

It is the opinion of this author that assessing the underlying cause of velopharyngeal (VP) dysfunction radiographically is the combined responsibility of the radiologist and the speech pathologist. Skolnick [62], recognizing that a fluoroscopic assessment of the VP port is frequently a new procedure for most radiologists, issued a plea for the development of a working relationship between radiologists and speech pathologists. Although Skolnick's plea was made more than a decade ago it would appear that there still exists too little interaction between the two specialties. For example, Schneider and Shprintzen [51] summarized the responses of approximately 600 speech pathologists, in the United States and Canada, to a survey in which the authors attempted to identify diagnostic and treatment strategies used

in managing patients with velopharyngeal insufficiency. These authors found that only 24 percent of the respondents use multiview videofluoroscopy; and only 11 percent of these respondents indicated that the radiologist was also a member of their cleft palate team. Although it is the speech pathologist who is likely to be the primary professional having the most extensive knowledge relative to the functional requirements of the VP port for normal speech, he or she typically has had little or no formal training in radiographic procedures. Skolnick [58], in recognizing this problem, has noted that although it is the speech pathologist who is expected to conduct the speech portion of the examination, it is the radiologist who is to perform the radiological portion.

The first use of x-ray in speech research was made by investigators whose primary interest was phonetic definition. The early work of such researchers as Scheier [50], Russell [48, 49], and Parmenter and Trevino [44] has been reviewed by MacMillian and Kelemen [35] and by Subtelny, Pruzansky, and Subtelny [68]. Through these early investigations it was established that certain consistent interrelationships exist between movements of the articulators and sounds in speech production.

Interest in defining the significance of variations of velar position for the production of speech was expressed early in the literature by Allen [1], Wardill and Whillis [71], and Bloomer [11]. Other investigators such as Kelly [31], West, Kennedy, and Carr [74], and McDonald and Baker [38] were among the first to direct attention to the relationship between VP closure and normal speech. The next major thrust of investigations was in defining the site, height, and amount of closure in normal VP valving. The intent was that this information could then be used for comparison with individuals with suspected structural or physiological abnormalities of the velar port. It is noted that although the literature appears to employ the terms "velopharyngeal incompetence," "velopharyngeal inadequacy" and "velopharyngeal insufficiency" interchangeably, the descriptor "insufficiency" appears to be most universally accepted as an encompassing term [33]. The term *velopharyngeal insufficiency* (VPI) will be used in this chapter as a generic descriptor unless otherwise defined.

Clinical tests of articulation skills, nasal resonance, and nasal emission provide the speech diagnostician with valuable information concerning both the overall profile and the specific speech characteristics of the patient's speech. If the patient's speech has been identified as demonstrating consistent hypernasality and inappropriate nasal air emission, we can assume that there is VPI. Without looking at the VP port radiographically, however, we cannot adequately determine the factors that are contributing to the VPI. Still, too often clinicians attempt to assess adequacy of velar length and movement, and even the overall functional integrity of the palatal port, from an oral examination. Unless there is an obvious oral defect, such as an unrepaired palatal cleft, a palatal fistula, or a velum with gross tissue deficiency or extensive scarring, it is *not* possible to determine VP competency for speech from an oral inspection [25]. This is not to negate, of course, the importance of conducting a thorough oral examination, as it is possible to determine such potentially contributing problems as hypertrophied tonsils, palatal fistulae, asymmetry in velar elevation, and submucous palatal clefts. It is not possible, however, to determine from oral inspection alone whether the soft palate, when it elevates while the patient produces an /ah/ sound, is or is not making contact with the posterior pharyngeal wall. As will be discussed later in more detail, VP closure typically takes place with the middle third or third quarter of the velum, which is at a level above and behind that which can be observed orally. Neither the speech evaluation nor the oral examination (in most cases) will provide clinical insight as to the exact nature of the insufficiency if one exists. We would agree with Skolnick, McCall, and Barnes [60] that "it is vital to know these precise defect(s) in a given patient's velopharyngeal closure mechanism prior to undertaking procedures to correct the abnormalities producing the deviant speech,

whether by surgery, prosthetic devices or speech therapy." It is the opinion of the present author that videofluorography is currently the optimal technique for defining physiological components underlying the VPI.

My intent in this chapter is to show how research that uses radiographic techniques to define normal VP closure has clinical applications in diagnosis and treatment of VPI. Although this chapter is directed to the technique of radiography, it must be noted that the information obtained is limited, providing only part of the required information relative to the functioning of the VP port. It is imperative that the clinician have an equally thorough working understanding of nasopharyngoscopy — a technique which involves the use of a small-diameter flexible fiberoptic scope which is inserted into the nose, providing the examiner with additional information on the functioning of the VP port unobtainable by radiography. Dr. Shprintzen has provided a thorough review on the use and clinical value of nasopharyngoscopy in Chapter 13.

SINGLE-EXPOSURE X RAY AND SPEECH RESEARCH

Single-exposure techniques have been used in the study of speech since Scheier's first application in 1897. In 1931 Broadbent [15] presented a technique that standardized lateral still single-exposure roentgenograms of the head. This was the beginning of cephalometric roentgenology, in which factors are controlled to enable exact comparison of subjects over time. Establishment of standardization not only permitted the comparison of one patient with another but made possible the accumulation of measurements of the velum and pharyngeal structures relative to age. For a more detailed historical development of cephalometry, see Brodie [17]. Specific applications of cephalometry in speech have been discussed by Subtelny et al. [68].

A second important technique employing single-exposure x ray is laminography. This process allows only the desired anatomical plane to come into focus, with a blurring of adjacent planes. Therefore only those structures, bony or soft tissue, that are within the determined anatomical plane will be sharp enough in detail to permit analysis. Subtelny [65], who employed laminography in a physiological study of sustained vowels, found that the overall maxillary dimensions were smaller in patients with cleft palate and that the soft palates were smaller and shorter than those in normal subjects. She also found the speakers with cleft palate to demonstrate abnormal lingual positions as compared to normal speakers. Hagerty et al. [27] used laminography in studying the posterior pharyngeal wall movement during velopharyngeal valving for speech and concluded that this movement is insignificant. Subtelny and Subtelny [69] reported a laminographic study of the articulatory mechanism and intelligibility of postoperative cleft palate speakers. They were unable to determine the existence of any direct relationship between the amount of velopharyngeal opening and the patient's total speech intelligibility score.

From the numerous studies involving the single-exposure x-ray technique has come most of the information known today about site, height, amount of closure, and interrelationships of structures involved in VP valving. For example, Aram and Subtelny [2] investigated the approximate level of VP closure by using lateral cephalometric roentgenograms. They found that the site of closure changed with an increment in age and that the level of closure was closely related to the palatal plane, being slightly below from 4 to 8 years of age and consistently above the level of the palatal plane thereafter. This information has immediate application in the positioning of speech bulbs and in determining the base site for the pharyngeal flap or pharyngeal wall implant. Other clinical information such as growth patterns of the face and pharynx as it develops in a forward and downward direction has also been reported [16, 32]. As this forward and downward growth occurs, the bony plates of the hard palate move down from the cranial base. Perhaps one of the most significant findings in abnormal facial morphology is the higher incidence of enlarged adenoids concomitant with cleft palate [18]. That this adenoid tissue has a role in VP closure has been shown by Subtelny and Baker [67] and Calnan [20]. Knowledge of this fact has provided a brake against indiscriminant adenoidectomy.

This information from the single-exposure process is invaluable to the current understanding of VP closure. There are certain advantages in the use of this technique, particularly in the study of

structural integrity, chiefly that a clear resolution of the image is provided. There are, however, some very serious limitations in all single-exposure x-ray techniques relative to assessing movement patterns of soft tissue structures. The most important for speech physiology is that the exposure is generally made while the subject or patient produces a sustained speech sound; in this case the articulatory structures are held immobile during the exposure, causing both an artificial state of "speech" and a limited "speech" sample. And, as will be shown in the following section on "speech sample," considerable research has revealed that the functioning of the VP port during an individual's production of isolated sustained sounds is not necessarily predictive of how the VP port functions during connected speech.

VELOPHARYNGEAL CLOSURE AS A FUNCTION OF THE SPEECH SAMPLE FOR NORMAL SPEAKERS

The continued use by many speech clinicians of the single lateral still x ray for assessing closure of the VP port appears to have created some confusion concerning the interpretations and clinical significance that can be obtained relative to VP function. The confusion appears to be whether or not complete closure of the VP port is necessary for the production of normal nonnasal speech. Through their use of single still x rays, it would appear that some clinicians have concluded that normal nonnasal speech does not require complete VP closure. This conclusion seems to be based on the selection of single-sound production as the speech sample.

VOWELS

Typically the type of speech production that has lent itself to the single x ray technique has been the isolated sustained sound such as vowels and sibilants. A number of research studies, however, have identified the condition of incomplete VP closure for normal-speaking individuals producing sustained vowels. These reports concerning single-vowel phonemes have been interpreted to imply that complete seal of the nasopharynx is not necessary for normal speech production in general.

The fact that complete VP seal is not necessary for normal production of certain sustained non-nasal speech sounds is no longer an issue. For example, Moll [40], using the technique of cine-fluorography, found that 37 percent of his normal speakers produced the vowel /a/ with the palatal port opened. In addition, 14 percent of his subjects were observed to phonate the vowel /i/ and 11 percent phonated the vowel /u/ with incomplete VP closure. These findings are supported by Benson [4], who also assessed palatal port function for normal speakers producing sustained vowels. He found that for his subjects, 63 percent produced the vowel /a/ with an open port, while 23 percent produced the vowel /i/ and 9 percent phonated the vowel /u/ with incomplete VP closure. Mourino and Weinberg [42], in a study assessing velar stretch in normal-speaking children, noted that 20 percent of their 10-year-old boys and 50 percent of their girls failed to make closure during the production of /u/. It seems that it must be concluded from studies such as these that many normal-speaking individuals do, in fact, produce acoustically normal vowels with incomplete VP closure. It would appear inappropriate, therefore, to employ a sustained vowel as the speech sample if one is attempting to determine whether the VP port can achieve functional closure during connected speech.

CONSONANTS

Single sustained consonants have also been employed as a speech sample for assessing palatal port closure. Lubker and Morris [34] conducted a study to determine whether cinefluorographic measures of VP opening could be predicted from measures taken from lateral still x rays. They found that their measures of lateral stills of subjects' production of sustained /s/ had a higher correlation with measures taken from cinefluorographic films than did lateral stills of the subjects' vowel production. However, Shelton, Brooks, and Youngstrom [53], in a radiographic study assessing patterns of VP closure, noted that one of their normal-speaking subjects failed to achieve closure on sustained /s/ and on /s/ syllables, even though this subject demonstrated closure on

other sounds. Björk and Nylén [8] have also noted that some of their normal speakers of Swedish were observed to produce some oral consonants, including /s/, /v/, /t/, /b/, and /d/, with incomplete VP closure. Thus, there is further evidence indicating considerable variance among normal-speaking subjects relative to the occurrence of an open VP port during the individual's production of isolated oral sounds. With this available information, it would seem to be too risky, if not inappropriate, to employ single sustained consonant sounds such as /s/ as the speech sample to determine whether the palatal port can achieve functional closure during connected speech.

SYLLABLES

In an attempt to improve on the known limitations of using isolated speech sounds to predict VP function during speech, Bzoch [19] conducted a study to determine whether normal speakers demonstrated complete closure of the VP port while repeating oral consonant-vowel (CV) syllables. Each subject was required to repeat, using normal rate, intonation, and intensity, the syllables /pi/, /pa/, and /pu/ 7 times each. Analysis of the cinefluorographic films revealed that the VP port for all subjects was completely closed during all the syllable productions. This finding is in agreement with the earlier findings of Graber, Bzoch, and Aoba [26], in which their sample of 44 normal-speaking subjects were observed to demonstrate complete VP closure during the repetitive productions of /pi/, /bi/, /fi/, and /wi/.

The results of the studies on vowels, consonants, and syllables suggest that complete closure of the VP port is typical of normal speakers only during repeated oral CV syllables, but that vowel or single consonant production alone can give an accurate indication of VP function for speech. Williams and Bzoch [76] have concluded that repetitive syllable productions such as /pi/ or /pa/ provide a better clinical speech sample than isolated sound production when only the lateral still x-ray technique is available to the clinician.

It is to be noted that the studies just reviewed, which employed vowels, consonants, or syllables, were assessed using the lateral projection only. As will be described in the following section, although the lateral plane of view provides considerable information about velar function, it provides little insight relative to lateral wall function, a necessary component in affecting complete closure of the VP port. Consequently, this author does not advise using repetitive syllable production with the lateral still procedure in attempting to assess the dynamic functioning of the VP port for speech.

VELOPHARYNGEAL CLOSURE AS A FUNCTION OF THE SPEECH SAMPLE FOR IMPAIRED SPEAKERS

Although differences in VP closure relative to the speech sounds elicited have been demonstrated to exist for normal-speaking individuals, there has been little information available relative to the opening or sealing of the palatal port for specific speech sounds for individuals with suspected aberrations of the palatal port. Bowman and Shanks [13], however, have stated that "the use of static lateral cephalometric radiographs is a generally acceptable method adopted clinically to confirm or reject the perceptual suspicion of VP incompetence," even though they note that the speech sample produced is often only the /i/ and /s/ sounds. In defense of the use of the static lateral still technique, Bowman and Shanks [13] have noted that there were no available data reported on the existence of differences between x-ray techniques used for assessing VP function.

Recognizing this deficit in the literature of comparing the findings obtained from the lateral still technique with its limited speech sample to that obtained from lateral fluoroscopy in which the patient can produce samples of connected speech, Williams and Eisenbach [79] assessed the velar closure patterns of 30 patients with suspected palatal port dysfunctions in an attempt to determine whether a clinical population of this type would demonstrate differences of VP function relative to the production of sustained vowels, repeated syllables, and connected speech. Lateral 70-mm spots were obtained during subjects' production of the sustained vowel /i/, and during the middle of a series of repeated productions of the syllable /pi/. Lateral cinefluorographic records were obtained while the subjects produced a sample of connected speech. Evaluation was made in terms of whether VP closure occurred or did not occur during each of the given speech tasks. Twenty-four of these patients failed to make VP closure as seen on the 70-mm spot during the production of the sustained /i/ sound. However, only 18 of these demonstrated VP incompetency during their production of connected speech. The point to be made here is that if only the sustained vowel had been used as the speech sample, there would have been a misdiagnosis of VPI for six of the patients or an error rate of 25 percent. For the repetitive production of the syllable /pi/, 17 (57%) of the 30 patients failed to make VP closure, whereas only three of these failed to make closure during the connected speech sample. In addition, only seven of 13 subjects who demonstrated closure on the repeated syllables were found to demonstrate velar inadequacy during connected speech. If a judgment were being made as to the adequacy or inadequacy of the palatal port on the basis of the repeated syllable /pi/, nine of the 30 patients, or 30 percent of the patient sample, would have been misdiagnosed.

It seems that the potential magnitude of the predictive error (33–46%) in information gathered from lateral still x rays is too great to warrant any surgical decision about palatal port reconstruction based on this technique [79]. It would appear that the functional adequacy of the VP port for speech can only be determined while the patient produces a sample of connected speech while being viewed with videofluoroscopy or nasoendoscopy.

CINE- AND VIDEOFLUOROGRAPHY AND SPEECH RESEARCH

Cineradiography allows the observation of the speech structures in motion. Although restricted to observations on a two-dimensional plane, it does reveal the ongoing dynamics of motor speech production. It supplies information about the placement of the articulatory structures for the production of any sound and makes visible the sequencing and timing of the movement of the structures during the production of speech sounds. Movement of the structures also aids in the identification of a particular structure. Although such investigators as Astley [3] and Björk [7] had early recognized the importance of lateral pharyngeal wall movement in contributing to VP closure, there appears to have been little clinical acceptance of this information. However, in 1969, Skolnick [58] developed the technique of frontal view projection, and in 1970 he introduced the base view [59]. The clinical community quickly became convinced of the importance of the additional information that this new view could provide.

Historically, it is of interest to note that lateral cineradiography, in the study of VP action for normal or cleft palate speakers, has been extensively used since the mid-1950s. Carrell [22] was one of the first to apply the principle of image intensification to fluorography and to synchronize the roentgen generator with the movie frame. Berry and Hofmann [5, 6] have written thorough descriptions of the principle and application of image intensification. Ramsey et al. [46] give a good historical and technological review of the development of cineradiography.

Most centers that employ the technique of cine- and videofluorography use basically similar equipment and procedures for obtaining the recorded speech sample. The subject is positioned between the fluoroscope and the image intensifier and is comfortably seated in a normal upright position with the head held stable by some type of headrest or cephalostat. The obtained x-ray image is amplified by electronic intensification, making it bright enough to be recorded by a movie camera. An additional feature is the incorporation of a distributor unit, which permits the simultaneous movie recording and videotaping as well as being able to view the function of the structures on a television monitor. The kind of camera used is dependent on the nature of the information desired; it may be one of either normal or high speed, and can be equipped with a synchronized sound track. Moll [40] has provided the first formally worked-out methodology and description of such equipment for speech research. Berry and Hofmann [5] have described their arrangement at the Lancaster Clinic, and Björk and Nylén [9] and Henningsson and Isberg [28] have discussed the technique they use in Sweden.

As one might expect, there have been numerous technical and methodological problems — for example, establishing an adequate filming rate and developing procedures for quantitatively reducing the information from the films in a reasonable period of time. Filming rate has been considered in papers by Shelton et al. [52], Björk

and Nylén [9], and Sparrow, Brogdon, and Bzoch [63]. Moll [40] developed a technique of tracing and measuring the outline of the projected image, which has become the basis for procedures followed in structural measurement studies. Wildman [75] has reviewed some of the measurement strategies for radiological assessment. Figure 11-1 illustrates the typical kinds of measurements used in studies to define site, height, and amount of seal of the velar port. The major criticism of lateral cinefluorography is that one can only visualize the upward and backward movement pattern of the soft palate, and the anterior displacement of the posterior pharyngeal wall. If the closure mechanism of the velar port is sphincterlike, then it is not likely that the mesial movement of the lateral pharyngeal wall will be seen from the lateral view alone.

In the base view as described by Skolnick [59], the patient is placed in a prone position on the

Figure 11-1. Exemplary measurements made from a single (stopped) frame videofluoroscopic film illustrating the lateral view of the velopharyngeal port at rest and in function for speech. L = length of the soft palate at rest, as measured in a straight line from the posterior nasal spine to the tip of the uvula; DN = depth of the nasopharynx as measured along the palatal plane from the posterior spine to the posterior pharyngeal wall; H = height of the velum as determined by a perpendicular measure from the palatal plane to the highest point of the levator eminence; PNS = posterior nasal spine; ANS = anteriornasal spine.

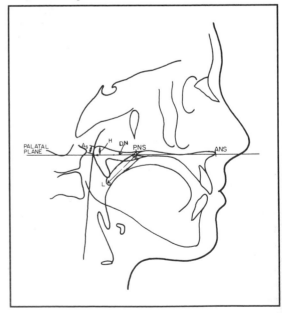

fluoroscopic table with the head and neck hyper-extended as in a "sphinx" position. In order to view the palatal port in this base position, the axis or plane of the port must be horizontal to the table which is, in turn, perpendicular to the x-ray beam. Skolnick notes that the plane of orientation of the palatal port varies between subjects primarily as a function of age, and he has identified the following factors on which optimal positioning of the plane is dependent: "(1) the level of the posterior pharyngeal wall that the velum either makes contact with or comes close to, (2) the contour of the posterior pharyngeal wall, and (3) the prominence of the adenoid pad." Skolnick [60] concludes that "the base view, which permits visualization of the velopharyngeal portal en face, shows the relationship of the velum and lateral-posterior aspects of the pharyngeal wall to each other and thus elucidates the mechanics of the entire sphincteric mechanism of velopharyngeal closure." This more complete picture of the VP port is not provided by the lateral view alone.

While the base view potentially provides for additional diagnostic information, certain inherent problems limit the objective use of this technique. Shelton and Trier [45] note that a problem encountered with the basal view is that of determining precisely the level at which the palatal port is being observed. They indicate that the base view may provide information about VP structures, but at a level different from the junction of the velum and the pharyngeal walls. Should this, in fact, occur, then the identification of VP closure could be overlooked. Shelton and Trier conclude that experimentation is needed in which radiopaque markers might be employed as an aid to identifying a system for locating the precise level at which the basal observation is being made. Bonnot [12] has provided some comparative data on measures of VP closure between the lateral and basal view for 20 cleft palate subjects. From seven different measures made of VP function, Bonnot found only the lateral measure of VP closure to be significantly related to the speaker's articulation and intelligibility scores. Bonnot concludes that the assessment of VP adequacy, in predicting speech proficiency, from a base view, is not better than that which is made from a lateral view.

A perpendicular orientation of the x-ray beam to the VP port can also be made by use of the Towne's view [23, 45]. Stringer and Witzel [64] have found that Towne's view provides for more valid registration of the VPI than does the base view. Both Towne's and the base projections require exaggerated extension or flexion of the neck. As McWilliams, Musgrave, and Crozier [39] have shown, flexion of the neck can result in atypical degrees of VPI. It seems prudent that until further evidence is available concerning the identification of closure patterns of the velar port when the patient is required to flex or extend the neck, the information obtained on basal films must be interpreted with considerable caution.

In addition to the several technical problems just described, other criticisms of cineradiography have been noted including the frequent lack of detail in the image projections, the expense of the equipment, delays in film processing, the inordinate amount of time required for data reduction, and the danger from radiation exposure. Some of these criticisms are no longer valid. For example, although the equipment is expensive, it is generally already installed in most hospitals and many clinics for other diagnostic purposes. Because of immediate playback capability with videotape, film processing delays are no longer a problem. Data reduction used to involve frame-by-frame analysis to measure site, height, and amount of closure. Because of the more extensive body of normative data available today, however, there is little clinical need for such extensive analysis. Assessment of the overall integrity of the VP port can now be made by examining the patterns of VP function. There still exists the danger of radiation exposure, but with proper selection of a speech sample (to be discussed below) and proper shielding of the body (particularly the eyes, thyroid glands, and gonads) radiation exposure can be minimized [30].

STANDARDIZATION

Some years ago concern was expressed that there was not enough standardization of normal speech patterns to allow clinical interpretations of the cineradiograph of abnormalities [76]. Over the past 20 years, however, considerable research has been done in defining normal parameters of speech physiology and the clinician is in a much better position to identify variation from the normal, both anatomically and functionally. Research has also been directed toward the identification of those factors that are meaningful to the actual dynamics of VP closure before attempting to standardize a particular measure. The measurement of velar length and the depth of the nasopharynx, for example, has been a subject of considerable study.

LENGTH OF VELUM AND DEPTH OF NASOPHARYNX

It is known that for VP closure to occur the soft palate must come into contact with the posterior pharyngeal wall. An adequate length, therefore, is one that allows the soft palate to span the depth of the nasopharynx and make closure. Warren and Hofmann [72] and Mazaheri, Millard, and Erickson [37] raised the question of whether a relationship existed between the length of the soft palate and the depth of the nasopharynx. In both these studies the length of the soft palate was defined as a straight-line measurement from the posterior nasal spine to the tip of the uvula with the velum *at rest.* They reported contradictory findings. It appears, as Simpson and Austin [57] have noted, that interest in the relationship between velar length and nasopharyngeal depth has been based on the assumption that both of these measures remain constant from rest position to function. Relative to the depth of the nasopharynx, there appears to be general agreement in the literature that this measure is essentially stable between physiological rest and function for normal speakers. As for a change in the length of the soft palate, it has been well documented that a significant increase in palatal length does occur for normal speakers. The increase in this "stretched" velum appears to range between 10 and 50 percent of its resting length [25, 55, 76]. This phenomenon appears to be, in part, a function of the subject's age [40]. The pull of the VP muscles as they act to elevate and approximate the velum to the pharynx thus increases the movement of what had appeared to be a finite length when the velum was at rest.

As it is easier to make a straight-line measurement, as in the at-rest position, than to measure along the total superior surface of the velum in functional position, Williams and Bzoch [76] tried to find a method of predicting velar length in the functional position for speech from its length at rest. They were unable, however, to identify an amount of increase that could be reduced to a constant or predictable factor. Simpson and Austin [57] also found a lack of any significant relationship between amount of velar stretch produced in function and velar length at rest, and were unable to establish any significant correlation between the measure of velar stretch with the measure of nasopharyngeal depth. The point to be made is that if a measure of velar length is to be "standardized," it would seem to be more meaningful if it were made with the velum in its functional position.

OTHER MEASURES

There have been numerous other radiographic studies concerned with an array of structural relationships attempting to define the normal mechanism. Much of the work has had significant application in the rehabilitation of patients with VPI. Rickets [47] and Brader [14] have analyzed the relationship of cranial base angulation and depth of the nasopharynx. Ricketts concluded that "cleft palate speech may be influenced by abnormal variation of the cranial base of the skull which provides the bony architecture for the drape of the pharyngeal musculature." Brader's [14] quantitative study, however, does not support the contention of abnormal angularity of the cranial base in subjects with cleft palate. Other investigators, such as Aram and Subtelny [2], Warren and Hofmann [72], and Mazaheri and Hofmann [36], have studied the relationship of the palatal plane to the height and site of velar closure. Establishing the limits of this relationship has aided in the identification of a more optimal position of prosthetic speech appliances.

PASSAVANT'S PAD

Since the original identification of a muscular bulge across the posterior pharyngeal wall at or near the level of the VP approximation by Philip Gustav Passavant in 1863 [29], there has been strong controversy and contradictory research findings concerning the significance of this "pad" for speech. Graber et al. [26] have noted the occurrence of a posterior wall bulge at the level of VP closure during speech for four of 44 normal speakers as determined by cephalometric analysis. Benson [4], however, observed a Passavant's pad for four of his 30 normal speakers but noted that its position was too low to be effective in aiding palatopharyngeal closure. Others [19, 26, 76] have noted minimal or insignificant posterior pharyngeal wall movement for normal-speaking individuals. Carpenter and Morris [21] and Townsend [70] have reported observing a velar-pharyngeal wall-pad closure mechanism to occur for their clinical population.

The classic clinical interpretation of the significance of this posterior pharyngeal wall displacement, or Passavant's pad, is that it is part of the VP closure complex. This bulging action has been interpreted as functioning similar to an adenoid pad which frequently aids in the closure of the nasopharynx, which otherwise would be too deep for palatal function alone. It is our experience, however, that most patients who demonstrate the existence of a pad do so at a level below where contact is being effected or attempted; therefore, explanations other than that of its possible assistance in reducing the VP port for all patients must be considered.

In our studies of VP function at the University of Florida for over 100 normal speakers, we have observed posterior wall movement that would approximate a Passavant's pad configuration in only one subject. Among our clinical cleft palate population and other individuals with congenital and acquired VPI, the occurrence of this pad is considerably higher. However, in those cases in which there is a noticeable and specific anterior bulging of the posterior pharyngeal wall, it generally has been at a level below where velar-pharyngeal wall contact is being attempted. In fact it is not uncommon to observe this discrete bulging of the constrictors across the posterior pharyngeal wall from an oral inspection alone. Knowing that VP closure normally takes place at or above the level of the palatal plane, which is not visible orally, the question is raised relative to the significance of this pad in VP physiology for speech. It has been documented through speech bulb reduction programs that compensatory movements of the lateral and posterior pharyngeal wall musculature do take place. Blakeley [10] and Weiss [73] have reported that some individuals develop such strong compensatory pharyngeal wall activity (both posterior and lateral wall) that this action becomes sufficient to close the gap between the speech bulb and the pharyngeal wall. However, it is not clear whether this buildup of

pharyngeal wall action with prosthetic stimulus is the same phenomenon as that which has been identified as Passavant's pad.

Hiramoto et al. [29] have noted from their assessment of 10 adult cleft palate patients with marked pharyngeal wall pad that the formation of the pad was not associated with the degree of VP closure but rather with lingual position for the production of specific sounds.

That many individuals with cleft palate and others with VPI develop articulation patterns significantly deviant is well-known. In cases in which pharyngeal fricatives and glottal stops are substituted for the pressure consonants, it is quite evident that unusual compensatory adjustments of the nasal, oral, and laryngeal structures occur. It seems plausible that displacement of the posterior wall may be the result of "overflow" activity of compensatory adjustments in laryngeal position, in lingual carriage, or in lateral pharyngeal wall activity. It is recognized that the relationship between posterior wall activity (Passavant's pad) and speech is not clear at this time and that further research is needed to identify not only the frequency of occurrence of posterior wall displacement, but the causal factor(s) that trigger this unusual physiological adjustment.

VELOPHARYNGEAL INSUFFICIENCY

Subtelny [66] has defined VPI as "a failure of the soft palate to contact the pharyngeal wall during speech and to separate the nasal cavity from the rest of the vocal tract." Williams and Bzoch [77] have extended this definition to include not only a failure of VP contact but also an inappropriate rate or closure sequence in which the ability to make an effective seal exists but the precision in timing of closure is off. It is only with the use of fluoroscopy (and nasoendoscopy) that detection of this inappropriate rate or closure sequence is possible. It may be possible for a patient to achieve closure physiologically but be unable to maintain appropriate rate of closure or appropriate sequencing of closure during speech. And this information is, of course, vital in the clinical evaluation of VP competency.

VIDEO- AND CINEFLUOROGRAPHY AS A DIAGNOSTIC TOOL — ANALYSIS OF VELOPHARYNGEAL CLOSURE PATTERNS

The following discussion covers some applications of video- and cinefluorographic data as they are currently being used in a situation in which there is collaboration of specialists from radiology, surgery, dentistry, and speech pathology for the preliminary diagnosis and treatment of VPI problems. It is the responsibility of the speech pathologist to not only analyze the fluoroscopic film in order to identify the factor(s) responsible for the VP dysfunction, but to then offer an opinion as to the best method of treating (surgical, prosthetic, or behavioral therapies) the dysfunction based on the observed and measured functional characteristics of the VP port during controlled samples of connected speech. Dixon-Wood and Williams [24] conducted a retrospective study of the medical records of 100 consecutive patients seen in the Craniofacial Center at the University of Florida to determine the rate of compliance of specific recommendations made by speech-language pathologists for the treatment of VPI. The primary question was whether the frequency of success in correcting symptoms associated with VPI was greater for those patients who received treatment recommended by the speech-language pathologist than for those patients who were treated in a manner other than that recommended by the speech-language pathologist. The specific recommendation for treatment for all patients made by the speech-language pathologist was based primarily on findings obtained from the lateral and frontal view fluoroscopic evaluation. These investigators found that 78 of the recommendations made by the speech-language pathologists on the team were in fact carried out. For this group, only eight (10%) continued to demonstrate a clinically significant residual speech problem associated with VPI. On the other hand, 22 of the recommendations made by the speech pathologist were not complied with. That is, the patients either received no treatment or received a treatment other than that

which was recommended. For these 22 patients, seven (32%) continued to demonstrate a clinically significant speech problem associated with VPI. There were records for only three of these 22 patients that explained why some other treatment was selected. The treatment of the other 19 patients appears to have been arbitrary. The point to be made from this study is that there were 3 times as many patients who were unsuccessfully treated when treated in a manner other than that recommended by the speech pathologist based on information obtained from the fluoroscopic assessment.

The cinefluorographic apparatus used in the Department of Radiology of the University of Florida Teaching Hospital has been described in a previous publication [63]. Briefly, we have had some modifications, of which the most important are the incorporation of a 16-mm movie film and synchronized sound tract, and the videofluoroscopy technique that permits television monitoring during the filming as well as rapid and easy playback capabilities. The analysis of the film has immediate application both clinically and in basic research.

NORMAL PATTERN

LATERAL

As noted earlier in this chapter, the lateral or midsaggital plane traditionally has been the primary plane of reference for assessing velar function in that it allows for subjective as well as objective measurement of several important parameters. For example, subjectively, the clinician can make an appraisal of the occurrence of velar mobility, the appropriateness of velar elevation relative to the speech samples being produced, and the existence of VPI if the velum fails to make contact with the posterior pharyngeal wall. In addition to this subjective analysis, there are several important objective measures that can be made of the VP port. Subtelny [66] has provided normative data by age for the following measures: (1) the length of the velum in its physiological rest position as measured from the posterior nasal spine (PNS) to the tip of the uvula; (2) the thickness of the velum as measured across its thickest point while at physiological rest; (3) the depth of the nasopharynx as measured along the palatal plane from PNS to the posterior pharyngeal wall (see Fig. 11-1). In addition to these standardized measures, a quantifiable measure of the lateral

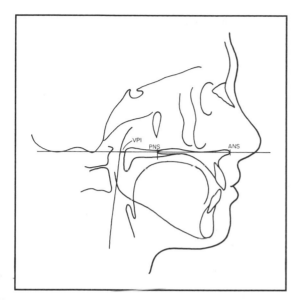

Figure 11-2. A lateral view illustrating a condition of velopharyngeal insufficiency (VPI) which occurs during the patient's production of connected speech involving nonnasal speech sounds. PNS = posterior nasal spine; ANS = anterior nasal spine.

dimension of the gap between the velum and the posterior pharyngeal wall can be obtained. Figure 11-2 illustrates these lateral measures.

We have analyzed the velopharyngeal closure patterns of 100 normal young adults speaking the same sentence [78]. Figure 11-3 shows a graph of a sample pattern in which time is plotted along the abcissa and opening (in millimeters) is shown

along the ordinate. For the sentence, "In the evening Connie watches TV with me," the pattern of opening and closing of the velar port was essentially identical for all subjects. That is, four openings, which occurred on the nasal consonants, and three points of closure, associated with oral consonants, were invariably found. Although the overall pattern was the same, certain variations existed among these speakers: (1) the slope of closure and opening curves indicating variations in amounts of assimilated nasality; (2) the amount of velar port opening for the nasal sounds, suggesting possible overall anatomical differences; and (3) the total time lapse for the production of the sentence, showing differences in speaking rate. This pattern for normal speakers is in agreement with the findings of Shelton et al. [53], who observed that for their normal subjects closure was maintained during speech except for breaks associated with nasal consonants and adjacent vowels. The desirability of assessing dynamic features of VP closure patterns during speech, such as these, has also been discussed by Moll [41], Björk [7], Nylén [43], and Skolnick et al. [61].

FRONTAL

As previously noted, Skolnick [58] identified the importance of the mesial movement of the lateral pharyngeal musculature (primarily the palatopharyngeus and salpingopharyngeus) muscle bundles in VP closure. A subjective assessment of several components of this side wall movement

Figure 11-3. The average open and closure pattern of the velopharyngeal (VP) port, measured from lateral cinefluorography, as demonstrated by 100 normal speakers producing the sentence "In the evening Connie watches T.V. with me." Time is plotted along the abcissa in terms of the number of movie frames (standard filming rate of 24 frames/sec). Openings of the velar port (gap between the velum and the posterior pharyngeal wall) are plotted in millimeters along the ordinate.

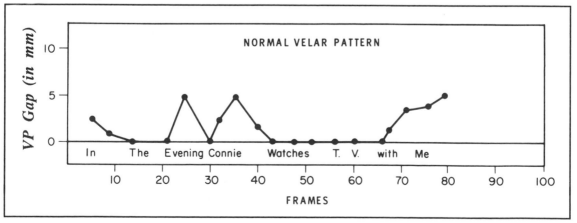

can be made including (1) the existence of identifiable lateral wall movement; (2) symmetry of the mesial movement between the two sides; (3) range or extent of movement toward the midline; and (4) the vertical position at which the maximal mesial excursion occurs relative to the point of attempted velar-pharyngeal wall contact.

VELOPHARYNGEAL INSUFFICIENCY

The uniform pattern of closure in normals illustrated in Figure 11-3 can be considered a standard against which to compare the patterns of defective speakers in similarly controlled studies. Figure 11-4, for example, shows the pattern of a deaf oral speaker who spoke the same sentence under the same conditions. It can be seen that the rate of speech as determined by the number of frames was much slower for the deaf subject and that although VP closure did occur, the pattern of closure was inappropriate. Although this individual sounded hypernasal, it can be noted from the graph that he did achieve VP closure several times during the speech sample. His abnormal pattern of rate and sequence led to hypernasal distortion of speech despite the existence of a potentially competent VP mechanism. It is clear that cinefluorography can aid the clinician in the identification of functional components underlying a patient's condition of hypernasality. Figure 11-5 illustrates the pattern of a speaker with a repaired cleft palate and reveals the consistent lack of closure during the production of this speech sample. It would appear that the initial palate repair did not provide an adequate VP mechanism, and the need for further surgical repair is clearly indicated. The graph that reflects the cinefluorographic analysis also shows the existence of velar mobility and demonstrates that the residual gap during the best attempt for closure in this sample was about 5 mm. This example illustrates well the factors we use for assessing velar function from a lateral view, as mentioned earlier: (1) whether there is velar movement, (2) if the movement pattern is appropriate to the speech sample, and (3) the depth of the residual gap. The identification of these factors aids us in selecting the optimal physical or behavioral management for each patient.

Intermediate between the kind of patient that shows an abnormal pattern due to functional causes such as deafness or faulty learning and the speaker that has an obvious organic deficit such as cleft palate or paralysis is the patient that can achieve closure but whose timing is inappropriate. Such a pattern is demonstrated in Figure 11-6. From this graph it can be seen that in the initial phase of the sentence the timing of the closure was late — that is, closure for the oral consonants was indeed being made but was too slow to coincide with the actions of the other articulators. Toward the end of the speech sample, the patient

Figure 11-4. Velopharyngeal (VP) dysfunction measured from lateral cinefluorography as demonstrated by an individual who is congenitally deaf and who consequently was unable to audibly monitor his speech production.

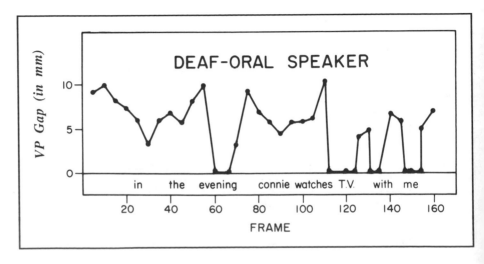

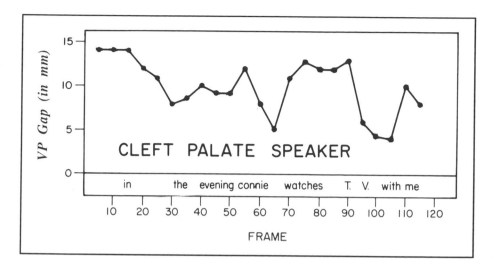

Figure 11-5. Velopharyngeal (VP) insufficiency measured from lateral cinefluorography as demonstrated by a postoperative cleft palate individual. The graph illustrates that although there is velar mobility, a consistent gap (5 mm or more) remained throughout the patient's production of the sentence.

was experiencing complete failure in making closure. With the causes of hearing loss and organic VP incompetency ruled out, the possibilities of learning, psychological, or neurological dysfunctions were indicated.

What the above cases had in common was a vocal quality symptom of hypernasality. The cause of each is not necessarily apparent from the usual chairside clinical tests. The analysis made possible by fluoroscopy, however, allowed for a differen-

tiation of etiological factors and subsequent selection of different treatment procedures.

Shprintzen, McCall, and Skolnick [55] have reported finding, through the use of multiview cine fluoroscopy, that speech, blowing, and whistling all share a common pattern of VP closure. They note that this pattern is significantly different from the closure mechanism identified for swallowing and gagging. From this observation the authors have suggested that the reason some individuals can achieve closure during blowing and whistling but fail to make closure for speech is that an error in learning has occurred. From this premise, Shprintzen et al. [56] have outlined an operant therapy procedure based on the strategy of starting from closure during blowing or whistling and proceeding through a series of succes-

Figure 11-6. Velopharyngeal (VP) dysfunction as demonstrated by an individual with a minor neurological disorder. Although this patient demonstrated the ability to achieve closure, it can be seen that the timing or pattern of closure is not appropriate and that he lacked the ability to sustain closure where required.

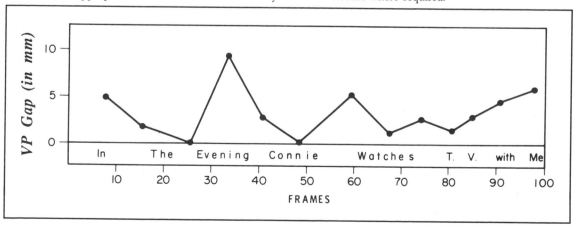

sive approximations that lead to closure for speech. Although these authors have reported considerable success in the employment of this operant modification program, there is still limited verification to date from other clinics relative to the efficacy of this technique.

SUMMARY

In summary, a review of the literature reveals that radiographic techniques have had application in the description of the articulation process and in defining patterns of normal velopharyngeal closure. This information has aided in the differential diagnosis of velopharyngeal insufficiency and in aiding in the identification of the optimal and specific treatment procedure including surgical, prosthetic, and behavioral therapies. It is apparent that inasmuch as we are dealing with a dynamic process, video- and cineradiography make an invaluable contribution to our task of defining the normal and of diagnosing the abnormal in speech performance.

REFERENCES

1. Allen, H. On a new method for recording the motion of the soft palate. *Trans. Coll. Physicians Phila.* 7, 1884.
2. Aram, A., and Subtelny, J. D. Velopharyngeal function and cleft palate prostheses. *J. Prosthet. Dent.* 9:149, 1959.
3. Astley, R. The movements of the lateral walls of the nasopharynx: A cine-radiographic study. *J. Laryngol. Otol.* 73:325, 1958.
4. Benson, D. Roentgenographic cephalometric study of palatopharyngeal closure of normal adults during vowel phonation. *Cleft Palate J.* 9:43, 1972.
5. Berry, H. M., and Hofmann, F. A. Cinefluorography with image intensification for observing temporomandibular joint movements. *J. Am. Dent. Assoc.* 53:517, 1956.
6. Berry, H. M., and Hofmann, F. A. Cineradiographic observations of temporomandibular joint function. *J. Prosthet. Dent.* 9:21, 1959.
7. Björk, L. Velopharyngeal function in connected speech: Studies using tomography and cineradiography synchronized with speech spectrography. *Acta Radiol.* 202:1, 1961.
8. Björk, L., and Nylén, B. The function of the soft palate during connected speech. *Acta Chir. Scand.* 126:434, 1963.
9. Bjork, and Nylén, E. O. Cineradiography with synchronized sound: Spectrum analysis. A study of velopharyngeal function during connected speech in normals and cleft palate cases. *Plast. Reconstr. Surg.* 27:397, 1961.
10. Blakeley, R. The rationale for a temporary speech prosthesis in palatal insufficiency. *Br. J. Disord. Commun.* 4:134, 1969.
11. Bloomer, H. Observations on palatopharyngeal movements in speech and deglutition. *J. Speech Hear. Disord.* 18:230, 1953.
12. Bonnot, J. A comparative study of two measures of velopharyngeal closure: Lateral and basal. Presented at Third International Congress on Cleft Palate, June 1977.
13. Bowman, S. A., and Shanks, J. C. Velopharyngeal relationships of /i/ and /s/ as seen cephalometrically for persons with suspected incompetence. *J. Speech Hear. Disord.* 43:185, 1978.
14. Brader, A. A. A cephalometric appraisal of morphological variations in cranial base and associated pharyngeal structures: Implications in cleft palate therapy. *Angle Orthodont.* 27:179, 1957.
15. Broadbent, R. H. A new X-ray technique and its application to orthodontia. *Angle Orthodont.* 1:45, 1931.
16. Brodie, A. G. On the growth pattern of the human head from the third month to the eighth year of life. *Am. J. Anat.* 68:209, 1941.
17. Brodie, A. G. Cephalometric roentgenology: History, techniques and uses. *Oral Surg.* 7:185, 1949.
18. Buck, M. Postoperative velopharyngeal movements in cleft palate cases. *J. Speech Hear. Disord.* 19:288, 1954.
19. Bzoch, K. R. Variation in velopharyngeal valving: The factor of vowel changes. *Cleft Palate J.* 5:211, 1968.
20. Calnan, J. Diagnosis, prognosis, and treatment of palatopharyngeal incompetence with special reference to radiographic investigations. *Br. J. Plast. Surg.* 8:265, 1956.
21. Carpenter, M. A., and Morris, H. L. A preliminary study of Passavant's pad. *Cleft Palate J.* 5:61, 1968.
22. Carrell, J. A cinefluorographic technique for the study of velopharyngeal closure. *J. Speech Hear. Disord.* 12:224, 1952.
23. Cotton, R. T., and Quattromani, F. L. Lateral defects in velopharyngeal insufficiency. *Arch. Otolaryngol.* 103:90, 1977.
24. Dixon-Wood, V. L., and Williams, W. N. Team compliance with speech pathologists' recommendations for treatment of VPI. *ASHA* 27:80, 1985.
25. Eisenbach, C. R., and Williams, W. W. Comparing the unaided visual exam to lateral cinefluorography in estimating several parameters of velopharyngeal function. *J. Speech Hear. Disord.* 49:136, 1984.
26. Graber, T. M., Bzoch, K. R., and Aoba, T. A functional study of the palatal and pharyngeal structures. *Angle Orthodont.* 29:30, 1959.
27. Hagerty, R. F., Hill, M. J., Pettit, H. S., and Kane, J. J. Posterior pharyngeal wall movements in normals. *J. Speech Hear. Res.* 1:203, 1958.
28. Henningsson, G. E., and Isberg, A. M. Velopharyngeal movement patterns in patients alternating between oral and glottal articulation: A clinical and cineradiographic study. *Cleft Palate J.* 23:1, 1986.
29. Hiramoto, M., Okazaki, N., and Honjo, J. Role of Passavant's ridge in cleft palate speech. Presented at Third International Conference on Cleft Palate, Toronto, June 1977.
30. Isberg, A., and Williams, W. N. Radiographic Examination of Velopharyngeal Function. In M. Delbas (Ed.), *Maxillofacial Imaging.* Philadelphia: Saunders, 1988.

31. Kelly, J. P. Studies in nasality. *Arch. Speech* 1:26, 1934.
32. King, E. W. A roentgenographic study of pharyngeal growth. *Angle Orthodont.* 22:23, 1952.
33. Loney, R. W., and Bloem, T. J. Velopharyngeal dysfunction: Recommendations for use of nomenclature. *Cleft Palate J.* 24:334, 1977.
34. Lubker, J., and Morris, H. Predicting cinefluorographic measures of velopharyngeal opening from lateral still X-rays films. *J. Speech Hear. Res.* 11:747, 1968.
35. MacMillian, A. S., and Kelemen, C. Radiography of the supraglottic speech organs: A survey. *AMA Arch. Otolaryng. (Chicago)* 55:671, 1952.
36. Mazaheri, M., and Hofmann, F. A. Cineradiography in prosthetic speech appliance construction. *J. Prosthet. Dent.* 12:571, 1962.
37. Mazaheri, M., Millard, R. T., and Erickson, D. M. Cineradiographic comparison of normal to noncleft subjects with velopharyngeal inadequacy. *Cleft Palate J.* 1:199, 1964.
38. McDonald, R., and Baker, H. Cleft palate speech: On integration of research and clinical observation. *J. Speech Hear. Disord.* 16:9, 1951.
39. McWilliams, B. J., Musgrave, R. H., and Crozier, P. A. The influence of head position upon velopharyngeal closure. *Cleft Palate J.* 5:117, 124, 1968.
40. Moll, K. L. Cinefluorographic techniques in speech research. *J. Speech Hear. Res.* 3:227, 1960.
41. Moll, K. L. Velopharyngeal closure on vowels. *J. Speech Hear. Res.* 5:30, 1962.
42. Mourino, A. P., and Weinberg, B. A cephalometric study of velar stretch in 8 and 10 year old children. *Cleft Palate J.* 12:417, 1975.
43. Nylén, B. O. Cleft palate and speech: A surgical study including observation on velopharyngeal closure during connected speech, using synchronized cineradiography and sound spectrography. *Acta Radiol.* 203:1, 1961.
44. Parmenter, C. E., and Trevino, S. N. Vowel positions as shown by X-ray. *Q.J. Speech* 18:351, 1932.
45. Quattromani, F. L., Benton, C., and Cotton, R. T. The Towne projection for evaluation of the velopharyngeal sphincter. *Radiology* 125:540, 1977.
46. Ramsey, C. G. S., Watson, J. S., Jr., Tristian, R. A., Weinbert, S., and Cornwell, W. S. *Cinefluorography.* Springfield, Ill.: Thomas, 1960.
47. Ricketts, R. M. The cranial base and soft structures in cleft palate speech and breathing. *Plast. Reconstr. Surg.* 14:47, 1959.
48. Russell, G. O. *The Vowel: Its Physiological Mechanism as Shown by X-ray.* Columbus: Ohio State University Press, 1928.
49. Russell, G. O. The mechanism of speech. *J. Acoust. Soc. Am.* 1:83, 1929.
50. Scheier, M. Ueber die Verwerthung der Rontgenstrahlen in der Rhino- und Laryngologie. *Arch. Laryngol.* 6:57, 1897.
51. Schneider, E., and Shprintzen, R. J. A survey of speech pathologists: Current trends in the diagnosis and management of velopharyngeal insufficiency. *Cleft Palate J.* 17:249, 1980.
52. Shelton, R. L., Brooks, A. R., Youngstrom, K. A., Diedrich, W. M., and Brooks, R. S. Filming speed in cinefluorographic speech study. *J. Speech Hear. Res.* 6:19, 1963.
53. Shelton, R. L., Brooks, A. R., and Youngstrom, K. A. Articulation and patterns of palatopharyngeal closure. *J. Speech Hear. Disord.* 29:390, 1964.

54. Shelton, R. L., and Trier, W. C. Issues involved in the evaluation of velopharyngeal closure. *Cleft Palate J.* 13:127, 1976.
55. Shprintzen, R. J., Lencione, R. N., McCall, G. N., and Skolnick, M. L. A three dimensional cinefluoroscopic analysis of velopharyngeal closure and non-speech activities in normals. *Cleft Palate J.* 11:412, 1974.
56. Shprintzen, R. J., McCall, G. N., and Skolnick, M. L. A new therapeutic technique for treatment of velopharyngeal incompetence. *J. Speech Hear. Disord.* 40:69, 1975.
57. Simpson, R. K., and Austin, A. A. A cephalometric investigation of velar stretch. *Cleft Palate J.* 9:341, 1972.
58. Skolnick, M. L. Video velopharyngography in patients with nasal speech, with emphasis on lateral pharyngeal motion in velopharyngeal closure. *Radiology* 93:747, 1969.
59. Skolnick, M. L. Videofluoroscopic examination of the velopharyngeal portal during phonation in lateral and base projections — a new technique for studying the mechanics of closure. *Cleft Palate J.* 7:803, 1970.
60. Skolnick, M. L., McCall, G. N., and Barnes, M. The sphincteric mechanism of velopharyngeal closure. *Cleft Palate J.* 10:286, 1973.
61. Skolnick, M. L., Shprintzen, R. J., McCall, G. N., and Rakoff, S. Patterns of velopharyngeal closure in subjects with repaired cleft palate and normal speech: A multiview videofluoroscopic analysis. *Cleft Palate J.* 12:369, 1975.
62. Skolnick, M. A. A plea of an interdisciplinary approach to the radiological study of the velopharyngeal port. *Cleft Palate J.* 14:329, 1977.
63. Sparrow, S. S., Brogdon, B. G., and Bzoch, K. R. The effect of filming rate and frame selection on cinefluorographic velopharyngeal analysis. *Cleft Palate J.* 1:419, 1964.
64. Stringer, D. A., and Witzel, M. A. A velopharyngeal insufficiency on videofluoroscopy: comparisons of projections. *Am. J. Radiol.* 146:15, 1986.
65. Subtelny, J. *Laminographic Study of Vowels Produced by Cleft Palate Speakers.* Dissertation, Northwestern University, Evanston, Ill., 1956.
66. Subtelny, J. D. Roentgenography Applied to the Study of Speech. In S. Pruzansky (Ed.), *Congenital Anomalies of the Face and Associated Structures.* Springfield, Ill.: Thomas, 1961. Pp. 314, 322.
67. Subtelny, J. D., and Baker, H. K. The significance of adenoid tissue in velopharyngeal function. *Plast. Reconstr. Surg.* 17:235, 1956.
68. Subtelny, J. D., Pruzansky, S., and Subtelny, J. The Application of Roentgenography in the Study of Speech. In L. Kaiser (Ed.), *Manual of Phonetics.* Amsterdam: North Holland Publishing Co., 1957.
69. Subtelny, J. D., and Subtelny, J. Intelligibility and associated physiological factors of cleft palate speakers. *J. Speech Hear. Res.* 2:353, 1959.
70. Townsend, R. H. The formation of Passavant's bar. *J. Laryngol. Otolaryngol.* 55:154, 1940.
71. Wardill, W. E. M., and Whillis, J. Movements of the soft palate, with special reference to the function of the tensor palati muscle. *Surg. Gynecol. Obstet.* 62:836, 1936.
72. Warren, D. W., and Hoffmann, F. A. A cineradiographic study of velopharyngeal closure. *Plast. Reconst. Surg.* 28:656, 1961.
73. Weiss, C. Success of an obturator reduction program. *Cleft Palate J.* 8:291, 1971.
74. West, R., Kennedy, L., and Carr, A. *The Rehabilitation of*

Speech. New York: Harper, 1947.

75. Wildman, A. J. Tongue, soft palate, and pharyngeal wall movement. *Am. J. Orthodont.* 47:439, 1961.

76. Williams, W. N., and Bzoch, K. R. Interrelationships of measurements in the dynamics of velopharyngeal valving as determined by cinefluorographic analysis. Presented at the Meeting of the American Cleft Palate Association, Mexico City, April 1966.

77. Williams, W. N., and Bzoch, K. R. Quantitative diagnos- tic procedures for assessing velopharyngeal closure. *Bull. Fla. Cleft Palate Assoc.* No. 4, 1972.

78. Williams, W. N., Bzoch, K. R., and Agee, F. Functional versus organic patterns of velopharyngeal insufficien- cy for speech. Presented at the Meeting of the Ameri- can Cleft Palate Association, Chicago, May 1967.

79. Williams, W. N., and Eisenbach, C. R. Assessing VP function: the lateral still technique vs cinefluorogra- phy. *Cleft Palate J.* 18:45–50, 1981.

CHAPTER 12

Nasopharyngoscopy

Robert J. Shprintzen

Among scientists who have advocated various diagnostic procedures for assessing velopharyngeal valving, there has been a tendency to tout a single procedure as being the "ultimate" in scientific technology. While it is the intent of this chapter to extol the magnificence of nasopharyngoscopy, and it is indeed a superb diagnostic technique, the reader must not be led into believing that it is *the only means* advocated for the diagnosis of velopharyngeal insufficiency. What should be stated, however, is that for the complete clinical diagnosis of velopharyngeal valving abnormalities, it appears to be absolutely essential to utilize both nasopharyngoscopy and multiview videofluoroscopy. Without these two methods of direct observation of the velopharyngeal valve, physical management recommendations for velopharyngeal insufficiency are only blind, and should not be undertaken if these more definitive studies are not available.

It is of interest to note for historical purposes that the initial descriptions of the clinical application of nasopharyngoscopy [16, 17] and multiview videofluoroscopy [32] occurred almost simultaneously in 1969. I am persistently asked the following question by colleagues: "If given a choice between nasopharyngoscopy and multiview videofluoroscopy, which would you use?" The answer actually is quite simple. I do have a choice, yet *I still use both.* Endoscopy and fluoroscopy are complementary examinations, but yield different types of information. Furthermore, the information provided does not always agree. Some specific data regarding this concept are provided later in this chapter; Dr. Williams described videofluoroscopy in Chapter 11. However, prior to the advocacy of nasopharyngoscopy, it was essential to let the reader know that no single diagnostic technique provides all necessary information.

CONCEPTUAL BASIS FOR NASOPHARYNGOSCOPY

The basic concept behind nasopharyngoscopy is to be able to directly visualize the velopharyngeal valve from above, without disturbing the normal flow of speech production. In order to fully appreciate the technique, certain features of velopharyngeal anatomy and physiology must be understood which will then guide the clinician's approach to endoscopic procedure and the choice of endoscopic equipment.

VELOPHARYNGEAL PHYSIOLOGY

When reference is made to the velopharyngeal valve, whether in the literature, in clinical discussion, or treatment planning, the majority of individuals picture a circular opening at some arbitrary point between the nasopharynx and oropharynx. In other words, velopharyngeal insufficiencies are described in terms of an "area." Actually, as pointed out in several recent publications [23, 24, 31], the velopharyngeal valve is not a two-dimensional "portal," but rather a three-dimensional tube with vertical depth in addition to cross-sectional length and width. Lateral pharyngeal wall motion very often will occur at a vertical level different than the height of velar elevation. If the clinician is able to understand that velopharyngeal physiology involves the motion and interaction of various moving parts (velum, lateral pharyngeal walls, and posterior pharyngeal wall) at several different vertical levels within the pharynx, then he or she will be able to understand how particular instrumentation can be applied.

INSTRUMENTATION AND TECHNIQUE

By definition, endoscopes are visual devices used inside the body. They must be able to convey light into a darkened space while returning a clear visual image to the examiner. There are three types of instruments currently in use to directly view the velopharyngeal orifice: a side-viewing rigid endoscope [18]; a side-viewing flexible endoscope [14]; and an end-viewing flexible endoscope [23, 24, 27]. Only the end-viewing flexible endoscope provides a view of both the horizontal and vertical aspects of pharyngeal structure and physiology [24]. The abilities of instruments to carry light, view images, yet be thin and easy to handle mean that certain characteristics must be traded off for others. These factors necessary for accurate and successful nasopharyngoscopic examinations are, in order of importance [24]:

1. Compliance, that is, easy passage of the endoscope without pain or discomfort
2. Visual access to as much of the upper airway as possible
3. Good light saturation (adequate illumination)
4. Good optical quality
5. Wide cone of acceptance, or the width of the visual field

It may seem odd that of the five points listed above, the first and most important one deals with patient cooperation while the other four deal with the instrumentation. But it should be obvious that even the finest of optics are of little value if the examination procedure is difficult to perform and compliance of patients is difficult to obtain because of the discomfort involved. Therefore, compliance is enhanced by thinner, more flexible endoscopes. Though the optics of a thin flexible endoscope cannot compare to that of a rigid endoscope, the rate of successful examination with the flexible instrument is far higher than with the rigid endoscope. Four-year-old children can routinely be examined successfully when using a 3-mm-diameter flexible nasopharyngolaryngoscope. My personal experience shows approximately 90 percent compliance for children ranging in age from 4 through 6 years. Above 6 years, there is near total compliance.

Using a rigid endoscope, examining children under the age of 8 years is extremely difficult. Personal experience with several hundred examinations using the rigid Storz-Hopkins instrument has resulted in a rate of successful examination near zero for children from 4 to 8 years of age and only slightly better than 50 percent for children over 8 years of age. Furthermore, after the first unsuccessful attempt with the rigid endoscope, the children were most reluctant to be examined a second time. It is unusual for an examination to be painless using a rigid endoscope, whereas with a flexible endoscope, the majority of examinations can be performed without discomfort. It is suggested that if both flexible and rigid instruments are available, that the flexible endoscope be used first so that compliance is assured.

The specific instruments currently in use for nasopharyngoscopy include the Storz-Hopkins side-viewing rigid nasopharyngoscope, the Olympus NPF Type S3 side-viewing flexible fiberoptic nasopharyngoscope, the Olympus ENF-P end-viewing nasopharyngolaryngoscope, the Machida 4L end-viewing nasopharyngolaryngoscope, the Machida 3L end-viewing nasopharyngolaryngoscope, and the Pentax FNL-10S end-viewing nasopharyngolaryngoscope.

The Storz-Hopkins instrument (Fig. 12-1A and B) has excellent optical characteristics. Housed in a rigid stainless steel sheath is the Hopkins rod lens system, which conveys an extremely clear image to the examiner. In the instrument typically used for the nasopharynx, the lens at the tip of the endoscope looks downward at a 70-degree angle. The viewing field covers a 105-degree angle of acceptance. The instrument is slightly elliptical and has a transverse diameter of slightly over 4 mm. The Storz-Hopkins instrument has gained wider acceptance in Europe, particularly Great Britain, than in North America and Asia.

Flexible fiberoptics received its initial impetus from Japan, and the earliest report of its use in the American literature came from Japan [14]. Miyazaki and his colleagues developed a flexible side-viewing endoscope specifically for use in the nasopharynx. Their intent was to have a slender (3.4 mm) instrument that would allow comfort while still providing good optics and light-carrying capabilities [14]. The concept was to position the instrument above the velopharyngeal orifice in the most favorable position for viewing the en-

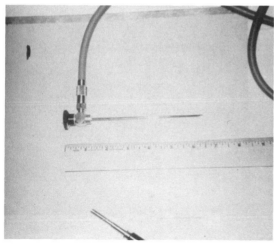

A

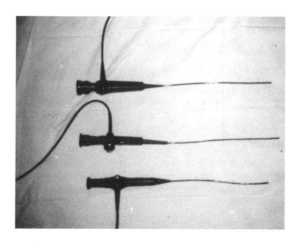

Figure 12-2. Comparison of the Pentax FNL-10S (top), Machida 3L (middle), and Olympus ENF P (bottom) nasopharyngolaryngoscopes. Note the smaller working length of the Olympus endoscope compared to the Machida and Pentax instruments.

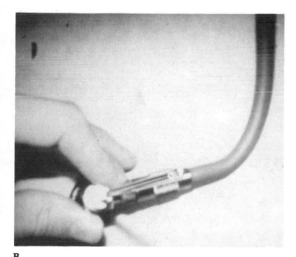

B

Figure 12-1. Rigid Storz-Hopkins endoscope, which looks downward at 70 degrees, showing the working length of the endoscope (A) and the lens (B).

tire portal during phonation. This instrument has been used more frequently in Japan than in North America or Europe.

The introduction of slender fiberoptic endoscopes in the mid-1970s prompted a rapid development of new instruments over the next decade. Initial reports of end-viewing flexible fiberoptic instruments for nasopharyngoscopy [5, 20, 21, 27, 28] described a variety of 4-mm diameter instruments from Machida, including the Machida ENT-US, ENT-US-25R, ENT-25 II, and 4L. Subse-

quently, thinner instruments with comparable optics became available, including the Olympus ENF-P (3.7 mm), the Machida 30P (3 mm), the Machida 3L (3 mm), and the Pentax FNL-10S (3.3 mm).

The most frequently used end-viewing flexible instruments as of this writing are the Machida 3L, the Pentax FNL-10S, and the Olympus ENF-P (Fig. 12-2). Each has certain characteristics which serve to differentiate it from its competitors. The Olympus instrument is the thickest of the three, but has excellent light-carrying capability and optics. The light-carrying fibers are arranged in two semicircular rows surrounding the objective lens (Fig. 12-3). It is the shortest of the instruments with a working length of 25 cm compared to 30 cm for both the Machida and Pentax instruments (see Fig. 12-2). The Pentax instrument has similar or superior optics. Its light-carrying fibers are arranged in a similar manner. It has a tapered configuration with a diameter of 3.3 mm at the distal tip which widens to 3.6 mm approximately 20 mm from the distal end. The fiberoptic portion of the endoscope is a bit stiffer with less yield than its competitors. The Machida 3L is the thinnest and most flexible of the instruments. The light-emitting characteristics are different from the Pentax and Olympus instruments in that the light-carrying fibers are arranged in two bundles above the objective lens, which generally results in slightly less overall brightness (Fig. 12-4). All three instruments have the capability of bending at the distal tip through an arc of approximately 180 degrees by using controls on the body of the endoscope (Fig. 12-5). The Pentax and Olympus instruments have thumb-operated levers (Fig. 12-6), while the Machida 3L has a full control wheel with a locking mechanism (Fig. 12-7) that allows the tip to remain deflected in a chosen position (Fig. 12-8).

Though the differences in diameters among the Machida 3L, the Pentax FNL-10S, and the Olympus ENF-P are less than 1 mm, this figure is somewhat misleading. It is the circular area of the instruments that should be calculated in order to see the actual volume of space that each will occupy within the nasal cavity. There is no doubt that the smaller the area of occupancy, the less discomfort. Thus, for the Machida 3L, the area of occupied space is 7.07 sq mm. For the Pentax FNL-10S, the value is 8.55 sq mm at the tip, but 10.18-sq mm further up the shaft of the instrument. For the Olympus ENF-P, the area occupied is 10.75 sq mm. Therefore, the Machida 3L has the smallest area of occupied space by over 3.0 sq mm. In younger children, this can made a difference in terms of compliance.

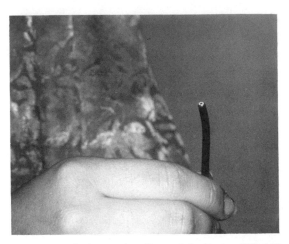

Figure 12-3. Light-carrying fibers of the Pentax FNL-10S endoscope arranged in a circular pattern.

Recently, a new generation of fiberoptic telescopes has been introduced which utilize quartz fibers to provide a very small-diameter endoscope (1 mm or less) with excellent optical characteristics. The Machida AG-1-60 is so slender (1 mm) that it can be inserted into the nose comfortably without anesthesia in the majority of people. The optics are excellent. At this point in time, this new generation of endoscopes are more fragile than the larger instruments and they do not have the same bending capabilities. However, it is certain that within the near future, nasopharygoscopy will benefit from constant improvements in the equipment. Therefore, it may be concluded that the technique of nasopharyngoscopy will remain a state-of-the-art technique for diagnosing velopharyngeal and laryngeal disorders, and improvements in diagnosis will come from advances in instrumentation rather than the use of other techniques which might supplant endoscopy.

Light is transmitted through the endoscope by means of a cold light source. "Cold light" refers to light which is generated by an external source (Fig. 12-9) and is then transmitted through the light-carrying fibers of the endoscope. Thus, the light emitted from the tip of the endoscope, whether rigid or flexible, does not generate heat and will not scorch the surrounding mucous

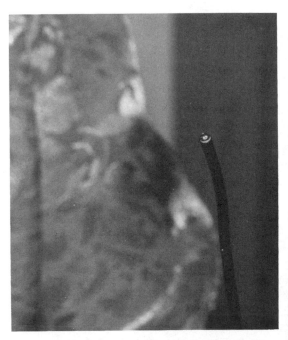

Figure 12-4. Light carrying fibers of the Machida 3L endoscope arranged in two light bundles over the lens.

membranes. There are numerous types of cold light sources which generate varying degrees of brightnesses and colors of light depending on the type of element used in the bulb. Halogen light sources tend to be the dimmest while xenon light sources are the brightest. For clinical examinations, a 150-W halogen light source is more than sufficient, but if the examiner wishes to videotape examinations, a far more intense light, such as a

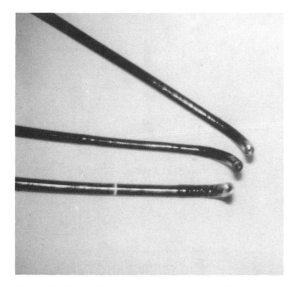

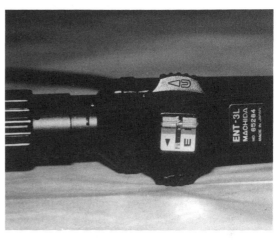

Figure 12-7. Control wheel on the body of the Machida 3L endoscope, which includes the lever for locking the angulation (middle).

Figure 12-5. Bending characteristics of the Pentax FNL-10S (top), Machida 3L (middle), and Olympus ENF-P (bottom) endoscopes.

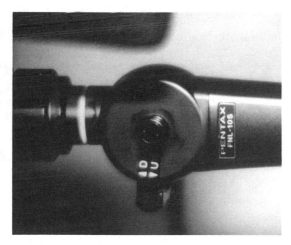

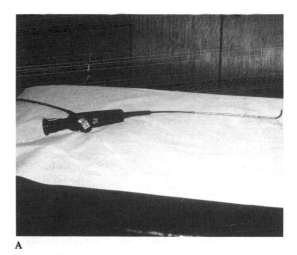

A

Figure 12.6. Thumb-operated control lever on the body of the Pentax FNL-10S endoscope.

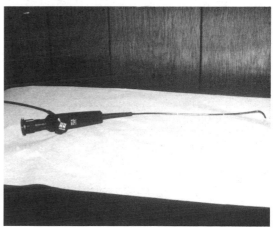

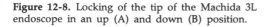

Figure 12-8. Locking of the tip of the Machida 3L endoscope in an up (A) and down (B) position.

B

mercury or xenon source, should be used. If cost is not a factor, the Pentax 75LX is an excellent small, portable xenon cold light supply. The Machida RG-400 supplies as intense a light supply for a much smaller price using a mercury halide bulb. The RG-400 is also relatively small and light in weight for easy portability.

Optically, there are some differences among the three endoscopes. Both the Olympus ENF-P and the Pentax FNL-10S have less magnification of the image (Fig. 12-10). As a result, there is a wider cone of acceptance. In other words, more of the pharyngeal diameter can be seen in a single field of view using the Pentax and Olympus instruments than the Machida, though what is seen will appear smaller, or further away. In terms of actual optical clarity of the image, I have personally found little appreciable difference among the three instruments.

One of the major drawbacks of flexible fiberoptic instruments, compared to rigid endoscopes, is the pattern of the image produced by the fibers which make up the optical bundle. Unlike the rigid endoscope, which is analogous to an observation through a telescope, a flexible fiberoptic image is actually an assemblage of many small "dots" of images, a kind of mosaic of small pictures. The fiberoptic image therefore cannot be as crystal-clear as the rod telescope image.

An important aspect of the examination technique and all of the accompanying optical parameters is the ease of recording examinations. A variety of recording techniques have been described in the literature utilizing expensive endoscopic television cameras, movie cameras, and still cameras. Adapting any camera to an endoscope is not difficult. But in order to study the movements of the velopharyngeal sphincter during speech, still photography is obviously of limited value. In any event, it is not difficult to lift single still pictures from a motion picture (film or video) if they are ever required. It is therefore recommended that all studies be recorded on a motion picture format. The easiest format is televised video.

There are a large number of television cameras specifically produced for endoscopes. Some have television tubes, others are so-called chip cameras in that they have no television tubes, but rather microchips which pick up the electronic signal. Endoscopic television cameras tend to be very expensive, the majority ranging from $5,000 to $10,000. It is actually easier and far less ex-

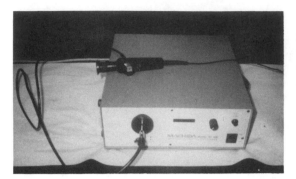

Figure 12-9. Machida RG-400 light source.

pensive to get an excellent television image using any of a number of consumer electronics television cameras. Many commercially available cameras or "camcorders" are able to record images in extremely low light, as low as 7 lux. This is actually far more light-sensitive than any of the cameras made specifically for endoscopes. Commercial television cameras can generally be purchased for $800, or less. Camcorders (cameras and video recorders combined in one unit) are generally slightly over $1,000. Using a flexible endoscope, the examination is quite easy to perform with a tripod-mounted camera or camcorder (Fig. 12-11). Depending on the endoscope used, adaptors are available which will screw into the lens of any video camera. Most of the endoscopic adaptors have diameters of 49 mm. The majority of television cameras have 58-mm diameters. It will therefore be necessary to purchase one or more step-down rings to adapt the 49-mm adaptor to the 58-mm lens (Fig. 12-12).

If the examiner wishes, still photography is possible through the nasopharyngoscope in much the same way as video recording (Fig. 12-13). It is best to use a 35-mm camera which has automatic exposure with the light being read directly off of the film. There are several excellent-quality cameras that function in this manner, such as the Pentax ME Super and the Olympus OM-2. The eyepiece of the camera will need to be fitted with a special endoscopic screen, but no other special modification is necessary. High-speed film should be used with as "fast" a lens as possible. As in videoendoscopy, both the camera and the endoscope should be focused at infinity so that the light rays enter the camera parallel to one another, rather than focused at a fixed point.

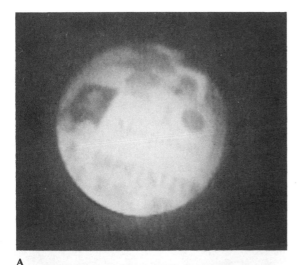

A

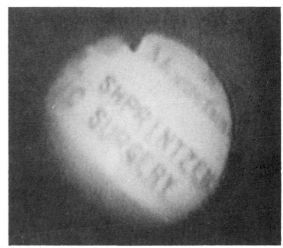

C

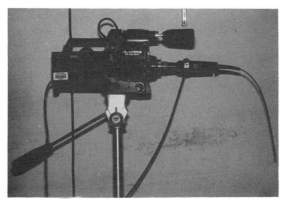

B

Figure 12-10. Photographed images of the author's identification badge through the Olympus ENF-P (A), Pentax FNL-10S (B), and Machida 3L (C) endoscopes taken from a similar distance at a similar light level. Note the increased magnification of the Machida 3L image.

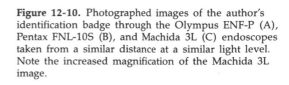

Figure 12-11. Machida 3L endoscope attached to a tripod-mounted Panasonic video camera.

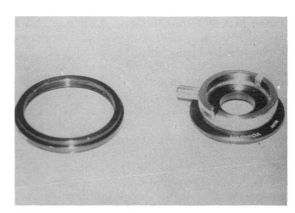

Figure 12-12. Machida C-mount adaptor with a 49 mm diameter (right) that fits into step-down rings will adapt to any camera lens.

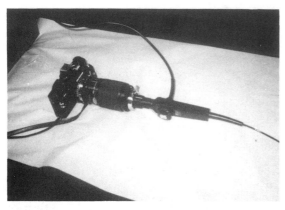

Figure 12-13. Machida 3L endoscope attached to a single-lens reflex 35 mm camera using the mounting device showin in Fig. 12-12.

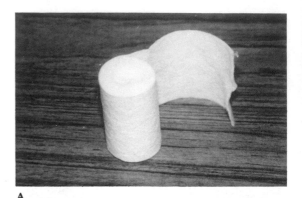

A

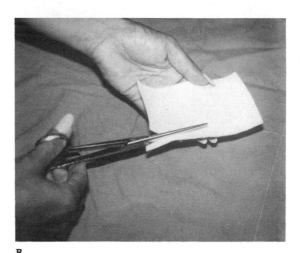

B

Figure 12-14. Webril cotton orthopedic bandage (A) being cut into a slender 3-mm-wide strip (B) to be used as a nasal packing for topical anesthesia.

PROCEDURAL RECOMMENDATIONS

TOPICAL ANESTHESIA

Extremely important to successful nasopharyngoscopic examination is the use of topical anesthesia in the nose. Personal experience has shown that careful administration of a mild topical anesthetic can assure a successful examination in even uncooperative children. The technique for the administration of anesthesia is as follows. First, it is essential to win the child's confidence. Therefore, begin by telling the child, "I am not going to hurt you." Follow this with an accurate and truthful explanation of what is to follow. Tell the child that he or she may feel some "tickling" in the nose, like a "sneezy" feeling, but that it will last for only a second and will not hurt.

The larger side of the nose should be determined. This can be done initially by direct visualization. The examiner can also have the patient inspire through each nostril while holding the other closed. The higher-pitched the noise made by the turbulence of air through the nostril, the smaller the nasal passage. Thus, the examiner will choose to anesthetize the side with the lower-pitched sound. In children with unilateral cleft lip–palate, the noncleft side should be the nostril of choice. The next step is to spray the nose with a mixture of ½% phenylephrine hydrochloride (Neo-synephrine hydrochloride) and a 2% aque-

nous tetracaine hydrochloride (Pontocaine) in equal parts. This spray will dilate and partially numb the turbinates. Following the spray, cotton packing moistened with 2% tetracaine hydrochloride should be inserted into the nose. The best material for the packing is Webril cotton orthopedic bandage (Fig. 12-14) cut into a slender strip 3 mm wide and approximately 7 or 8 cm long. After cutting the strip, it should be "twirled" (Fig. 12-15) for additional stiffness. It should then be doused liberally with tetracaine hydrochloride. The packing is then inserted into the nose using small bayonet forceps (Fig. 12-16). Care should be taken to make sure that the packing does not bunch up in the front of the nose. This packing is left in the nose for approximately 10 minutes. Patients will often report numbing of the maxillary incisors, which is a good sign that ade-

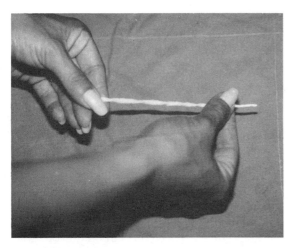

Figure 12-15. Strip of cotton packing being "twirled" into a stiffer packing for topical anesthesia.

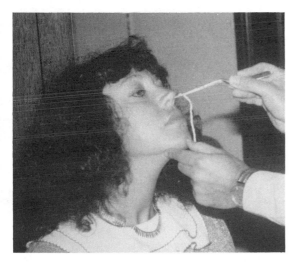

Figure 12-16. Cotton packing from Fig. 12-14 and 12-15 being inserted into the nose using a small bayonet forceps.

quate anesthesia has been attained. The cotton packing can then be removed and the examination can commence.

SPEECH SAMPLE

The speech sample for nasopharyngoscopy should include the same one suggested for videofluoroscopy (see Chap. 11), if only to compare the two studies for the same speech sample. However, because radiation exposure is not a concern in endoscopy, the examiner should feel free to

experiment as much as possible with the patient's speech. With adequate topical anesthesia, an examination can last for 20 minutes or more, when necessary.

The speech sample used during videofluoroscopy and repeated during nasopharyngoscopy is designed to provide the maximum information in the shortest period of time in order to limit radiation exposure. The speech sample used is as follows:

ma-ma-ma
pa-pa-pa
ta-ta-ta
ka-ka-ka
sssssss (sustained /s/)
kitty cat
Suzy sees Sally
Stop the bus
Catch a fish
Gerry's slippers
Popeye plays baseball
1-2-3-4-5-6-7-8-9-10 (counting to 10)

Of particular importance in this speech sample is the use of the sustained /s/ phoneme. In cases of inconsistent velopharyngeal closure, the phoneme most likely to be different from the others is the isolated /s/. That is, in cases of phoneme-specific velopharyngeal insufficiency, the /s/ is most often the phoneme that is insufficient. In cases where velopharyngeal closure is obtained on only one phoneme while all others show velopharyngeal insufficiency, the sustained /s/ is most likely to be the phoneme for which closure is achieved.

GUIDING AND POSITIONING THE ENDOSCOPE

Even with the nose well anesthetized, the examiner must be careful to guide the endoscope through the nasal cavity and into the pharynx without striking or impinging on the surrounding structures of the nose. Though the turbinates are sensitive to touch, if the nose is adequately anesthetized most patients should feel nothing in the area of the turbinates. Some patients may sneeze repeatedly if the turbinates are touched; others may feel an unpleasant pressure sensation in the nose. But once traversed, the turbinates are not problematical. The most sensitive structure within the nose is the base of the nasal septum in the area of the choanae. The examiner must avoid direct contact with the septum or the patient may feel pain, even with good anesthetic coverage.

Navigation of the endoscope through the nasal cavity is strictly a matter of common sense. The examiner knows that striking a sensitive part of the nose with the tip of the instrument will cause the patient pain or discomfort and will probably result in an unsuccessful examination in younger or uncooperative children. At the same time, the examiner has full control over the flexible fiberoptic endoscope in terms of complete maneuverability of the instrument from outside of the nose. The control wheel provides movement of the tip of the instrument through an arc of approximately 180 degrees. Movement of the tip from side to side can be provided in two ways. First, by rotating the body of the instrument clockwise or counterclockwise, the tip of the instrument will turn in a similar manner within the pharynx, thus providing a full view in both lateral directions. Also, the examiner should be grasping the instrument as close as possible to the patient's nose. This will allow the examiner to move the instrument from side to side within a range of several millimeters, which is usually sufficient to encompass the entire pharynx (Fig. 12-17).

Given the full range of movements the examiner can make with a flexible instrument, avoiding discomfort for the patient is not difficult. The best possible instrument for a painless examination is the end-viewing flexible fiberoptic instrument. The examiner can see exactly what is in front of the instrument and therefore avoid striking it. By maneuvering the instrument while traversing the nasal cavity, the examiner is able to see all of the structures within the nose so that they can be avoided with the appropriate maneuvers. In short, the examiner should think as though the tip of the instrument were analogous to the windshield of a car. With his or her hands on the steering wheel, if an obstacle appears in the road ahead, the examiner can steer the car in such a way as to avoid striking it head-on. This includes, of course, the ability to back up and try a different route if the one ahead is blocked by an obstacle. For example, it is usually preferable for an instrument to be passed through the middle meatus of the nose so that it is as high above the palate as possible and therefore not resting on the soft palate. Unfortunately, on occasion, the middle meatus may be too constricted for passage of the instrument. Therefore, the endoscope must be withdrawn and passed through the inferior meatus, which is often larger.

With the nose successfully traversed, the examiner now faces the task of getting the necessary information from the procedure. Some investigators have indicated that placing the endoscope in the most favorable position is critical to a successful examination. Both Miyazaki et al. [14] and Ibuki, Karnell, and Morris [9] describe the importance of correct position of the endoscope, though it should be pointed out that both of these authors were using the side-viewing flexible Olympus NPF instrument which must be positioned somewhere above the velopharyngeal sphincter in order to visualize any of the component movements. Pigott and Makepeace [18] indicate, in their description of the use of the rigid side-viewing Storz-Hopkins instrument, that the position of the endoscope is of great importance. However, as mentioned previously in this chapter, Shprintzen [23, 24] reported that fixating an endoscope in a single position is a mistake, especially when using a flexible end-viewing instrument. In fact, movement of the instrument is more important to a successful examination. It is most important to be able to pass the endoscope in and out of the velopharyngeal sphincter in order to appreciate that the velopharyngeal mechanism is not a simple "port" or "isthmus," but rather a volumetric tube with height, width, and depth that makes a variety of movements along the tube which contribute to velopharyngeal valving. If the view of the velopharyngeal sphincter is from a stable position above the tube, as with a rigid endoscope, the movements seen from a point of constriction and above may be interpreted as the only movements of velopharyngeal closure, but other movements may be occurring below, out of the sight of the endoscope. These movements may be as important to velopharyngeal valving as the movements seen at the level of the velum. Because rigid endocopes and side-viewing flexible endoscopes cannot be maneuvered to pass deeply into the velopharyngeal sphincter, these movements cannot possibly be appreciated. End-viewing flexible endoscopes can, however, examine the entire airway from choanae to glottis.

EXAMINATION INTERPRETATION

STRUCTURE

In the remediation of velopharyngeal insufficiency, the most valuable contribution of naso-

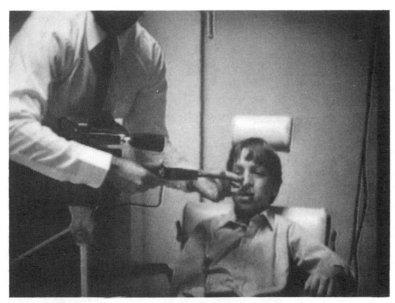

A

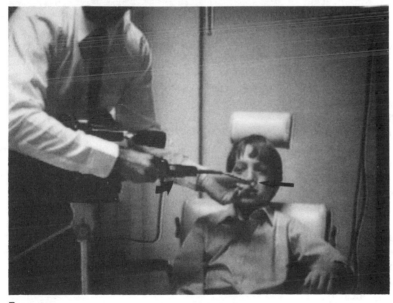

B

Figure 12-17. Rotational movement of the endoscope body (curved arrow) allowing side-to-side movement of the tip (straight arrow) for full viewing of the pharynx.

pharyngoscopy is the ability to see the complete in vivo structure of the nasopharynx, oropharynx, and hypopharynx. This is especially important because of data which indicate that the most frequent modality of treatment for velopharyngeal insuffi-ciency is surgery [19]. Endoscopy allows the surgeon to see every detail of the operating field, including the appearance of the mucous membrane, the presence of scarring, lymphoid tissue (tonsils and adenoids), abnormal growths or structures, airway size, and vasculature. It seems incomprehensible that with the ability to directly view the velopharyngeal structures prior to surgery, that surgeons would not wish to have a look.

Two conditions which may lead to velopharyngeal insufficiency and are directly related to structural abnormality are best-diagnosed using endoscopy. In fact without nasopharyngoscopic views of the nasopharynx, these diagnoses would be nearly impossible. These conditions are the occult submucous cleft palate and tonsillar hypertrophy.

"Occult submucous palate" is a term coined by Kaplan [10]. In his 1975 report, Kaplan described a series of patients in whom hypernasal speech was present in the absence of any stigmata of cleft palate or the stigmata of submucous cleft palate as described by Calnan [4], including bifid uvula, notching of the posterior border of the hard palate, and a zona pellucida indicative of muscular separation within the velum. While performing pharyngeal flap surgery on these patients, Kaplan discovered that the orientation of the muscle fibers within the soft palate was identical to that seen in patients with overt or submucous palatal clefts. Because the peroral examinations of these patients were completely normal in spite of the abnormal musculature, Kaplan used the term "occult" to describe the hidden nature of the defect, though still labeling the anomaly as a submucous cleft palate because of the abnormal anatomy. Kaplan did not utilize nasopharyngoscopy to visualize the velopharyngeal mechanisms of his patients and therefore concluded that the only way to conclusively identify occult submucous clefts was by surgical dissection.

In 1978, Croft and his colleagues [5] described the nasopharyngoscopic appearance of the velum in patients with occult submucous cleft. Similar reports followed [11, 12]. These authors are all faculty at the Center for Craniofacial Disorders of Montefiore Medical Center (Bronx, New York) where both nasopharyngoscopy and multiview videofluoroscopy are applied to all patients with velopharyngeal insufficiency. They reported that the endoscopic appearance of the velum in patients with the peroral stigmata of submucous cleft palate showed a deep central concavity, or groove, which is in contrast to the appearance of the velum in noncleft (normal) subjects. In normals, the velum has a large convex mound in the midline [5, 11, 21, 22] representing the bulk of the musculus uvulae (Fig. 12-18). In the occult submucous cleft, the nasal surface of the velum has either a midline concave depression (Fig. 12-19), or a totally flat surface (Fig. 12-20) signifying the absence or hypoplasia of the musculus uvulae combined with a diastasis of the palatal musculature. Croft et al. [5], Lewin et al. [11], and

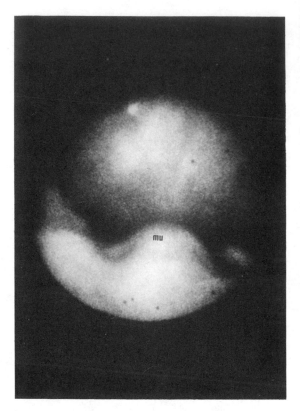

Figure 12-18. Midline bulge of the soft palate showing the large convex bulge of the musculus uvulae (mu).

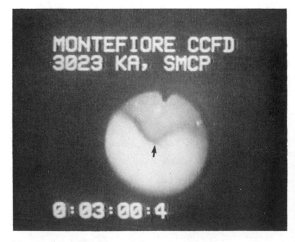

Figure 12-19. Midline of the soft palate in an individual with submucous cleft palate showing a deep V-shaped groove (arrow), indicative of the absence of the musculus uvulae and diastasis of the velar musculature.

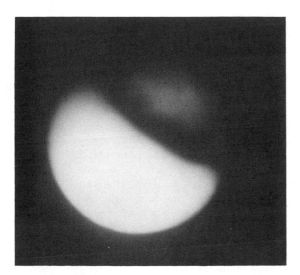

Figure 12-20. Midline of the soft palate in an individual with occult, submucous cleft palate showing a flattened nasal surface, indicative of the absence of the musculus uvulae.

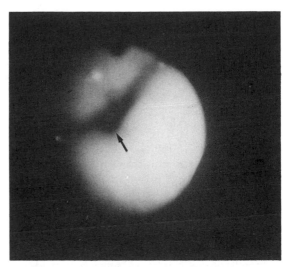

Figure 12-21. A small midline velopharyngeal gap during speech in the patient in Fig. 12-20, caused by the absence of the musculus uvulae. Note the V-shaped groove (arrow) in the center of the velum.

Shprintzen [21, 22] all concluded that occult submucous cleft palate could be accurately diagnosed nasopharyngoscopically in all cases. During phonation, patients with occult submucous cleft palate often have small central gaps in the velopharyngeal sphincter located where the bulk of the musculus uvulae should be (Fig. 12-21).

A warning commonly reinforced by all clinicians involved with children who have hypernasal speech is "never remove tonsils and adenoids." This is in recognition of numerous data which have demonstrated the importance of the adenoids in normal velopharyngeal closure in both cleft and noncleft children [3, 6, 13, 15, 29, 33–35]. Also, there have been reports in the literature on the development of velopharyngeal insufficiency following adenotonsillectomy [6, 7, 35]. However, generically lumping together tonsils and adenoids is not warranted. The removal of adenoids can cause the development of velopharyngeal insufficiency in individuals with anatomically abnormal palates or physiologically abnormal velopharyngeal mechanisms [6] because of their strategic location within the nasopharynx. The tonsils, however, are located in the oral cavity between the faucial pillars and do not normally extend into the pharynx or the velopharyngeal valve.

In some individuals, the tonsils extend beyond the tonsillar pillars and into the pharyngeal airway (Fig. 12-22). Occasionally they will extend up

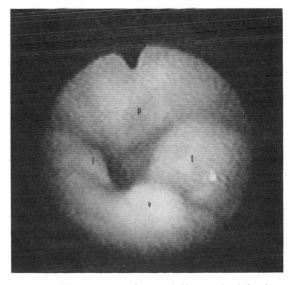

Figure 12-22. Intrusion of a tonsil (t) into the left of the velopharyngeal valve (l) between the velum (v) and the posterior pharyngeal wall (p).

into the nasopharynx. These individuals often present with abnormal resonance balance. Part of this resonance abnormality is related to a muffled oral resonance caused by the obstruction of the oropharynx and oral airway. Otolaryngologists have typically referred to this problem as "potato-in-the-mouth" voice quality. But a more interesting yet generally unknown speech problem related to the tonsils is hypernasality. On occasion, the tonsils may be so hypertrophic as to interfere with elevation of the lateral aspects of the velum, the medial movements of the lateral pharyngeal walls, or both. This diagnosis can only be made using flexible fiberoptic nasopharyngoscopy. Endoscopically, the tonsils can be seen in the pharyngeal airway (Fig. 12-23), and during phonation the velum may contact the posterior pharyngeal wall centrally, but show air leaks around its lateral aspects. In some cases, the insufficiency may be intermittent. Hypernasality is often perceived as being variable. In such cases, tonsillectomy without adenoidectomy is indicated. The majority of cases resolve with tonsillectomy alone, though in some cases it is necessary to follow tonsillectomy with speech therapy.

Tonsillar hypertrophy must also be considered prior to pharyngeal flap surgery. Nasopharyngoscopic studies prior to pharyngeal flap surgery will provide evidence that the tonsils sit in a position which would contribute to postoperative airway obstruction. When sitting posteriorly in the oropharynx, the tonsils could prompt the development of obstructive sleep apnea following pharyngeal flap surgery in the following ways:

1. Following pharyngeal flap surgery, the pharynx heals by circular contraction, thus narrowing the entire pharyngeal circumference in the oropharynx, the flap donor site. The tonsils occupy a relatively larger portion of the airway and they are drawn closer together making upper airway collapse more likely.
2. The tonsils may sit directly under the lateral ports of the flap, thus fully compromising the nasal airway as well. The combination of oropharyngeal and nasopharyngeal compromise could be potentially dangerous, if not lethal.

Another important use of the nasopharyngoscope prior to pharyngeal flap surgery is the ability to see the vasculature of the nasopharynx. In several recent publications [12, 26] an abnormal coursing of the internal carotid artery has been detected nasopharyngoscopically in the velocardiofacial syndrome. The artery has been displaced medially, thus increasing the risk of a serious surgical complication. Other vascular abnormalities may also be detected endoscopically, as might other tissue abnormalities, such as polyps, neoplasms, and other sources of airway obstruction.

FUNCTION

Velopharyngeal physiology was discussed earlier in this chapter. With this in mind, the examiner should have all of the information necessary to perform a successful examination and to interpret the results. The examiner must be cognizant of the tubelike nature of the pharynx and that there are movements at several different vertical as well as horizontal locations [23, 24, 31]. The examiner must also vary the speech sample so that the consistency of velopharyngeal valving can be observed across a variety of phonemic tasks. The importance of having sustained voiceless continuants (e.g., /s/ and /f/) cannot be overemphasized. The majority of the speech sample should be as close to conversational speech as possible.

Of course, the interpretation of the nasopharyngoscopic study is dependent on the treatment options available to the patient. There are several different levels on which decisions can be made:

TO TREAT, OR NOT TO TREAT

Once a speech pathologist has a question regarding resonance balance, it is certainly imperative to view the velopharyngeal sphincter directly during speech in order to determine if the abnormality is in fact related to an abnormality in velopharyngeal valving. This is especially of importance in cases of uncertainty when the speech pathologist may note an abnormality of resonance, but is not certain that it is truly hypernasal resonance. There can be other resonance problems which may be confused for hypernasality. These include an unusual oral resonance caused by lymphoid obstruction as mentioned above. In some cases, hyponasality can be confused with hypernasality, especially when it is accompanied by tonsillar hypertrophy. A variety of articulation impairments may also be difficult to differentiate from hypernasality, such as dysarthria (even though many dysarthrics also have hypernasal speech).

Therefore, the first decision must relate to the presence or absence of velopharyngeal insufficiency. The examiner should maneuver and manipulate the endoscope in order to observe the degree of velar movement, the degree and vertical level of maximal lateral pharyngeal wall movement, the presence or absence of posterior pharyngeal wall movement, and the anatomical nature of the palate and surrounding nasophar-

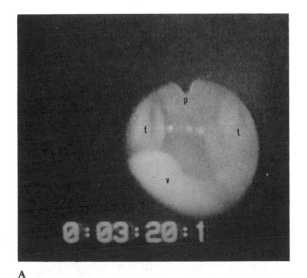

A

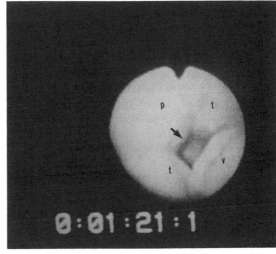

C

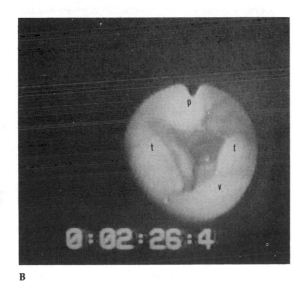

B

Figure 12-23. Sequence of an endoscopic view of velopharyngeal insufficiency caused by tonsillar hypertrophy. A. The tonsils (t) can be seen against the lateral pharyngeal walls. B. they are drawn into the plane of velopharyngeal closure by movements of the lateral pharyngeal walls resulting in a small velopharyngeal gap (C). p = posterior pharyngeal wall; v = velum.

ynx. If velopharyngeal insufficiencies occur, the examiner should note if they are consistent in size and shape. If they do vary, it should be noted if the variation is phoneme-specific, or if there is variation on repeated trials of the same phonemic context. If the insufficiency is large, it should be obvious to the examiner. If the insufficiency is very small, the examiner should be alert for the presence of air bubbles seen in the mucus lining the nasopharynx. Structurally, the examiner should be especially sensitive to midline deficiencies in the velum (whether secondary to a repaired cleft, a submucous cleft, or an occult submucous cleft

palate) and the presence of tonsils in the pharyngeal airway. All of these abnormalities would be strong indications for some type of physical management, unless the insufficiency is inconsistent, in which case speech therapy may be indicated. However, if no velopharyngeal insufficiency is observed, then obviously no treatment is indicated. This seems like an absurdly simple point to make, but the author has personally seen many patients who had been scheduled for pharyngeal flap surgery at other institutions based on perceptual judgment alone who had no sign whatsoever of abnormal velopharyngeal function.

SURGERY, PROSTHESIS, OR SPEECH THERAPY

The decision regarding the type of treatment is made on the basis of the consistency of the velopharyngeal insufficiency. Inconsistency provides an excellent prognosis for success with speech therapy, especially when the insufficiency is phoneme-specific. Inconsistent insufficiencies may also respond well to a speech bulb reduction program. Consistent insufficiencies may also be treated prosthetically if surgery is contraindicated by either the patient's preference, or for medical reasons. However, if there is no variability in velopharyngeal valving for different phonemic contexts, surgical intervention is usually the treatment of choice.

One difficult type of velopharyngeal insufficiency which can only be observed with a direct observation of the velopharyngeal valve is the "pulsing" phenomenon. This type of insufficiency may be observed in individuals with clefts, in patients with neurological or neuromuscular disorders, or in otherwise normal individuals. However, it is certainly most common in neurologically impaired individuals. In this type of velopharyngeal insufficiency, the velopharyngeal sphincter is observed to close and open on several occasions during a single nonnasal production. This phenomenon may occur on each syllable or only where there is a voiced-voiceless junction. For example, in the phrase "stop the bus," an individual without velopharyngeal insufficiency will close the velopharyngeal sphincter immediately prior to the initiation of the /s/ in "stop" and not release closure until the cessation of the /s/ in "bus." However, individuals with the pulsing phenomenon will open and close the velopharyngeal sphincter as often as 3 times during this one phrase. The resulting speech is perceived as continuously hypernasal even though closure is achieved intermittently.

IF SPEECH THERAPY, WHAT TYPE?

Though many clinicians still believe that speech therapy cannot improve problems of velopharyngeal insufficiency, certain types of insufficiency respond extremely well, and sometimes extremely quickly, to speech therapy. The most easily treated type of velopharyngeal valving abnormality is the phoneme-specific insufficiency. This can really be regarded as a simple articulation disorder. It could respond to the use of acoustic feedback, feedback with some type of air flow or pressure device, or even to techniques designed to "trick" the patient. It is not uncommon in phoneme-specific insufficiencies to find patients who on endoscopic examination achieve a tight velopharyngeal seal for all speech tasks with the exception of /s/, /z/, /f/, and /v/. On occasion, affricates are also symptomatic. By using the /t/ phoneme in therapy to have the patient achieve velopharyngeal closure with the same tongue placement in a voiceless production, the therapist can use a slender applicator stick to groove the center of the tongue during the production of /t/. This will cause air to escape through the center of the tongue resulting in /s/ with the same velopharyngeal closure as achieved on /t/.

A newer approach recently described in the scientific literature is the use of nasopharyngoscopic biofeedback therapy [8, 30]. By using video-endoscopy, the patient can see his or her own velopharyngeal valving mechanism and alter the valving pattern during a 20- to 30-minute session. Data [8] suggest that this treatment modality can be a rapid and effective method of treating phoneme-specific insufficiencies. The use of nasopharyngoscopic biofeedback obviously depends on the logistics of having instrumentation and qualified personnel to perform the procedure. While still in its infancy, the technique may have tremendous value in the future. It is still not clear, for example, if changes in consistently abnormal velopharyngeal valving can be affected with nasopharyngoscopic biofeedback. To date, only patients with inconsistencies in valving have received well-documented treatment [8]. The ability for some individuals to improve even consistently poor velopharyngeal valving with nasopharyngoscopic biofeedback could potentially save many patients from surgery or prosthetic intervention.

IF A PROSTHESIS, WHAT TYPE?

Though less common today than it was 20 years ago, prosthetic management of velopharyngeal insufficiency still has a place in the treatment battery which can best be suited to the patient based on nasopharyngoscopic examination. Nasopharyngoscopic evidence of inconsistent or weak velar elevation in the presence of some lateral pharyngeal wall movement is a good indication for the use of a palatal lift prosthesis. However, palatal lifts are best for passively pushing the velum into the nasopharynx in order to obturate it. It must be regarded in most cases as a permanent solution unless it is being used temporarily until surgery is performed. Palatal lifts may often be applied to dysarthrics who have the incoordinated velar movements referred to above as "pulsing."

Nasopharyngoscopy is particularly well suited to the placement of speech bulbs. In cases where physical obturation of the velopharyngeal valve is required, the speech bulb must be placed appropriately to make the best use of the available medial motions of the lateral pharyngeal walls and posterior pharyngeal walls at the most appropriate vertical level. One major advantage of speech bulbs and fitting by nasopharyngoscopy is that the endoscopic information can be used to adjust the bulb as often as necessary until there is an airtight fit during speech. Material can be added to the bulb, or shaved off the bulb, and the bulb can be elevated or lowered. In short, using a nasopharyngoscope to guide bulb placement, speech bulbs should essentially always eliminate velopharyngeal insufficiency. Palatal lifts may be altered in much the same way.

Temporary speech bulb appliances used to stimulate lateral pharyngeal wall movement can be modified endoscopically in a bulb reduction program. At the Center for Craniofacial Disorders, an active bulb reduction program is currently under way which shows great promise. The concept is to take children who have observable velopharyngeal insufficiency, and fit them with a temporary speech bulb endoscopically until it provides complete velopharyngeal closure. The patient uses this appliance continuously for approximately 3 months. Then, under endoscopic guidance, the bulb is shaved down until velopharyngeal closure is barely marginal. The patient then returns a month or so later to see if velopharyngeal closure is being maintained. It is then shaved down again. This continues on a monthly basis either until the bulb cannot be reduced further without a persisting velopharyngeal insufficiency, or the bulb is completely eliminated and velopharyngeal closure fully maintained.

IF SURGERY, WHAT TYPE?

As mentioned above, one advantage of prosthetic appliances is the ability to modify them until they provide an airtight fit. Surgery, on the other hand, should be a one-time treatment with a high success rate. Literally hundreds of reports have appeared in the literature describing myriad procedures for resolving velopharyngeal insufficiency. Generically, pharyngeal flaps, secondary

palatoplasties (i.e., push-backs), posterior wall implants or augmentations, and sphincter pharyngoplasties have all been touted as near total cure-alls. But in spite of many claims of near 100 percent success, new procedures continue to appear. Within each of the generic categories, many variations of these operations have been described. The number of different types of pharyngeal flaps are far to numerous to cite. Implant materials ranging from parrafin to Teflon have been described. In all of the reports describing specific operations, the emphasis has always been on the surgery itself. But recently, it has been shown that the success or failure of operative approaches is more dependent on the diagnostic workup and less dependent on the operation itself. Many reports from our center [1, 2, 20, 24, 25, 28] have described how the combination of nasopharyngoscopy and multiview videofluoroscopy could be used to vary the operative approach on an individual basis so that pharyngeal flaps and other operative procedures could be tailored to fit the velopharyngeal gap. In other words, if the surgeon can be shown the exact nature of the size and shape of the velopharyngeal insufficiency, it becomes more likely that he or she will be able to find the best operation for closing it.

At the beginning of this section, it was stated that the way in which diagnostic information is interpreted has much to do with the way it is used. The more sophisticated the treatment options, the more important it is to interpret the diagnostic information appropriately. For example, if the surgeon on a particular team does only one operation for all patients with velopharyngeal insufficiency and there is no input from the prosthodontist, the diagnostic information obtained from endoscopy may only be used at the most primary level. The decision will be made to treat or not to treat based on the presence or absence of an insufficiency. But once it is decided to treat the problem, only one treatment would be available. However, if all prosthetic, speech therapy, and surgical treatments can be offered to the patient, then the diagnostic information must be very specific as to the size, shape, and consistency of the insufficiency.

SUMMARY

The treatment of velopharyngeal insufficiency is absolutely dependent on accurate diagnostic information. There is no denying that the direct visualization of the deficiencies of velopharyngeal valving are the most valuable asset in the description of the problem. Measuring artifacts of the act of velopharyngeal closure cannot be as valuable as seeing it for oneself. Nasopharyngoscopy is the only method which lets the examiner see both the anatomy and physiology of the velopharyngeal valving. It's advantages include:

1. The absence of radiation exposure.
2. It may be repeated as frequently as necessary.
3. Its relative ease of examination.
4. It is generally painless.
5. It is easy to record.
6. The equipment is not prohibitively expensive.
7. The equipment is easily accessible.
8. The equipment is portable.
9. It has therapeutic applications.
10. It is a multipurpose tool and can be used for laryngeal examinations, airway analysis, in the search for neoplasms, and even by anesthesiologists for the guidance of difficult intubations.

One caveat must be offered, however. In a comparison of nasopharyngoscopy and multiview videofluoroscopy in the same patients, disagreement between the two diagnostic techniques in approximately a third of the cases has been reported [23]. Specifically, it was reported that nasopharyngoscopy tends to underestimate the full extent of lateral pharyngeal wall motion in cases where the view of the lower portion of the pharyngeal tube is obscured by movements occuring higher in the nasopharynx. Therefore, for a complete assessment of the movements in the velopharyngeal valve, it is strongly recommended that both nasopharyngoscopy and multiview videofluoroscopy be utilized and compared prior to treatment recommendations. Furthermore, the use of an end-viewing flexible fiberoptic instrument attached to a video camera is recommended. Finally, treatment, especially surgical treatment, should never be recommended unless both the speech pathologist and surgeon have had the benefit of seeing the velopharyngeal valve directly through the use of endoscopy and fluoroscopy. In all other fields of surgical endeavor, this is certainly the case, and it should be no different in surgery for speech.

REFERENCES

1. Argamaso, R. V. Physical management of velopharyngeal incompetence. *J. Child. Commun. Dis.* 10:67–74, 1986.
2. Argamaso, R. V., Shprintzen, R. J., Strauch, B., Lewin, M. L., Daniller, A. I., Ship, A. G., and Croft, C. B. The role of lateral pharyngeal wall movement in pharyngeal flap surgery. *Plast. Reconstr. Surg.* 66:214–219, 1980.
3. Calnan, J. S. Movements of the soft palate. *Br. J. Plast. Surg.* 5:286–296, 1953.
4. Calnan, J. S. Submucous cleft palate. *Br. J. Plast. Surg.* 6:164–168, 1954.
5. Croft, C. B., Shprintzen, R. J., Daniller, A. I., and Lewin, M. L. The occult submucous cleft palate and the musculus uvulae. *Cleft Palate J.* 15:150–154, 1978.
6. Croft, C. B., Shprintzen, R. J., and Ruben, R. J. Hypernasal speech following adenotonsillectomy. *Otolarygol. Head Neck Surg.* 89:179–188, 1981.
7. Gibb, A. G. Hypernasality (rhinolalia aperta) following tonsil and adenoid removal. *J. Laryngol. Otol.* 72:433–451, 1958
8. Hoch, L., Golding-Kushner, K., Sadewitz, V. L., and Shprintzen, R. J. Speech therapy. *Semin. Speech Lang.* 7:311–323, 1986.
9. Ibuki, K., Karnell, M. P., and Morris, H. L. Reliability of the nasopharyngeal fiberscope (NPF) for assessing velopharyngeal function. *Cleft Palate J.* 20:97–104, 1983.
10. Kaplan, E. N. The occult submucous cleft palate. *Cleft Palate J.* 12:356–368, 1975.
11. Lewin, M. L., Croft, C. B., and Shprintzen, R. J. Velopharyngeal insufficiency due to hypoplasia of the musculus uvulae and occult submucous cleft palate. *Plast. Reconstr. Surg.* 65:585–591, 1980.
12. MacKenzie-Stepner, K., Witzel, M. A., Stringer, D. A., Lindsay, W. K., and Munro, I. R. Abnormal carotid arteries in the velocardiofacial syndrome: A report of three cases. *Plast. Reconstr. Surg.* 80:347–351, 1987.
13. Mason, R. M. Preventing speech disorders following adenoidectomy by preoperative examination. *Clin. Pediatr.* 12:405–414, 1973.
14. Miyazaki, T., Matsuya, T., and Yamaoka, M. Fiberscopic methods for assessment of velopharyngeal closure during various activities. *Cleft Palate J.* 12:107–114, 1975.
15. Morris, H. L., The speech pathologist looks at the tonsils and the adenoids. *Ann. Otol. Rhinol. Laryngol.* 84(Suppl. 19):63–66, 1975.
16. Pigott, R. W. The nasoendoscopic appearance of the normal palatopharyngeal valve. *Plast. Reconstr. Surg.* 43:19–24, 1969.
17. Pigott, R. W., Benson, J. F., and White, F. D. Nasoendoscopy in the diagnosis of velopharyngeal incompetence. *Plast. Reconstr. Surg.* 43:141–147, 1969.
18. Pigott, R. W., and Makepeace, A. P. Some characteristics of endoscopic and radiological systems used in elaboration of the diagnosis of velopharyngeal incompetence. *Br. J. Plast. Surg.* 35:19–32, 1982.
19. Schneider, E., and Shprintzen, R. J. A survey of speech pathologists: Current trends in the diagnosis and treatment of velopharyngeal insufficiency. *Cleft Palate J.* 17:249–253, 1980.
20. Shprintzen, R. J. The Use of Multiview Videofluoroscopy and Flexible Fiberoptic Nasopharyngoscopy as a

Predictor of Success with Pharyngeal Flap Surgery. In R. Ellis and F. C. Flack (Eds.), *Diagnosis and Treatment of Palato-Glossal Malfunction.* London: College of Speech Therapists, 1979. Pp. 6–14.

21. Shprintzen, R. J. Hypernasal Speech in the Absence of Overt or Submucous Cleft Palate: The Mystery Solved. In R. Ellis and F. C. Flack (Eds.), *Diagnosis and Treatment of Palato-Glossal Malfunction.* London: College of Speech Therapists, 1979. Pp. 37–44.

22. Shprintzen, R. J. Palatal and pharyngeal anomalies in craniofacial syndromes. *Birth Defects* 18:53–78, 1982.

23. Shprintzen, R. J. An invited commentary on the preceding article by Ibuki, Karnell, and Morris. *Cleft Palate J.* 20:105–107, 1983.

24. Shprintzen, R. J. Evaluating velopharyngeal insufficiency. *J. Child. Commun. Dis.* 10:51–66, 1986.

25. Shprintzen, R. J. Surgery for Speech: The Planning of Operations for Velopharyngeal Insufficiency with Emphasis on the Preoperative Assessment of Both Pharyngeal Physiology and Articulation. In M. Ferguson (Ed.), *Proceedings of the British Craniofacial Society.* Manchester: University of Manchester Press, 1989.

26. Shprintzen, R. J. Velo-cardio-facial Syndrome. In *birth Defects Encyclopedia.* New York: Alan R. Liss, 1989.

27. Shprintzen, R. J., Croft, C., Berkman, M. D., and Rakoff, S. J. Pharyngeal hypoplasia in Treacher Collins syndrome. *Arch. Otolaryngol.* 105:127–131, 1979.

28. Shprintzen, R. J., Lewin, M. L., Croft, C. B., Daniller, A. I., Argamaso, R. V., Ship, A. C., and Strauch, B. A comprehensive study of pharyngeal flap surgery: Tailor-made flaps. *Cleft Palate J.* 16:46–55, 1979.

29. Shprintzen, R. J., Schwartz, R. H., Daniller, A., and Hoch, L. Morphological significance of bifid uvula. *Pediatrics* 75:553–561, 1985.

30. Siegel-Sadewitz, V. L., and Shprintzen, R. J. Nasopharyngoscopy of the normal velopharyngeal sphincter: An experiment of biofeedback. *Cleft Palate J.* 19:194–200, 1982.

31. Siegel-Sadewitz, V. L., and Shprintzen, R. J. Changes in velopharyngeal valving with age. *Int. J. Pediatr. Otorhinolaryngol.* 11:171–182, 1986.

32. Skolnick, M. L. Video velopharyngography in patients with nasal speech, with emphasis on lateral pharyngeal motion in velopharyngeal closure. *Radiology* 93:747–755, 1969.

33. Skolnick, M. L., Shprintzen, R. J., McCall, G. N., and Rakoff, S. J. Patterns of velopharyngeal closure in subjects with repaired cleft palate and normal speech: A multi-view videofluoroscopic analysis. *Cleft Palate J.* 12:369–376, 1975

34. Subtelny, J. D., and Koepp-Baker, H. The significance of adenoid tissue in velopharyngeal function. *Plast. Reconstr. Surg.* 17:235–250, 1956.

35. Witzel, M. A., Rich, R. H., Margar-Bacal, F., and Cox, C. Velopharyngeal insufficiency after adenoidectomy: An 8-year review. *Int. J. Pediatr. Otorhinolaryngol.* 11:15–20, 1986.

CHAPTER 13

Aerodynamic Assessment of Velopharyngeal Performance

Donald W. Warren

The development of instruments capable of measuring aerodynamic performance during speech has led to improved, more objective methods for assessing palatal function. These tools range from simple sensing devices [5–8, 11, 14] to elaborate combinations of pressure transducers and air flow meters [19–27, 33, 34, 38]. While the former are only capable of gross determinations of palatal function, the latter provide acceptable estimates of velopharyngeal port size.

In the past clinicians have used a number of devices to provide a gross indication of nasal escape. These included U-shaped manometers, mirrors which recorded nasal fogging, and various blowing devices, such as the oral manometer [1, 2, 4, 10, 40].

In most instances the measurements obtained with such devices related more to respiratory effort than to palatal closure [26, 29]. Also, response times were extremely slow and errors in measurement often occurred. In addition, these measurements were usually made during nonspeech activities such as blowing or sucking, and as Morris [10] has pointed out, individuals with incomplete palatal closure can sometimes perform these activities satisfactorily utilizing lingual-palatal contacts. Thus, nonspeech tasks may not reflect the true capability of the velopharyngeal mechanism.

The deficiencies associated with simple manometric instruments have led to the development of more elaborate, complex, and expensive tools for objective evaluation of palatal function [29]. The basic components of these aerodynamic measuring systems are flowmeters, which record volume rates of air flow, and pressure transducers, which record airway pressures within the vocal tract.

MEASUREMENTS OF PRESSURE AND AIR FLOW

AIR PRESSURE DEVICES

The pressure transducers presently in use are either variable resistance, variable capacitance, or variable inductance gauges [30]. Resistance wire strain gauges respond to changes in pressure with a change in resistance when the strain-sensitive wire is exposed to stretch. A metal bellows is compressed by pressure within the chamber. This action results in a resistance imbalance in a Wheatstone bridge that is proportional to the applied pressure. The resulting output voltage from the bridge is amplified and recorded.

The electrical capacitance transducer is a condenser formed by an electrode separated from a stiff metal membrane by a carefully adjusted air gap. Movements of the membrane in relation to the electrode vary the capacitance, which can be measured by a radiofrequency circuit. Membrane displacement is extremely small, and therefore the frequency response is excellent. However, this device is more temperature-sensitive than the strain gauge manometer.

The capacitance-type pressure transducer is distinguished from other types by its exceptional accuracy, high level outputs, and built-in signal conditioning. Typically, these transducers are connected directly to data instrumentation and are used for pressure measurement without need for additional signal conditioning.

These studies were supported in part by Grants DE07105 and DE06957 from the National Institute of Dental Research.

Variable inductance pressure gauges can be made so small that they can be placed directly on the site to be measured. The tranducer utilizes a soft iron slug placed within two coils of wire and fastened to the center of an elastic membrane. Pressure moves the iron slug, and this movement results in a change in magnetic flux. The change in inductance of the coils is then recorded through an appropriate bridge circuit.

It is common practice to amplify the signal from transducers to provide power to drive galvanometers. The mechanical intertia of some direct-writing galvanometers is so great that the frequency response is limited, and amplification is required to produce any measurable response at all. Usually a carrier wave amplifier is used in combination with a strain gauge tranducer. An oscillator supplies an alternating current, and the amplitude is continuously affected by the varying resistance of the Wheatstone bridge. The output of the transducer enters a capacitance-coupled amplifier, which amplifies the modulated carrier wave. Then the signals are rectified and the carrier wave is filtered out, leaving a DC voltage which powers the recording instrument.

AIR FLOW DEVICES

The most accepted air flow device is the heated pneumotachograph which consists of a flowmeter and a differential pressure transducer [5]. This device utilizes the principle that as air flows across a resistance the pressure drop which results is linearly related to the volume rate of air flow. In most cases, the resistance is a wire mesh screen that is heated to prevent condensation. A pressure tap is situated on each side of the screen, and both are connected to a very sensitive differential pressure transducer. The pressure drop is converted to an electrical voltage that is amplified and recorded either on tape or on a direct writing instrument. Pneumotachographs are valid, reliable, and linear devices for measuring ingressive and egressive air flow rates. In addition, they are easily calibrated with a rotameter.

ORAL PRESSURE MEASUREMENT

Pressure devices have been used in a variety of ways to measure the aerodynamics of speech production. Usually, measurements are made of oral pressures, nasal pressures, or both. Intraoral pressure can be recorded by placing a catheter in the mouth and attaching it to a pressure transducer and recorder. Pressures in the oral cavity vary from 3 to 8 cm H_2O for nonnasal consonants in normal conversational speech.

Voiceless consonants usually demonstrate pressures about 20 percent higher than their voiced cognate pairs [20, 28]. This apparently relates to the need for greater aerodynamic energy for voiceless sounds since they are not reinforced with acoustic energy from the vocal folds. Additionally, there is a difference in energy loss across the glottis between the two consonant types [28].

More importantly, in spite of what many believe, consonantal intraoral pressures generally remain above 3.0 cm H_2O even in individuals with gross palatal incompetency [37]. Table 13-1 lists mean intraoral air pressures according to degree of velopharyngeal closure for the plosive /p/ in /hamper/.

A number of factors are involved in maintaining intraoral pressures above 3.0 cm H_2O. Perhaps the most important factor is resistance of the nasal airway. The cleft nasal airway is often approximately 25 percent smaller [27, 35] in cross-sectional size than the noncleft airway. This is due to maxillary growth deficits and nasal abnormalities such as vomerine spurs, alar collapse, and septal deformities. A smaller nasal cross-sectional area increases resistance to air flow and helps maintain intraoral pressures during speech. Approximately 60 to 70 percent of intraoral pressure can be maintained by nasal airway resistance alone. In addition, the nasal valve in the anterior part of the nose can function dynamically and further reduce the size of the nasal airway [3].

Another strategy to maintain an adequate level of intraoral pressure is the use of increased respiratory air flow and volumes. Individuals with palatal incompetency increase respiratory effort

TABLE 13-1. INTRAORAL PRESSURES ACCORDING TO COMPETENCY OF CLOSURE

	Adequate	Adequate-Borderline	Borderline-Inadequate	Inadequate
Area	0–0.049 sq cm	0.05–0.099 sq cm	0.10–0.19 sq cm	>0.2 sq cm
Pressure	6.4 cm H_2O ±2.2	5.0 cm H_2O ±1.9	4.3 cm H_2O ±1.8	3.7 cm H_2O ±1.9

about two- to threefold. Air flow rates as great as 800 cc per second have been observed [26].

Since intraoral pressures are usually maintained at levels above 3.0 cm H_2O, regardless of the degree of incompetency, it is obvious that measurements of intraoral air pressure will not provide a valid estimate of palatal function and therefore should not be used for this purpose.

NASAL PRESSURE MEASUREMENT

Nasal pressures have also been used as an index of velopharyngeal competency [4]. This has usually involved the placement of a nasal olive against a patent nostril while having the subject produce nonnasal consonants within test sounds or phrases. This approach will provide a gross estimate of incompetency since nasal pressures should be negligible or zero for competent closure and in the 1 to 6 cm H_2O range for incompetency. However, the technique does not differentiate borderline incompetency from gross incompetency and can be inaccurate in instances where the nostril is not patent. These serious limitations have restricted the use of this approach.

DIFFERENTIAL
PRESSURE MEASUREMENT

A more valid approach to screening velopharyngeal competency involves measuring oral and nasal pressures simultaneously. Warren [31] described a technique which measures the pressure difference across the velopharyngeal port for rating competency. The instrument, called PERCI,* is a simple and reliable tool when used correctly. The validity of the instrument depends on its ability to separate the effects of velopharyngeal function from the activities of other speech structures. Otherwise, an assessment of the velopharyngeal mechanism is easily confounded by misarticulations not directly related to the mechanism.

Closure of the palatopharyngeal orifice creates a pressure difference between the nose and mouth. When complete closure occurs, as during the consonant /p/, pressure in the mouth is determined by respiratory effort and will vary from about 3 cm H_2O to 8 cm H_2O [20, 30]. Pressure in the nose will be atmospheric or zero since no air leaks into the nasal chamber. However, if there is an opening, the difference in pressure will vary

with the size of the opening. The production of plosive sounds creates a stagnant column of air in the mouth which eliminates the effects of tongue position. That is, with no air flow the tongue does not produce a pressure drop. Since a difference in oral and nasal pressures is used, the effect of respiratory effort is cancelled out when the orifice is not completely closed.

The speech sample should include voiceless plosive consonants in such contexts as /papa/ and /hamper/. The efficiency rating is based on the use of the voiceless plosive /p/ because this sound provides an aerodynamic state which varies directly with the degree of velopharyngeal closure. The /p/ is produced by closing the lips and velopharyngeal orifice and stopping air flow for a period of time. If closure is complete, the pressure measured by the PERCI is equal to intraoral pressure. Any opening results in air flow into the nose which reduces the pressure difference between the nose and mouth. The result is a lower PERCI rating. Also, when air flow is stopped in the oral cavity, placement of the tongue does not affect pressure within the stagnant air column. Improper tongue placement is therefore eliminated as a potential problem. This is not true for other sounds. For example, fricative sounds are produced with oral air flow. If tongue-palatal contacts occur, an additional pressure drop would result. This could cause spurious values. Voiced sounds are not used because they often have lower, more inconsistent pressure patterns [31].

The nasal-plosive combination, as in the word /hamper/, is used to stress the palatal mechanism. Pressure flow studies have demonstrated that some individuals can close adequately for plosives in nonnasal contexts but cannot for those with adjacent nasals [31]. These same individuals also tend to be inadequate on fricative sounds and in continuous speech. Therefore, the nasal-plosive combination is used to determine closure ability under more difficult circumstances.

Catheter placement is shown in Figure 13-1. The catheters are attached to a differential pressure transducer connected to the PERCI. The difference in pressure between nose and mouth is converted to an electrical signal which is read directly on the PERCI as in the actual ΔP measurement.

The PERCI is calibrated against a water manometer so that the digital read-out is in actual pressure values. The criteria used for estimating competency from ΔP measurements are:

* Microtronics, Inc., Carrboro, N.C.

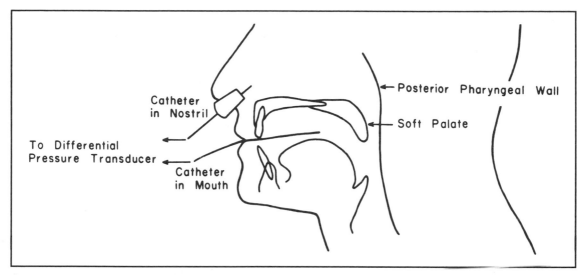

Figure 13-1. Catheter placement for measuring the difference in pressure between the mouth and nose, or for measuring orifice differential pressure.

>3.0 cm H_2O Adequate
1–2.9 cm H_2O Borderline closure
<1.0 cm H_2O Inadequate closure

These values were obtained from a study of 75 cleft palate patients [31] and later confirmed in a study of 518 patients [9]. Patients with velopharyngeal orifice areas of less than 0.10 sq cm demonstrated pressure readings greater than 3.0 cm H_2O on the PERCI. Those with areas between 0.10 sq cm and 0.2 sq cm had readings of 1.0 to 2.9. Individuals with palatal incompetency greater than 0.2 sq cm had readings less than 1.0.

It should be stressed, however, that the difference between competency and incompetency is not a point but, rather, a limited range which will vary from individual to individual. The efficiency rating obtained by this instrument is based on a physiological definition of competency, and the validity of the data depends on an understanding of this.

The PERCI efficiency rating is based on data generated from pressure and air flow studies which define competency in terms of respiratory parameters. An opening greater than 0.2 sq cm during nonnasal consonant productions is inadequate for normal speech [29]. Individuals with orifice openings of this magnitude usually impound lower intraoral air pressure unless the nasal cavity is grossly obstructed. Similarly, nasal emission of air is excessive and audible, and resonance is hypernasal. The efficiency rating under these circumstances is less than 1.0 and more than likely zero.

Competency therefore has a range that is less than 0.2 sq cm. When the opening is less than 0.05 sq cm, voice quality, except in extremely rare instances, should be within normal limits. Speech performance is determined by accuracy of articulation rather than palatal closure. The efficiency rating is above 3.0 for plosive consonants in these instances.

Openings between 0.05 and 0.10 sq cm are in the adequate-borderline range and may not interfere with an individual's ability to impound intraoral pressure. However, nasal emission will occur. Under certain circumstances it may be audible.

If the nasal airway is obstructed, turbulence will produce audible air flow which will be most noticeable during fricative productions since respiratory effort is increased. Otherwise, resonance will be within normal limits or slightly hypernasal, provided that articulatory performance is reasonably correct.

Individuals who speak with an overclosed oral airway, that is, with teeth close together, will sound hypernasal even with this small degree of opening. Oral airway impedance under such circumstances may be high enough to shunt a greater amount of acoustic energy into the nasal cavity, producing slightly hypernasal speech. Undoubtedly, this is an instance where tight, complete closure is necessary.

Openings between 0.10 and 0.20 sq cm represent borderline incompetency, and the efficiency rating is less than 3.0, usually between 1.0 and 2.5. Again, the term "borderline" represents a physiological determination based on the respiratory requirements of speech. Its acoustic analog may differ slightly. That is, in most instances, the listener will recognize slight-to-moderate audible nasal emission and hypernasality. However, there will be infrequent instances where speakers will sound normal in spite of borderline respiratory inadequacy.

AIR FLOW MEASUREMENT

Measurements of nasal emission frequently have been used to assess velopharyngeal competency [6, 8, 14, 18, 20]. Since there should be little or no nasal emission for all sounds except /m/, /n/, and /ng/, *nasal emission during the production of other sounds usually denotes palatal incompetency.* While nasal emission of air generally does increase with increased incompetency, a number of factors influence the outcome enough to result in a low correlation between the two variables [22]. Respiratory effort and nasal airway resistance are factors which influence nasal air flow during speech when tight velopharyngeal closure cannot be attained. For example, an individual with high nasal resistance to air flow will generate a sufficient intraoral pressure for nonnasal consonants with less respiratory effort than another individual with the same degree of incompetency but lower nasal resistance. Less respiratory effort means less air flow from the lungs and therefore less subsequent nasal emission as well.

At best, measurements of nasal emission or nasal air flow should be limited to gross judgments of velopharyngeal competency. That is, it is safe to consider peak nasal air flow rates above 150 cc per second during nonnasal consonant productions to be indicative of incompetent closure. However, the converse may not always be true. Flow rates of less than 150 cc per second may occur in spite of sphincter incompetency if there is nasal obstruction or decreased respiratory effort.

> # APPLICATION OF AERODYNAMIC PRINCIPLES FOR MEASUREMENT OF VELOPHARYNGEAL FUNCTION

* PERCI-PC, Microtronics Corporation, Carrboro, N.C.

In general, measurements of pressure and air flow alone have not provided the definitive diagnostic information required by most clinicians. These deficiencies have led to the development of more elaborate approaches for evaluating velopharyngeal competency. The techniques involve the application of hydrokinetic principles. Upper airway structures such as the tongue, teeth, lips, and palate form numerous constrictions which influence air flow and pressure. Hydraulic equations are used to estimate the resistance or size of these constrictions.

There is a self-contained software and related hardware package* available for aerodynamic assessment of speech and breathing. This system is used to collect pressure-flow data and the software provides analysis modes for measuring the pressure, air flow, volume, sphincter area, resistance, conductance, and timing variables associated with palatal closure and breathing.

AREA MEASUREMENT

Constrictions that form along the vocal tract, such as the velopharyngeal sphincter, produce an orifice-type of air flow pattern. The pressure drop which results is expressed as

$$P = \frac{d}{2k^2}\left(\frac{\dot{V}^2}{A}\right)$$

where k is the discharge coefficient which depends on the sharpness of the edge of the orifice and on Reynold's number. It has a value of 0.6 to 0.7 in the speech and breathing air flow range [19].

The relationship of pressure to air flow across the vocal tract constrictions has led to the application of hydrokinetic principles to estimate the size of the velopharyngeal orifice. The basis for this measurement can be explained in terms of air flow through simple pipes. The size of the constriction in a pipe can be calculated by measuring the air flow through the pipe $(\dot{V})$ and the pressure drop across the pipe $(P_1 - P_2)$. The area of constriction is then calculated from the equation

$$A = \dot{V}/k \ (2\Delta P/d)^{-2}$$

where $k = 0.65$ and d = density of air. Figure 13-2 illustrates catheter placement and instrumentation for estimating velopharyngeal orifice size.

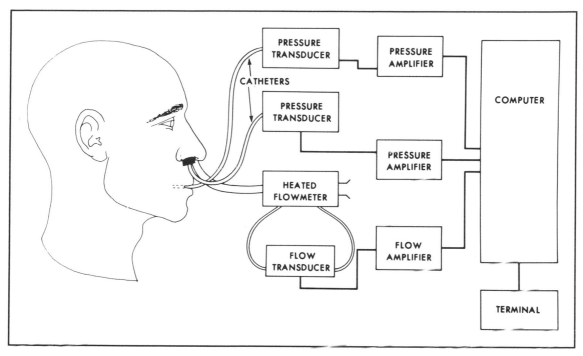

Figure 13-2. Catheter placement and apparatus for estimating velopharyngeal orifice size. The oral catheter is held by the patient and placed within the oral cavity.

Briefly, the pressure drop across the palatopharyngeal orifice (oral pressure minus nasal pressure) is measured by placing one catheter in the left nostril and another in the oropharynx. The nasal catheter is secured by a cork which blocks the nostril, creating a stagnant column of air. Both catheters measure static air pressures and transmit these pressures to a pressure transducer. Nasal air flow is measured by a heated pneumotachometer connected by plastic tubing to the subject's right nostril [30]. As discussed previously, voiceless plosive sounds should be used in the speech sample.

The same approach can be used for measuring oral port size during fricative productions. This port is the space between the tongue, teeth and palate and is approximately 0.06 sq cm during the production of /s/ [17, 32]. Figure 13-3 illustrates catheter placement. One catheter is placed within the oral cavity and the other within a well-fitting face mask. This measures the pressure drop across the oral port. Oral air flow is measured by a pneumotachograph attached to the oral mask. Figure 13-4 illustrates pressure and air flow data for calculation of the oral port area.

RESISTANCE MEASURMENT

Resistance to air flow is opposition to air motion caused by friction (viscous drag). Friction dissipates mechanical energy in the form of heat as air moves through the respiratory tract. This energy is supplied by the respiratory muscles which require more forceful contractions as airway resistance increases.

The measurement of velopharyngeal and nasal resistance involves the simultaneous recording of the rate of air flow and the pressure drop across the orifice and nose. The rate of air flow is measured by a pneumotachograph and the pressure drop is measured by a differential pressure transducer. The resistance to air flow is explained by analogy to Ohm's law for electrical currents and air flow and is given by:

$$R = \frac{\Delta P}{\dot{V}}$$

Where R = Resistance
ΔP = Pressure drop
$\dot{V}$ = Airflow

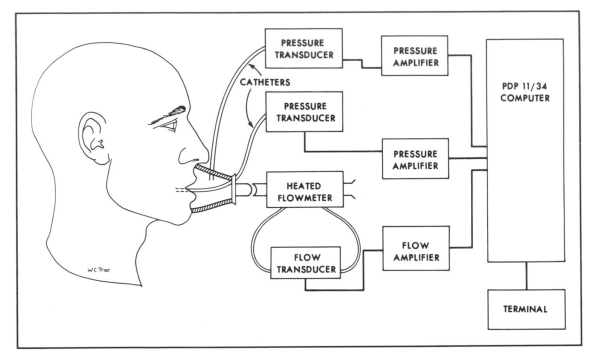

Figure 13-3. Instrumentation and catheter placement for estimating oral port size during fricative productions.

Since air flow through the vocal tract is partly laminar and partly turbulent, measurements must be made at comparable rates of flow if comparisons are to be meaningful [27].

The pressure drop is measured with the differential pressure transducer connected to two catheters. The first catheter is positioned in the subjects' oropharynx and the second catheter is placed within a nasal mask in front of the nose. Both catheters are occluded at their tips but have side holes for measurement of static pressures.

Nasal air flow is measured with a heated pneumotachograph connected to a well-adapted nasal mask. Particular attention is given to positioning the mask so that it does not contact the nostrils. Figure 13-5 illustrates this procedure.

The subject is then asked to produce test phrases using plosive consonant sounds. Resistance can then be calculated from the parameters of pressure and air flow. This measurement includes velopharyngeal resistance and nasal resistance. If velopharyngeal resistance alone is desired, the subject is then asked to breathe in and out through the nose. The resulting pressure-flow data can be used to calculate nasal resistance values. Subtraction of nasal resistance values from total resistance values will provide an estimate of velopharyngeal resistance.

Again, if comparisons among subjects are to be made, resistance measurements must be made at comparable rates of air flow. This is because resistance values are flow-dependent when there is turbulence in the airway (Fig. 13-6).

Thus, when air flow is laminar, $P = k_1 \dot{V}$. The pressure required to move the air is directly proportional to the viscosity of the air. The constant k_1 includes viscosity as well as length and radius. Air flow is usually not laminar during speech, however, because of the branching, irregular shape of the upper airway. Eddying occurs at bifurcations or when the surface is rough or constricted. When air flow is turbulent the pressure necessary to produce a given amount of air flow varies with the square of the flow, or $P = k_2 \dot{V}^2$ where k_2 is related to density, length, and radius. Turbulence occurs when the relationship of density $\times$ velocity $\times$ diameter/viscosity exceeds 2000, which is Reynold's number.

NASAL CROSS-SECTIONAL SIZE MEASUREMENTS

Clefts of the lip and palate frequently produce significant nasal deformities such as deviated sep-

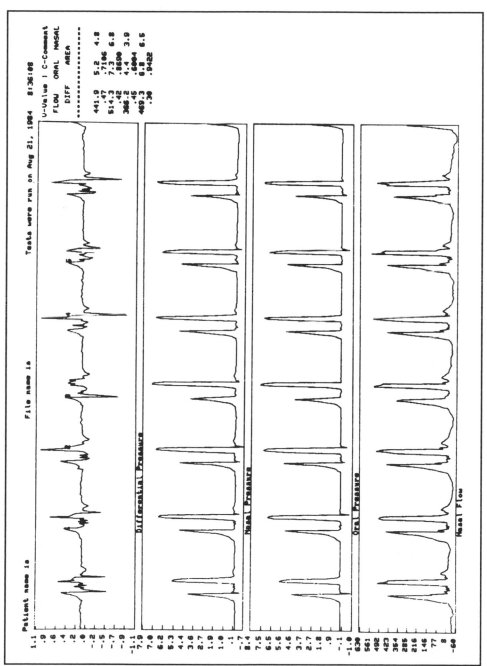

Figure 13-4. Data from a patient with gross palatal incompetency. The lower record demonstrates peak airflow rates of 350–500 cc/second. Intraoral pressures are greater than 4.0 cm H$_2$O, but differential pressures are approximately 0.4 cm H$_2$O. Orifice size is greater than 0.2 cm².

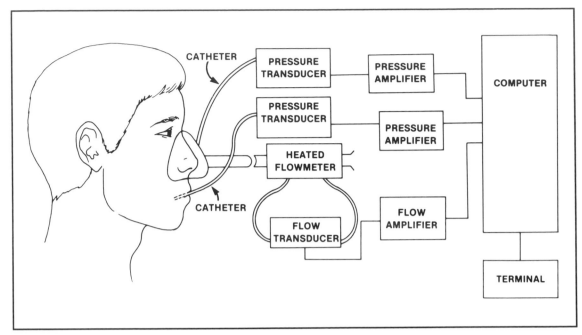

Figure 13-5. Instrumentation for estimating nasal airway size and nasal resistance.

tum, vomerine spurs, and atresia of the nostrils, as well as maxillary growth deficits which alter the nasal floor. These abnormalities tend to reduce the size of the nasal airway and increase nasal airway resistance [27]. High nasal resistance has implications for individuals with cleft palate since compensatory speech strategies in response to velopharyngeal incompetency may be influenced by nasal impairment. If nasal resistance is high, certain maneuvers, such as increased respiratory effort, may not be required to maintain an adequate level of intraoral pressure. Therefore, measurements of nasal cross-sectional area are frequently useful in assessment of cleft palate speech.

Structures such as the nose are basically tubes which offer resistance to air flow. The basis for measurement again can be explained in terms of air flow through simple pipes. The size of a constriction in a pipe can be calculated by measuring the air flow through it ($\dot{V}$) and the pressure drop across it ($P_1 - P_2$). Area of the constriction is then calculated in the same manner as velopharyngeal port size. Briefly, the pressure drop across the nose is measured by placing one catheter in the mouth and the other in the nasal air mask. Catheters are attached to pressure transducers.

Air flow is measured by a heated pneumotachograph attached to the nasal mask (see Fig. 13-5). Each subject is asked to inhale and exhale as nor-

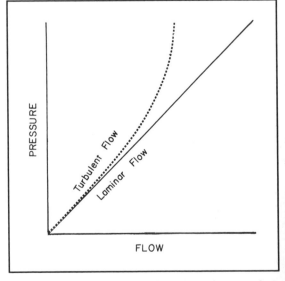

Figure 13-6. The relationship between pressure and air flow for laminar flow and turbulent flow. Measurements of resistance must be made at specific rates of flow for accurate comparisons within and among patients.

mally as possible through the nose. The resulting pressure and air flow patterns are transmitted to a recorder for analysis.

Figure 13-7 illustrates a hard-copy record of a cleft palate subject with an impaired airway. A

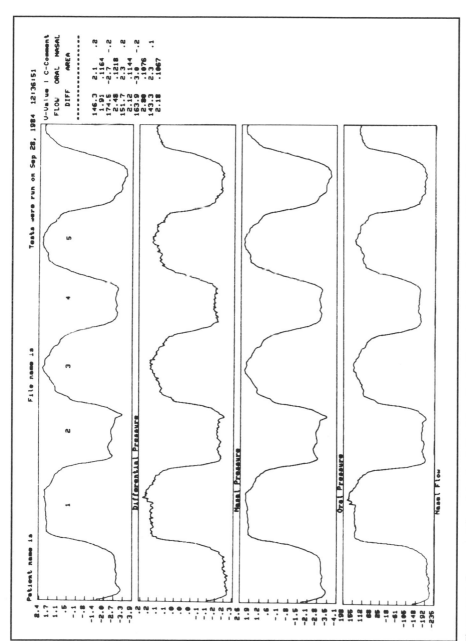

Figure 13-7. Pressure-airflow data of a cleft palate patient with an impaired nasal airway of 0.11 cm². In adults, an airway less than 0.4 cm² is impaired and obligatory mouth breathing results.

computer system was utilized for generating these data. The top line is nasal airway differential pressure, the second line is mask pressure, the third line is oral pressure, and the bottom line is nasal air flow. The data are printed out in the same order in the upper right. The impaired airway in this instance is 0.11 sq cm. The numbers 1 to 5 represent points on the cursor at which measurements were made.

AREA OF THE VELOPHARYNGEAL ORIFICE AND VELAR RESISTANCE

There is evidence that the aerodynamics of speech generally follow the rules of a regulating system [36, 37]. The essential feature of a regulating system (i.e., cardiovascular, respiratory) is the ability to respond to changing situations and maintain relatively steady-state conditions.

Certain responses of speech articulators are similar to regulating system behaviors. For example, there appears to be some control of airway resistance along the vocal tract during speech [33]. While resistance of such structures as the vocal folds, velopharyngeal sphincter, and tongue may vary according to phonetic context, total airway resistance remains fairly high. This maintains subglottal pressure at a somewhat stable level during speech [36]. Thus, in normal speech, vocal fold resistance for a vowel is approximately 40 to 80 cm $H_2O/L/S$ [36] but is only 25 cm $H_2O/L/S$ for voiced fricatives. However, oral port resistance for fricatives is approximately 75 cm $H_2O/L/S$, thus providing a total resistance across the vocal tract about equal in magnitude to vowel productions (Fig. 13-8).

Velopharyngeal resistance is usually infinite for nonnasal consonants. Figure 13-9 illustrates that the relationship between velopharyngeal area and velopharyngeal resistance is inverse and nonlinear [21]. Since a loss in velar resistance would result in low intraoral pressures, individuals develop compensatory behaviors in response to incompetency in an attempt to increase intraoral pressure.

The drop in pressure resulting from air moving across a structure is proportional to the reciprocal of the fourth power of the radius. Reducing the radius of an airway by one half increases the pressure drop 16-fold [39]. The pressure drop is also proportional to volume rate of air flow. Thus, airway resistance is an important factor in maintaining stable speech pressures. The actual relation-

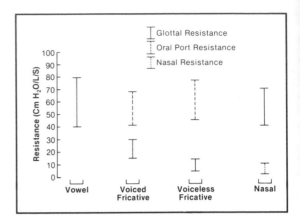

Figure 13-8. Resistance across the vocal tract is maintained at a high level regardless of the phoneme produced. One or more structures may contribute to total airway resistance.

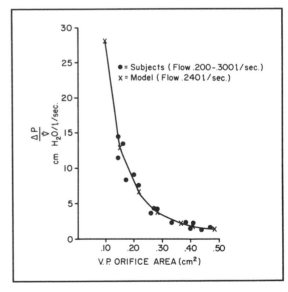

Figure 13-9. The relationship between velopharyngeal orifice area and velopharyngeal resistance based on model studies and human studies. The relationship is nonlinear and demonstrates that resistance is high when orifice size is less than 0.2 sq cm.

ship between velopharyngeal orifice size and velopharyngeal resistance can be described in mathematical terms using a resistance-area conversion equation. This equation

$$R = 1.9 + \frac{.03 + (0.009 \times flow)}{A^2}$$

is derived from data generated in breathing studies [39] and is valid for a velopharyngeal area range of 0 to about 0.6 sq cm. Since nasal resistance becomes a factor when velar resistance falls below about 10 cm $H_2O/L/S$, this equation includes both velar and nasal resistance. Since resistance is flow-dependent, the two- to three-fold increase in air flow rate generally observed in individuals with velar incompetency usually provides enough resistance to maintain intraoral pressures at appropriate levels for speech.

TIMING STUDIES

Aerodynamic assessment techniques can also be used to evaluate timing patterns associated with palatal function [34]. Individuals with competent, borderline, and incompetent velar function can be differentiated on the basis of specific timing parameters such as the onset, peak, and end of pressure and air flow patterns. Each closure group manifests certain unique timing features. Figure 13-10 illustrates the pressure-flow patterns of an individual with adequate velopharyngeal function producing the word /hamper/. Air flow for the /m/ ends prior to the pressure peak for /p/. Figure 13-11 illustrates the change which occurs with palatal incompetency. The entire air flow record shifts to the right.

Timing studies also discriminate between individuals with hypernasality due to delayed, but adequate, velopharyngeal closure and those with hypernasality due to incompetent closure. Figure 13-12 illustrates an individual with a lag in closure. Nasal air flow for the /p/ in /papa/ is shown to occur during the pressure-rise phase. There is no air flow at the pressure peak. This suggests the presence of assimilative nasality since in conversational speech the delay in closure would nasalize preceding vowels. Timing problems should always be considered when pressure-flow assessment indicates adequate or adequate-borderline closure, but listening suggests hypernasality.

EFFECTS OF FISTULAE

Recent studies suggest that fistulae associated with cleft palate repair adversely influence speech performance [16]. Richtner [15] experimentally manipulated size and location of openings through

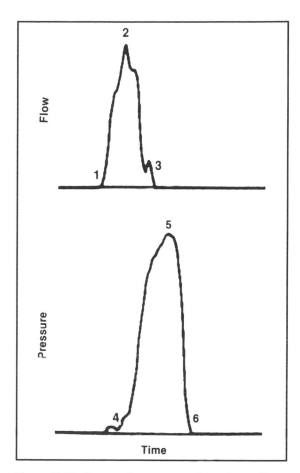

Figure 13-10. Pressure-flow pattern of a patient with competent velopharyngeal closure phonating the nasal-plosive blend /mp/ in /hamper/. Note that the flow peak (2) is approximately at the beginning of the pressure rise (4) point. End of flow (3) occurs before the pressure peak (5).

a subject's prosthetic palatal applicance and measured the effect on speech articulation, resonance quality, and pressure and air flow. Her findings revealed that both hole size and location of the fistula determine the degree of speech impairment. The greatest distortion of articulation and resonance quality was perceived when the fistula was located in the velar port and near the incisive foramen. Size of the fistula was also a significant variable with greater distortions occurring with increased openings. Even the smallest fistula of 0.05 sq cm caused mild distortion. At 0.1 to 0.2 sq cm, articulation proficiency and nasality were significantly affected. These findings are in agreement for those reported by others for velar incompetency [31].

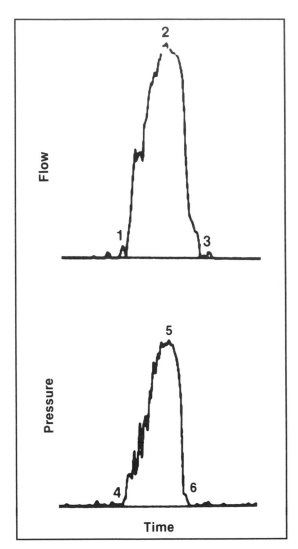

Figure 13-11. The pattern of a patient with incompetent closure. Note that the flow peak (2) is near the pressure peak (5). End of flow (3) is near the end of pressure (6).

DO'S AND DON'TS
OF AERODYNAMIC MEASUREMENT

The hydrokinetic equation provides acceptable estimates of orifice size when used correctly. The determination of port areas rests on some simplifying assumptions and incorporates some empirically derived, but nonetheless ad hoc, corrections. The most important of these relates to the constant k which is introduced into the equation. Warren and DuBois [19] have emphasized (on the basis of physical models) that k may vary from

0.59 to 0.72 and they recommend a mean k of 0.65. Indeed, Muller and Brown [13] argue strongly for great caution in the choice of k, pointing out its dependence on unverifiable assumptions about the geometry of the velopharyngeal port.

While k does vary with size, the error produced is very small over the port sizes and air flow values associated with speech. The Muller and Brown [13] observation concerning geometry of the velopharyngeal port is theoretically correct. However, Warren and DuBois [19] used circular ports in modeling studies. Rectangular ports were also studied and no significant difference was found in terms of k [21]. The point to be made is that the hydrokinetic equation has limitations and accuracy must be maximized with a very careful approach to details. There are several key factors in maximizing accuracy. Although many appear to be minor points, if not followed inaccuracies would result. Attention to details is essential.

Transducers must be balanced prior to each study. Most transducers have input voltages which vary slightly. Usually there is a zero suppression, balance button, or screw adjustment to assure a null point. If balancing is not done, an error will be introduced, with the magnitude varying with the degree of unbalance of the transducer.

Calibration of the transducers must be accomplished prior to each study and at least on each day of data collection. Calibration of pressure transducers is accomplished with a water manometer. Calibration of the pneumotachograph requires a rotameter. It should be noted that when calibrating a pneumotachograph, the air supply should be regulated so that variations in flow rate do not occur. Usually a central source of air without a regulator is unacceptable because of pressure drops in a multiuser system. A cylinder of compressed air with a regulator is an ideal source.

Finally, an additional and important validation of the system involves checking it against a known orifice size. A simple tube with a plastic cylinder having a known orifice area should be used. Measurement of pressure drop across the cylinder simultaneously with air flow through it should provide a constriction size equivalent to the model when the hydrokinetic equation, or a simplified method for estimating area from pressures and air flow [12], is used.

The speech sample used in testing is extremely important. The plosive /p/ provides an aerodynamic environment which assures greater accuracy than other sounds. Voiced plosives are often

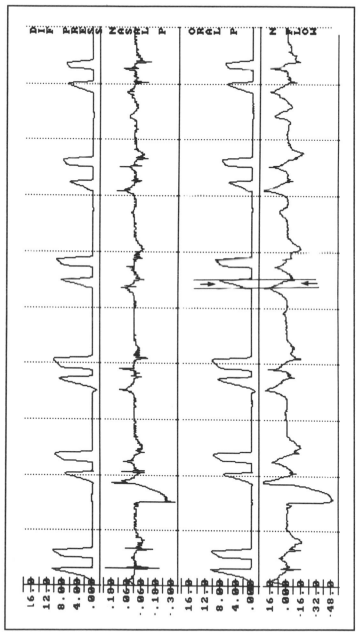

Figure 13-12. Pressure flow patterns of a patient with assimilative nasality. Although this patient achieves adequate velopharyngeal closure (0.01 cm²), it is late, thereby nasalizing the preceding vowel. The lower arrow points to the presence of nasal airflow during the pressure buildup phase of consonant production (upper arrow).

produced with lower pressures and although in most instances intraoral pressure would be greater than 3.0 in normals, in some cases it would not. Sounds such as /t/ should not be used because the airway is occluded where the catheter is placed. Similarly, fricative sounds such as /s/ should not be used because improper tongue placement (e.g., palatal-lingual contacts) could result in a spurious reading, as explained previously.

The use of the test words which contain combinations of the nasal /m/ and voiceless plosives such as in /hamper/ is helpful in determining whether a patient has a problem achieving closure rapidly enough. There are individuals who demonstrate timing problems and although they can achieve adequacy in time, the pressure-rise phase of the consonant is slow and nasal emission occurs because of late palatal closure. The nasal /m/ and plosive /p/ combination stresses the mechanism and aids in identifying those individuals who often sound hypernasal. Also, more importantly, this phonetic combination more nearly approximates the degree of closure which occurs during fricative productions or continuous speech. Some individuals will show adequacy on isolated sounds and plosives but only borderline closure in conversational speech or with words containing fricatives.

Another point that should be emphasized is that individuals with severe open bites or lip incompetency may not always have labial closure on plosives and this would produce a false low reading if it were not detected. The lips must be closed for plosives and the patient should be watched during phonation of the test sounds.

OTHER SOURCES OF ERROR

The measurement of velopharyngeal orifice size requires that both nostrils be patent. It has been our experience that less than 5 percent of the cleft palate population has one nostril completely obstructed. However, if this is the case, there are two alternatives. One is to use the patent nostril for air flow measurement and the obstructed nostril for nasal pressure measurement. Since nasal pressure will be zero, the orifice size calculations will understimate area. This still may provide useful data. For example, if orifice size is recorded as 0.15 sq cm under these conditions, the actual size would be greater than 0.15 sq cm. Thus, the data would reveal incompetent closure.

The other alternative is to use the differential pressure measurement as an index of velopharyngeal function. The patent nostril would be used for nasal pressure measurement in this circumstance.

Another source of error is a leak in the system. If the nasal olive, cork, or tubing does not fit properly, or the catheter connection to the transducer is not tight, a leak will occur and the data will be spurious. One quick test of the system involves connecting the water manometer to the pressure transducer and introducing 2 to 4 cm H_2O pressure. If a leak is present, the pressure will fall to zero. Another source of error involves kinks in the tubing, especially in the tubing connecting the flow meter to the transducer in the pneumotachograph. Adjustments of the pneumotachograph to fit the patient can produce a kink in the tubing and this must be corrected for an accurate air flow measurement. The ideal test of the entire system is to run a calibration study using a cylinder with a known orifice size as described earlier.

THE EQUATION

The estimate of orifice size decreses in accuracy considerably at areas above 0.8 sq cm during speech. Since the nasal airway produces a more significant resistance to air flow during speech than the velopharyngeal sphincter at a size greater than 0.2 sq cm, larger sphincter sizes have little effect on pressures and air flow. For this season we report any orifice size greater than 0.2 sq cm as greater than 0.2 sq cm and incompetent. This maximizes accuracy.

Another point that should be stressed is that the orifice equation is most accurate when measurements are made at the flow peak of an utterance. That is, where the rate of change of flow is zero. Measurements at the rise or fall portion of the flow peak are considerably less accurate.

Finally, it must be reiterated that pressure-flow testing does not evaluate speech performance. It provides an objective assessment of a structure's activity in terms of the respiratory requirements of speech.

REFERENCES

1. Buncke, H. J. Manometric evaluation of palatal function in cleft palate patients. *Plast. Reconstr. Surg.* 23:148–158, 1970.
2. Chase, R. A. An objective evaluation of palatopharyngeal competence. *Plast. Reconstr. Surg.* 26:23–39, 1960.

3. Hairfield, W. M., Warren, D. W., Hinton, V. A., and Seaton, D. Inspiratory and expiratory effects of nasal breathing. *Cleft Palate J.* 24:183–189, 1987.

4. Hess, D. A., and McDonald, E. T. Consonantal nasal pressure in cleft palate speakers. *J. Speech Hear. Res.* 3:201–211, 1960.

5. Lubker, J. F. Aerodynamic and ultrasonic assessment techniques in speech-dentofacial research. *American Speech and Hearing Association Reports* 5:207–223, 1970.

6. Lubker, J. F., and Moll, K. L. Simultaneous oral-nasal air flow measurements and cineflurorgraphic observations during speech production. *Cleft Palate J.* 2:257–272, 1965.

7. Lubker, J. F., and Schweiger, J. W. Nasal airflow as an index of success of prosthetic management of cleft palate. *J. Dent. Res.* 48:368–375, 1969.

8. Machida, J. Air flow rate and articulatory movement during speech. *Cleft Palate J.* 4:240–248, 1967.

9. Morr, K. E., Warren, D. W., Hinton, V. A., and Hairfield, W. M. Orifice differential pressure: an index of velopharyngeal function. *ASHA* 28:103, 1986.

10. Morris, H. L. The oral manometer as a diagnostic tool in clinical speech pathology. *J. Speech Hear. Disord.* 31:362–369, 1966.

11. Moser, H. M. Diagnostic and clinical procedures in rhinolalia. *J. Speech Hear. Disord.* 7:1–18, 1942.

12. Moon, J. B., and Weinberg, B. Two simplified methods for estimating velopharyngeal orifice area. *Cleft Palate J.* 22.1–10, 1985.

13. Muller, E. M., and Brown, W. S., Jr. Variations in the Supraglottal Air Pressure Waveform and Their Articulatory Interpretation. In N. Lass (Ed.), *Speech and Language: Advances in Basic Research and Practice*. New York: Academic Press, 1980. Vol. 4, pp. 317–389.

14. Quigley, L. F., Shiere, F. R., Webster, R.C., and Cobb, C. M. Measuring palatopharyngeal competence with the nasal anemometer. *Cleft Palate J.* 1:304–313, 1964.

15. Richtner, V. E. M. Effects of experimental palatal fistulas on speech and resonance. Dissertation, University of Florida, Gainesville, 1986.

16. Shelton, R. L., and Blank, J. F. Oronasal fistulas, intraoral air pressure and nasal air flow during speech. *Cleft Palate J.* 21:91–99, 1984.

17. Smith, Z. H., Allen, G., Warren, D. W., and Hall, D. J. The consistency of the pressure-flow technique for assessing oral port size. *J. Acoust. Soc. Am.* 64:1203–1206, 1978.

18. Subtelny, J. D., Worth, J. H., and Sakuda, M. Intraoral pressure and rate of flow during speech. *J. Speech Hear. Res.* 9:498–518, 1966.

19. Warren, D. W., and DuBois, A. B. A pressure-flow technique for measuring velopharyngeal orifice area during continuous speech. *Cleft Palate J.* 1:52–71, 1964.

20. Warren, D. W. Velopharyngeal orifice size and upper pharyngeal pressure-flow patterns in normal speech. *Plast. Reconstr. Surg.* 33:148–161, 1964.

21. Warren, D. W., and Devereux, J. L. An analog study of cleft palate speech. *Cleft Palate J.* 3:103–114, 1966.

22. Warren, D. W. Nasal emission of air and velopharyngeal function. *Cleft Palate J.* 4:148–156, 1967.

23. Warren, D. W., and Ryon, W. E. Oral port constriction, nasal resistance, and respiratory aspects of cleft palate speech: an analog study. *Cleft Palate J.* 4:38–46, 1967.

24. Warren, D. W., and Mackler, S. B. Duration of oral port constriction in normal and cleft palate speech. *J. Speech Hear. Res.* 11:391–401, 1968.

25. Warren, D. W., and Wood, M. T. Respiratory volumes in normal speech: a possible reason for intraoral pressure differences among voiced and voiceless consonants. *J. Acoust. Soc. Am.* 45:466–469, 1969.

26. Warren, D. W., Wood, M. T., and Bradley, D. P. Respiratory volumes in normal and cleft palate speech. *Cleft Palate J.* 6:449–460, 1969.

27. Warren, D. W., Duany, L. F., and Fischer, N. D. Nasal pathway resistance in normal and cleft lip and palate subjects. *Cleft Palate J.* 6:134–140, 1969.

28. Warren, D. W., and Hall, D. Glottal activity and intraoral pressure during stop consonant productions. *Folia Phoniatr.* 25:121–129, 1973.

29. Warren, D. W. The Determination of Velopharyngeal Incompetency by Aerodynamic and Acoustical Techniques. In M. Hogan (Ed.), *Clinics in Plastic Surgery*. Philadelphia: Saunders, 1975. Pp. 299–304.

30. Warren, D. W. Aerodynamics of Sound Production. In N. Lass (Ed.), *Contemporary Issues in Experimental Phonetics*. Springfield, Ill.: Thomas, 1976.

31. Warren, D. W. Perci: a method for rating palatal efficiency. *Cleft Palate J.* 16:279–285, 1979.

32. Warren, D. W., Hall, D. J., and Davis, J. Oral port constriction and pressure airflow relationships during sibilant productions. *Folia Phoniatr.* 33:380–394, 1981.

33. Warren, D. W. Aerodynamics of Speech. In N. J. Lass, L. V. McReynolds, J. L. Northern, and D. E. Yoder (Eds.), *Speech, Language and Hearing*. Philadelphia: Saunders, 1982.

34. Warren, D. W., Dalston, R. M., Trier, W. C., and Holder, M. B. A pressure-flow technique for quantifying temporal patterns of palatopharyngeal closure. *Cleft Palate J.* 22:11–19, 1985.

35. Warren, D. W., Hairfield, W. M., and Hinton, V. A. The respiratory significance of the nasal grimace. *ASHA* 27:82, 1985.

36. Warren, D. W. Compensatory speech behaviors in cleft palate: a regulation/control phenomenon? *Cleft Palate J.* 23:251–280, 1986.

37. Warren, D. W. The velopharyngeal sphincter: a control factor in the speech regulating system. *ASHA* 28:103, 1986.

38. Warren, D. W., Hairfield, W. M., Seaton, D., Morr, K. E., and Smith, L. The relationship between nasal airway size and nasal-oral breathing. *Am. J. Orthod. Dentofacial Orthop.* 93:289–293, 1988.

39. Warren, D. W., Hairfield, W. M., Seaton, D., and Hinton, V. A. The relationship between nasal airway size and nasal airway resistance. *Am. J. Orthod. Dentofacial Orthop.* 92:390–395, 1987.

40. Weinberg, B., and Shanks, J. C. The relationship between three oral breath pressure ratios and ratings of severity of nasality for talkers with cleft palate. *Cleft Palate J.* 8:251–256, 1971.

CHAPTER 14

Cleft Palate Speech Assessment Through Oral-Nasal Acoustic Measures

Samuel G. Fletcher
Larry E. Adams
Martin J. McCutcheon

Nasal consonants are found in virtually every language of the world and nasalized vowels in about one out of five [5, 19]. This reflects the fact that nasal resonance is a highly distinctive, readily perceived acoustic quality which may be mixed with orally produced sounds to invoke specific phonetic contrasts. The penetrating quality of nasality as an acoustic property is unacceptable to listeners when it is injected dominantly and nonphonetically into speech.

Despite its easily recognized presence, the degree of excessive nasality in speech has been shown to be notoriously difficult to establish perceptually [2, 3, 25]. Since the nasal chambers may be activated by any acoustic vibrations that reach the nasal cavities, a certain degree of nasality is normal in all vocalizations. Even in the presence of a closed velopharyngeal port, nasal resonance may be instigated by vibrations from surrounding bony and soft tissue structures. The ciliated walls of the respiratory tract tend to dampen the vibrations and reduce acoustic transmission in this condition, however.

When nasal resonance exceeds some as yet undetermined level, it is noticed. At some point above this level of detection it is perceived to be abnormal. The voice is then judged to be "hypernasal." Different listeners vary in where they would locate the boundaries between normal, noticeably nasal, and hypernasal voice quality [8]. Perhaps because of the variable, possibly fluctuating, baseline that listeners apply in judging perceived nasality, establishing normal limits for this vocal quality has presented a serious challenge in diagnosis and management of cleft palate speech.

The ultimate purpose of instrumentation is to improve measurement accuracy and repeatability in difficult diagnostic and treatment tasks. When instrumental devices are used to assist clinicians, an important criterion is that the measures obtained agree rather closely with what humans discern to be the essential problem. In this instance, the scores should agree as closely as possible with the degree of nasality perceived by listeners as they hear a person talk.

Since hypernasality is one of the criterion features of cleft palate speech, both its presence and magnitude are important diagnostically and therapeutically. How to measure these facets of nasality has occupied clinical and experimental interest for several decades. McDonald and Koepp-Baker [20] speculated that nasal voice quality is somehow identified auditorily by discerning a "balance or ratio" between acoustic resonances associated within the oral and nasal cavities. Moser, Dreher, and Adler [21] claimed that the perception of nasality was instigated by extra resonances added to the speech spectrum. House and Stevens [15] used an electrical analog of the vocal trace with variable cross-sectional dimensions to model nasalization in vowel production in their efforts to isolate those acoustic properties. They concluded that changes in the region of the first formant were likely the primary source of perceived nasality. This agreed with experimental findings by Hattori, Yamamoto, and Fujimura [14] who identified an antiresonance effect at about 500 Hz in the spectrum of the oral signal from all five Japanese vowels when they introduced a nasal side branch from the oral cavity.

Andrews [1] manipulated the degree of coupling between the oral and nasal cavities by changing the dimensions of an aperture in a prosthetic bulb located between the soft palate and the pharyngeal wall and studied the effect on the acoustic spectrum of the response and on the degree of nasality perceived by three listener judges. The only parameter he found to be consistently related to the acoustic attributes was a reduction in the third and seventh harmonics of the signal. In the responses of a male talker this would place resonances at around 400 and 1000 Hz.

Fletcher and Bishop [12] compared acoustic output from the nasal and oral chambers and judgmental ratings of nasality in the Zoo Passage [8] spoken by twenty 5- to 19-year-old subjects with velopharyngeal insufficiency following repaired palatal clefts. Agreement between the judgmental scores of the 10 listeners and nasal-oral measurements of the speech output was greatest when the signals were limited to a frequency band centered near 500 Hz. Further experiments indicated that this agreement was optimized with a 300 Hz bandwidth around the 500 Hz central frequency. Finally, Lindqvist and Sundberg [18] reported that when the paranasal sinuses were included as shunting cavities in a twin-tube model of the nasal tract, the response curve peaked in the 400 to 600 Hz range.

The conclusion from the converging series of experiments cited above is that perceived nasality reflects specific acoustic differences in the speech spectrum, with the major effect on the output evidenced in a 100- to 150-Hz band around a 500-Hz central frequency.

The device called *TONAR* was designed to measure oral and nasal sound signals and calculate a score which represented the ratio of the two signals within the 500 ± 150 Hz bandwidth. In *TONAR II*, which was manufactured commercially, the following equation was introduced for calculating the ratio of nasal and oral acoustic output. The resultant score was labeled "percent nasalance" to distinguish it from judged nasality:

$$\text{Nasalance} = \frac{N}{N + O} \times 100$$

In the above formula N refers to nasal sound pressure and O to oral sound pressure in the 350 to 650 Hz band. The resultant sound energy ratio is multiplied by 100 to convert it to a percentage score. This equation has several advantages. First, the comparison between nasal output and the combined nasal-plus-oral outputs seems intuitively close to how listeners likely process the nasalized speech signals as they discern the degree of nasality. Second, the formula establishes absolute limits at each end of the nasalance continuum. Speech produced with no nasal sound would generate a nasalance score of 0. Speech in which all sound is from the nose would produce a 100 percent nasalance score. Third, percentage scores are common and thus likely to be immediately meaningful to both an evaluator and a person whose speech is evaluated.

The TONAR II and the pressure-flow device described originally by Warren and Dubois [24] are among the most widely used noninvasive instruments that do not involve radiation [23]. Dalston and Warren [4] studied interrelations among these devices and listener judgments of hypernasality in the speech of 124 child and adult subjects seen for evaluation. They reported that in general larger velopharyngeal orifice areas from pressure-flow measures were associated with higher TONAR II scores and judged hypernasality. In fact, the three measurement procedures produced highly complementary data. Only one individual would have undergone unnecessary treatment if it were done only when both TONAR II and pressure-flow findings indicated a need for it, and only five of 118 would have had such treatment withheld for at least a trial period when the joint assessments indicated it should have been given.

THE NASOMETER

The TONAR II instrumentation was replaced by the Nasometer. The nasometer is similar in principle to TONAR II, but significantly different in structure, function, and practical features. The schematized diagram in Figure 14-1 illustrates the essential characteristics of the instrument. It consists of three major subunits: (1) a sound separator, or baffle, that partitions the outputs from the nasal and oral cavities and contains microphones for tranducing the acoustic signals emitted, (2) electronic circuits for frequency band–limiting and processing the microphone signals and transmitting them to a computer, and (3) a personal computer for receiving data, processing the information, calculating nasalance values, and display-

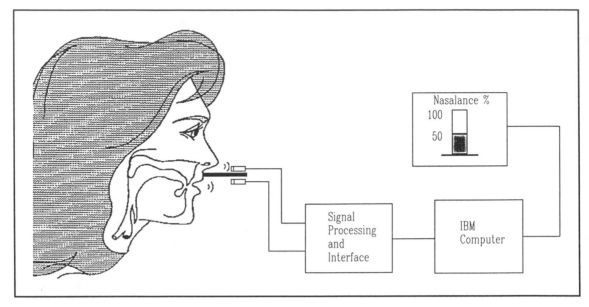

Figure 14-1. Functional elements of the nasometer.

ing the nasalance scores along with other parameters in printed or graphic (e.g., "nasogram") form. The sound separator design and electronics are based on a prototype by one of the authors (M.J.M.). Improvements and refinements were made in the current manufactured version, but the basic elements are the same. These elements will now be considered in greater detail.

SOUND SEPARATOR

The sound separator assembly consists of a metal plate or baffle, headgear to support the baffle, and two microphones that transduce the separated nasal and oral acoustic signals. Anthropomorphic data were used to establish the shape and size of the plate so it would fit a wide range of faces, and in particular that of a young adult. During use, the plate is oriented perpendicular to the frontal plane of the face and centered on the prolabium approximately midway between the nose and upper lip. A disposable soft plastic lining covers the portion of the plate that contacts the face. This lining helps form a seal and makes the baffle plate contact more comfortable to the user. The baffle is supported by a dual arm with an adjustable linkage attached to a plastic headband. Adjustment straps at the sides of the headband and the baffle enable the baffle position to be fixed vertically and horizontally. This permits the

plate to be established at right angles to the frontal plane (see Fig. 14-1).

The acoustic amplitude of the signals from the nose and mouth is transduced to proportional electrical signals by the microphones mounted above and below the separator plate. The microphones are unidirectional, close-speaking, and dynamic. They have a 50 to 15,000 Hz frequency response with a 66 dB sensitivity. The unidirectional response characteristic of these microphones increases the acoustic separation of the nasal and oral signals and helps reject potentially contaminating environmental noise. Under these conditions the nasal-oral signal separation is about 25 dB.

ELECTRONIC SIGNAL PROCESSING

The block diagram in Figure 14-2 shows the electronic signal processing in identical nasal and oral channels. Each microphone signal is amplified by a preamplifier circuit with a gain of nearly 900. This output is fed to bandpass filters with fourth-order Butterworth characteristics centered at 500 Hz and a − 3 dB bandwidth of 300 Hz. This captures the critical portion of the oral and nasal signals in the lower frequency region, as discussed above, and rejects high- and low-frequency ambient noise. The output from the bandpass filters is fed to an RMS-DC conversion circuit that

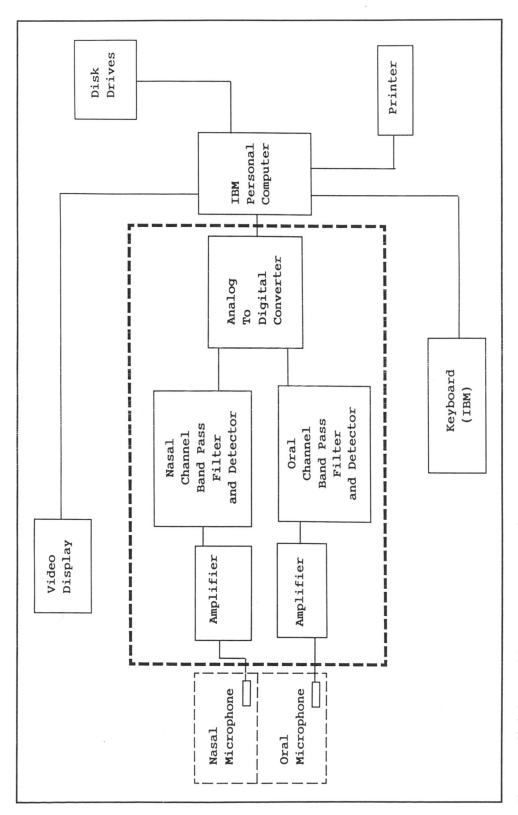

Figure 14-2. Block diagram of the nasometer instrumentation.

produces a DC output proportional to the RMS value of the input signal. This stage also contains an averaging-smoothing circuit with a settling time of approximately 35 msec. This smoothing time was chosen to give a relatively fast response to changes in the nasal-oral output.

The smoothed output of the RMS-DC circuit is further amplified to match the input range of an eight-bit, multichannel analog-to-digital (A/D) converter. An internal oscillator circuit drives a small loud-speaker that provides an acoustic signal to the separator microphones. This signal is used by an operator to "calibrate" the system. This is done by selecting the calibration mode that gives a continuous display of the channel balance and then using a potentiometer to adjust the gain balance between the nasal and oral channels.

The advantages of the current design include natural speech acoustics without injection of competing cavity resonances and without impedance loading present in a more closed system. It also allows talkers to self-monitor their speech with minimal distortion. The lighter, portable headgear and separator plate can be easily worn by subjects confined to beds or wheelchairs. This increases the utility of the instrumentation. Finally, the parts of the system that come into contact with the user are easily sterilized.

SOFTWARE

The Nasometer is microcomputer-based and software-driven. This permits several features not available in TONAR II. The major functions of the software, based on prototype software by one of the authors (L.E.A.), include data acquisition, data editing and analysis, stimulus presentation, display generation, file management, and various utilities. Each of these functions will be described in detail.

Data acquisition routines form the central core of the software. They sample the nasal and oral signals at a rate of 120 Hz, extract the nasal and oral A/D values, and calculate percent nasalance scores. The values are proportional to the RMS signal level in each channel, not instantaneous waveform values. The results of the computations may be viewed on the computer monitor or plotted as printed nasograms with information pertinent to date, time, stimulus materials, and subject identification added in response to standard queries. The data may also be stored on a disk drive for later retrieval and analysis.

Considerable flexibility is available in the software for data editing and analysis. In the data editing mode the user can control placement of both left and right vertical cursors. The subroutine then displays the nasalance value under each cursor and enables the blanking of data either between or outside the cursors. This feature is useful for deleting data from extraneous noise in the environment. It also permits selection of another subroutine which calculates statistics for the data between the cursors. These statistics include the mean and standard deviation of the nasalance, the minimum and maximum nasalance values in the sample, and the time range of the sample along with the values of both the left and right cursors. The nasalance slope value may also be calculated when short time periods are specified in the data window.

The nasalance scores are displayed in real time following either a time history or bar "thermometer" display option. When the time option is selected, the x-axis represents time and the y-axis represents percent nasalance. The amount of time represented along the x-axis is variable. This permits the user to select data analysis periods of 2, 4, 6, 8, 20, 40, 60, 80, or 100 seconds. The ability to examine different time segments of the data provides opportunity to examine both the overall pattern of nasalance and the details of nasalance variability within small segments of the response. This is particularly helpful in evaluating special functions such as possible neurological disturbance effects on velar timing. It also permits indepth assessment of subtle changes in nasalance, such as that which accompanies disintegration of velar control across speaking time. The time history display, utilizing various time segments, is also useful in assessing the degree and stability of change in velopharyngeal valving in response to standard or experimental treatment regimens instituted to alter abnormal nasal resonance.

The bar, or thermometer, display option represents dynamic nasalance on the y-axis of the video screen. The display includes a peak holding cursor which identifies the highest-occurring nasalance value during a response. This display is particularly useful as feedback to younger patients. It also serves an important role in instrument calibration.

Both the time history and the bar displays permit the selection of a nasalance goal threshold value. This is shown as a reference value on the screen as a guide for assessing the potential for improved velopharyngeal valving. It may also be used as a concrete, quantitative, biofeedback index or goal level during therapy aimed at nasalance reduction.

INTERPRETING NASALANCE REDUCTION

Fletcher [10] examined the relationship between perceived nasality and instrumental measures of nasalance through a series of comparisons between instrumentally derived and listener judgmental scores. His basic data consisted of sound-field and nasal-oral sound–separated tape recordings of 23 children speaking the Zoo Passage. The speakers, drawn from a random sample of 70 children with repaired palatal clefts from throughout Alabama, displayed a wide range of nasality. Twenty listeners served as judges of their speech. A series of listening tasks were used which progressed from rating the speech as simply "normal" or "abnormal" in nasality to a paired comparison routine where the sound field recordings were compared and recompared until the listeners arrived at a systematic progression from least to most nasality perceived in the paragraphs spoken by the different talkers. They then sorted the responses into five groups according to "normal," "mildly nasal," "moderately nasal," "severely nasal," and "very severely nasal" classifications of the perceived nasality in the responses of the talkers. Finally, each response was assigned an absolute magnitude score which represented the listener's impression of precisely how much nasality was present in each talker's speech relative to that of all other talkers.

As the listeners progressed through the tasks described above, listener-to-listener agreement increased. This suggests that they were "tuning in" to a common acoustic element in the spoken patterns. Of particular importance was that as the listener's perceptual ratings became more closely aligned, agreement with the instrumentally derived nasalance scores systematically increased. That is, greater precision in listener observations led to correspondingly higher agreement with the instrumental scores, suggesting that the perceptual and instrumental observations had a common basis.

It is important to note that the instrumentation provided explicit information with respect to certain ranges of nasal resonance that were particularly difficult for listeners to resolve. For instance, in the initial task a subgroup of talkers was identified which the listeners consistently judged as having normal nasality. These talkers had low nasalance scores. Another group was consistently judged as abnormally nasal. They had high nasalance scores. In the midrange where listener-to-listener variability was high and interjudge agreement comparatively low in classifying and explicitly rating the responses, the instrumentation provided particularly meaningful differentiation of the degree of nasal resonance in talker's responses.

A key point in the above discussion is that as the listeners in Fletcher's experiment gained experience in judging nasality, and as the listening tasks demanded greater judgmental precision, interjudgmental agreement increased systematically. The judgmental scores also moved systematically toward the instrumental measures. In light of the many factors that influence listener nasality judgments, the final correlation of 0.91 between nasality and nasalance scores suggests that for most purposes the instrumental measures may be used as a valid estimate of the degree of nasality likely to be derived from pooled observations from listener judges.

FACTORS RELATED TO NASALANCE IN IN CLEFT PALATE SPEECH

For the most part, attention has been given to velopharyngeal valving as the primary factor of speech disability in cleft palate talkers. This has obscured the role of other factors such as coordination between articulation and velopharyngeal valving actions, patency of nasal passageways, and extent of physical damage in the early developmental processes as contributers to speech disabilities. In an effort to overcome that limitation, Fletcher [10] used a maximum R^2 multivariate statistical modeling routine with nasalance as a dependent variable to extract a set of measures from a potential pool of 103 items that could provide a broader base for interpreting malfunctions related to disturbed nasal resonance in speech. The nasalance scores were from recorded utterances of the Zoo Passage by 70 child talkers who ranged from 6 to 13 years old with a mean age of 9.8. They had varying degrees of velopharyngeal competency following primary cleft palate surgery at around 19 months of age.

The degree of velopharyngeal closure during cephalometrically observed production of the /i/

and /a/ vowels emerged as the most important factor in Fletcher's multivariate analysis. Those who achieved "firm" closure had normal nasalance; those with "touch contact" (i.e., less than 5 mm contact between the soft palate and the pharyngeal wall) had borderline normal nasalance; those with "near approximation" (0–2 mm velopharyngeal gap) were abnormally nasalant; and those with velopharyngeal gaps greater than 2 mm were severely nasalant. The degree of velopharyngeal closure alone could account for only 30 percent of the variance in nasalance, however.

The second major variable that emerged in Fletcher's multifactorial model of nasalance was sex of the speaker. The mean nasalance of the 31 girls in the study was significantly lower than those for the boys. This paralleled higher speech articulation and intelligibility scores for girls.

The third major variable that emerged in Fletcher's multifactorial model was maximum rate at which the talkers could repeat polysyllable utterances (e.g., pata, taka, pata, pataka). Rapid syllable repetition tasks have traditionally been used as a measure of oral motor control. If a talker can execute a series of syllables rapidly and rhythmically, it is assumed that he or she has the physiological capability of producing the rapid, integrated sequences of articulatory movements demanded in speech (but see Kent, Kent, and Rosenbeck [16] for cautions in interpreting maximum performance speech production tests). Fletcher's model suggested that those with less skill in rapid syllable repetition were in fact less skillful, or less coordinated, in controlling both speech articulation and nasal versus oral resonance. Those with lower rates of syllable repetition also had lower speech articulation and intelligibility scores. In other words, higher nasalance scores were associated with poorer general oral motor control as well as higher nasality.

The acoustic affect of oral and nasal coupling was also influenced by other factors, such as the position of the tongue within the oral cavity For example, disadvantageous compensatory tongue-positioning and reduced jaw-opening during sound production can impede the flow of the soundstream through the oral cavity. These effects would be expected to be multiplied with the spread of the original congenital anomaly to encompass more and more structures. That is, the types of compensatory activities that a talker may use would be expected to increase with the extent and degree of anomalous malformation and malformations associated with the palatal cleft [7]. The

combination of 10 unique factors in Fletcher's final multidimensional model could account for 70 percent of the nasalance variance in the speech of the 23 talkers. Other factors, such as three-dimensional velopharyngeal valving characteristics and patency of the nasal chambers [13, 22], might be expected to contribute the remaining 30 percent of the variance. Being able to obtain stable, valid instrumental nasalance measures is an important step toward deeper understanding of fundamental anatomical and physiological properties that regulate or impinge on nasal resonance in speech.

As indicated earlier, the nasometer instrumental system differs substantially from the earlier Tonar system. This being so, a new set of normative data was needed. Data were drawn for this purpose from a group of 117 children enrolled in kindergarten through the fifth grades in a suburban Birmingham, Alabama public school. The children were 5 years, 7 months to 12 years, 8 months old at the time of the study. They averaged 8.5 years in age with a standard deviation of 1.8 years around that mean. All of the children had previously passed speech and hearing screening tests administered by the school speech pathologists and been judged to be normal in both respects.

To collect the nasalance data, the child was seated in a quiet office in the school. The sound separator assembly was placed on the head with the separator approximately parallel to the Frankfort plane. Care was taken to assure firm contact between the nostrils and the separator and sufficient space between them for the child to breathe easily through the nose.

The kindergarten and first-grade children repeated each set of stimuli as they were modeled by an examiner. All others read the passages aloud. The children were occasionally prompted on particular words. The Zoo Passage and the Rainbow Paragraph were produced once; the Nasal Sentences twice.

The responses were processed in real time by the Nasometer under control of an IBM XT computer. They were also stored on floppy disks. This resulted in three data files for each subject. Each of these files was later loaded into an IBM AT-compatible computer and reanalyzed utilizing the Nasometer software.

The mean scores from each set of data were subjected to a $2 \times 3 \times 8$ (sex $\times$ stimulus $\times$ age) multivariate analysis of variance to determine *if there were significant main effects or interactions.* This analysis revealed no significant age or sex effects

TABLE 14-1. NASOMETER MEASURES OF NASALANCE DURING PRODUCTION OF THE ZOO PASSAGE, THE RAINBOW PASSAGE, AND FIVE SENTENCES WITH A HIGH PROPORTION OF NASAL CONSONANTS BY 117 5- TO 12-YEAR-OLD NORMAL SPEAKING CHILDREN

	Mean Nasalance	SD
Zoo Passage	15.53	4.86
Rainbow Paragraph	35.69	5.20
Nasal Sentences	61.06	6.94

but a highly significant ($p<.01$) effect for the different stimulus materials. The means and standard deviations for these data are shown in Table 14-1 and portrayed graphically in Figure 14-3.

The mean nasalance score for the talkers during production of the Zoo Passage, which had no nasal consonants, was 15.5 $\pm$ 4.9 percent. During production of the Rainbow Paragraph the nasalance scores rose to 35.7 percent. Consistent with earlier findings with Tonar, this represented a doubling in the nasalance when the speakers moved from the Zoo Passage to the Rainbow paragraph, and a doubling again when the Nasal Sentences were produced.

TRANSPOSING SCORES FROM THE NASOMETER AND TONAR II

PHONETIC ATTRIBUTES OF NASALANCE

Many investigators have shown that the degree of nasal resonance in the speech of normal talkers varies systematically with the phonetic content of the utterance. Fletcher used the Zoo Passage [8, 10], the first paragraph of Fairbank's phonemically balanced Rainbow Paragraph, and a set of five sentences with a high proportion of nasal consonants to study the effects of phonetic content in connected speech on nasal resonance. In the 75-word Zoo Passage, all of the consonant and vowel sounds except the /m/, /n/, /ŋ/ nasal consonants appear in approximately the same proportion as in spoken English. The mean nasalance as this paragraph is spoken may therefore be used as an index of the usual balance between nasal and oral resonance when the phonetic content of the utterance does not dictate an open velopharyngeal valve. In earlier TONAR measures of speech from normal talkers the resultant scores were in the 5 to 15 percent range. In current Nasometer measures from normal production of the Zoo Passage, these scores range from 10 to 20 percent nasalance (see Fig. 14-3).

The Rainbow Paragraph was developed by Fairbanks to represent the typical phonetic content of the English language. All sounds are represented in proportion to their frequency in normal speech. Eleven percent of the phonetic elements are nasal consonants. The effect of these nasal consonants is not limited to the moment of their utterance, however. Rather, a co-articulatory "spread of nasalization" is found in which the nasal consonants are anticipated by opening of the velopharyngeal valve prior to the onset of the nasal element in the speech output. Kent, Carney, and Severeid [17] reported, for example, that a

Figure 14-3. Normative nasometer scores for school-age children.

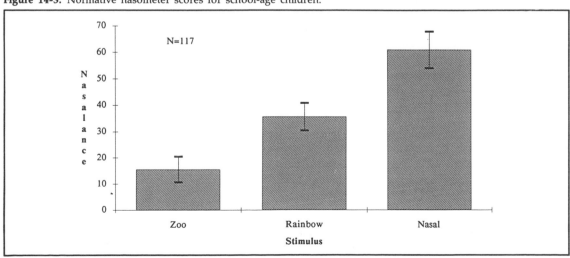

speaker they studied dropped the palate to its lowest point during production of the /a/ vowel preceding the nasal consonant when the word *contrast* was spoken. The palate was rising during production of the /n/ in anticipation of the upcoming /t/. The generalized effect of nasal consonants in the Rainbow Paragraph on the nasal-versus-oral acoustic ratio results in an average nasalance score of 36 ± 5 percent in current nasometric measures.

One of the common means of testing the intactness of a system is to stress the processes involved and observe the effect on performance. In measures of velopharyngeal sufficiency this may be done by choosing stimuli with an unusually high proportion of nasal consonants. The nasal sentences described by Fletcher [10] fit this requirement. Thirty-five percent of the phonetic elements in the five Nasal Sentences are nasal consonants. The mean nasalance for this type of material in current nasometric measurements from the child normative population was found to be 61 percent. Normal talkers producing sentences with an unusually high proportion of nasal consonants seem to follow different strategies. Some individuals continue to restrict the nasal resonance to the location of the nasal consonants in the material spoken. The graphic representation then shows sharp bursts of energy in the plot just at the time of nasal consonant production. Other talkers seem to indicate that the spoken material has a high proportion of nasal consonants by increasing the general level of nasalance throughout the utterance. They overlay the oral articulatory gestures onto a generally nasalized soundstream. The nasalance scores of this group tends to be somewhat higher than those of the first group.

PATTERNS OF NASALANCE

The nature of the measurement procedure dictates that the degree of nasalance in speech will be proportional to the acoustic energy of the signal as it exits from the nasal and oral chambers. This proportion is controlled by the physical characteristics of the oral and nasal chambers, the integrity of the velopharyngeal valve, postures of the lips and tongue, and by the phonetic demands of the sounds spoken. Each of these multidimensional factors influences the graphic pattern of nasalance.

One of the characteristics of speech by persons with excessive nasalance is a lower degree of association between the phonetic content of an utterance and the nasalance in their speech. This was particularly evident in a comparison of mean nasalance in the speech of talkers with repaired palatal clefts by Fletcher [10]. A mean score of 17 percent was found during production of an isolated /a/ vowel, 23 percent during the Zoo Passage, 36 percent during the Rainbow Paragraph, and 48 percent during the Nasal Sentences. This compares with 5 percent, 8 percent, 19 percent, and 36 percent nasalance during production of the same materials by their normative peers. It may be seen that the differences between the groups lessened with changes in the phonetic content of the utterances.

The degree of nasalance in speech is also directly related to the auditory acuity and general motor skills of the talker as well as the intactness of the speech mechanism, the physiological integrity of the motor system, the positions of the articulators during speech production, and the relative energy a talker is willing or able to expend in speaking. The importance of auditory monitoring in controlling the degree of nasal resonance in speech has been shown in studies of hearing-impaired talkers. Children with severe-to-profound hearing impairment have had nasalance scores greater than 2 SDs above the mean of the normative group of talkers. Plots of the nasalance in their speech showed frequent spikes of nasalance during normally nonnasalized periods of speech production, and occasional prolonged bursts of nasalance not associated with the presence of nasal consonants. Neither of these phenomena are found in the responses of the normal subjects.

Mentally retarded children also show erratic changes in nasal resonance [11]. In this instance, the variations seem to reflect less awareness of nasal resonance in their speech and perhaps reduced motor control in articulator positioning and velopharyngeal valving.

Persons with velopharyngeal insufficiency from structural impairments, such as palatal clefts, show yet a different pattern. Those with marginal ability to achieve velopharyngeal closure are particularly challenging. They may produce speech that is essentially normal by effortfully monitoring and controlling the nasality in their speech during therapy periods but be hypernasal in less controlled situations. The price they must pay in physical effort to achieve normal levels of nasal resonance in their speech may simply be too high to maintain in less demanding situations. This is particularly apparent during the early stages of speech therapy. In such instances, the nasalance will typically rise as the speaking context becomes less demanding or as the talker tires.

As the degree of velopharyngeal valving insufficiency rises, the peak nasalance levels and the mean nasalance score tend to rise concomitantly and systematically. This relationship can be used effectively in charting benefits from surgical or prosthetic intervention aimed at improving the potential for normal nasal resonance. Although sharp spikes of nasalance are occasionally found, prolonged bursts of nasalance which signal dramatic changes in velopharyngeal control are unusual in talkers with anatomical deficiencies of the velopharyngeal valving mechanism.

Fletcher, Sooudi, and Frost [12] presented data from 36 patients with hypernasality incident to congenital palatal insufficiency, acquired anatomical defects following surgery for neoplastic growths, and neurogenic disturbances that highlight the importance of previous speech experience. They charted changes in nasalance for each of the subjects. All except one patient, who had a neurological degenerative disease, showed significantly lower scores in response to the prosthetic assistance provided. They observed further that except in extreme cases with massive tissue removal, the patients with acquired anatomical defects regained essentially normal speech competency, either when they were fitted with the speech prosthesis or after a relatively short period of usage. Those with congenital velopharyngeal incompetencies, however, had no built-in reference to draw on for taking advantage of the prosthetic assistance. In this instance, the initial reduction in nasalance when the prosthesis was first used was often followed by a period of increased nasalance. In most instances this regression to higher nasalance was temporary, but in the responses of two of the 20 subjects it returned to essentially the preprosthesis level and remained there until an instrumental feedback and shaping program was instituted. The postprosthesis nasalance rise was interpreted as evidence of a highly habituated repertoire of physiological control that governs the degree of nasality in speech.

These talkers with many years of pathological speech experience had apparently circumvented the prosthesis and regained a perceptual feedback reference which included hypernasality. Lack of other descriptions of this relationship likely reflects the paucity of physical measurement in prosthetic management rather than the rarity of nasalance regression in the speech of individuals with congenital speech impairment. The patterns of the nasalance shown on a Nasogram, as well as changes across time, can thus provide rather subtle indices of underlying disturbance in perceptual monitoring, physical integrity of the mechanism, and present or potential motor control of the resonance system.

Nasalance may also be a sensitive indicator of the presence and progress of neuromuscular disease. An example of this relationship was described by Fletcher [11]. He produced data that showed a person with myasthenia gravis had essentially normal nasalance during a single production of the Zoo Passage. As the person was involved in continuous speaking, however, the neuromuscular strain on velopharyngeal valving became evident. The graphic displays of nasalance first showed an increased number of sharp bursts in nasal resonance, then more prolonged periods of nasal escape, and finally heightened nasalance throughout the response. A history of variable nasality should be carefully noted as possible evidence of underlying neurological disturbance. The presence of a congenital palatal cleft should not cause one to ignore other possible disturbances. Nasalance measures may provide meaningful information related to the presence, degree, and possible progression of parallel disorders when they are suspected.

NASAL RESONANCE REDUCTION

At least three fundamental questions must be answered when hypernasality is identified in speech.

1. Can the talker produce speech that is within normal or near-normal resonance limits?
2. Can nasal resonance be reduced by the talker without excessive physical effort?
3. Can reductions in nasal resonance be habitualized?

Each of these questions has direct clinical ramifications. None yields easy answers. Answers to the first question may be gleaned in part from examination of pretreatment nasograms. Plots of nasalance in utterances by normal speakers show time-varying changes that are generally in the 0 to 20 percent range. Only rarely do more than a few of the nasalance peaks exceed 25 percent nasalance levels.

The provision for rapid, accurate biometric feedback provides opportunity to probe the modifiability of nasalance systematically. Fletcher

[10] used this capability to examine the modifiability of nasal resonance in the speech of 19 talkers with hypernasality following childhood post–cleft palate surgery. Nasalance during production of the Zoo Passage was used to establish the pretreatment baseline level of nasal resonance in the speech of these talkers. The stimuli used in the shaping routines progressed systematically from sentences with a phonetic content that places comparatively little demand on velopharyngeal closure (approximant consonants with low vowels) to a phonetic content with stringent phonetic demands (sibilant consonants with high vowels). Each subject received 13 treatment sessions. The materials used in the training varied somewhat according to the needs of the particular subject.

The results obtained in Fletcher's biometric nasalance management study were found to vary considerably from subject to subject. Certain common learning patterns were identified, however. One group of eight subjects with pretreatment Zoo Passage mean nasalance scores of 27 ± 5 percent showed rapid reduction of nasalance on all sets of stimulus materials and maintenance of the performance attained. This finding suggests that a substantial number of individuals with hypernasality have the potential for achieving essentially normal nasal resonance through use of systematic, biometric monitoring and shaping routines alone.

A second group of five subjects in Fletcher's study had pretreatment mean nasalance scores of 28 ± 5 percent. This group showed rapid nasalance reduction to within normal limits for one of the sets of stimulus sentences but not the others. Their nasalance rose higher when the more demanding stimuli were introduced, and failed to descend to the normal nasalance range when the feedback and shaping program was applied. They also evidenced less ability than those in the first group to maintain the degree of nasalance control achieved. It was uncertain whether these subjects could eventually attain normal nasality in their speech without additional surgical or prosthetic assistance.

The third group of four subjects had a mean nasalance score of 52 ± 10 percent, and the final subject had a nasalance score of 37 percent. These five individuals showed erratic performance in their efforts to reduce the nasal resonance and poor maintenance of the reductions attained. These findings suggest that individuals with Tonar II nasalance scores above about 35 percent would

be unlikely to achieve normal nasal resonance without additional physical management such as secondary surgery or a prosthesis. This cutoff score should be viewed as predictive, not prescriptive, however. Other measures would be needed to confirm an assumed physical inability to achieve normal nasal resonance in speech.

REFERENCES

1. Andrews, J. R. A study of the contribution of nasally emitted sound to the perception of nasality. Presented at the Annual Meeting of the American Speech and Hearing Association, Chicago, 1967.
2. Bradford, J. L., Brooks, A. R., and Shelton, R. L., Jr. Clinical judgments of hypernasality in cleft palate children. Cleft Palate J. 1:329–335, 1964.
3. Counihan, D. T., and Cullinan, W. L. Reliability and dispersion of nasality ratings. Cleft Palate J. 7:261–270, 1970.
4. Dalson, R. M., and Warren, D. W. Comparison of Tonar II, pressure-flow, and listener judgments of hypernasality in the assessment of velopharyngeal function. Cleft Palate J. 23:108–115, 1986.
5. Ferguson, C. A. Assumptions about Nasals: A Sample Study in Phonological Universals. In J. H. Greenberg (Ed.), Universals of Language. Cambridge, Mass.: M.I.T. Press, 1963. Pp. 53–60.
6. Fletcher, S. G. Hypernasal voice as an indication of regional growth and developmental disturbances. Logos 3:3–12, 1960.
7. Fletcher, S. G. Cleft palate: A broader view. J. Speech Hear. Disord. 31:3–13, 1966.
8. Fletcher, S. G. Contingencies for bioelectric modification of nasality. J. Speech Hear. Disord. 37:329–346, 1972.
9. Fletcher, S. G. "Nasalance" vs. listener judgments of nasality. Cleft Palate J. 13:31–44, 1976.
10. Fletcher, S. G. Oral-nasal resonance. In Diagnosing Speech Disorders from Cleft Palate. New York: Grune & Stratton, 1978. Pp. 92–157.
11. Fletcher, S. G., and Bishop, M. E. Measurement of nasality with Tonar. Cleft Palate J. 7:610–621, 1970.
12. Fletcher, S. G., Sooudi, Il, and Frost, S. D. Quantitative and graphic analysis of prosthetic treatment for "nasalance" in speech. J. Prosthet. Dent. 32:284–291, 1974.
13. Graber, T. M. Cited by Counihan, D. T. A clinical study of the speech efficiency and structural adequacy of operated adolescent and adult cleft palate persons. Dissertation, Northwestern University, Evanston, Ill., 1956.
14. Hattori, S., Yamamoto, K., and Fujimura, O. Nasalization of vowels in relation to nasals. J. Acoust. Soc. Am. 30:267–274, 1958.
15. House, A. S., and Stevens, K. N. Analog studies of the nasalization of vowels. J. Speech Hear. Disord. 21:218–232, 1956.
16. Kent, R. D., Kent, J. F., and Rosenbeck, J. C. Maximum performance tests of speech production. J. Speech Hear. Disord. 52:367–387, 1987.
17. Kent, R. D., Carney, P. J., and Severeid, L. R. Velar movements and timing: Evaluation of a model for binary control. J. Speech Hear. Res. 17:470–488, 1974.
18. Lindqvist, J., and Sundberg, J. Acoustic properties of the nasal tract. Speech Trans. Lab. Q. Rep. 1972. Pp. 13–17.

19. Maddieson, I. *Patterns of Sounds.* Cambridge: Cambridge University Press, 1984. Pp. 59–72, 130–132.
20. McDonald, E. T., and Koepp-Baker, H. K. Cleft palate speech: An integration of research and clinical observation. *J. Speech Hear. Disord.* 16:9–20, 1951.
21. Moser, H. M., Dreher, J. J., and Adler, S. Comparison of hyponasality, hypernasality, and normal voice quality on the intelligibility of two-digit numbers. *J. Acoust. Soc. Am.* 27:872–874, 1955.
22. Pruzansky, S. Description, classification, and analysis of unoperated clefts of the lip and palate. *Am. J. Orthod.* 39:590–611, 1953.
23. Schneider, E., and Shprintzen, R. J. A survey of speech pathologists: Current trends in the diagnosis and management of velopharyngeal insufficiency. *Cleft Palate J.* 17:249–253, 1980.
24. Warren, D. W., and Dubois, A. B. A pressure-flow technique for measuring velopharyngeal orifice area during continuous speech. *Cleft Palate J.* 1:52–71, 1964.
25. Watterson, T., and Emmanuel, F. Observed effects of velopharyngeal orifice size on vowel identification and vowel nasality. *Cleft Palate J.* 18:271–285, 1981.

CHAPTER 15

Acoustic Analysis of Velopharyngeal Dysfunction in Speech

Raymond D. Kent
Julie M. Liss
Betty Jane Philips

Speech is a fleeting event. Just milliseconds after a word is uttered it is gone. Researchers and clinicians strive to capture the speech signal so that it may be examined. Those who work with individuals with cleft palate often seek to derive specific information about the speech signal. Is it hypernasal? How pervasive is the hypernasality? Are there other articulatory manifestations of velopharyngeal dysfunction such as nasal snorts? And is the infant with cleft palate developing speech sounds normally in spite of the orofacial defect?

Techniques used to address these issues include aerodynamic measures, radiography, accelerometry, fiberoptics, and acoustic analysis. Each of these techniques offers clues. None is sufficient in itself to give a full description of resonance, articulatory accuracy, or velopharyngeal function for speech.

Studies in recent years have evaluated the potential utility of acoustic analysis of nasality and cleft palate speech [1–4, 6, 8]. In spite of varied interpretations, this body of literature indicates that spectrographic analysis does reveal a fairly consistent set of acoustic characteristics associated with nasality, hypernasality, and articulatory manifestations of velopharyngeal incompetency. This chapter addresses the diagnostic and clinical use of acoustic analysis with cleft palate speakers.

SOURCE-FILTER THEORY

Before we can adequately discuss the measurement and analysis of speech by acoustic methods,

it is essential to understand how the acoustic speech signal is produced. The most widely used theory for this purpose is the source-filter theory of speech production [2]. This theory proposes that the acoustic energy arising from a source (vibrating vocal folds) travels through the vocal tract. The vocal tract has a certain varying shape determined by the articulatory configuration, that is, the positions of the tongue, lips, jaw, pharynx, and palate at instants in time. The shape of the vocal tract determines which frequencies of the glottal source spectrum will be enhanced or resonated.

This property of the vocal tract is known as the *transfer function* or *filter*. Filter is a general term for any frequency-selective system. The filtered sound is then passed out of the mouth and into the atmosphere where it can be heard by a listener or sensed by a microphone.

SOURCE

The energy source for speech can be of three types: (1) voicing energy, or the puffs of air produced by vibrations of the vocal folds; (2) noise energy, or the aperiodic sound generated as air is forced through a narrow constriction; and (3) transient energy, or the short burst of energy produced when a stop consonant is released. A voiced vowel sound is an example of voicing energy; the fricative /s/ as in *see* is an example of noise energy, and the release burst of /t/ in *tea* is an example of transient energy.

These three sound sources provide the acoustic energy that is shaped into the recognizable sounds of speech by filtering or resonance. For the sake of brevity, we will take voicing energy for vowel production as the main example in this discussion.

FILTER

The vocal tract, formed of the pharyngeal, oral, and nasal cavities, is a resonant system. This means that the vocal tract will resonate to applied sound energy at certain frequencies. The resonant frequencies of the vocal tract are called *formants*. There are theoretically an infinite number of formants in vowel production, but only the first three are necessary for recognition of a particular vowel. These first three formants, abbreviated F1, F2, and F3, constitute the *filter function* (or *transfer function*) of the vocal tract. That is, the filter function represents the combined effect of the primary formants (F1, F2, and F3 for present purposes).

These three formants are sometimes called the main vowel formants. Typically, F1 is the most intense formant (it contains the largest amount of acoustic energy) and it therefore determines the perceived loudness of most vowels. The frequency of F1 relates primarily to the height of the tongue. F1 frequency is low for vowels with a high tongue position, like /i/ in *heat* or /u/ in *new*, and F1 frequency is high for vowels with a low tongue position, like /æ/ in *hat*.

The frequency of F2 is determined mostly by the position of the tongue in the front-back dimensions. Back vowels like /u/ in *who*, have a low F2 frequency. Front vowels, like /i/ in *he*, have a high F2 frequency.

The frequency of F3 varies in a more complex fashion with vowel articulation related to adjacent consonants. It is sufficient for the purposes of this chapter to note that (a) F3 frequency tends to be low for lip-rounded vowels, like the vowel in *boot*, and for vowels with /r/-coloring, like the vowel in *bird*, and (b) F2 is high and close to F3 for front vowels.

However, the nasal cavity also is a resonant system. When this cavity is coupled to the pharyngeal-oral cavities by velopharyngeal opening, the resonant properties of the nasal cavity are added to the resonant properties of the pharyngeal-oral cavities. The coupling of cavities is illustrated in Figure 15-1. The result of this coupling is a nasalized vowel. The filter function for a nasalized vowel is more complicated than for an oral (non-

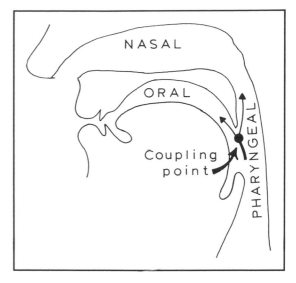

Figure 15-1. Vocal tract showing the possibility of coupling of the oral and nasal cavities. The circle represents the coupling point.

nasalized) vowel because the nasalized vowel has a filter function composed of:

1. The formants of the pharyngeal-oral cavities involved in oral vowel production.
2. The formants of the pharyngeal-nasal cavities which form a resonating tube extending from the larynx to the nares.
3. Antiformants (or antiresonances) produced by the bifurcation or division of the vocal tract into oral and nasal branches. Antiformants are essentially opposite in effect to formants and reduce the transmission of acoustic energy in affected frequencies. Nasalized vowels are further reduced in energy compared to oral vowels by the sound-absorbing properties of the nasal cavities. The sound absorption, technically called *damping*, results from the convoluted and highly vascularized mucous passages of the nose.

THE SPECTROGRAM

Because the acoustic signal of speech changes almost continuously with time, it is desirable to have a visual display that shows these time-related changes. The standard display for this purpose is the *spectrogram*. This is a three-dimensional display in which changes in the speech signal are shown for time, frequency, and intensity.

Figure 15-2 depicts these dimensions of the spectrogram and shows spectra for two time points in the spectrogram. On the spectrogram, time is represented on the horizontal axis, frequency on the vertical axis. The intensity is represented on the gray scale (variations in blackness). With the spectrogram, any acoustic signal can be visualized as a pattern in time, frequency, and intensity. The spectrum shows an intensity by frequency analysis for a selected point in time. Figure 15-2 illustrates spectra for two time points: the midpoint of a vowel (a) and the midpoint of a fricative (b).

Spectrograms are shown in Figure 15-3 for some major classes of speech sounds. Vowels appear as horizontal bands of energy corresponding to the formants. The center of each band is the formant frequency, and the width or thickness of each band reflects the formant bandwidth. Fricatives (Fig. 15-4) are represented as diffuse noise energy that has a random "salt and pepper" appearance. The exact distribution of this noise energy over frequency depends on the particular fricative under study. For example, the noise energy for the /s/ as in *see* is higher in frequency than the energy for /ʃ/ in *she*.

Glides (Fig. 15-5) are seen as bands that bend or curve in frequency. These bends, called *formant transitions*, are produced as the vocal tract changes in shape. The changes in shape are reflected as changes in formant pattern. In general, whenever the vocal tract changes in shape, the resonances or formants also change. *Stops* (Fig. 15-6) are a sequence of acoustic events including (1) a stop gap, or silent interval corresponding to articulatory closure for the stop; (2) burst, or brief explosion of noise that occurs as the articulatory closure is released; and (3) formant transitions, or changes in the formant frequencies that reflect changes in vocal tract shape as the stop is followed by another sound, especially a vowel.

Spectrograms reveal many speech characteristics. However, the appearance of these characteristics can vary with the analyzing bandwidth that is selected to make the spectrogram. Conventionally, the analyzing bandwidths are 300 Hz (*wide band*) and 45 Hz (*narrow band*). The wide-band analysis is better suited to show brief acoustic events, like stop bursts, or to show formant patterns. The narrow-band analysis is preferred for

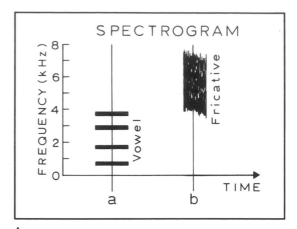

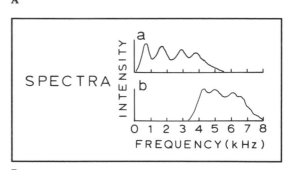

Figure 15-2. A. The three dimensions of a spectrogram — time, frequency, and intensity. B. Two spectra (intensity by frequency analysis) are shown for time points in a vowel and a fricative.

applications requiring a finer frequency resolution, such as the depiction of laryngeal harmonics. There is no single analyzing bandwidth that is ideal for all speakers. Unfortunately, the 300-Hz bandwidth that is generally satisfactory for men's voices does not always work well for women's and children's voices. As a rule of thumb, the wideband analyzing filter should be 2 to 3 times the vocal fundamental frequency.

Wide-band and narrow-band spectrograms are two different ways of representing a particular speech utterance. For example, Figure 15-7 shows a wide-band (top) and narrow-band (bottom) spectrogram of a vowellike babble of an infant. The formants are marked by the labeled arrowheads in the wide-band spectrogram. Formants appear in the narrow-band spectrogram as a strengthening or reinforcement of certain harmonics. In the first vowel segment, the harmonics in the vicinity for the first formant (F1) are the fifth and sixth harmonics. When the fundamental

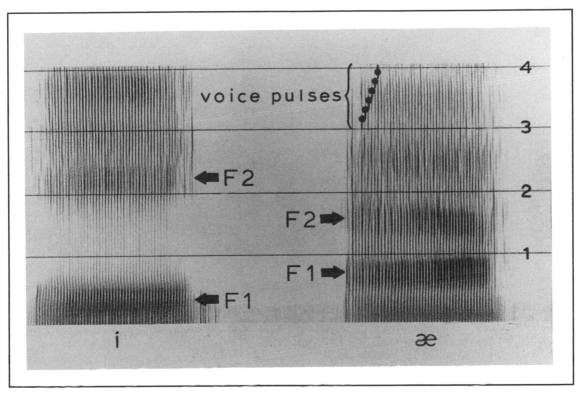

Figure 15-3. Sample spectrogram of vowels. The sounds shown are /i/ (*heat*) and /æ/ (*hat*).

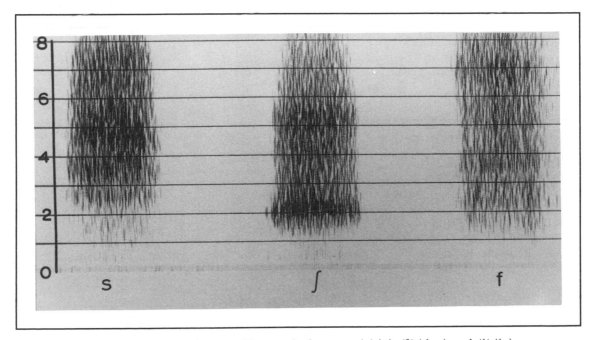

Figure 15-4. Sample spectrogram of fricatives. The sounds shown are /s/ (*so*), /ʃ/ (*show*), and /f/ (*foe*).

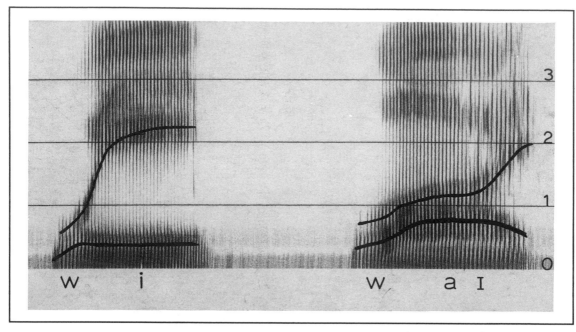

Figure 15-5. Sample spectrogram of glides. The glides are /w/ as in *we,* /wi/, and /wɑɪ/, pronounced *why.* Note the gliding formant movements for /w/.

frequency is higher than about 75 Hz, vocal fold vibration is represented on the wide-band spectrogram as finely spaced vertical striations and in the narrow-band spectrogram as horizontal bands. However, when the fundamental frequency falls below 75 Hz, vocal fold vibration tends to appear as vertical striations in both the wide-band and narrow-band spectrograms. The interval labeled *C.V.* is creaky voice or laryngealized phonation.

THE ACOUSTICS OF NASALIZATION

The individual with velopharyngeal dysfunction cannot either adequately or consistently close the velopharyngeal port during speech. Therefore sound energy directed orally escapes through the nasal cavity. When too much of the energy travels through the nasal passage, listeners perceive the speech as hypernasal. The degree of oral or nasal resonance in speech can be gauged by acoustic analyses. The following section considers some possibilities for such analysis.

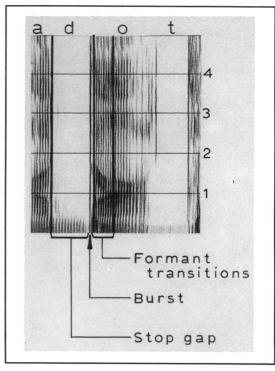

Figure 15-6. Sample spectrogram of a stop consonant, /d/, as in the phrase *a dot.* The acoustic sequence contains (1) a stop gap or silent interval, (2) release burst, and (3) formant transitions.

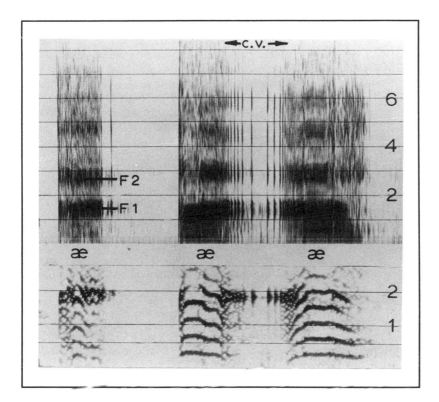

Figure 15-7. Wide-band and narrow-band spectrograms of an infant's babble. The first two formants, F1 and F2, are labeled and an interval of "creaky voice" is marked as *c.v.*

The acoustic effects of nasalization vary somewhat across speakers, across phonetic contexts, and with the sound that is under examination. In addition, these effects are not easily quantified with conventional analyses such as spectrograms. Despite these difficulties, the primary acoustic correlates of nasalization can be described fairly simply. One way to understand nasalization is in terms of phonetic and acoustic contrasts, for example, a nonnasal vowel versus a nasal consonant, an oral (nonnasalized) vowel versus a nasalized vowel, and a stop consonant versus a nasal consonant.

The contrast of nonnasal vowel versus a nasal consonant is shown in Figure 15-8. The spectrum for the vowel has several peaks, or formants. The spectrum of the nasal consonant /m/ also has several peaks but only the lowest of these (the *nasal formant*) has an amplitude that rivals that of the vowel formants. All of the higher spectral peaks for /m/ are substantially lower (weaker) than the spectral peaks for the vowel. In other

words, the nasal consonant has a dominant low-frequency resonance whereas the vowel has several strong resonances. It follows, then, that non-nasal vowels are typically more intense (therefore louder) than nasal consonants but that the energy of the two sounds is nearly equivalent in the low frequencies.

The acoustic contrast between an oral and nasal vowel is depicted in Figure 15-9. Both the oral vowel and nasal vowel have several spectral peaks, but the peaks for the nasal vowel are broader and lower in amplitude. In particular, F1 for the nasal vowel is less prominent than for the oral vowel and is surrounded by shallow valleys [7]. The effect is that the F1 region for the nasal vowel is less intense and flatter. These effects reflect the greater damping (absorption of energy) for the nasal vowel and the addition of nasal formants and antiformants.

Another fairly consistent consequence of vowel nasalization is a raising of the F1 frequency. The nasal vowel typically has a low-frequency resonance (the nasal formant) below F1. The other formants and antiformants attributable to nasalization are not as consistent in their appearance as the preceding characteristics, but they can be important indicators of nasalization.

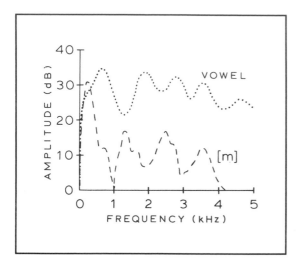

Figure 15-8. Spectra for a nonnasal vowel and the nasal consonant /m/. Note the reduced amplitude for /m/ compared to the vowel, except in the very low frequency region.

Figure 15-10A and B illustrates the acoustic contrast between a stop consonant and a nasal consonant in the syllable-initial position. The release of the stop is marked spectrographically by a transient called the burst (b), which is followed by the interval of formant transition (t). As the formant frequencies of the vowel are assumed, the formant pattern stabilizes in a steady-state (ss) interval. The nasal consonant does not have a release burst but rather a nasal murmur (m) segment of at least 40 msec duration. The murmur is followed by formant transitions (t) that are highly similar to those of a stop consonant with the same place of articulation. The formant transition interval is followed by the vowel steady state (ss).

Perceptual experiments indicate that the identification of nasal consonants involves an integration of two acoustic cues: the *nasal murmur* and the *formant transitions*. A distinct nasal consonant has a murmur of adequate duration and a set of formant transitions into or out of the adjacent sounds. A distinct stop consonant in syllable-initial position has a release burst and a set of formant transitions. If the intended stop is nasalized, the interval of oral closure may sound like a nasal murmur as acoustic energy travels through the nasal cavity. Some individuals with severe velopharyngeal dysfunction lose the stop-nasal contrast such that /b/ sounds like /m/, /d/ like /n/, and /g/ like /ŋ/.

EFFECTS OF VELOPHARYNGEAL DYSFUNCTION

The primary effects of nasalization are summarized in Table 15-1 for major sound classes and for common strategies that a speaker might use to reduce nasalization. The table lists the perceptual and acoustic effects of nasalization and also describes the anatomical and physiological correlates of these effects.

Figure 15-9. Spectral (amplitude by frequency analysis) for a nonnasal /a/and its nasal counterpart /ã/. Note the flattening of the spectrum in the F1 region of the nasal vowel.

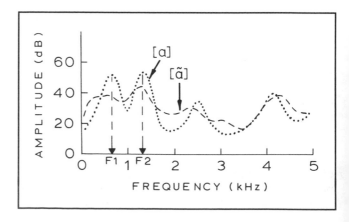

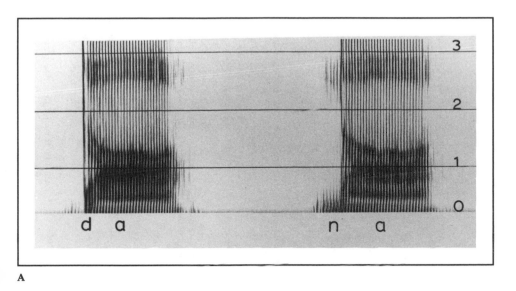

A

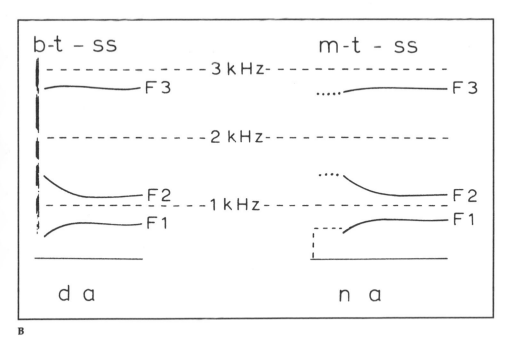

B

Figure 15-10. A. Spectrogram of an oral consonant /d/ and a nasal consonant /n/ in the nonsense syllables /da/ and /na/. B. Stylized version of *A* showing the principal acoustic features of the stop-nasal contrast.

TABLE 15-1. EFFECTS OF VELOPHARYNGEAL DYSFUNCTION

Sound class	Perceptual effects	Acoustic effects	Anatomical-physiological correlates
Vowels and glides	Resonance imbalance may be perceptible —"talking through one's nose" Nasalized vowels may be less contrastive than nonnasal vowels In VP-disordered speakers, the high vowels tend to sound more nasal than the low vowels ("reed" vs. "rod")	In a spectrogram, the following cues of nasalization may be noted: (1) Increase in formant bandwidth—formant energy appears broader or more diffuse (2) Decrease in overall energy (3) Introduction of low-frequency nasal formant F_N around 250–500 Hz (below F_1) for adult males (4) Slight raising of F_1 frequency with slight lowering of F_2 and F_3 frequencies (5) The presence of one or more antiresonances The nasalized vowel or glide looks weaker and more diffuse than its nonnasal counterpart, with low frequency being more intense	For vowels adjacent to nasal consonants the VP port does not close, thereby "nasalizing" the vowel. In VP-disordered speech, the VP port may remain open for vowels regardless of context The tongue is high in the oral cavity for high vowels. This may obstruct air flow and direct it to the path of least resistance into the nasal cavity
Obstruents	Normally obstruents are produced by closing off the nasal cavity so that air flow is directed through the oral cavity In the disordered speaker who can't close off the nasal cavity sufficiently: (1) Stops may sound like their nasal cognates ("bad" may sound like "man") (2) Voiceless sounds may be perceived as voiced ("ta" like "da") (3) Nasal snorts, nasal emission may occur	In severe hypernasality, there may be little or no energy above 1 kHz. However, when the disordered speaker can achieve or approximate velopharyngeal closure intermittently, the acoustic cues include: (1) Weak or absent F_2 (2) Strong low-frequency resonance (3) Weak formats at high frequencies (4) Broad bandwidths (5) The presence of one or more antiresonances Nasalized stop gaps Evidence of voicing during voiceless obstruent segments Noise energy superimposed on the spectrum	Normally for stops, fricatives and affricates the VP port closes completely allowing air flow to pass only orally. Then the oral cavity offers some obstruction (either complete closure as in the stop or partial as in the fricative) to the air flow. When the VP port does not close sufficiently, it prevents the speaker from impounding enough oral pressure to produce the sound The open VP port allows air flow meant for oral passage into the nasal cavity Nasal air escape during articulatory closure affects the suppression of voicing Air flow through the nose generates noise

(4) May evidence compensatory articulation or strategies to decrease hypernasality		
(a) Increase or decrease pitch	As fundamental frequency F_0 increases so does the perception of pitch	F_0 corresponds to the rate of vibration of the vocal folds
(b) Increase or decrease in loudness	The darker the gray scale on the spectrogram, the more intense the signal	With increasing vocal effort (loudness), the subglottal air pressure and average air flow increase
(c) Alter place of articulation for stops, fricatives, and affricates	Spikes or transients represent glottal stops; spirantization corresponds to weak closure or articulatory contact; an unexpected F_2 locus may be evidence of unusual place of articulation	Compensatory place of articulation for stops including glottis, pharynx, palate; and for fricatives, the glottis, pharynx, velum, palate
(d) Omission of consonants	Silence or lengthening of adjacent segments	Omission of normal obstruction
(e) Adjust duration of spondees to provide important acoustic cues	Timing of articulation and voicing may not be similar to the normal population in terms of VOT and durations of segments, transitions, etc.	The disordered speaker may develop timing and movement strategies to accommodate abnormal structure and function.

Key: VP = velopharyngeal; VOT = voice onset time.

A spectrographic comparison of normal speech and velopharyngeally incompetent speech is given by Figures 15-11A and B and 15-12. Figure 15-11A and B shows spectrograms of a normal speaker's production of the sentence *Mama made apple jam*. The actual spectrogram is shown in Figure 15-11A. A stylized spectrogram in Figure 15-11B is shown to highlight the F1-F2 formant pattern, nasal murmur (labeled with the numeral 1), stop gap (labeled with the numeral 2), and frication noise (labeled with the numeral 3).

Wide-band and narrow-band spectrograms of the same sentence produced by a speaker with cleft palate (see Fig. 15-12) have much less acoustic contrast than that evident in the spectrogram of normal speech. The utterance in Figure 15-12 has pervasive nasalization (as shown by the nasal formant circled in the figure), weakened formant energy and poorly formed or missing stop gaps and frication intervals. The comparison of Figures

Figure 15-11. A. Spectrogram of the sentence *Mama made apple jam*, produced by a normal speaker. B. Stylized representation of A showing the F1 and F2 formant patterns, nasal murmur (1), stop gaps (2), and frication noise (3).

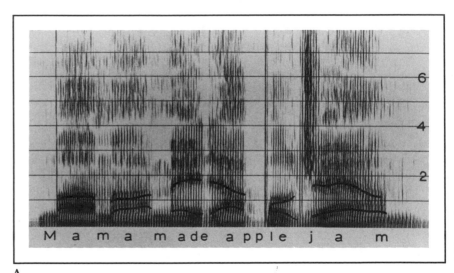

A

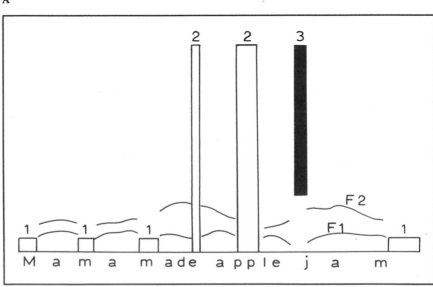

B

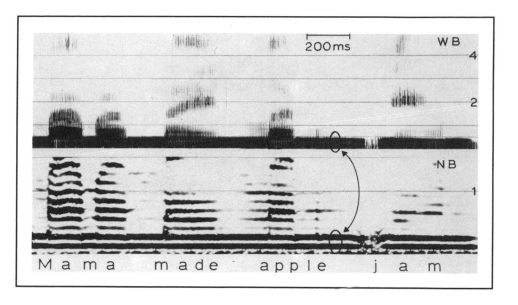

Figure 15-12. Spectrogram of the sentence *Mama made apple jam*, produced by a speaker with cleft palate, showing resulting velopharyngeal dysfunction. Compare with spectrogram of a normal speaker in Fig. 15-11. (Reprinted with permission from Philips, B. J., and Kent, R. D. Acoustic-Phonetic Descriptions of Speech Production in Speakers with Cleft Palate and Other Velopharyngeal Disorders. In N. J. Lass [Ed.], *Speech and Language: Advances in Basic Research and Practice*, Vol. II. New York: Academic Press, 1984.

15-11 and 15-12 indicates why velopharyngeal dysfunction can seriously impair speech intelligibility.

When nasalization occurs or when atypical articulatory productions are used, the temporal features of the phonemes and also the total phrase or sentence may be altered. Forner [3] reported that 5- and 6-year-old children with cleft palate demonstrate a significant increase in duration of both syllables and sentences as compared with noncleft children when nasal phonemes were present in the utterances. Figure 15–13 provides an illustration of the differences in duration for a phrase produced by a child, age 9, who had a surgically repaired cleft palate, and a noncleft adult. Discrepancies between the speech of an adult who has had a cleft palate and a noncleft adult may be subtle residual temporal and suprasegmental differences. Such characteristics are difficult to identify perceptually and difficult to remediate.

APPLICATIONS OF ACOUSTIC ANALYSIS

Acoustic analysis of the speech patterns used by speakers who have had palatal clefting adds significant information that enhances our understanding of the effects of velopharyngeal function. Spectrographic data extend the knowledge gained from perceptual and aerodynamic studies that demonstrate results of physiological response to disruption of velar function. As the study of the subtle effects of velopharyngeal incompetency on speech and the efficacy of management options is pursued, acoustic analysis will be a valuable tool for researchers.

Procedures for remediation of speech problems associated with cleft palate and velopharyngeal incompetency have received relatively little attention compared with those for evaluation of the speech disorders. Nor has there been much study of the effectiveness of remedial speech services. Acoustic phonetic analysis is a viable approach to the definition of remedial objectives and procedures, and offers a means of comparative analysis of speech before and after remediation. The usefulness of spectrographic study for "registration" of speech characteristics prior to initiation

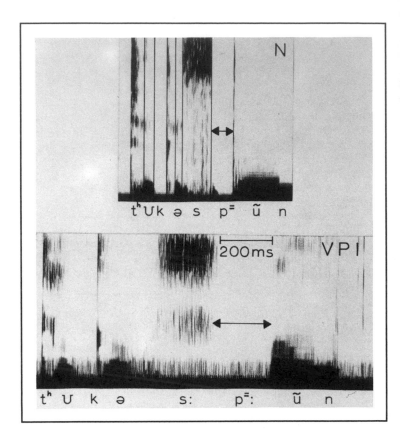

Figure 15-13. Spectrograms for the phrase *took a spoon,* produced by a normal adult woman (N) and a 9-year-old child with velopharyngeal dysfunction (VPI). Note that the child's production has a longer overall duration, a longer duration of /s/ frication, and a longer duration of closure for /p/. (Reprinted with permission from Philips, B. J., and Kent, R. D. Acoustic-Phonetic Descriptions of Speech Production in Speakers with Cleft Palate and Other Velopharyngeal Disorders. In N. J. Lass [Ed.], *Speech and Language: Advances in Basic Research and Practice,* Vol. II. New York: Academic Press, 1986.)

of speech pathology services as well as comparative studies of pre- and postremediation changes, have been described for diagnostic and therapeutic applications in this population at high risk for velopharyngeal function–related speech problems.

REFERENCES

1. Curtis, J. F. Acoustics of Speech Production and Nasalization. In D. C. Spriesterbach and D. Sherman (Eds.), *Cleft Palate and Communication.* New York: Academic Press, 1968.
2. Fant, C. G. M. *Acoustic Theory of Speech Production.* The Hague: Mouton, 1960.
3. Forner, L. Speech segment durations produced by 5 and 6 year old speakers with and without cleft palate. *Cleft Palate J.* 20:185, 1983.
4. Horii, Y., and Lang, J. C. Distributional analysis of an index of nasal coupling (HONC) in simulated nasality. *Cleft Palate J.* 18:279, 1982.
5. Philips, B. J., and Kent, R. D. Acoustic-Phonetic Descriptions of Speech Production in Speakers with Cleft Palate and Other Velopharyngeal Disorders. In N. J. Lass (Ed.), *Speech and Language: Advances in Basic Research.* New York: Academic Press, 1984. Vol. II.
6. Schwartz, M. Influence of utterance length upon bilabial closure duration for /p/. *J. Acoust. Soc. Am.* 51:666, 1972.
7. Stevens, K. N. Spectral prominences and phonetic distinctions in language. *Speech Commun.* 4:137, 1985.
8. Watterson, T., and Emanuel, F. Effects of oral-nasal coupling on whispered vowel spectra. *Cleft Palate J.* 18:24, 1982.

III.

HABILITATIVE AND REHABILITATIVE ASPECTS

CHAPTER 16

Rationale, Methods, and Techniques of Cleft Palate Speech Therapy

Kenneth R. Bzoch

An ounce of prevention is worth a pound of cure.
Anon.

RATIONALE

If it is important to correct the abnormal characteristics of cleft palate speech at some time in the lives of our patients, then it is even more important to do this before the scars of rejection or the feeling of abnormality and difference are formed in their developing personalities. A general criticism of cleft palate therapy, as still practiced in some communities today, is that (1) it is still too often made available too late in a child's life to be meaningfully effective; (2) the usual methods of speech therapists working on mastery of misarticulation by one sound element at a time are inappropriate for most of the error patterns of children and adults with cleft palates; and (3) postponing decisions for secondary surgical reconstruction of the palate over the critical years, or failing to refer for surgical correction when clinical evidence persists of an underlying problem of velopharyngeal insufficiency to support clear speech production, further diminish the efficacy of speech therapy for children born with clefts of the palate and related disorders.

It has always seemed to me that not all speech disorders are equally handicapping to the individuals we serve. Cleft palate speech with its several categorical differences from normal speech is very handicapping in the lives of these clients. However, hypernasal voice distortion, a gross sound substitution articulation error pattern with velar fricatives, lisping, a developmental dyslalia at 5 years of age, and articulation disorders limited to /w/for /r/ substitutions in speech do not each carry the same psychosocial stigma. The significance that a given type of speech disorder has to a particular person is also related to the person's age, sex, geographic environment, and socioeconomic status.

Suther [9] has presented some objective evidence that severely negative interpersonal attributes evidenced by low ratings on all dimensions of the Semantic Differential are associated with hypernasal voice distortions in comparison to hyponasality or to defective articulation with normal voice quality. Although further research is needed to verify the impression, it seems that of the 11 categories of cleft palate speech, the problems of (1) hypernasality, (2) gross substitution error patterns, and (3) delayed speech and language development are the most stigmatic of the speech disorders present in children born with cleft palates.

Effective means of focusing on the prevention or early correction of these serious problems have been developed and refined over the past 10 years. They are presented in this chapter along with actual case study examples of their application to different problems frequently managed by cleft palate teams. The remaining chapters in Part II cover the underlying oral sensory functions related to effective speech therapy, the techniques for guiding a pragmatic home language stimulation program of infants born with cleft palate, direct language stimulation management programs for infants and toddlers with cleft palate, and techniques tried and evaluated for palatal training procedures.

Although effective means are known, they are often not available in many communities. It would probably be accurate to state that a large percentage if not a majority of the infants born in the United States with clefts involving the soft palate still most often exhibit the stigma of cleft palate speech abnormalities throughout most of their important formative and early school-age years.

Only in an optimally effective cleft palate team program can treatment result in some 95 percent of all newborn infants obtaining speech patterns completely free of any categorical aspects of speech disorders. Counseling of parents on early language development from the earliest contact with each infant, a home speech and language stimulation program directed by a speech pathologist, and direct speech therapy made available for each child when indicated, as early as age 2 or 3 years, in a team approach with the plastic surgeons and dental specialists available *in each community*, appears to be necessary to reach this goal. Under such optimal treatment programs the speech and language of children with cleft palate can be made identical or even superior to that of their peers without cleft palate before school age (5–6 years) is reached. This optimistic goal of prevention and early total correction of speech disorders in a clinical population is not possible in other organic areas of speech pathology practice such as working with cerebral-palsied children. Empirical knowledge indicates today that this challenging goal is attainable in the preschool years for 95 out of 100 children born with cleft palate if certain conditions for treatment and functional training are met.

The *basic rationale* that has evolved through three decades of work with speech problems at cleft palate centers can be stated simply as follows: *To be maximally effective, speech therapy and language stimulation training, along with parental counseling, should be instituted in early infancy for each cleft palate child. Direct and individual therapy should be provided as indicated by clinical tests of developing speech and language behavior. Therapy should incorporate methods of training that are as directly related to the definable categories of speech abnormalities as possible, with techniques appropriate to the specific error patterns found, and to the age and personality of the patient.*

municative disorders were discussed in Chapters 1, 5, and 8. Chapter 1 reviewed the basic principles and scientific information regarding the abnormal anatomy, embryology, and congenital anomaly classification systems needed for understanding the presenting physical problems and for counseling parents as to the medical, surgical, dental, and behavioral treatments available to offset the otherwise severely handicapping sequelae presented by the birth of a child with a cleft of the primary or secondary palate structures. It included a set of recently approved statewide guidelines for the care and treatment of children born with cleft lip and palate with specific recommendations for speech and hearing services. Chapter 5 reviewed the causes, in addition to congenital velopharyngeal insufficiency, that are related to the frequent development of cleft palate speech disorders in this population. Chapter 8 reviewed the clinical tests and introduced the instrumental tests available today to measure the the several categorical aspects of cleft palate speech. The remainder of this book focuses on what you *can* do after you have evaluated cleft palate speech disorders; that is, the focus will be on speech therapy.

The oral sensory basis for changing speech behavior is covered in Chapter 17. Chapter 18 discusses how a speech clinician can guide the speech and language development of a cleft palate child in private practice related to cleft palate team management. A direct speech and language therapy program for cleft palate infants and toddlers is described in Chapter 19 and the potential success and limitations of therapeutic techniques directed toward correcting symptoms of velopharyngeal insufficiency are covered in Chapter 20.

CASE STUDIES — I.

METHODS

The basic methods for achieving prevention and early correction (effective management) of com-

Perhaps the juxtaposition of one early case study with later and then recent examples will best illustrate the reasons for the rationale and methods described earlier in this book and at the same time introduce and illustrate the techniques of speech and language therapy that have proved most effective with the special problems of children and adults with cleft palate speech disorders.

CASE 1 (1956)

A 56-year-old woman was referred to a cleft palate center with the major complaint of "a severe speech disorder." Medical history indicated that she was born with an isolated cleft involving the hard and soft palates only. The cleft had been surgically repaired at age 4 years. She had no pronounced dental or facial cosmetic problems or hearing difficulties. She was led to understand by the surgeon that nothing further could be done for her condition. She had therefore never before consulted a speech pathologist or been evaluated by a cleft palate team.

Her speech reportedly had always been severely distorted and characteristically "cleft palate speech." Examination by the cleft palate team indicated severe velopharyngeal insufficiency for normal speech production due to a scarred and immobile palate, with a mimimal gap of 1 cm between the soft palate and the pharyngeal wall at its nearest approximation from cephalometric studies during repeated pressure consonant syllables. Clinical tests indicated that her speech was distorted by hypernasality, by audible nasal emission on some pressure consonant sounds, and by an articulation error pattern of substitution of glottal stops for the majority of the bilabial and lingua-alveolar plosive and fricative consonant sounds. These sound elements were regularly produced as glottal stops or with glottal co-articulation accompanying labial and lingual articulation gestures.

Her velopharyngeal incompetency was successfully treated with a prosthetic speech appliance at that time. Speech intelligibility was somewhat improved, but her speech remained extremely abnormal and defective due to the strong glottal stop error pattern. She was an intelligent and gray-haired woman who had quit school in the sixth grade, reportedly because of teasing about her speech disorder. She had worked hard, later married, and developed a successful business which she managed. She raised two children through high school and in most ways appeared to be successful. When asked why, after 56 years of living, she still wanted to be completely rehabilitated, if this were possible, she said: "I'm happy. I'm married. I have two children and I've more or less accepted it. But yet, when you meet people, and you don't want people to look at you . . . people are cruel, people are mean, and I don't know why! When you live in a world where you might get along if people understand you and tried to help one another, and yet it's hard for people to be good and help one another, and I can't understand it. So I feel that if my speech could improve I could contribute not only to my family's well-being but also to myself. I would like to be like other people. I'd like to go to school. I haven't had much education."

She worked diligently each week over a period of 2 years to improve her speech habits. She made some improvements in the strongly habituated gross articulation error pattern, but she was never completely able to eliminate the years of habit of glottal articulation for sounds such as the /k/, /s/, and /z/ and their blends in her connected speech. She still lived with the stigma of cleft palate speech, when everything that could be done for her had been tried, and she was unable to continue further efforts at speech training. Her speech was no longer nasal. It was more correctly articulated. However, her speech pattern would still be identified as cleft palate speech. She resigned herself to being different due to the remaining problems, which were now limited to *strongly habituated* functional articulation disorders of speech.

DISCUSSION

The majority of school-aged and adult clients at a metropolitan cleft palate center with whom I worked at that time (1956) presented with voice and speech diagnostic findings similar to those of Case 1. Many had received up to 8 years of speech therapy in the public schools with limited success. Children and young adult patients who were diagnosed as having velopharyngeal insufficiency, making it impossible to support normal speech production, as in Case 1, could only have such problems corrected through carefully fitted prosthetic appliances [7] at a few specialized cleft palate centers. Later, such corrections became routine through an improved secondary surgical technique utilizing a carefully constructed, broad obturating epithelialized pharyngeal flap [1]. While both of these procedures eliminated the hypernasality, the nasal emission distortions of pressure consonant sounds, and the occasional accompanying nasal and facial grimacing problems, the physical management treatments were too late to have any effect on the other strongly habituated categories of defective cleft palate speech (i.e., the phonatory, resonance, and articulation compensations learned over many years).

This center's speech clinic program supported a year-round outpatient speech therapy service focused on eliminating these remaining "functional" problems. The experience of directing this clinic over a period of years led to the development of speech therapy techniques effective in changing cleft palate speech error patterns. However, the effectiveness of such programs was clearly related directly to the age of the client after adequate correction of the underlying problems of velopharyngeal insufficiency, dental abnormalities, and hearing. The number of hours of direct training required and the time required to reach acceptable or normal levels of speech production was directly correlated with the age of the client. Like the woman in Case 1, too many elementary school, high school, and young-adult patients were unable to invest enough time and effort to modify their gross sound substitution error patterns and related speech compensation habits to achieve levels of normal speech production. Similar problems, however, were usually successfully eliminated in 2 to 3 years of speech therapy for patients aged 4, 5, 6, and even 7 years, following correction of velopharyngeal incompetency. Marked improvement in the speech behavior of the younger patients was often achieved in less than 1 year.

Most of the older cleft palate patients had received up to 8 years of speech therapy in the public schools for similar error patterns with little improvement and obvious remaining stigmata of cleft palate speech. This seemed in part to be due to the delayed and isolated approach that was generally employed at that time. Speech therapists then worked mainly in public school programs and focused therapy goals at improving perceived levels of hypernasality and correcting articulation error patterns by working on only one speech sound element at a time. In our specialized clinic program, by developing speech therapy drills involving all sound elements similarly substituted for by glottal stops or pharyngeal fricatives (i.e., the entire gross substitution error pattern), we succeeded where previous attempts had failed. Case 2 describes the technique that was developed then and used since for the early correction of a developed gross sound substitution error pattern.

CASE 2 (1957)

Michael, a cooperative 4-year-old born with a left unilateral complete cleft of the primary and secondary palates, was seen for the first time in private practice in November 1957. His lip and nasal floor had been repaired at 5 weeks of age. His soft palate had been closed at 18 months of age. The remainder of the cleft of the hard palate was not closed until 36 months of age although a palatal obturator was repeatedly modified to provide velopharyngeal adequacy before final surgical reconstruction. Surgery had been delayed to prevent possible growth problems of the maxilla from "early surgery." Michael, who had just passed his fourth birthday, was an outgoing boy, and easy to test.

Table 16-1 shows the articulation test error pattern for the pressure consonants recorded at our first meeting, limited to the plosive and fricative sounds as they occurred in initial, medial, and final word positions. The responses reveal a strongly habituated pattern of substituting a glottal stop for almost all plosive or fricative sounds. However, the fact that the initial-position /p/ response was made correctly without nasal emission indicated that the child probably had adequate velopharyngeal function to support normal speech. This was confirmed by the articulation error pattern profile changes (shown in Table 16-2) recorded 3 weeks later following three speech therapy visits. The same articulation test was again administered at the start of his fourth weekly visit for a half-hour speech therapy lesson and resulted in the improved profile recorded in Table 16-2.

The three therapy lessons are described here to illustrate the general method called *multiple sound articulation training* which has been found to be effective for correcting a gross sound substitution error pattern. In general, the method is to teach directly and to quickly reinforce by home practice supervised by a parent or concerned family member the normal production of sets of four or more sound elements per lesson. This can be most often accomplished by using

TABLE 16-1. INITIAL ARTICULATION TEST ERROR PATTERN PROFILE OF PRESSURE CONSONANTS FOR CASE 2, A 4-YEAR OLD MALE WITH SURGICALLY RECONSTRUCTED CLEFT LIP AND PALATE AS DETERMINED ON 11/16/57

Test Sound	Test Response		
	Initial	Medial	Final
p	+[a]	G[b]	O
b	I m/b	I m/b	m/b
t	G	G	O
d	n/d	n/d	n/d
k	G	G	G
g	G	G	G
f	G	G	G
v	I b/v	I b/v	O
θ	G	G	G
ð	I n/ð	I n/ð	—
s	G	G	G
z	G	G	G
ʃ	G	G	G
tʃ	G	G	G
dʒ	G	G	G

[a] + = correct production
[b] G = glottal strop substitution /ʔ/.

TABLE 16-2. ARTICULATION TEST ERROR PATTERN PROFILE ON PRESSURE CONSONANTS FOR CASE 2 ON 12/21/57 AFTER FOUR SPEECH THERAPY LESSONS

Test Sound	Test Response		
	Initial	Medial	Final
p	+[a]	+	+
b	+	+	+
t	+	+	O
d	n/d	+	+
k	G[b]	G	G
g	G	G	G
f	+	+	+
v	b/v	I	f/v
θ	G	G	θ
ð	n/ð	I	—
s	G	G	G
z	ʃ/z	G	G
ʃ	+	G	+
tʃ	G	G	G
dʒ	G	G	G

[a] + = correct production.
[b] G = glottal stop production.

strong, direct, motor-kinesthetic, tactile, and visual cues for the correct rewarded production of target sound elements associated with their alphabetic letters in isolation. No "ear training" techniques are used initially. Techniques using the air paddle, feather-on-card, or feeling the egressive airstream on the back of the hand assure that the airstream is released at the glottis and impounded or constricted at the correct place of articulation. During initial practice on sounds in isolation and in nonsense syllable drills, the sounds are associated with alphabet letters. These are usually printed on 3 × 5-in. index cards and copied by the client for daily review during home practice exercises and games. The client's parents, siblings, and friends are shown how to supervise daily practice and participate in games and activities at home to reinforce what is taught by the therapist each week.

In Michael's case, the following techniques were employed during the first month: The /p/ sound element was taught by demonstration and imitation of first blowing down and then popping an air paddle, as described in Chapter 8, which was held up to the closed lips. The letter *P* was then printed on an index card. The sound, called the "pee sound," was demonstrated again. Michael's hand was guided to write a *P* on a second card. Both therapist and Michael then produced another pee sound 2 more times, printing two more *P* cards before going on to a second sound.

Next the /m/ sound was taught by the strong stimulus-response technique of humming loudly with lips closed and placing Michael's hand on the bridge of my nose to feel the vibration. Michael was then asked to produce the same sound and feel it with his hand on the bridge of his own nose. He did, and the letter *M* in capital form (looking like two mountain peaks) was written on an index card and called the "mmm sound" as in *mountain*. The same procedure as with /p was then followed until four cards with the letter *M* had been written. All eight cards were then shuffled and turned face down on the table. The top cards were turned over one at a time with the associated sound being produced by both therapist and client at each turn. The paddle was routinely placed at the lips and bent by the puff of air as each "good" pee sound was made. The bridge of the nose was routinely felt for each /m/ sound.

Next the /b/ sound element was introduced as the "noisy sister sound to /p/," using a strong stimulus-response method and a view of the air paddle at the lips in a mirror to assure prior glottal release. The capital letter *B* was written on an index card and the similarity to the closed lips at the initiation of /b/ was noted. The syllable /bə/ was shouted very loudly to initiate an imitation response. Four cards were prepared with the noisy sister sound /bə/ shouted each time by the therapist and then by Michael. All 12 cards were now shuffled and turned face down, then turned over one at a time and the sounds produced in isolation with their appropriate visual and tactile sensory cues of glottal release.

Next the /f/ sound was taught by placing the extended index finger over the lower lip, pressing the lower lip inward against the upper incisors with the jaw slightly opened, and blowing a sustained /f/ sound. Michael imitated the "wind sound," and the letter *F* was written on four cards, repeating the procedure as with the other isolated sound elements. Feeling the tickle of the airsteam on the hair of the back of the hand was the technique used to assure glottal release on the /f/ sound element. Only about 20 minutes had elapsed at this point during the first lesson.

The 16 cards were shuffled and the game "speech-sound canasta" was introduced. To play this game, two players take turns taking one card from the top of the deck, turning it over, and making the sound for the letter symbol found. The first to get three cards with the same letter wins. Michael's parents were brought in and shown how to play the game with the visual and tactile cues needed to assure glottal release of the airstream. They were asked to play the game at least 3 times each day and to return in 1 week. The therapy session was completed in a half-hour.

At the second session *key words* were introduced, initiated by each of the four sound elements taught in the first lesson. Next the /t/, /d/, and /s/ sounds were taught in isolation by techniques similar to those used with the /p/, /m/, /b/, and /f/ sounds. Four cards for each of the three new sounds were added to the canasta deck. The requirement for saying the key word following the sound in isolation for the first set of four elements was added. The parents were instructed in the expanded speech sound canasta game and asked to continue daily practice.

For the third lesson the seven sounds were reviewed again. Ten practice words each for the /p/ and /f/ and /b/ and /m/ were introduced and practiced. Single key words for /t/ and /d/ and /s/ were given. The /th/ and /v/ and /n/ were taught as new sounds in isolation and added to the canasta deck. Parents were taught how to play the expanded game using words for the first two sets of sounds. They were asked to start a scrapbook of magazine pictures, with two pages of illustrations of words for each of Michael's new sounds.

On the following week the sound articulation test profile (shown in Table 16-2) was recorded at the beginning of the lesson. A nonsense syllable drill was added that followed the vowel triangle initiated or closed off by the sounds taught in isolation and being practiced at home. The /k/, /g/, /v/, and /ʃ/ sounds were next taught in isolation. Four cards for each of this new set of four sounds were added to the speech-sound canasta game. Practice in phrasing in short sentence utterances with the words containing the first set of sounds taught was added the following week. Lessons were expanded to include all sounds previously involved in the gross sound substitution error pattern. Table 16-3 shows the articulation test–pressure consonant sound error pattern changes accomplished by January 1958. Table 16-4 shows the remaining limited pattern of occurrence of gross substitution errors in March 1958. The articulation test profile obtained in April 1958 and shown in Table 16-5 is actually somewhat superior to what one would expect of most of Michael's 4-year-old peers without clefts.

These changes in speech behavior were accomplished in only 5 months' time through 20 speech therapy lessons facilitated by daily practice at home. This method of therapy has since been used successfully for shaping the speech behavior of hundreds of children with cleft palate and similar problems of deviant speech behavior. The comparative effectiveness of the general method probably lies mainly in its approach of working to modify the entire underlying habit pattern of glottal and pharyngeal constrictions rather than a limited part of the error pattern evidenced by clinical articulation tests. If 4 or 5 months were

TABLE 16-3. ARTICULATION TEST ERROR PATTERN PROFILE ON PRESSURE CONSONANTS FOR CASE 2 ON 1/11/58

Test sound	Test Response		
	Initial	Medial	Final
p	+[a]	+	+
b	+	+	+
t	+	+	+
d	n/d	+	+
k	+	G[b]	+
g	k/g	+	+
f	+	+	+
v	m/v	+	+
θ	+	G	+
ð	+	+	—
s	+	G	t/s
z	j/z	G	d/z
ʃ	+	+	+
tʃ	ʃ/tʃ	G	G
dʒ	I	G	n/dʒ

[a] + = correct production.
[b] G = glottal stop substitution

TABLE 16-4. ARTICULATION TEST ERROR PATTERN PROFILE ON PRESSURE CONSONANTS FOR CASE 2 ON 3/8/58

Test sound	Test Response		
	Initial	Medial	Final
p	+[a]	+	+
b	+	+	+
t	+	+	+
d	+	+	+
k	+	G[b]	+
g	+	+	+
f	+	+	+
v	+	+	+
θ	+	+	+
ð	+	+	—
s	G	G	O
z	I	G	I d/z
ʃ	+	+	+
tʃ	+	+	+
dʒ	+	G	t/ʃ/dʒ

[a] + = correct production.
[b] G = glottal stop substitution

TABLE 16-5. ARTICULATION TEST ERROR PATTERN PROFILE ON PRESSURE CONSONANTS FOR CASE 2 ON 4/12/58

Test sound	Test Response		
	Initial	Medial	Final
p	+[a]	+	+
b	+	+	+
t	+	+	+
d	+	+	+
k	+	G[b]	+
g	+	+	k/g
f	+	+	+
v	+	+	+
θ	+	t/θ	+
ð	+	+	+
s	+	I	+
z	+	+	+
ʃ	+	+	+
tʃ	+	+	+
dʒ	+	+	+

[a] + = correct production.
[b] G = glottal stop substitution

spent at establishing rapport, ear training, and direct therapy for bringing only /p/, /b/, and /f/ articulations into running speech, the other glottal substitution errors would work against a basic change in speech behavior. The continuing glottal errors on the remaining sound elements would keep the gross substitution error pattern strongly entrenched in propositional speech.

CASE 3 (1967)

A 2-year-old boy was examined for the first time in the Communicative Disorders Division of the Teaching Hospital at the University of Florida. He had been referred by the family pediatrician and a plastic surgeon for recommendations regarding preschool speech and language development. As in Case 1, the congenital cleft involved only the hard and soft palate. He had been referred to the plastic surgeon at age 1. The child was followed for 1 year to see if palatal growth would develop sufficiently for a simple closure of the defect to suffice. The judgment of the surgeon was that there was a gross inadequacy of tissue. The primary closure was therefore not performed until 20 months of age and included a broad pharyngeal flap procedure.

The speech evaluation consultant's report, when the child was 2 years, 1 month old, included the following statements: "The patient was cooperative in testing. He displayed a beginning speech pattern indicating the early habituation of substitutions of glottal and pharyngeal constrictions in place of labial and lingual articulations in his speech efforts. Language development and estimated intelligence are about average as indicated by the findings on the Mecham Verbal Language Development Scale and by his ability to name words from picture stimuli, and by his ablity to name some words on the Peabody Picture Vocabulary Test, Form B correctly.

"All of the pressure consonant sounds which require the use of the palate were misarticulated due to the substitution of glottal stops and, more frequently, pharyngeal fricative sounds. Considerable time was spent with Mrs. J., who was an elementary school teacher, explaining principles of a home training program for the patient and demonstrating some methods and techniques for motivating him to produce sounds normally in isolation and to associate them with movements of air through the mouth or nose by the use of various games and devices. The mother will start him on a home training program beginning with blowing, speech sound stimulation and early word training activities." (A monthly appointment to check progress and train the mother in new techniques and methods for home training was scheduled.)

"Examination of the palatal area indicated a very healthy-looking, wide pharyngeal flap attachment. The patient demonstrated ability to impound interoral air pressure in blowing, in imitating a /p/ sound, and occasionally on producing a /b/ sound in words."

Prognosis was considered good for habituation of normal speech patterns in the preschool years and for maintenance of velopharyngeal adequacy.

The following month he received his first direct speech therapy lesson. After reviewing with his mother the progress in the home language stimulation program, which emphasized games for practice of producing pressure consonant articulations on /p/ and /b/ from blowing activities to sounds to words, the following observations and recommendations were made:

"S. demonstrated clear articulation of /b/ in words such as boy, big, and baby, with correct bilabial articulation, with release of pressure at the lips, indicated by air paddle and feather-on-card techniques, and without nasal escape or glottal constriction accompanying the production of these sounds in words."

He also demonstrated clear articulation on /p/ in initial and final word positions and on the /g/ and /k/ sounds in final word position. "Stimulation on fricative sounds was introduced after a review of plosives and blowing activities. This led to good imitation of a prolonged /f/ sound and to clear production of a sustained /ʃ/ in isolation and in the word show.

"The mother was directed to review daily practice of the sounds /b/, /p/, /g/, /f/, and /ʃ/, first in sounds, then with words, and then used in simplified shortened sentences. The patient is beginning to use more speech and sometimes talked in five- to ten-word utterances." The phonic card association method was used.

In a visit in April 1967, a review of all target sounds indicated they were correctly carried out, with the father observing techniques. Index cards, 3 × 5 in., were used, and letters representing the sounds practiced in the previous lesson were associated, mixed up, hidden, found, and produced in phonic association training techniques that were demonstrated to the father. The appointment in May was cancelled, so in June 1967, the mother attended the next speech stimulation session.

Again, direct speech therapy training techniques led to excellent imitation and initiation of clear articulation on several pressure consonant sounds. Rapport was excellent. The mother reported, however, that the family had to move to Miami unexpectedly. She was therefore given a picture drill book and instructions on reinforcement and carryover exercises to eliminate the glottal stop and pharyngeal fricative error substitution habit. These were no longer present in the practice sessions and occurred only occasionally in connected speech.

Referral was made by telephone and correspondence to another state cleft palate team program. The patient was seen again with both parents, following training in Miami, in December 1967, for a speech and language reevaluation. The report at this time indicated: "Velopharyngeal function for clear speech production following primary pharyngeal-flap procedure remains excellent. Home language training program and direct articulation therapy have already effected a complete reversal of the pharyngeal fricative and glottal stop articulation error pattern found at age 2."

Language development on the Mecham Verbal Language Scale was now approaching the 4-year-old level. Articulation mastery was essentially normal, with no remaining errors in single consonants in single words. Connected speech was intelligible and was not distorted. Sentence length was averaging five to six words. This appeared to be an excellent result. Recommendation to taper off therapy to occasional visits was made to the Miami cleft palate center program.

CASE 4 (1976)

A 2-year, 8-month-old white female without overt cleft palate but with intelligible, hypernasal speech was referred by the Children's Medical Services Division for initial evaluation studies and recommendations. The same five tests used in the cleft palate team clinic can be used for clinical speech evaluations of hypernasally distorted speech. Following complete administration of all five tests and using the standard recording form discussed in Chapter 8, these findings indicated that she most probably presented with congenital velopharyngeal insufficiency without overt cleft palate and therefore needed physical management, as in cases of overt clefts, before any benefit would be gained from speech therapy.

Her initial clinical study indicated that the glottal stop or pharyngeal fricative had been substituted for seven of the 30 test sound elements on the 30-element error pattern screening articulation test. Only the /m/, /n/, and /l/ were judged to be correctly produced. An /m/ or /n/ was substituted for the other 20 target speech sound elements. However, the nasal emission ratio, determined from 10 repeated /pi/ syllables after a period of diagnostic therapy, remained at a high 10/10 ratio, indicating probable consistent velopharyngeal incompetency. The clinical diagnosis based on these findings was clearly congenital velopharyngeal insufficiency. This was later confirmed by cinefluorographic x-ray studies. A palatal push-back combined with a pharyngeal flap operation was carried out in January 1977 to correct this basic physical problem. The patient was started on a direct speech therapy program 3 times a week in early April after some otological treatment and surgery were completed. She was 3 years, 5 months old before effective speech therapy could be undertaken.

The following excerpts from the speech and language clinician's notes in the medical record describe the form and content of the multiple-sound direct articulation therapy program that was carried out at that time:

4/11/77 — One hour of speech therapy. Reviewed the /p/ and /b/ sounds previously learned in diagnostic therapy. Taught the /f/ and /m/ in isolation and started on the speech-sound canasta game with these four elements. Grandfather to review daily at home..

4/8/77 — Practiced acquired sounds in isolation and in words. New sound /ʃ/ was introduced in isolation and tried in several words — successfully in *shoe*. Patient is highly stimulable.

4/11/77 — One hour of therapy today. Sound contrasts of /m/, /f/, and /s/ in word sequences. Faster word drilling on /b/, /p/, and today's /m/ and /f/ words. The /t/ sound was introduced quite successfully at syllable level.

4/13/77 — Client was introduced to /k/ sound element this morning. She could produce it inconsistently in isolation but should master it by the next session. Reviewing /s/, she was able to produce it in initial word positions. Same for /m/, /p/, /b/, /d/, and /t/. /f/ is still inconsistent.

4/15/77 — Client was introduced to the /t/ sound this morning. We also worked on the /k/ and /s/. She is still having difficulty with the /k/ sound. However, /m/, /p/, /b/, /t/, and /f/ are now consistent in isolation and words. Played speech sound canasta and also went through the pictures in her speech book.

4/27/77 — [After 4 other therapy sessions] She worked really hard today. We drilled /d/ in inital and final word positions and reviewed all other sound elements she was previously given. The sound elements /t/, /p/, and /b/ were stabilized initially and almost consistent in final position. This will be the next session's goal. Phrasing with /p/, and /b/, and /d/ words is also being drilled, using contrasting phonemes in each phrase.

5/13/77 — [After five more therapy sessions] She worked on endings again today and achieved the 85 percent criteria level for all sound elements. The /s/ is still unstable but she can produce it correctly after stimulation. She began using it in words such as *sea, saw, sing*, etc., with more consistency.

5/25/77 — [After four more lessons] She reviewed all pictured words in her speech book and phrased each one with "I see a . . ." and was very successful except on the /y/ words. The /k/ productions are still not fully stable, but well over the 80% level. She has overgeneralized it to some initial /t/ words, but self-corrects easily.

6/8/77 — After four more therapy sessions, this patient was reevaluated and found to have only occasional simple substitutions common for her chronological age group. There were no findings of any gross sound substitutions or omissions remaining on the complete Bzoch Error Pattern Diagnostic Articulation Test of 100 elements. Speech was already intelligible, nonnasal, and age-appropriate.

DISCUSSION

The last three case studies emphasize the contrast between earlier clinical experience and what could then be achieved in a coordinated cleft palate team approach to similar developmental problems with cleft palate patients. Approaching similar clinical problems such as the gross substitution error pattern at an opportune age has consistently proved to be more effective. Although cases were unusually successful and were completed about a year earlier than some others treated similarly, the experience has been repeated in over 200 similar cases with excellent results, with patients younger than 5 years of age.

Over the last 10 years of clinical practice, methods to prevent delayed language and avoid development of the cleft palate speech articulation disorders typical of the past have demonstrated that these problems can be prevented effectively as well as treated.

RECENT PREVENTIVE THERAPY TECHNIQUES

Since the introduction and use of the *REEL Scale* in 1971 it has been easier both to conduct and to study the effects of language stimulation training programs for infants with cleft palate. As reported in Chapter 8, initial scale studies on 25 consecutive cleft palate infants revealed a common pattern of lowered expressive language quotients of varying degrees for all. Whenever possible, a home language stimulation program was carried out. There was counseling, teaching, and directing of the parents in methods of language reinforcement training designed to elicit the responses that the child had failed to give on the expressive language items, or on which he had fallen below his chronological or receptive language age. The derived language quotients obtained over time allowed for the measurement of changes in language skills for individuals and groups with and without such language training programs.

Table 16-6 presents the findings of changes in language quotients for eight infants with cleft palate whose parents were enrolled in a parental counseling and direct language therapy training program. The program involved monthly visits to the clinic by one or both parents and child, with a careful review of home routines and the language items that should next emerge in the child's behavior.

It is apparent from Table 16-6 that the average delay in receptive language development and the greater delay in expressive language development found at the mean age of 19 months were

TABLE 16-6. MEAN LANGUAGE QUOTIENTS FOR EIGHT PATIENTS WITH CLEFT PALATE BEFORE AND AFTER PROGRAM OF PARENTAL COUNSELING AND DIRECT LANGUAGE THERAPY

Mean age	RLQ	ELQ	CLQ
19 mo. (before)	95	79	88
25 mo. (after)	110	103	107

Key: RLQ = receptive language quotient; ELQ = expressive language quotient; CLQ = combined language quotient.

TABLE 16-7. CASE STUDY (K.G., BORN 3/18/70) SHOWING CHANGES IN LANGUAGE QUOTIENTS OVER PERIOD OF DIRECT LANGUAGE THERAPY PROGRAM

Age (mo.)	RLQ	ELQ	CLQ
8	100	83	92
8	100	88	94
14	114	114	114
19	116	116	116

For abbreviations, see footnote, Table 16-6.

TABLE 16-8. CASE STUDY (L.H., BORN 12/14/69) SHOWING INCREASE IN LANGUAGE DELAY OVER PERIOD OF NO CONTACT OR THERAPY PROGRAM

Age (mo.)	RLQ	ELQ	CLQ
15	93	73	87
23	87	52	70

For abbreviations, see footnote, Table 16-6.

eliminated over an average 6-month period of language training for these eight infants with cleft palate.

Table 16-7 shows the changes in language quotients for K.G., enrolled at 6 months of age after a finding at a team clinic of a depressed expressive language quotient of 83. The table shows that by 19 months of age that quotient had risen to 116 and the receptive language quotient improved to the same level. At 19 months K.G.'s language skills were actually better than the average of her normal peers despite cleft lip and palate and chronic otitis media.

Table 16-8 shows a case study revealing the type of increase in delayed language development that is often found when no language intervention program is initiated. Note that even the receptive language quotient was significantly lowered by 23 months of age, due probably, in this case, to a severely deprived home environment.

Table 16-9 presents the more common pattern of increased delay in expressive language levels with essentially normal receptive language functions, the situation most frequently found when a parental counseling and language stimulation program cannot be carried out due to lack or inability of parental cooperation.

The general methods of procedure involved for correcting these problems require early counseling and education of parents for early direct or indirect articulation, vocabulary, and language stimulation through daily pragmatic language-mediated interactions at home. The material covered in the counseling and training sessions usually also includes the topics and types of information covered in the booklets *Bright Promise* [5], *Your Cleft Lip and Palate Child: A Basic Guide for Parents* [8], *Assessing Language Skills in Infancy* [4], and the newer parent information references listed in the Appendix to Chapter 4.

The actual techniques used by therapists vary. Some workers, like myself, prefer to focus on phonic association articulation developmental activities. Others work with more indirect articulation training through such techniques as those described by Dr. Hahn in Chapter 18 and by Dr. Scheuerle in Chapter 19.

The rationale, methods, and techniques discussed in this chapter are the model for a cleft palate center in a metropolitan area where excellent early medical and dental treatment are available. It must be recognized, however, that this is the ideal rather than the common situation for most clinicians and patients needing cleft palate therapy services. Only a small portion of today's cleft palate population are being treated in well-organized cleft palate and craniofacial team programs. The remainder requires professional services through local community-based programs for multiply handicapped and high-risk children which are being developed as mandated under Public Law 99-457. The following more recent group and individual case studies are presented to illustrate how both language delay problems and the early modification and correction of developing abnormal articulation and voice production disorders can be managed successfully in the preschool years.

CASE 5 (1980)

This case study illustrates the success that can be achieved almost routinely in managing lan-

TABLE 16-9. CASE STUDY (P.F., BORN 9/18/70) SHOWING INCREASED DELAY OVER PERIOD FROM 20 MONTHS TO 34 MONTHS WITH NO CONTACT OR THERAPY

Age (mo.)	Receptive language	Expressive language	Difference	Combined language scores
20	20 mo.	11 mo.	9 mo.	15 mo.
34	36 mo.	14 mo.	12 mo.	25 mo.

guage, speech and hearing development of children born with cleft palates. The tests described above assisted in verifying the essentially normal speech and language developmental status over time and facilitated the counseling of parents, communication with team members, and writing professional reports in the medical records.

J.T. was a female patient born with a cleft of the secondary palate only and limited to the soft palate. She was first seen by the entire team at 4½ months of age. At that time, the speech pathology report in the team record was as follows:

"Initial speech, language, and hearing evaluations were completed on this date. Mother was counseled at some length regarding the first year of speech development. J.T. is apparently an alert and well-developed child who at 4 months of age scored at the 5-month level on the REEL Scale. She responds to both live voice and sounds during diagnostic play therapy. Early surgical reconstruction of the soft palate is planned by plastic surgery at 7 months of age. J.T.'s status should be reviewed by the entire team at 2-3 months postsurgery."

Surgery was carried out at 7 months of age, and J.T. was seen again with both parents present for two outpatient language stimulation visits in the first year of life as well as team visits at 6-month intervals. The speech pathology report at a team visit when she was 17 months old included the following reference to her language skill development:

"Early speech and language stimulation was initiated through parent counseling in the past. J.T. continues to develop on schedule with good evidence of velopharyngeal adequacy. She is in a jargon stage of speech development and her /p/ and /b/ sound elements in syllables appear clear and oral. She also contrasts nasal syllables in utterances. On the REEL Scale, she reaches 18 months for both receptive and expressive language at 17 months chronological age."

A problem of recurrent otitis media detected through audiological assessments at cleft palate team meetings was treated by pressure-equalizing (PE) tubes on two occasions when J.T. was between 17 and 41 months of age; her speech and language skill development remained at normal levels over the first 3 years. At 3 years, 5 months of age, her team speech pathology report read as follows:

"This child talks intelligibly in 10-word sentences with excellent articulation skills. Speech skill is above her chronological age level, with consonant blends and sibilants normally articulated. There is no evidence of velopharyngeal incompetency. Nasal emission ratio 0/10; hypernasality ratio 0/10; hyponasality ratio 0/10. Had surgery at 7 months of age and seems to have excellent normal language development. On her single word Screening Articulation Test,

the /str/ and /sk/ and other difficult blends were perfectly articulated. Vowels in words were not aspirate or hoarse."

This young child's situation as regards cleft palate speech and language development through the preschool and into the early school-age years remains essentially the same. She was one of 50 consecutive cases over a 5-year period of cleft palate team–managed treatments that achieved normal and good developmental levels of both speech and language skills.

CASE 6 (1981)

The case of H.F. illustrates the management techniques based on standardized clinical tests for indicating the need for early secondary palatal reconstructive surgery while maintaining essentially normal language skill development.

H.F. was a white female cleft palate patient born with a cleft limited to the posterior two thirds of the secondary palate. The plastic surgeon elected to perform a complete primary reconstruction of the cleft palate at 5 months of age. Following primary surgery and due to low scores on the REEL Scale in the first year of life, H.F. was also enrolled in a language stimulation therapy program with her mother in the second year of life. By 20 months of age, her language quotients had changed from the 70s to over 100. From that time to the present, H.F. has presented with essentially normal and above-normal language development quotients on several language tests despite her development of later velopharyngeal insufficiency needing secondary palatal reconstruction. At 2 years, 6 months of age, her team speech pathology evaluation was as follows:

"Her parents report H.F. appears to have excellent receptive and expressive speech and language development. She is talking in sentences, sometimes 7-8 words long. She had complete closure of congenital cleft since 5 months of age, which is unusually early. It is not possible from her clinical speech testing alone to determine whether the velopharyngeal mechanism is totally adequate to support normal speech. However, a nasal emission index of 0/8 was obtained on this date. There appear to be no nasal distortions of speech utterances observed on this visit. An early recall is recommended in view of the early surgery and need for better determining postsurgical status of the palate function."

Following this visit, the speech test battery administered at two cleft palate team reevaluations at 6-month intervals indicated she then had essentially normal velopharyngeal function to support further normal speech production (e.g., she presented with 0/10 indices on tests 1, 2, and 3). However, on a later team reevaluation, when the patient was 4 years of age, her test evaluation record read as follows: "Patient's speech has regressed to lateralizations with nasal distortions and nasal emission developing very strongly over the past six-month period. Examination of the palate indicates the palate is somewhat short but remains mobile. Repeated observations of connected speech and recent case history indicates development of velopharyngeal incompetency (probably due to the downard and forward growth of the hard and soft palate). Nasal emission index was 10/10, hypernasality index 10/10, hyponasality index 0/10. Articulation shows either distortions due to nasal emission, nasal substitutions, or gross substitutions now predominate in running speech. These signs are all strong enough to recommend surgical reconstruction of the velopharyngeal mechanism as soon as possible."

Following this team report and after confirmation by cinefluoroscopy, a pharyngeal flap operation was carried out. Correction of developmental secondary velopharyngeal incompetency was verified in the following team reevaluation, and language and speech parameters have remained essentially normal since.

GROUP DATA FROM 50 CONSECUTIVE CASE STUDIES (1980–1983)

An assessment of the clinical test battery data described above to evaluate the efficacy of a team program focused on prevention of communicative disorders in 50 consecutive infants born with clefts has been reported in some detail [2, 3]. The following is a brief presentation and discussion of this study:

Our recent experience up to 1983 as compared to past studies using similar clinical indices is presented in Table 16-10. Whereas in the past, cleft palate speech disorders were present in an estimated 75 percent of the population, only 20 percent of this group were found to have any form of speech disorder, and most of these were mild forms of developmental dyslalia or dental-related articulation disorders.

It can be seen from Table 16-10 that the most unusual speech problem related to cleft palate, that of *gross sound-substitution error pattern*, was found in only three, or 6 percent, of the 50 case studies, as compared to 56.4 percent of a previous sample diagnosed in a similar manner. Two of these cases showed evidence of continued velopharyngeal incompetency for speech following primary reconstructive surgery, and were already scheduled for further palatal reconstruction. The third had had a successful secondary palatal reconstruction and was making rapid progress in breaking the gross substitution error pattern through speech therapy.

The problem of hypernasal distortion of syllabic elements in speech was found to be present in only two of the subjects judged through the clinical speech test battery to have velopharyngeal incompetency. These same two subjects also presented with a glottal stop error pattern (the other subject with a glottal stop error pattern showed no evidence of hypernasality by the base 10 cul-de-sac resonance test used to judge the presence or absence of hypernasal distortion of voice). Under the limits of this clinical investigation, therefore, it appears that operationally defined hypernasality was reduced from 43.1 per-

TABLE 16-10. COMPARISON OF THE FREQUENCY OF OCCURRENCE OF SPECIFIC TYPES OF CLEFT PALATE SPEECH DISORDERS FOLLOWING PAST AND PRESENT MANAGEMENT PROCEDURES

Categorical speech defects	Past studies (N = 1000) (%)	Present study (N = 50) (%)
1. Gross sound-substitution error pattern	56.4	6.0
2. Hypernasal distortion of voice	43.1	4.0
3. Distortion of articulation from nasal emission	42.3	8.0
4. Developmental dyslalia	34.0	10.0
5. Aspirate voice	31.3	10.0
6. Hoarse voice	15.0	0.0
7. Dental-related articulation disorders	12.8	8.0
8. Hyponasal voice	12.0	2.0
9. Distraction from nasal grimacing	4.2	0.0

cent under previous team management to 4 percent under the present system.

Distortions of pressure consonant sounds from nasal emission were found in only four cases (8%) in the present study as compared to 42.3 percent in previous studies. Two of these four cases were the same two as presented with hypernasality, gross sound-substitution error pattern, and velopharyngeal incompetency confirmed by speech cinefluorography and diagnostic therapy. One of the remaining cases presented with a mild nasal emission problem in the index range of 2/10 to 5/10 on the base 10 nasal emission test. The cause was determined to be a fistula in the anterior hard palate. This was confirmed both by temporary obturation of the fistula, which then yielded a 0/10 index, and by the fact that no nasal emission occurred on the syllable /ki/ as compared to /pi/ on repeated clinical testing. A dental obturator was placed until such time as surgical closure or spontaneous closure over time could eliminate the problem. The remaining case with nasal emission findings were mild, with indices of 2/10 to 0/10 on repeated testing without evidence of hypernasality on the cul-de-sac test or perceived hypernasality in running speech by listener judgment. This was thought to be a case of borderline-adequate velopharyngeal valving, to be managed by further speech therapy and frequent diagnostic testing.

Developmental dyslalia (functional articulation disorder) is a problem reported in approximately 10 percent of the beginning school-age population. It can be seen from Table 16-10 that developmental dyslalia was found in five subjects, or 10 percent, of the study group, as compared to 34.0 percent in previous studies. The limitation of functional articulation disorders was thought to be accomplished mainly through routine counseling of parents during cleft palate clinics or through home speech and language stimulation techniques and the prevention of functional delayed speech and language development.

The frequency of findings of *aspirate voice* characteristics was also limited to five subjects, or 10 percent, as compared to 31.3 percent in the past studies. The determination was made from test IV, the phonation test of our clinical test battery, and was limited to subjects who were unable to sustain phonation for 10 seconds on three tries for each vowel; who sounded aspirate in running speech to the speech pathologist; and whose parents confirmed that this phonatory quality was generally typical of speech at home. It is not known what percentage of a normal population sample of similar preschool-age children would be judged to have aspirate voice.

Hoarse voice (as operationally defined for this and our previously reported studies) is generally of more serious concern because of the frequent finding of vocal nodules. None of the 50 subjects presented with hoarse voice abnormalities, whereas it occured in 15 to 25 percent of previously reported cleft palate samples [4, 6].

It can be seen from Table 16-10 that *dental-related articulation disorders* remained at a fairly similar level (8% compared to 12.8%) to that found in a previous, larger population sample. This type of speech disorder may be similar in difficulty of management to the problem of otitis media from poor eustachian tube function. An aggressive early pedodontic and orthodontic program in the first 4 years of life would probably be necessary to replace missing lateral incisor teeth and alveolar cleft areas and to move collapsed buccal segments before mixed dentition if this problem were to be totally prevented.

In the past, *hyponasal voice* distortions were found to be present in 12 percent of a larger, and generally older, cleft palate population sample. This voice abnormality was generally a temporary sequela to the frequent use of the broad obturating pharyngeal flap surgical procedure most frequently used in the past to correct persistent velopharyngeal insufficiency following unsuccessful primary cleft palate surgery. This finding was present for only one (2%) of the 50 more recent case studies reported here. This subject was one of three presenting with a previously developed gross sound substitution error pattern, and was now making good progress with therapy following a recent pharyngeal flap secondary operation. As the hyponasality index was in the range of 2/10 to 5/10 and the 5-year-old patient was less than 1 year postsurgery, this finding of mild hyponasality was judged to be a tolerable problem.

It can be seen from Table 16-10 that the final problem of *distraction from nasal and facial grimacing* was not found in the present sample. It occurred in 4.2 percent of past studies and appears to develop only when prolonged development of speech with velopharyngeal insufficiency occurs.

EVALUATION OF LANGUAGE DEVELOPMENT DATA

The REEL Scale norms and specific items of achievement of both receptive and expressive language skills are based on the actual achievement of healthy, "normal" infants from linguistically enriched environments. The original validity studies [4] showed that 90 percent of well-baby infant population samples scored within 1 age interval on this scale, and that sample normal well-baby populations should have average language quotients of slightly over 100. The average combined language quotient for both male and female normal sample groups was 105.

The available data from 116 REEL Scale evaluations of the language development status of 43 of our 50 subjects is presented in Table 16-11. Five of the seven subjects not tested on the REEL Scale were over 3 years of age when first seen, and two were not tested because of time limitations and lack of a knowledgeable informant.

Inspection of Table 16-11 reveals that the average combined language age quotients were as high or higher than those of the well-baby samples reported in the validity studies for this scale. Table 16-11 also shows that 46 REEL Scale evaluations were given to 32 different subjects in our year-1 sample, and that calculation of the mean combined Language Age Score yielded a quotient of 111.67 with a standard deviation of 23.02. Twenty of these 32 subjects (63%) had a combined language quotient of 90 or above, and 19 subjects (59%) scored above 100. Only five (16%) scored between 80 and 90 in the first year of life, and two subjects (6%) had combined language quotients below 80.

In the second year of life, a mean combined language quotient of 107.32 with a standard deviation of 13.49 was obtained from 50 REEL Scale evaluations on 32 subjects. In year 2, 30 of the 32 subjects (94%) had quotients of 90 or above, with 21 (66%) of these scoring above 100. One subject (3%) scored between 80 and 90 and one had a quotient below 80.

In the third year of life, a mean combined language quotient of 105 with a standard deviation of 12.42 was found for 20 tests given to 16 subjects. Fifteen of the 16 subjects (94%) measured on the REEL Scale in year 3 had quotients of 90 or above, with 10 of these (63%) scoring above 100. Two subjects (13%) scored between 80 and 90, and none below 80.

Test results were also evaluated according to receptive, expressive, and combined language skills by sex, cleft type, age at primary closure, and socioeconomic status. We were also interested in changes in language skills durng the first 3 years of life. Results were evaluated using the

TABLE 16-11. REEL SCALE COMBINED LANGUAGE QUOTIENTS BY MEAN AND STANDARD DEVIATION FOR THE FIRST 3 YEARS OF LIFE

	N	Number of tests	$\bar{X}$	SD
Year 1	32	46	111.67	23.02
Year 2	32	50	107.32	13.49
Year 3	16	20	105.00	12.42

TABLE 16-12. MEAN COMBINED QUOTIENTS BY SEX FOR THE FIRST 3 YEAR OF LIFE

	N	Number of tests	$\bar{X}$
First year			
Male	19	29	113.86
Female	13	17	108.64
Second year			
Male	19	29	101.72
Female	13	21	110.76
Third year			
Male	10	10	107.40
Female	6	10	102.60

mean receptive, expressive, and combined language quotients.

Inspection of Table 16-12 reveals that both groups had essentially normal language achievement levels for each of the first three years of life. Although there were no substantial differences between the means, males scored slightly higher in the first and third years and females in the second years.

Table 16-13 presents the findings of the mean average receptive language quotient, expressive language quotient, and combined language quotient, as well as the receptive-expressive quotient (difference) scores for subgroups of four different types of clefts for each of the first 3 years of life. Table 16-13 reveals some trends related to type of cleft, particularly for achieving a small receptive-expressive (R-E) language difference. One subject with a cleft of the primary palate only had a substantial R-E language level difference accounting for most of the negative difference in score in years 1 and 2 for this small subgroup.

Such differences in some children with isolated cleft lip only indicate a functional delayed expressive language use that is related to environmental rather than physical causes. Since previous research found similar delayed expressive language problems in children with cleft lip only,

TABLE 16-13. MEAN RECEPTIVE LANGUAGE QUOTIENTS (RLQ), EXPRESSIVE
LANGUAGE QUOTIENTS (ELQ), COMBINED LANGUAGE QUOTIENTS
(CLQ), AND RECEPTIVE-EXPRESSIVE LANGUAGE DIFFERENCE (R-E DIFF.)
FOR FOUR TYPES OF CLEFT SUBGROUPS IN THE FIRST 3 YEARS OF LIFE

	Quotients	Primary palate only (N = 13)	Secondary palate only (N = 13)	Unilateral complete (N = 9)	Bilateral complete (N = 7)
Year 1	RLQ	150.0	107.2	115.5	108.2
	ELQ	125.0	97.6	105.4	94.0
	CLQ	137.5	102.4	110.1	101.2
	R-E Diff.	−25.0	−9.6	−10.0	−14.2
Year 2	RLQ	127.5	117.4	115.3	101.5
	ELQ	85.0	101.9	103.7	90.0
	CLQ	106.5	109.6	109.7	95.7
	R-E Diff.	−42.5	−15.5	−11.6	−11.5
Year 3	RLQ	100.0	98.3	101.5	107.5
	ELQ	110.0	94.0	90.0	100.3
	CLQ	109.0	96.7	95.7	103.8
	R-E Diff.	+10.0	−4.3	−11.5	−7.2

this possibility should be anticipated and language counseling and home stimulation programs initiated for this subgroup. Interestingly, the one child with oblique facial cleft in this subgroup had above-average language scores at 12 months of age. Subjects with clefts of the secondary palate only (N = 13) revealed normal language scores for the first 2 years of life but had large R-E language level differences. Children in this subgroup tested in the third year had slightly lower but normal language scores and a marked decrease in the R-E difference.

The children with unilateral complete clefts of the primary and secondary palates (N = 19) had normal and above-normal scores for all 3 years. Children with bilateral complete clefts of the primary and secondary palates (N = 7) showed lower expressive scores than the other cleft types in the first 2 years, although the scores were near normal. The R-E differences decreased but did not disappear in the third year. Expressive and receptive quotients remained in the normal range.

Two final factors thought to be related to delayed language development are (1) age at which complete primary reconstructive surgery is completed, and (2) family socioeconomic level. No statistically significant differences were found for either factor. However, a trend based on the small sample subgroups for timing of surgery is worth describing. The children in our sample who had clefts involving the secondary palate and complete reconstructive surgery between 7 and 12 months of age (N = 26) all had excellent lan-

guage level scores with small R-E language differences. Subjects who had their surgery completed between 13 and 18 months all had excellent (>100) receptive language quotients, but decreased (although within the normal range) expressive language scores. They tended to have large R-E language differences in each of the first 3 years. Both a slight decrease in receptive language quotients and a more marked decrease in expressive language quotients were characteristic of the group (N = 7) who had primary palatal reconstructions after 19 months of age.

CASE STUDIES II

The following most recent case studies were provided by our present team coordinator, Mrs. Virginia Dixon-Wood, M.A., co-author of Chapter 4. These case studies exemplify how cleft palate infants referred after prior treatment in other communities might still be satisfactorily managed for often severe presenting problems before school age is reached.

CASE: A.K.

Allen came to our center at 27 months of age. He was born with a bilateral cleft of the primary palate with complete cleft palate. The lip had been repaired at 2 months of age and the palate at 11 months in another state.

Our initial speech evaluation revealed (1) nasal substitutions for stops (/m/ for /p/, /m/ for /b/, /n/ for /d/, and /n/ for /t/); (2) severe glottal articulation pattern for velar stops and all fricatives; (3) no clear clinical evidence of velopharyngeal incompetency or adequacy from nasal emission or hypernasality tests because Allen was using nasal phonemes or glottalizing which prevented oral or nasal air flow; (4) language levels that were age-appropriate or normal according to his mother's responses on the REEL Scale. This set of initial clinical findings led to the recommendation of a period of diagnostic speech therapy as described below:

Goals. Our goals for therapy were not to eliminate or reduce velopharyngeal insufficiency for speech, but rather to (1) improve speech intelligibility by reducing glottal articulation, and (2) condition Allen so that further testing of the velopharyngeal port (including videofluoroscopy and/or nasoendoscopy) could be accomplished.

Methods. Children who develop glottal articulation patterns do so in an effort to compensate for their inability to produce oral breath pressure required for oral articulation of consonants. Because of this, Allen had to relearn articulation patterns. In his case, this meant learning how to produce oral breath flow. Due to his age, we incorporated many visual and tactile cues in simple tasks below the word or even the syllable level of production, including (1) a "sigh" with body movement which later developed into /h/; (2) gentle blowing of a paper paddle to watch it move (this was often accompanied by nasal air flow which was accepted and acceptable for the goals of diagnostic therapy); and (3) putting an index finger to his rounded lips as he blew to create an /s/-like sound.

Once the concept of producing oral breath flow was understood and any of these three tasks could be done consistently, the next step was to use oral flow to produce the bilabial stops /p/ and /b/. These sound elements were chosen because they are highly visible sounds and can be taught with the aid of an air flow paddle. We were most successful with vowel-consonant-vowel (VCV) nonsense syllables with oral air flow and /p/ or /b/ consonant approximations first. After some time, Allen could produce VCVC bisyllables. At that point, the initial vowel was dropped in imitative repetitions to obtain productions of initial position oral consonants in syllables.

Nonsense syllable drills were next used, initiated by his learned bilabial stop initiation pattern. These syllable drills led to word productions of true words initiated by /p/ or /b/ and shortly thereafter by other phonemes as generalization began to occur through the multiphonemic syllable drill approach.

After 4 months of diagnostic therapy, Allen could model the therapist's articulatory placement for /b/, /p/, /w/, and /f/. After 1 year of therapy, he was using correct articulatory placement for these phonemes spontaneously. However, oral breath pressure remained weak, nasal substitutions for plosives in running speech continued, and nasal emission distortions and hypernasality were now perceived during speech efforts with oral air flow.

The clinical impression of an underlying problem of velopharyngeal insufficiency was verified at age 3 years, 9 months through a speech videofluoroscopic evaluation of the functioning of the velopharyngeal mechanism. A valid test was accomplished then because (1) Allen had eliminated glottal articulation in single test words, a condition

affecting palatal movements and the reliability of instrumental tests, and (2) better cooperation had been obtained from Allen through frequent visits for therapy. This procedure can be frightening for a child, but engaging him in familiar activities and repeating familiar words put him at ease. The videofluoroscopy showed appropriate palatal movement patterns, but only occasional touch closure occurred. A specific surgical reconstruction of the velopharyngeal port was recommended and performed.

A speech reevaluation at 6 months postoperatively revealed the following: (1) Allen's nasal emission ratio was now 0/10, his hypernasality ratio, 0/10, and his hyponasality ratio, 0/10, all indicating essentially normal velopharyngeal function to support normal voice and articulation. (2) He was already producing all of the plosive sounds correctly in initial, medial, and final word positions. (3) His language skills were age-appropriate. (4) His remaining cleft palate speech disorder was now limited to a gross substitution error pattern of using pharyngeal fricatives for sibilants and affricates. Prognosis for correction of this problem before regular school age was reached was considered good.

CASE: J.J.

Effective speech therapy techniques for correcting the occasional problems from phoneme-specific nasalance distortions (which are considered as having a functional rather than an organic basis and which may be distinguished from cleft palate speech problems directly related to velopharyngeal insufficiency through the short clinical test battery) are reviewed below.

J.J. first presented at 2 years, 9 months of age with nasal emission, gross sound substitution, and distraction from facial grimacing disorders, but in a pattern that was phoneme-specific. Nasal emission distortions occurred only for the sound elements /p/, /b/, /t/, and /d/. Pharyngeal fricatives occurred only for /s/ and /z/, while other fricatives were normally produced. In addition, nasal grimacing, poor eye contact, and echolalia were all observed.

J.J. was therefore enrolled in a direct speech therapy program. Therapy was based on the assumption that adequate velopharyngeal function was demonstrated by his error pattern. His hearing and language tests were all within normal limits, but he was immature and for several weeks his mother had to be present in the therapy room at all times.

Goals. J.J.'s goals were different from Allen's in that (1) his nasal emission and glottal articulation were phoneme-specific, (2) he had already produced other sounds with good oral air flow and pressure, and (3) he was stimulable for correct production of error sounds. None of these were characteristic of Allen's initial speech evaluation findings.

Methods. The goal of decreasing nasal emission distortions was begun by using strong visual and tactile feedback cues for nasal emission on bilabial plosives (a simple clinical biofeedback technique). J.J. was encouraged first to use a whisper or soft onset voice during which no nasal emission occurred as indicated by visual or tactile cues. Next, this was contrasted to production with a voice of normal intensity. In addition, we slowed the speaking rate to create more "get ready time." In J.J.'s therapy, we began directly with syllables and words rather than sounds because he had a very limited gross substitution error pattern.

After 5 weeks of therapy, correction of nasal emission was generalizing to the alveolar plosives. At 10 weeks, he was able to use both bilabial and alveolar plosives correctly without nasal emission in phrases like "Eat the [pie, bread, tasty tarts, darn good dandelions, etc.]."

The glottalization pattern was approached by pairing production of the /s/ with the /t/, which has the same place of articulation. By first repeating the /t/, which had no pharyngeal fricative substitution, and then the /ts/ blend in imitation of the therapist, and then /t/ followed immediately by a prolonged /s/, and finally an /s/ in isolation J.J. over time was able to produce an /s/ at will without gross substitution taking place. After 12 months of therapy, J.J. could produce /s/ in words and phrases in drills like "See the ____ ." By 14 months of therapy, he had begun to use /s/ and /z/ spontaneously in connected speech with the ability to self-correct occasional errors. Intelligiblity was 89 percent. Nasal emission errors no longer occurred. Pharyngeal fricatives or glottals no longer occurred. Resonance was normal. No further therapy was recommended except for a 6-month checkup by a speech pathologist as the family was moving from our area.

RECENT GROUP STATISTICS

The achievement of normal and good language development skills and the avoidance or early management of gross sound substitution error patterns and nasalance distortions, both nasal emission and hypernasality, is demonstrated again in the grouped case studies of the next 20 cases following the 50 case study evaluation and managed as described above. It takes 3 to 4 years to accumulate and analyze the test and clinical evaluation records of an additional group of 20 consecutive cleft lip and palate patients. As in the prior study, patients were limited to patients presenting with isolated clefts exclusive of syndromes with retardation or deafness. However, by chance, the eight male subjects classified under Cleft of the Secondary Palate II as in Table 16-14 were all diagnosed as having Pierre Robin sequence (micrognathia with wide U-shaped clefts of the hard and soft palate structures), presenting some difficult-to-manage problems for early surgical correction.

It can be seen from Table 16-14 that the next 20 cases treated involved a sampling of the usual variations of cleft lip or palate malformations but not in as close a representation of the overall cleft population as in the 50 case studies discussed earlier. The sample included nine cases with clefts of the secondary palate only, three with primary palate clefts, and eight with combined clefts, of which five were unilateral and three bilateral. Atypically, eight of the nine cases presenting with clefts of the secondary palate only and diagnosed as having the Pierre Robin sequence had wide U-shaped clefts of the hard and soft palate. Such cases are often postponed for primary surgery for this and other complications of respiration and hearing. Despite the large number of wide clefts of the secondary palate, the mean age for completed primary reconstruction of the clefts in this sample was 10.5 months; the range was from 6 months to 15 months. The modal age was 11 months, indicating a skew to the right in the distribution; that is, surgery is usually done at about 11 months in current practice, rather than from 18 to 26 months as in the past.

Table 16-15 presents the mean, mode, and range of REEL Scale language quotients taken from 50 REEL Scale measures on the 20 subjects in this continuing clinical demonstration study. Quotients that were correct for age were used because, as in the earlier study, essentially normal receptive and expressive language development was maintained in the population sample over each of the 3 years covered despite the many high-risk factors concomitant with cleft lip and

TABLE 16-14. DESCRIPTION OF THE POPULATION SAMPLE (N = 20) BY SEX AND TYPE OF CLEFT

	Cleft of primary palate, I	Cleft of secondary palate, II	Combined unilateral, III	Combined bilateral, IV
Males (16)	3	8[a]	3	2
Females (4)	0	1	2	1
Total	3	9	5	3

[a] Pierre Robin sequence.

TABLE 16-15. THE MEANS, MODES, AND RANGES OF 50 REEL SCALE LANGUAGE QUOTIENTS ON A RECENT GROUP OF 20 CONSECUTIVE CASE STUDIES OF CHILDREN BORN WITH CLEFTS

	RLQ	ELQ	CLQ
Means	109.6	102.5	106.0
Mode	115.0	105.0	110.0
Range	86–157	83–157	83–157

For abbreviations, see footnote, Table 16-6.

palate. The language scores averaging above 100 indicate that the language development of this group was comparable to healthy normal infants from stimulating home environments whence the norms of the scale derive.

Table 16-16 presents a percentage comparison of the frequency of each of nine categorical aspects of cleft palate speech compared to recent findings in a similar age population sample and earlier findings in a much older population sample. It can be seen from this table that only one or two of the subjects under five years of age (e.g., in the range 5–10%) had any remaining problems formerly common in this population. Each of these problems was well diagnosed and appropriate therapy already instituted before school age. Similar findings were demonstrated in the recent study initiated about 1980.

I have tried to demonstrate in this chapter that the state of the art of cleft palate management and cleft palate speech therapy is at a level for almost routine prevention or early correction of the com- municative disorders that plagued this large population of children in the past. The challenge to our profession in every community is to realize this goal for all newborn children with cleft palate and to improve the care and development of children with the many even more challenging problems involved in craniofacial disorders.

REFERENCES

1. Bzoch, K. R. The effects of a specific pharyngeal flap operation upon the speech of forty cleft-palate persons. *J. Speech Hear. Disord.* 29:111–120, 1964.
2. Bzoch, K. R. Clinical Evaluation and Management of Problems of Speech, Language, and Hearing. In F. W. Pirruccello (Ed.), *Cleft Lip and Palate.* Springfield, Ill.: Thomas, 1987. Chap. 11.
3. Bzoch, K. R., Kemker, F. J., and Wood, V. D. The Prevention of Communicative Disorders in Cleft Palate Infants. In N. J. Lass (Ed.), *Speech and Language: Advances in Basic Research and Practice.* San Francisco: Academic Press, 1984. Vol. 10, pp. 59–110.
4. Bzoch, K. R., and League, R. *Assessing Language Skills in Infancy.* Austin, Texas: Pro-Ed, 1971.
5. McDonald, E. T. *Bright Promise.* Chicago: National Society for Crippled Children and Adults, Inc., 1959.
6. McWilliams, B. J., Lavorato, A. S., and Blueston, C. D. Vocal cord abnormalities in children with velopharyngeal valving problems. *Laryngoscope* 83:1745, 1973.
7. Rosen, M. L., and Bzoch, K. R. The prosthetic speech appliance in rehabilitation of patients with cleft palate. *J. Am. Dent. Assoc.* 57:203–210, 1958.
8. Snyder, G. D., Berkowitz, S., Bzoch, K. R., and Stool, S. *Your Cleft Lip and Palate Child: A Basic Guide for Parents.* Evansville, Ind.: Mead Johnson Laboratories, 1969.
9. Suther, J. A. Listener's social perception of the cleft palate speaker. Thesis, University of Florida, Gainesville, 1974.

TABLE 16-16. COMPARISON OF THE FREQUENCY OF OCCURRENCE OF NINE SPECIFIC TYPES OF SPEECH DISORDERS IN PAST, RECENT, AND CURRENT CLINICAL STUDIES.

Categorical speech defects	Present study (N = 20) (%)	Recent study (N = 50) (%)	Past study (N = 1,000) (%)
1. Gross sound substitutions	10.0	6.0	56.4
2. Hypernasality	5.0	4.0	45.1
3. Nasal emission	5.0	8.0	42.3
4. Developmental dyslalia	5.0	10.0	34.0
5. Aspirate voice	0.0	10.0	31.3
6. Hoarse voice	0.0	0.0	15.0
7. Dental-related articulation	10.0	8.0	12.8
8. Hyponasal voice	0.0	2.0	12.0
9. Nasal grimacing	0.0	0.0	4.2

CHAPTER 17

Oral Sensory Function in Speech Production and Remediation

Ralph L. Shelton

He crossed the courtyard with a kind of military precision, as if each step he took, each movement of his arms, was separately controlled by orders sent down from on high.

Ross McDonald [103a]

Speech pathologists serving patients with cleft palate are interested in the physiological mechanisms that mediate awareness of the sound and feel of one's own speech and with how that sensory information contributes to the control of skilled speech movements. Clinicians have recommended that patients be taught to monitor movements and contacts in attempts to improve velopharyngeal function [9, 163]. and articulation [102]. This chapter focuses on *somesthesis,* which refers here to the senses of movement, position, touch-pressure, and pain, and to muscle sense (awareness of muscle tension) and an associated sense of effort. The physiology of somesthesis is introduced and several viewpoints about the control of speech movements are reviewed. We wish to know what oral sensory information is available to the cleft palate patient in speech therapy and about concepts from speech motor control theory that might contribute to the conceptualization of speech therapy for the patient with cleft palate. Measures of oral sensory function are described, and their use in studies of persons with disordered speech is reviewed. That information pertains to our ability to assess variability in oral sensory function among persons with disordered speech. Finally, information is reviewed that pertains to speech somesthesis and other variables in the correction of speech disorders in persons with cleft palate.

SOMESTHESIS

Kinesthesis refers to awareness of the movement of body parts [51] and sometimes to position sense as well [65]. *Kinesthesis* and *proprioception* are sometimes used interchangeably and kinesthesis has been said to be knowledge of proprioception [12]. However, Boring [16] used *proprioception* to refer to certain afferent phenomena that do not reach consciousness and *kinesthesis* to refer to movement sensation available for introspection.

Gibson [47] used *kinesthesis* to refer to the awareness of the movement of one's own body regardless of what systems, including articular, vestibular, and visual, are used to register the knowledge. He described the importance to perception of active exploration of stimuli, and he said that a person "feels an object relative to the body and the body relative to an object." Somewhat similarly, a talker can shift attention between conveyance of a message and movements and contacts of the articulators in speech [35].

In this chapter, *kinesthesis* and *proprioception* are used as employed by the authors cited. Otherwise, *kinesthesis* refers to awareness of movement regardless of the source of the information underlying that awareness. *Proprioception* refers to sensory information that does not reach consciousness. Similarly, *tooth-pressure* refers to sensory cues that are available for introspection, and *taction* and *tactile* refer to neural impulses that do not reach consciousness [53].

PHYSIOLOGY OF SOMESTHESIS

Most knowledge of somesthesis and movement control [96] was obtained by study of movements not involving speech, and it is still uncertain how valuable that information is to understanding operation of the speech mechanism [23]. Speech is unique in that it involves movement of articulators within the body [33], and generalization from study of one articulator to another may be erroneous [38]. Nonetheless, Abbs and Kennedy [3] observed that there are findings which indicate that speech and nonspeech movements are controlled in comparable fashion.

MECHANORECEPTORS

Somesthetic percepton appears to involve interaction among several types of mechanoreceptors [98] which are sensitive to muscle length

Figure 17-1. The muscle spindle consists of nuclear bag and nuclear chain intrafusal muscle fibers. Primary endings from group Ia afferent nerve fibers contact both bag and chain muscle fibers, whereas secondary endings from group II afferent nerve fibers lie predominantly on nuclear chain intrafusal muscle fibers. The nuclear bag muscle fibers are innervated by dynamic gamma motor nerve fibers, which are sensitive to phasic stretch, whereas the nuclear chain muscle fibers are innervated by static gamma motor nerves, which respond to static stretch. (Adapted from Matthews [97].)

and rate of change in length, muscle tension, position of bones around a joint, vibration and deep pressure, velocity of joint movement, skin stretch, skin indentation, two-point discrimination, pain, temperature, touch, hair movement, and air pressure below the vocal folds [33–69]. The primary and secondary afferent muscle spindle endings and the Golgi tendon organs are especially important to kinesthesis and position sense.

Golgi tendon organs are in series with muscle fibers and are located at the junctions of muscles and tendons. They sense tension or force produced by muscle contraction. Muscle spindles are located within muscles and are parallel with extrafusal muscle fibers which accomplish bodily movements [48, 55]. They sense stretch and detect change in muscle length and rate of change in length.

The muscle spindle includes intrafusal muscle fibers that make no detectable contribution to muscle tension [34] but that do influence the output of afferent receptors in the spindle. Also included are (1) gamma motor neurons that activate the intrafusal muscle fibers, and (2) sensory neurons that detect the movement of those muscle fibers (Fig. 17-1). Extrafusal muscle fibers may be activated through either direct or spinal level loop connection with the spindles. They may also be directed by higher brain centers that either work through the muscle spindles or that send signals directly to extrafusal muscle fibers via alpha

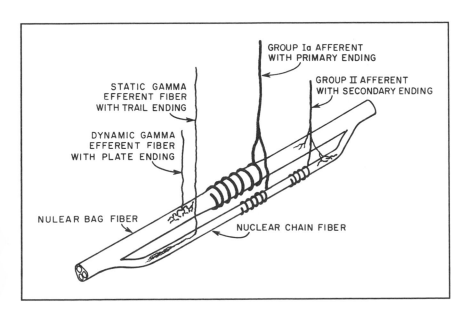

GROUP Ia AFFERENT WITH PRIMARY ENDING

GROUP II AFFERENT WITH SECONDARY ENDING

STATIC GAMMA EFFERENT FIBER WITH TRAIL ENDING

DYNAMIC GAMMA EFFERENT FIBER WITH PLATE ENDING

NULEAR BAG FIBER

NUCLEAR CHAIN FIBER

motor neurons. Borden [12] wrote that feedback from spindles precedes movement whereas touch-pressure and auditory cues follow movement initiation.

A viewpoint that muscle receptors are involved in motor control but not in kinesthesis was held for a time. Henneman [56] indicated that knowledge of joint position is lost when joint receptors are anesthetized but is retained when muscles are denervated. However, Matthews [98] reported a return to an earlier view that muscle afferents do contribute to kinesthesis. This return was based in part on the observation that little kinesthesis is lost with the surgical replacement of joints with prostheses. Furthermore, Schmidt [137] reported that cortical representation has been identified for Ia afferents and that stimulation of muscle spindles produced illusions about joint position.

UNJOINTED ARTICULATORS

Much research in somesthesis has been directed to muscles controlling the limbs which are jointed. Since the tongue, lips, and palate are unjointed, their somesthesis may be unique. Cooper [28] wrote that while the tongue lacks a joint and hence joint receptors, it is well endowed with touch endings which can serve a guidance function. Kawamura [66] commented that the tongue is controlled primarily by surface exteroceptors. Bowman [22], however, noted that surface receptors are not activated until a contact has been made and that lingual spindles differ from one another in sensitivity to stretch stimuli from different directions. He hypothesized that the transverse, vertical, and horizontal arrangement of muscles within the tongue allows lingual spindles to signal movement. That is, the anatomy of the tongue is such that its movement can be signaled by muscle spindles even though no joint receptors are activated. See Lowe [86, 87] for reviews of neural control of tongue movements.

Sussman [159] wrote that both kinesthetic and touch-pressure information are needed for the control of tongue movements. Also, the close relationship between movements of mandible and tongue adds another possibility for transmission of kinesthetic information from receptors to cortex. This reasoning does not extend to the velum and pharyngeal walls which are not well endowed with touch receptors [49] nor associated with jointed structures. The velum does not perform as skillfully as the tongue even though it presents timing and range-of-motion performances

suitable to contextual co-articulation in the achievement of closure [70]. Control of the velum may be more dependent on mechanisms that are not available to introspection than are movements of the tongue and jointed structures. Research regarding velar awareness is summarized later.

OTHER NEURAL CONTRIBUTORS TO SOMESTHESIS

Mechanoreceptors function in conjunction with other components of the nervous system; the basal ganglia, the cerebellum, and the cerebral cortex are important to motor control [12, 23, 24, 90, 115]. Angevine [5] cited a hypothesis that the basal ganglia store movement programs that are probably activated and sustained by widespread regions of the cerebral cortex. Program execution is monitored and modified by sensory feedback. Angevine hypothesized that the cerebellum is involved in rapid movements and the basal ganglia in slow movements. Semmes [143] reviewed literature regarding the role of the lemniscal system in somesthesis.

Signals from mechanoreceptors may be variable in reaching brain areas that mediate perception. Spindle receptors may discharge at different rates for the same movements and positions depending on signals being sent to the spindles from the neurons that innervate them [110]. The brain must decode the overall pattern. Guyton [51] wrote that tendon organs and muscle spindles send signals to the spinal cord, cerebellum, and cerebral cortex and that they function at an unconscious or nearly unconscious level in the reflexive contraction of muscles. Despite their unconscious level of operation, spindles and tendon organs transmit great amounts of information into the nervous system, thus helping CNS centers control muscle contraction.

Kennedy and Abbs [69] reported that receptors show differential sensitivity; that is, the sensation that is received appears to be a function of where in the CNS the impulses arrive. Hardy [53] noted that signals from a given receptor might contribute to the operation of more than one control loop and that some of the signals might reach conscious levels and others not. Abbs and Kennedy [3] indicated that motor control involves interactions among cascaded neural pathways in a hierarchical fashion. There are multiple pathways — some automatic and some voluntary — and loops within loops. Different circuits control different kinds of movement, and experience, instruction, and other variables influence how control is conducted. For example, movement dynamics, novelty of task, and subject intention may be involved in the programming and conduct of motor gestures. Abbs and Kennedy [3] referred to a redundancy of control programs, and they stated [3] that in controlling voluntary motor performance the nervous system employs different modes of functioning, including tight feedback control, central programming of movement, and combinations. Mountcastle [110] said that awareness of position and movement may depend on CNS integration of visual and vestibular as well as somesthetic sensory information. He indicated that the integration appears to be performed in the brain's parietal lobe. For speech, hearing would, of course, be of critical importance.

It seems likely that damage to sensory pathways or cortical centers, rather than damage to mechanoreceptors, would impair oral somesthesis. MacNeilage, Roots, and Chase [94] described a 17-year-old girl who misarticulated and presented oral and nonoral nonspeech movement difficulties. Neurological examination suggested that the girl's disability was primarily somesthetic rather than motor in origin. She failed several somesthetic measures but did not show evidence of motor abnormalities of peripheral, cerebellar, or extrapyramidal origin. Hearing and speech perception were described as normal. Oral sensory receptors and nerves appeared normal at biopsy, and no lesion or group of lesions was found that might account for the girl's disability.

Corollary Discharge

Signals from motor areas of the brain contribute to somesthesis. These signals have different names including *corollary discharge* and *efference copy*. As Guyton [51, p. 599] put it, muscle sense probably involves information about the intensity of motor signals to the muscles as well as impulses from receptors in deep tissues. Mountcastle [110] wrote that people appear to be "able to sense the 'central effort' exerted in a motor act independently of peripheral input." Schmidt [137] wrote about a "carbon copy" of neural activities that is sent from the central motor centers to centers involved in deep sensibility. He said that these signals provide information about forthcoming muscular activity and associated movements. These efference copies may be used to eliminate ambiguity in information arising from somesthetic and exteroceptive sources. Mount-

castle wrote that there is little direct evidence concerning the corollary discharge [110]. Semmes [143] cited Gibson's [46] observations that active exploration of objects provides more information than does passive contact with a stimulus. She conjectured that interaction between sensory and motor systems could be such that a lesion of the motor cortex could have a detrimental effect on sensory function and that the mechanism of this change might involve a loss of the corollary discharge.

The concept of corollary discharge is pertinent to communication disorders. Writing about hearing-impaired children, Ling [83] cited "a simultaneous efferent discharge . . . to the motor system . . . and to the associated sensory system." He wrote, "Only if there is a mismatch between the sensory patterns derived from the movements executed and the sensory patterns forecast by feedforward does conscious feedback occur." Netsell [111] said that the stored representation of the external world postulated in feedforward control models may for speech take the form of a vocal tract analog. "There may also be a provisional or initial command ('corollary discharge' . . .) that (1) accounts for the peripheral state of the vocal tract . . . and (2) makes online changes in its controlling signal to the muscles." Both state of the vocal tract and past experience would be involved in this control adjustment.

Movement Initiation

Requirements for the control of movement initiation are different from those for the control of ongoing movement. Initiation of voluntary movement may employ direct cortical activation of alpha motor neurons and extrafusal muscle fibers, or the cortex may first activate the muscle spindles via their gamma motor nerve fibers. In the latter instance, afferent impulses from the spindles collaborate with and facilitate cortical impulses to alpha neurons (Fig. 17-1). The two sources of neural impulse may work together to activate muscle fibers [21]. Corollary discharges may also play a role in the initiation of movement.

Speech clinicians and others [68] have expressed concern that neural transmission time may limit one's ability to use kinesthesis and touch-pressure to correct speech movements [164]. However, Netsell [111] reported that speech, which is relatively slow compared to the fast movements made by the eyes, may benefit from different forms of control and that mode of control may change with change in rate of speech.

He also suggested that central neural processes may partially compensate for feedback limitations imposed by neural transmission time.

The literature reviewed above indicates that much sensory information about motor performance is sent from mechanoreceptors into the nervous system. While that information contributes to motor control, much of it is not available to consciousness. Information that does reach consciousness may vary in precision from a sense of effort to precise awareness of position and movement. Structures differ in somesthesis, and it is likely that the velopharyngeal mechanism is less well equipped for kinesthesis than are other articulators. The operation of the sensory system in motor performance is highly complex. Sensory function is influenced by experience, and somesthetic impulses associated with a given speech act vary depending on numerous conditions. Next, we consider theoretical viewpoints about how speech motor control is achieved.

CONTROL OF SPEECH MOVEMENTS

In this section, we consider selected control hypotheses that are more focused on speech movement than was the information cited above. Open- and closed-loop control hypotheses are introduced. Then sensorimotor control of speech movements is related to the expression of meaning, and flexibility and plasticity are described and related to velopharyngeal function. Finally, the regulation and control of aerodynamic variables in speech is cited. These viewpoints were selected for study because they are relevant to speech therapy [164] and to the function of the velopharyngeal mechanism. Little attention is given to learning in most control models [71].

OPEN- AND CLOSED-LOOP CONTROL

Servosystem models have been used to describe and explain the role of sensory feedback in speech [3, 35, 157, 164]. MacNeilage [92] and MacNeilage and MacNeilage [93] differentiated between closed- and open-loop theory. Closed-loop theory formulates speech production in terms of idealized target positions for speech units. Feedback that permits moment-to-moment monitoring of ongoing movement is presumed to guide the articulators toward those targets. Feedback involves the transmission of information about muscle and movement to the neural cen-

ters that regulate motor performance [111]. Closed-loop control at a spinal or cerebellar level would make no provision for awareness mediated by muscle receptors. MacNeilage concluded that some form of closed-loop control is involved, at least in the initiation of speech. Kelso and Tuller [68] wrote that closed-loop control has been overvalued for biological systems. They said that deafferented humans perform too well for a closed-loop control system to be plausible, at least for some performances.

Open-loop theory postulates control of the production of speech units in terms of invariant motor commands. Open-loop systems control movements that are not subject to feedback modification once they are initiated. Preprogrammed performance that is oblivious to the senses probably contributes to speech [111]. This is not to say that repetitions of movements used in a particular skill must involve invariant neural commands or stereotyped execution. Welford [172] wrote that utilization of movements involves a delay between movement command and execution. The command must involve a prediction of the state of the organism at the time the command will be executed, and this prediction will involve computation that takes into account the immediate stimulus to action, future goals, past experiences, and concurrent factors such as posture. Thus movements processed by open-loop control mechanisms can be influenced by learning.

Speech control is not limited to either closed-or open-loop mechanisms. Both appear to be involved; many variables influence the lower motor neurons that activate muscles. Next we consider three viewpoints regarding speech motor control.

SENSORIMOTOR CONTROL AND THE EXPRESSION OF MEANING

Netsell [111] described speech as a motor-acoustic means of expressing language. Speech motor control involves "the motor-afferent mechanisms that direct and regulate speech movements." Mechanisms include the motor speech apparatus that produces the acoustic patterns of the speaker's language and the auditory and somesthetic apparatus that guides it. Speech movement achieves phonetic units and their acoustic and perceptual consequences. The acoustic events must be compatible with the language spoken and the message to be conveyed. Daniloff, Schuckers, and Feth [33] noted that articulatory models must accommodate both the biomechanics of articulatory movement and the phonological level of language. Articulation must serve the expression of meaning.

Netsell [111] also wrote that to produce an acoustic signal that is meaningful as speech, the speaker must precisely achieve and time satisfactory vocal tract shapes. Speech development involves feeling speech movements and hearing the speech that one producees. These perceptual images "become yoked to the motor and somatoafferent patterns used to generate them . . . ." Tight coupling of sensorimotor and auditory variables is necessary to the refinement of speech and contributes to the development within the nervous system of internal representations of the sensorimotor activities of speech. Nonetheless, flexible motor actions are used.

MacNeilage [91] hypothesized that sequences of movement are not stored for independent execution but are guided by a space coordinate system postulated by Lashley [77]. The speaker must reach spatial targets but may do so in different ways. Daniloff, Schuckers, and Feth [33] wrote that rules "governing conversion of vocal tract shape to acoustic patterns" seem to reflect flexibility in operation of the articulatory mechanism. Thus, "a wide variety of shapes can be, and often are, used to create a single acoustic target."

In summary, the control of speech movements is tied to linguistic abstractions, and the expression of a given meaning may be achieved by a variety of motor performances.

FLEXIBILITY AND PLASTICITY

Speech sounds perceived by listeners lack one-to-one correspondence with articulatory movements as observed cinefluorographically or with acoustic measures [29, 89]. Theory must account for variability in movements associated with repetition of phone-sized units in different speech contexts. Netsell [111] indicated that storage of internal representations — in contrast to storage of fixed movement routines and muscle contractions — permits flexibility in the achievement of speech goals. The speaker can employ a highly flexible motor program to achieve a highly consistent acoustic product. Spatial-temporal goals can be achieved by different motor acts. This achievement of a goal by different means has been termed *motor equivalence.* Initially, the nervous system specifies goals and then works out the means to achieve those goals.

The concept of motor equivalence is related to the concept of coordinative structures [38]. The latter involves the idea that action units are functionally but not anatomically specific. Kelso [67] differentiated between coordinative structure hypotheses and viewpoints that formulate motor control in ways that offer less flexibility. He wrote that multiple motor components are assembled "softly" and that they are flexible — not machinelike — in function. Kuehn and colleagues [74, 75] theorized that coordinative structures involve interdependencies among muscles and that such a structure sends parallel signals to the musculus uvulae and the levator veli palatini muscles which work together in the accomplishment of velopharyngeal closure.

Lubker [88] discussed a theory that holds that the speaker has freedom in production so long as the speech perceived by the listener is intelligible and acceptable. That which the listener receives must bear a close relationship to linguistic abstractions such as phonemes even though the speaker's motor performance does not.

Netsell [111] acknowledged limits to flexibility. While speech does not involve strings of stereotyped articulatory gestures, "the speech motor acts of a given language, once learned, are not infinitely flexible, but quasi-fixed, in that certain tightly coordinated movements cannot be broken up except by neurologic lesion, and others are extremely difficult to learn or unlearn beyond a certain age."

Folkins [37] reviewed and rejected co-articulatory models of speech motor control. Those models concern how phonetic units (phone, allophone, feature, syllable, etc.) are sequenced to achieve speech goals. From a co-articulatory perspective, oral sensory information is related to the production of speech units and their patterning in running speech.

Folkins [37] viewed a speaker's goal as a perceptually adequate output that may be achieved in different ways. The speaker develops motor strategies that permit achievement of perceptually acceptable speech. "After a speaker has used the sound system of the language to decide what to say, there is no reason to insist that the motor system be constrained by the order of phonetic units in producing the desired holistic percept" [37]. Folkins attributed variablity in the achievement of perceptually acceptable speech to flexibility and plasticity.

Flexibility takes two forms, each of which works within the individual's linguistic rule system. One form is free variation whereby there are alternative paths to a goal and no reason need be offered for the choice made. The other form is forced-variation flexibility. Here an obstruction such as a dental appliance forces the talker to alter the physiological parameters used in talking. One path is closed, but an alternative may be taken within the linguistic system. Speech mechanism adjustments reflecting flexibility are immediate.

Something may happen to a speaker, such as prosthetic or operative treatment, that precludes achievement of perceptual goals within the individual's lingusitic system. Flexibility is insufficient to permit the individual to produce perceptually acceptable speech. However, over time the individual may reacquire the ability to talk in a perceptually acceptable way. From Folkins' perspective, that adaptation — which he termed plasticity — reflects a change in the person's rule system.

Folkins [37] and Lubker [88] each applied a perceptual model of speech motor control to velopharyngeal requirements for speech. According to Folkins, the speaker may use different combinations of velopharyngeal variables to achieve perceptually acceptable speech. For example, area of velopharyngeal opening, movement patterns, timing, and oral opening may be combined in different ways to achieve acceptable speech. That is, the talker may take advantage of flexibility and plasticity to achieve acceptable speech even in the presence of a velopharyngeal mechanism that is — to a degree — lacking normal structure or needed range of motion. These hypotheses encourage the viewpoint that persons with velopharyngeal deficits can learn good speech through compensatory performance. Specific clinical applications should be submitted to experimental test.

AERODYNAMIC REGULATION AND CONTROL

The motor control theories cited so far are directed to the accomplishment of speech acceptable to listeners. Warren [167] wrote that speech motor control is directed more to aerodynamic performance than to acoustic accuracy. He cited literature which indicates the importance of the control of subglottal air pressure, intraoral air pressure, and other aerodynamic variables during speech. He wrote that in motor control terms, production of obstruents requires hypothetical respiratory and articulatory systems that form a coordinative structure that regulates speech pressures.

Warren discussed the regulation and control of aeromechanical variables. Regulation refers to the maintenance of a parameter at a steady level, and control is the means whereby regulation is achieved. From this perspective, compensatory articulations shown by the patient with velopharyngeal incompetency serve a control function in the regulation of intraoral air pressure. Warren cited tongue carriage and speech-timing variables as examples of compensatory speech. He noted that his regulation-control hypothesis explains the origin of compensatory articulations. Those articulations are maintained after surgery because the surgery does not change the control used by the patient.

This section has contrasted open- and closed-loop control, and selected theoretical perspectives have been presented that are compatible with physiological information introduced in earlier sections. Much worthy writing on this topic has not been cited, but the information presented indicates that within limits, a given speaking goal may be achieved in different ways. It should not surprise us that individuals respond in different ways to inability to achieve velopharyngeal closure. Also, there is some potential for compensation for physiological disabilities including those involving the velopharyngeal mechanism. If we are to understand that potential at the empirical level of clinical management, we must deal with somesthesis operationally and we must test means of using somesthesis and other sensory information in speech teaching. Next we turn to the psychophysics of somesthesis.

THE PSYCHOPHYSICS OF SOMESTHESIS AND SPEECH MOTOR CONTROL

Let us shift attention back to the assessment of oral sensory capability. Feedback during speech has been disrupted in many ways. For example, auditory feedback has been delayed, filtered, amplified, and attenuated [12, 154]. Here we review studies of the disruption of oral somesthetic function in speech by anesthetization. Also, we review psychophysical measures and oral sensory tests that have been employed or developed for the quantification of oral sensory function and the identification of oral sensory variables important to speech production and remediation.

ORAL ANESTHETIZATION

Oral sensory anesthetization has been utilized to determine the function of the sensory apparatus in speech production, and the data obtained have been interpreted in terms of capabilities a servosystem would require to control known speech phenomena [53, 121]. Studies have varied in the administration of anesthetization and in dependent variables studied. Both nerve block and topical anesthetization have been employed in this research.

INFLUENCE OF ANESTHETIZATION ON SPEECH

Much information has been gathered regarding speech function under different anesthetic conditions. This work began with the research of McCroskey and colleagues [100, 101]. Gammon and colleagues [42] used nerve block anesthesia in a study of articulation and stress-juncture. A 2% lidocaine (Xylocaine) solution was used in bilateral infraorbital, bilateral inferior alveolar, nasopalatine, and bilateral posterior palatine blocks that affected the lips, alveolar ridges, teeth, palate, and anterior two-thirds of the tongue. The authors found that stress-juncture distinctions between word pairs like *redcoat* and *red coat* or *impact* (verb) and *impact* (noun) were not destroyed by nerve block anesthesia. Rhythm and voice quality become progressively worse under the following conditions: auditory masking, nerve block anesthesia, and masking and anesthesia combined. Rhythm irregularities consisted of the intrusion of pauses within sentences. Few vowel articulation errors were observed in the study, but other articulation errors were common — especially for fricatives and affricates with labial or alveolar place of articulation. Coleman and Schliesser [27] reported that under anesthetic conditions similar to those used in the Gammon study their subjects became deprived of any kinesthetic or positional sense of the tongue, in that subjects were oblivious of gross but passive tongue movements produced by use of a forceps to manipulate the tongue. Gammon and colleagues [43] replied that anesthetized subjects appear to be aware of their own active tongue movements. Corollary discharge may have been a factor in the observations they reported.

Scott and Ringel [140] commented that the study by Gammon and colleagues was addressed to phonemic errors of voicing, manner, and place of articulation and that information was needed regarding nonphonemic changes that might result from oral anesthetization. From their own research, which involved close phonetic transcription supplemented by spectrographic analysis of some recorded speech events, the authors concluded that most articulatory changes under anesthesia were nonphonemic in nature and involved less close fricative constrictions, retracted place of articulation, and loss of retroflection. In a related study Scott and Ringel [141] reported that sensorily deprived speakers tended to retract intended alveolar and velar stops.

Hardcastle [52] studied one subject by means of spectrographic and electropalatographic techniques while the individual was under various combinations of masking noise, topical anesthesia, and unilateral lingual nerve block anesthesia. Altered auditory and tactile feedback was associated with overshooting of target articulation, especially for the /s/ and /ʃ/, greater area of tongue-palate contact, higher fricative frequency, and more frontal place of articulation. Fletcher [36] noted that the groove used for air passage in the articulation of sibilant fricatives may be narrowed under anesthetization.

Putnam and Ringel [118] found that stop portions of /sp/ clusters lacked complete closure of the oral cavity and the area of lip opening tended to be much less for the release phase of /p/ in *peat* and *speed* under anesthesia than in normal speech. Horii and colleagues [61] observed reduction in high-frequency spectral components, temporal disorganization manifested as decreases in rate of utterance and prolongation of voiced syllabic nuclei, and higher and more variable fundamental frequency. Hutchinson and Putnam [63] reported elevated intraoral air pressure and air flow rate which they interpreted to indicate adjustments made in the interest of obtaining increased sensory data to guide articulators to appropriate targets. Prosek and House [117] reported that subjects moved the tongue carriage posteriorly and spoke at a slower rate. Altered lip and tongue activity resulted in minor articulatory imprecision. Intraoral air pressure was slightly greater during consonants.

Borden, Harris, and Oliver [15] found speakers to be highly variable in their response to bilateral mandibular nerve blocks, but a high degree of intelligibility was retained by all speakers. Kramer and colleagues [73] studied co-articulation under nerve block anesthetization in two normal adult subjects. The frequency of the second formant was taken as an index to the positions of the lips and tongue. Stop gap duration and other variables were measured from spectrograms. Anesthetization had little effect on the measures studied, and the authors concluded that oral sensory feedback is not critical to co-articulation and that co-articulation is probably controlled by central mechanisms. In a related study, Kelso and Tuller [68] studied the frequencies of the first and second formants of /i/, /ɑ/, /u/ in isolation and consonant-vowel-consonant (CVC) syllables under auditory masking, bite-block perturbation, topical anesthetization of the oral mucosa, bilateral nerve block anesthetization of the temporomandibular joints, and combinations. The subjects were normal adults. According to a closed-loop control model, distortion of the formant frequencies would be expected but little occurred even when the several disruptions were presented simultaneously. The authors rejected closed-loop control models in favor of a model that "argues that functional groupings of muscles, sometimes called synergies . . . or coordinative structures . . . exhibit behavior qualitatively similar to a (nonlinear) mass-spring system." A target is achieved regardless of starting conditions.

Siegel, Pick, and Garber [154] reviewed data which indicate that altered auditory and somesthetic feedback have greater effect on suprasegmental variables (intensity, pitch, and quality) than on articulation.

LIMITATIONS OF ANESTHETIZATION TECHNIQUES

Several investigators have noted that nerve block anesthetization may influence motor as well as sensory nerves [2, 54, 84, 93, 118, 140], and Borden, Harris, and Catena [14] indicated that anesthetization may cause drowsiness and central compensatory reorganization. Thus anesthetization as a method for the study of oral sensation and its role in speech is somewhat confounded. Abbs and Kennedy [3] wrote that anesthetization studies give subjects opportunity to use conscious and unconscious adaptation strategies. They recommended study of perturbations unexpected by the subject in studies of speech motor control. Bite-blocks and palatal plates have been used in such research [38, 68, 120].

Hardcastle [52] used a unilateral nerve block because a dental consultant advised him that bilateral blocks could be hazardous. While Borden, Harris, and Catena [14] noted that oral anestheti-

zation provides one of the few available means to alter the speech of normal adults, the technique should be used with care.

INTERPRETATION OF THE ORAL ANESTHETIZATION DATA

This research has been interpreted in different ways. Prosek and House [117] considered the possibility that sensitivity to air pressure contributes to control. They concluded that an open-loop mechanism is of primary importance in the control of articulation and that language rules direct the open-loop mechanism. Scott and Ringel [141] inferred that autonomous commands (target specifications) direct the speech mechanism in open-loop fashion but that closed-loop feedback contributes to refinement where especially precise articulation is required.

Hardcastle [52] concluded that auditory rather than touch-pressure feedback is important to the temporal control of those articulations involving small areas of contact with the palate, and Hutchinson and Putnam [63] stated that the temporal sequencing of speech appears to be independent of feedback. Borden, Harris, and Catena [14] noted that trigeminal nerve block anesthesia did not seem to influence temporal relationships among electromyographic (EMG) signals; they stated that disruption of temporal relationships by anesthesia should have more devastating effects on speech than they observed. They commented that oral sensory monitoring of speech movements may be important during speech learning but not later in life.

Abbs [1] studied jaw movements directly in place of acoustic or perceptual phonetic variables. He stated that because the latter two classes of variables are "removed from the actual motor output of the system by several transfer functions, they are very likely confounded by several levels of physical and perceptual distortion."

Putnam and Ringel [119] discussed the role of nervous system disorganization, reorganization, and compensation in speech anesthetization studies (see also Borden et al. [14]). Subjects may respond to oral anesthetization by use of various adjustments involving the CNS. Different individuals may compensate for sensory loss in different ways, and idiosyncratic articulatory adjustments may result. This is compatible with ideas of nervous system flexibility discussed earlier.

The several studies cited demonstrate that oral anesthetization disrupts many speech measures, but the disruptive effect is weak. While subjects differ in their speech responses to anesthetization, speech remains intelligible. The contribution of somesthetic feedback to speech skill is complex and flexible. Findings that hold for one subject or speech condition do not necessarily hold for others, and combinations of open- and closed-loop circuits are probably involved in speech.

Next let us consider work that has been directed to the measurement of oral sensibility and to the relationship of that sensibility to articulation and other variables. We are particularly interested in what speech somesthetic information is available to the patient with cleft palate and with its possible use in therapy. Also, can we measure individual differences in that sensibility? Tests and psychophysical measures have been used to assess touch-presure sensitivity, two-point discrimination, oral sensitivity to vibrations, the ability of subjects to answer questions about the location of their articulators during the production of different sounds, and other variables. Tests of oral stereognosis — sometimes called form recognition — have received extensive investigation.

MEASURES AND TESTS OF ORAL SOMESTHESIS

Ringel and colleagues [122, 123, 125, 126, 128, 129] developed a battery of procedures for use in assessment of oral somesthesis. Their measures included an index of sensitivity to the texture of sandpaper, mandibular kinesthesis, two-point discrimination, and oral form discrimination. Their two-point esthesiometer permitted control of force of presentation of points to tissue. Rutherford and McCall [134] described tests of tactile acuity, tactile localization, tactile pattern recognition, and kinesthetic pattern recognition.

Findings obtained through the use of the Ringel esthesiometer indicated that discrimination was most precise in the tongue tip and progressively less precise from finger tip through lip, soft palate, alveolar ridge, and thenar region of the hand. Thresholds were lower for midline than for lateral regions of a structure.

Oral two-point discrimination studies were reported by numerous authors [50, 80, 81, 99, 104]. The two sides of the tongue were observed by several authors to differ in two-point discrimination.

Threshold for sensitivity to touch-pressure is measured by stimulation with Frey's hairs, which are graduated relative to the pressure they will withstand before bending. This measure has been used to study recovery of tactile sensitivity in persons recovering from skin flaps [177].

Weiffenbach [168] and Weiffenbach and Thach [169] inferred oral sensitivity in infants from observation of reflexive tongue movements in response to tactual stimulation of the tongue with a nylon filament. Study of two infants with cleft palate indicated that one performed similarly to normal individuals and the other did not.

Siegenthaler and Hochberg [156] compared tongue tip reaction time to touch-pressure and auditory stimuli. The authors assumed that reaction time reflected the efficiency of the sensory channel. Lingual reaction times were shorter for touch-pressure than for the auditory stimuli studied.

The sensory system can be studied by observation of movements if other variables are kept constant. For active movements, somesthesis has been studied by judgments of position and by measurements of movement accuracy. Movement direction, distance, speed, and also accuracy of pressure production have all been studied [62, 152]. Several studies reported information about the ability of children and adults to report articulatory somesthetic information associated with the production of speech sounds [31, 32, 138]. Ruscello, Moreau, and Sholtis [133] found that misarticulating and normal-speaking children did not differ in their awareness of articulatory gestures, but that individual children may depart from the group mean and demonstrate poor skills on such tasks.

Fucci and associates [29, 39–41] developed and tested instrumental means for measuring the threshold of vibrotactile stimulation. The structure to be tested — often the anterior region of the tongue — is contacted with a vibrating probe. The frequency and amplitude of vibration are controlled by use of a sine wave generator and an amplifier. A clamp is used to prevent the spread of mechanical vibrations beyond the target area, and noise masks auditory information. These authors found that persons who misarticulate tend to have poorer oral sensory abilities than those who articulate normally. They found the tongue to be more sensitive than the lip but less so than a thumb site. They compared thresholds obtained with ascending and descending techniques, with pulsed and continuous stimuli, and with different psychophysical techniques. From a study of threshold and suprathreshold measures, Fucci,

Harris, and Petrosino [40] concluded that peripheral (threshold) and central (suprathreshold) somesthetic processing are independent. However, they noted that function may be different during threshold testing where the tongue is constrained and during speech where it moves. They also discussed the viewpoint that taction may involve external feedback that conveys information about the consequences of movement and internal feedback which is proprioceptive in nature. A thorough review of the work of Fucci and colleagues is beyond the scope of this chapter.

ORAL STEREOGNOSIS TESTING

Oral stereognosis, or form recognition, has been studied extensively [17, 18]. It has been described as a complex perception dependent on touch-pressure, kinesthesis, and other bodily senses and as reflecting overall oral sensory function [65, 174]. Semmes [142], however, differentiated between tests of object recognition and measures of sensory function. Her study of manual stereognosis in patients who had suffered penetrating wounds of the brain indicated that impairment of manual stereognosis results from sensory deficits but may occur in their absence. Impaired manual stereognosis was also associated with poor spatial awareness. Semmes noted that oral stereognosis is less likely than manual stereognosis to be impaired by brain lesions. Oral structures are in body midline and should obtain sensory information from at least one side of the brain.

Tests have been developed that require the matching of forms explored orally with forms or drawings studied visually [6, 7, 103, 144] (Fig. 17-2). This oral-to-visual matching procedure has been termed *intersensory matching* [82]. Reliability and item homogeneity data were reported for different test versions. Visual, oral, and manual exploration of forms was studied by Weinberg, Lyons, and Liss [171].

Ringel, Burk, and Scott [124] described an oral form discrimination procedure in which subjects studied orally first one test form and then a second (see Fig. 17-2B). Subjects were to report whether the forms were the same or different. This test procedure, which removed the visual system from the testing, was termed a *form discrimination task* [42]. Ringel and his associates initiated the same-different procedure partly because intersensory matching studies had not shown strong test score differences between persons with good articulation and those with poor

articulation. Two classes of items were used in this test: (1) those wherein both items in a pair were similar in geometric configuration, and (2) those wherein the two forms were from different geometric classes. Triangular, rectangular, oval, and biconcave items were used to tap different levels of discrimination activity. The test used 10 forms (see Fig. 17-2B). Fifty-five pairs were presented. Ten involved comparison of a form with itself (same), and 45 involved comparison of a form with a second form (different). The authors found the test differentiated to a statistically significant level between good and poor articulators in studies of both adults and children.

No item analysis of the item pairs in this test has been published; so, item homogeneity is not well understood [144]. An imbalance between the number of same and different pairs on a same-different measure can lead to an expectancy effect that biases the results [166]. Bishop, Ringel, and House [10] used a form discrimination (same-different) task wherein equal numbers of same and different item pairs were used in order to minimize subject response bias. Research using the same-different or form discrimination procedure was conducted by a number of investigators [78, 79, 82, 162, 178]. Much of this research was directed to test procedure issues. Landt and Fransson [76] studied speed as well as accuracy of form recognition.

Other oral form recognition or stereognosis test variations have employed geometric forms that varied in size, shape, thickness, and surface characteristics [59, 109, 176].

ORAL STEREOGNOSIS (FORM RECOGNITION) TEST FINDINGS

Some studies reported that subjects with cleft palate differed from normal individuals on oral form recognition measures [59, 116] and others found no difference [26, 96]. Andrews [4] reported that cleft palate subjects with poor articulation scores differed in oral stereognosis from normal subjects. However, cleft palate subjects with better speech did not differ from their age-matched controls. Covering the palate with a dental appliance did not influence stereognosis scores [112].

On the basis of an item factor analysis of their intersensory matching test, McDonald and Aungst [103] inferrred that oral form recognition is a general ability.

Arndt and his co-workers [6, 7] reported normative data for one intersensory match test

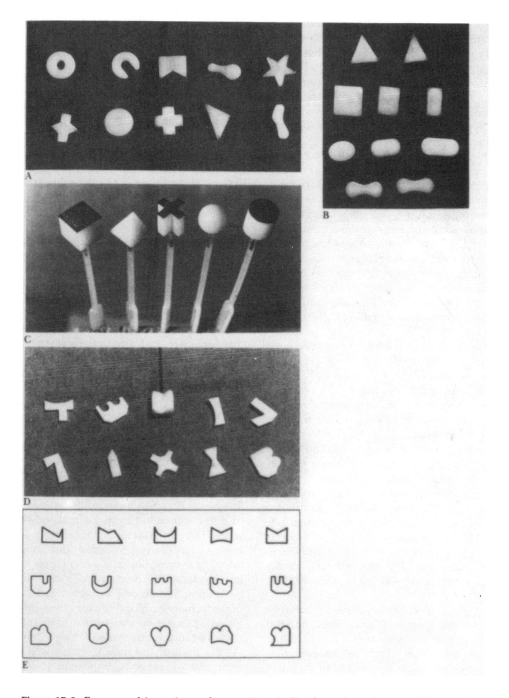

Figure 17-2. Forms used in testing oral recognition. A. Ten forms from the set of 20 sometimes called the NIDR (National Institute of Dental Research) 20. These forms were among the 25 used by McDonald and Aungst [103]. B. The remaining 10 forms from the NIDR set. These were also used in Ringel's [124] form discrimination test. C. The 5 forms that complete the set of 25 used by McDonald and Aungst. D. Ten forms added by Arndt et al. [7] to the preceding 25 items to produce a 35-item test. E. Multiple choice items employed in the test developed by Arndt et al. Multiple choice items were developed for each of the 35 items shown in A–D.

version. They did not find a significant correlation between form recognition and articulation in a sample of 15 children who made developmental articulatory errors [6]. However, in a subsequent cluster analysis study [7], some subject clusters were characterized by modestly poor performance on the Arndt oral form recognition measure. It was one of the few measures that differentiated between 26 children who misarticulated /r/ and 47 children who misarticulated /s/.

Thirteen- and 14-year-old children who spoke normally or who misarticulated /s/ or /r/ were compared by McNutt [105]. The /s/ children did not differ from the normal children on measures of oral stereognosis on a two-point discrimination, but they were slower on a diadochokinetic task. The /r/ children were inferior to the normal children on all three measures and to the /s/ children on between-class oral stereognosis items.

Numerous other investigators have used oral-to-visual or oral-to-oral form recognition measures in the study of misarticulating children [41, 85, 124, 127, 158, 170].

Oral form recognition has been correlated with tests of speech-sound discrimination [95, 107] and diadochokinesis [113, 114]. The only statistically significant result [95] involved a negative correlation between Ringel form discrimination scores and Wepman auditory discrimination scores in first-grade children.

Dental patients administered an oral form recognition test while under the influence of oral nerve block anesthetization functioned at a chance level [136] whereas dental students performed as well following bilateral mandibular block anesthesia as they did in the unanesthetized state [96]. Oral form recognition has been measured in stutterers and in persons with cerebral palsy, blindness, deafness, apraxia, dysarthria, and edentulousness [10, 11, 109, 130, 135, 161, 176].

The validity of these tests as bases for inferences about patients is not well established, and the differences among the tests make it difficult to interpret results. Arndt et al. [6] showed that many first-grade subjects responded to their test at a chance level, which indicates that the test is not suitable for them. Oral form recognition scores may help sort misarticulating children into subgroups, but they will not predict children's further articulation behavior. The inference that poor oral form recognition causes misarticulation does not seem warranted considering the descriptive-correlational nature of the research. A study involving subjects with cleft palate showed oral stereognosis to account for little speech variance. Pressel and Hochberg [116] noted that even though their children with surgically repaired clefts did differ in oral form recognition from children free from clefts, "the difference between group performance was dependent upon only 3.5 percent of inter-group variance." They concluded that the difference was not meaningful. This study and those of Arndt and colleagues [6, 7] suggest that oral form recognition probably accounts for very little variance that is clinically significant to the speech pathologist. On the other hand, if oral form recognition is independent of other variables related to disordered speech and captures speech variance that they miss, that could be a favorable outcome. Perhaps poor oral form recognition performance is associated with a particular type of misarticulation.

Schliesser [135] interpreted his study of speech and oral sensory variables in children with spastic hemiplegia to support the hypothesis that CNS organization of speech differs from that for other oral motor performance. He also concluded that oral sensory deficits may interfere with the automatization of skilled speech production movements.

This section has reviewed the influence of oral anesthetization on speech, means of measuring oral somesthesis, and somesthetic findings in different subject groups. Many means have been used to measure oral stereognosis or form recognition, touch-pressure threshold, two-point discrimination, and oral vibrotactile thresholds. Subjects with speech disorders have been found to differ somewhat from normal individuals on somesthetic measures but validity remains elusive — particularly predictive and construct validity. Oral sensation and articulation are probably moderately correlated. Relationships have been identified among variables, but knowledge of performance on oral sensory measures has not found a place in treatment planning. Information reviewed in this chapter so far also indicates that (1) the back of the mouth is less well endowed with sensory capacity important to articulation than is the front of the mouth; (2) the mouth is better at some sensory tasks than the eyes or hands but poorer at others; (3) a subject who demonstrates oral sensory deficit on one task may have other oral sensory resources that he can use to guide his motor performance; and (4) the palate appears to lack a mechanism for kinesthesis or position sense.

Next we turn to oral somesthesis and related matters as they pertain to speech therapy for the patient with cleft palate. We begin with consideration of development as it relates to oral sensation and to the treatment of patients.

DEVELOPMENT — MATURATION AND LEARNING

Witkop and colleagues [175] showed that a protein deficiency disease, kwashiorkor, is associated with poor oral stereognosis performance, communication disorder, and other problems of interest to the speech pathologist. This study reminds us that adequate nutrition and health underlie communication maturation and learning and the biological integrity on which they rest.

Bosma [19, 20] discussed mechanisms and processes of neurological development of the pharynx, larynx, and mouth. Motions evolve in conjunction with neurological maturation, and bulbar function, the cerebellum, hypothalamus, thalamus, and cerebrum are linked as the brain develops. Bosma noted that development is associated with loss of sensory neurons. He wrote [20] that inhibition is important to the development of skilled performance: "The superior quality of more mature motions is achieved by restraint." Bowman [23, 24] wrote that in early life exploratory tongue movements contribute to the establishment of a reciprocal relationship between lingual sensation and movement. "The reciprocal matching of sensory and motor processes occurs at a cortical level and forms an essential substrate for a central representation of oral function in which sensory transforms can specify motor events and vice versa" [24].

The role of different forms of feedback in speech control probably changes as the individual matures. Siegel and co-workers [154] cited views that auditory feedback may give way over time to somesthetic feedback relative to importance in speech. Speech in the normal individual may be gradually freed from some dependence on feedback.

Children may develop idiosyncratic patterns of velopharyngeal movement in speech. Netsell [111] described a boy who showed velopharyngeal opening during a string of /pa/ syllables but who achieved closure during such words as *puppy* and *puffy*. A boy with a repaired cleft palate whom we evaluated presented a similar pattern. He showed little or no velopharyngeal movement during strings of CV, VC, or CVC syllables, but approximated closure during [pap+apap+pap] uttered as a phrase. These observations were made with oral videoendoscopy.

Neurological differences may account for inconsistent velopharyngeal closure in some individuals with cleft palate [58, 106], and the inconsistency is probably orderly. Delay in physiological maturation may be involved in the disordered speech presented by some of these individuals. Netsell [111] referred to developmental dysarthrias in the form of subtle neuromotor delays, and he discussed differences in rates of development of cortical and subcortical regions of the brain. He wrote that orofacial maturation is sufficient at birth to serve vegetative functions, but further maturation is needed for speech. In the early years, children establish the neural schemata that will govern their speech. "Care should be taken in presenting phonetic stimulus materials to maximize early success as the children are forming perhaps the single most important mechanism of the speech motor system — that is, the internal associations of what it feels like to make the movements that generate the acoustics just produced" [111].

The following anecdote illustrates possible lingual sensorimotor maturation during a period of speech therapy. We provided therapy to a preschool boy who was born with a bilateral complete cleft. At 3½ years of age, this child drooled and was unable to elevate his tongue tip voluntarily. When asked to do so, he rolled his tongue to the side. Later, he used his fingers to elevate the tip. In a few months the drooling and rolling motion disappeared, and he developed the ability to use the tongue muscles to elevate the tongue tip. A portion of his therapy did involve his use of his tongue to remove sugar from the central alveolar ridge; initially he used the tongue blade to perform that task.

Jordan and colleagues [65] fitted normal and misarticulating first-grade boys with palatal plates equipped with touch-sensitive electrodes. The subjects performed nonspeech tongue positioning tasks under topical anesthetization and unanesthetized conditions. Performance was thought to reflect deep sensibility and kinesthesis since receptors mediating touch-pressure were anesthetized. The good-articulating boys performed better than those with poor articulation. However, the poor articulators improved their performance, thus indicating that they were not deficient in kinesthesis. The authors concluded that those boys made inefficient use of their sensory mechanisms but that it was unlikely that they presented mild neuroanatomical defects.

Folkins [37] considered the role of development as it pertains to plasticity and motor performance. He differentiated between maturation and cumulative learning. From a cumulative learning perspective, how a person responds to a learning task is in part a function of what was learned earlier. Earlier learning may impair later learning: "... once the motor system becomes more and more organized through learning, it may become progressively more difficult to reorganize some of the earlier levels." This contrasts with the maturation model which posits sensitive periods. Here what the person is ready to learn is a function of maturational readiness rather than past learning. Folkins discussed the implications of these two views for therapy planning: "The cumulative learning approach might lead one to investigate the motor processes that a patient has already learned and to relate them to ideas of how motor tasks are developed."

We know relatively little about changes that may occur in physiological readiness for speech on the part of preschool children with articulatory or sound patterning speech differences.

THERAPY

Some speech therapy for the correction of articulation errors involves conscious utilization of somesthetic senses and vision as well as auditory information. For example, McDonald's [102] sensorimotor therapy requires the patient to sense contacts and movements that occur during speech. Use of touch-pressure and kinesthetic cues is integral to the motor-kinesthetic method of speech therapy [165], and the speech clinician may attempt to improve palatal function by use of training intended to increase somesthetic awareness of the palate [9, 163]. Hodgson [69] reviewed use of vibrotactile stimulation in communication function and training for the deaf.

In a recent expression of a sensory facilitation therapy philosophy, Borden [13] advocated therapy to heighten kinesthesis. She likened this to learning auditory detection of allophonic variability that is normally ignored. To help clients make such distinctions, she uses amplification, selective filtering, and transduction of output into visual displays. She also said that pinching of the tongue enhances sense of position and movement. Borden noted that French *orthophonistes* (speech pathologists) use oral probes to increase oral tactile sensation. Vaughn and Clark [165] also described the use of sensory probes in speech therapy.

The practice of calling sensory cues to a patient's attention in therapy is not without controversy. Netsell [111] wrote that adults unconsciously generate speech movements and that children may develop speech movement control in a similar unconscious fashion. Therapy techniques that establish visual or somesthetic awareness of speech movements may be incompatible with control processes associated with normal speech development. Ling [83] commented that use of feedback devices in therapy is not easily made compatible with the complexities of the feedback processes reflected in the literature. Klein and Posner [72], in a review addressed to visual and kinesthetic components of skills, reported that the presence of a visual pattern can disrupt the acquisition of a kinesthetic pattern. Some speech pathologists recommend biofeedback for velopharyngeal function as a routine matter. Such advocacy begs a number of questions. Important among them are the matters of just what is the therapy, what characteristics must a patient present to be a candidate for such therapy, and precisely what outcome can be anticipated from it? If improved function is established through use of instrumental feedback, can it be maintained when that feedback is withdrawn?

The operation of closed-loop mechanisms in speech control appears to be limited. Neural impulses associated with position and movement may not reach the talker's awareness. If somesthetic cues are to be used in therapy, consideration should be given to the sorts of cues that are available to the learner and to how they might be employed. The clinician should not ask the patient to tune in nonavailable information. Early somesthetic monitoring therapy focused on the velum much more than the pharyngeal walls because the importance of pharyngeal wall movement was not appreciated. Pharyngeal wall movements intruded on the consciousness of few, if any, clinicians as they attempted to develop improved velar movements in their patients or research subjects.

The literature cited relative to motor control, flexibility, and plasticity does suggest that the patient has potential to perform articulatory compensation for disability. A case study by Fletcher [36] demonstrated that a patient with an unrepaired cleft palate had relatively high intelligibility and appeared to compensate for velopharyngeal opening by narrowing the oral groove used in the production of sibilant fricatives. The patient was successful at establishing lingual-palatal contacts in a nonspeech task — especially when biofeedback was provided. Fletcher discussed this patient's success in terms of motor control theory and observed that, "Adaptive possibilities are rarely driven to their limits." Shelton and McCauley [148] described skilled performance in the use of a hinged obturator demonstrated by an adult with an unrepaired cleft palate. The authors inferred that the individual had learned the performance.

In the next sections we examine data pertaining to the use of oral sensory information in therapy for the improvement of articulation and then for velopharyngeal function.

ORAL STEREOGNOSIS TRAINING AND ARTICULATION

Three studies were addressed to the influence of oral stereognosis training on articulation or vice versa. Wilhelm [173] used the oral form recognition test materials of Arndt and colleagues [6, 7] as training stimuli to teach form recognition to misarticulating children. Articulation improved. However, in a near replication [151], results were negative. Ruscello [131] reported that form recognition scores improved in children undergoing speech therapy. Studies have also tested treatments intended to increase velopharyngeal movement, awareness of velar position and movement, or both. Some of this work involved biofeedback.

VELOPHARYNGEAL MOVEMENT TRAINING: SOMESTHESIS AND BIOFEEDBACK

Shelton and colleagues [145, 147] conducted two training studies concerned with palatal kines-

thesis and movement. The first study [147] involved the ability of normal children and adults to learn to produce and report voluntary nonspeech palate elevations. Responses were described to subjects as they attempted velar elevation, and they observed their efforts in a mirror. Palate elevation was learned quickly, and most elevations following the command to elevate were reported. Unfortunately, subjects also reported elevations not evident to observers and failed to report 60 percent of the elevations that occurred prior to the command to elevate. Some subjects said that they could sense palatal movements, and others said that they could not. Muscle sense awareness of tension but not of position or movement [44], corollary discharge, or both may have been involved.

In a related study [145], two normal adults were instructed to produce nonspeech palate elevations to different heights on command. Maximal elevation was to be produced in response to the command "seven," and smaller elevations were to be produced for lower numbers. Information analysis of EMG data indicated that the subjects were able to raise the palate reliably to about two categories of elevation. Pain cues associated with surface EMG electrodes may have contributed to performance. The two studies suggest that somesthetic information about the palate is available but that it is not very precise. It seems unlikely that the training studied would contribute to the improvement of skilled, automatic use of the velopharyngeal mechanism during speech.

Other research has used biofeedback for the improvement of velopharyngeal movements and perhaps for the establishment of velopharyngeal competency [132]. Biofeedback employs instrumental display of visual or auditory information to guide motor performance. Instrumental sources of information substitute for or supplement bodily sensations.

Shprintzen, McCall, and Skolnick [153] used display of nasal emission to establish velopharyngeal closure for speech in individuals who closed during blowing but not during speech. Siegel-Sadewitz and Shprintzen [155] used videonasoendoscopy feedback to teach a normal adult subject to alter the contribution of her lateral pharyngeal walls to velopharyngeal closure. They inferred that there is physiological plasticity in the velopharyngeal sphincter and that learning has a role in the treatment of velopharyngeal disorder.

Shelton and colleagues [146, 149] used an oral panendoscope coupled to a television system to teach nonspeech palate elevations to two individuals with velopharyngeal disability. The improved performance by the latter two persons during training trials did not carry over to spontaneous speech.

Hoch and colleagues [146 149] referred to the use of tactile and kinesthetic cues in speech therapy for patients with cleft palate. Explicit techniques were not described except for palpation of the breathstream and closure of the nares to assist in oral direction of the airstream. What the patient was to sense during that maneuver was not explained. However, we have noted in some patients that closure of the nares blocks air and sound emission as though articulatory gestures were directing the airstream entirely through the nose. Closure of the nares combined with instruction seems to help these individuals learn to direct the airstream out the mouth.

Hoch and colleagues [58] also described use of videonasoendoscopy to train velopharyngeal function in patients who ranged in age from 6 through 29 years and who presented different types of inconsistent velopharyngeal closure —in some cases phoneme-specific openings. The subjects reportedly improved velopharyngeal function, perhaps through discovery or insight. In some cases pharyngeal flap operations followed treatment, and in other cases closure problems were resolved. The only failure among the nine patients involved an individual with a neurological disorder. Neither the articulation, the aeromechanical performance, nor the velopharyngeal movements of any of these patients were described in any detail. This therapy may have a place in service for patients who continue to present nasal air leakage after primary surgery and receipt of articulation-oriented speech therapy in the preschool years. However, it seems unlikely that it could be successfully delivered to younger subjects. It is important to note that the therapy required only four to nine sessions. An open-ended number of lessons is not justified.

The scheduling of therapies for velopharyngeal structure and function is another issue. Development of sound production skills and their phonemic patterning is enhanced by the availability of velopharyngeal competency. Some clinicians advocate surgical repair of palate clefts earlier than 18 months at which age theory has the child shifting from a word-based phonology to one that employes rule-governed use of sound segments [139]. If early repair is critical to speech development, then early delivery of any secon-dary services should also be considered. Perhaps obturation should be used between primary and secondary surgery when velopharyngeal insufficiency or incompetency is suspected in young children. There are no data to guide the scheduling of behavioral therapy for improved use of existing velopharyngeal structures.

DISCUSSION

The literature on therapy involving either somesthetic monitoring or instrumental biofeedback for patients with clefts is small, and support for use of oral sensory cues in either articulation therapy or velopharyngeal training is more a matter of advocacy than evidence. Instrumental biofeedback therapy may be justified in part by poor somesthetic awareness of velopharyngeal position and kinesthesis. Speech pathologists have recommended use of touch-pressure and kinesthesis in therapy, but they have also recognized that the application of these stimuli has limitations [35]. Regarding the palate, Morley [108] wrote that while a person may be able to control the palato-pharyngeal sphincter consciously during exercises, this control is seldom possible during speech.

The speech pathologist does wish to take advantage of somesthesis, motor control, flexibility, and plasticity to teach articulatory and prosodic skills and phonological patterning that will result in speech that is intelligible, acceptable, and meaningful to the listener. However, while respecting the ideas of equivalence, flexibility, and plasticity and their role in normal performance, discussed earlier in the chapter, we would not abandon the goal of standard production of sound segments in conversational speech unless the talker appeared to lack the wherewithal to achieve such production. By standard production we refer to phonetic textbook information about how most persons articulate consonants, vowels, and diphthongs. Articulatory gestures accepted as compensations may generalize to sounds where they are unneeded and unwanted. Cinefluoro-graphic observation of an adolescent patient with cleft palate showed him to use the tongue dorsum to obturate the velopharyngeal port and to use the tongue dorsum in the posterior place of articulation of many sounds: /t/, /d/, l/, /ʃ/, /s/. All but one of these sounds were acceptable to the ear during spontaneous conversation. The exception was /s/, which was noticeably distorted. The articulatory pattern described continued into the patient's adulthood. The /s/ was troublesome to him, and a short period of therapy at that time was not successful. Perhaps acceptance of posterior placement for /t/, /d/, /l/ and /ʃ/ generalized to intefere with /s/ learning.

We expect to teach oral articulation to the child with a normal velopharyngeal mechanism who for some reason has learned to direct one or a few sounds out the nose. Determination of the relative value of endoscopic feedback and articulation training for the resolution of this problem is a matter for research. In planning therapy for patients with cleft palate, one should determine whether they have the physical capability needed to benefit from the service. Velopharyngeal structural defects do constrain speech performance, and we do not expect therapy to solve the closure problems of individuals with gross velopharyngeal structural deficits or of persons who use substantial range of motion of velum and pharyngeal walls but fall short of the closure needed for good aeromechanical function. The latter persons may fall in a borderline closure competency category. We hypothesize, on the basis of the literature reviewed in this chapter and from clinical observation [150], that some patients with clefts do improve velopharyngeal function over time. This hypothesis should be tested through longitudinal observations based on instrumental measurement. Claims of treatment effectiveness must stand the tests of experimental control and replication.

Perhaps sensory facilitation of motor performance deserves more serious applied study than it has received in speech pathology to date. Questions include whether one's oral somesthesis can be heightened and, if so, if benefit accrues. How might one compensate for substandard somesthesis? Sensory techniques used in phonetic training can be tested experimentally. One such technique requires the patient to feel the tongue against the lateral maxillary teeth as part of positioning instruction for teaching /ɝ/ or for correcting a lateral lisp [45].

Progress in understanding somesthesis is almost miraculous. It was not until 1861 that the muscle spindle was first described [97], but since then remarkable technological developments have allowed elegant histological and electrophysiological investigation. Progress has also been made in the conceptualization of the role of somesthe-tic mechanisms in human functions, including speech. This progress is a source of satisfaction to persons sensitive to order and understanding. Much remains to be learned, however, if oral somesthesis, instrumental feedback, or a combination is to be employed effectively in therapy intended to improve velopharyngeal function. Experimental research is needed more than test development at this time. The speech pathologist looks to the speech scientist and the physiologist for leads to testable clinical hypotheses pertinent to articulatory-phonological therapies for the individual with developmental misarticulation and for the cleft palate patient with articulatory disability, velopharyngeal function deficit, or both. The applied work must involve the acquisition of skills and their patterning at an automatic level within the language system of the patient.

REFERENCES

1. Abbs, J. H. The influence of the gamma motor system on jaw movements during speech. *J. Speech Hear. Res.* 16:175, 1973.
2. Abbs, J. H., and Eilenberg, G. R. Peripheral Mechanisms of Speech Motor Control. In N. J. Lass (Ed.), *Contemporary Issues in Experimental Phonetics.* New York: Academic Press, 1976.
3. Abbs, J. H., and Kennedy, J. G. III. Neurophysiological Processes of Speech Movement Control. In N. J. Lass, L. V. McReynolds, J. L. Northern, and D. E. Yoder (Eds.), *Speech, Language, and Hearing.* Philadelphia: Saunders, 1982. Vol. 1.
4. Andrews, J. R. Oral form discrimination in individuals with normal and cleft palates. *Cleft Palate J.* 10:92, 1973.
5. Angevine, J. B. Basal Ganglia. In J. B. Angevine and D. G. Stuart (Eds.), *Neurosciences Course Syllabus.* Tucson: College of Medicine, University of Arizona, 1985.
6. Arndt, W. B., Elbert, M., and Shelton, R. L. Standardization of a Test of Oral Stereognosis. In J. F. Bosma (Ed.), *Second Symposium on Oral Sensation and Perception.* Springfield, Ill.: Thomas, 1970.
7. Arndt, W. B., Gauer, J., Shelton, R. L., Crary, D., and Chisum, L. Refinement of a Test of Oral Stereognosis. In J. F. Bosma (Ed.), *Second Symposium on Oral Sensation and Perception.* Springfield, Ill.: Thomas, 1970.
8. Arndt, W. B., Shelton, R. L., Johnson, A. F., and Furr, M. L. Identification and description of homogenous subgroups within a sample of misarticulating children. *J. Speech Hear. Res.* 20:263, 1977.
9. Berry, M. F., and Eisenson, J. *Speech Disorders.* New York: Appleton-Century-Crofts, 1957. P. 329.
10. Bishop, M. E., Ringel, R. L., and House, A. S. Orosensory perception in the deaf. *Volta Rev.* 74:289, 1972.
11. Bishop, M. E., Ringel, R. L., and House, A. S. Orosensory perception, speech production, and deafness. *J. Speech Hear. Res.* 16:257, 1973.
12. Borden, G. J. Use of feedback in established and developing speech. *Speech and Language: Advances in Basic Research and Practice* 3:233, 1980.
13. Borden, G. Consideration of Motor-Sensory Targets and a Problem of Perception. In H. Winitz (Ed.), *Treat-*

ing Articulation Disorders: For Clinicians by Clinicians. Austin: Pro-Ed, 1984.

14. Borden, G. J., Harris, K. S., and Catena, L. Oral feedback: II. An electromyographic study of speech under nerve-block anesthesia. *J. Phonetics* 1:297, 1973.

15. Borden, G. J., Harris, K. S., and Oliver, W. Oral feedback: I. Variability of the effect of nerve-block anesthesia upon speech. *J. Phonetics* 1:289, 1973.

16. Boring, E. G. *Sensation and Perception in the History of Experimental Psychology.* New York: Appleton-Century-Crofts, 1942.

17. Bosma, J. F. (Ed.). *Symposium on Oral Sensation and Perception.* Springfield, Ill.: Thomas, 1967.

18. Bosma, J. F. (Ed.). *Second Symposium on Oral Sensation and Perception.* Springfield, Ill.: Thomas, 1970.

19. Bosma, J. F. Anatomic and Physiologic Development of the Speech Apparatus. In E. L. Eagles (Ed.), *The Nervous System.* Vol. 3, *Human Communication and Its Disorders.* New York: Raven, 1975.

20. Bosma, J. F. Postnatal ontogeny of the pharynx, larynx, and mouth. *Am. Rev. Respir. Dis.* 131(Suppl. 10): 1985.

21. Bouman, H. D. Some considerations of the physiology of sensation. *J. Am. Phys. Ther. Assoc.* 451:573, 1965.

22. Bowman, J. P. *The Muscle Spindle and Neural Control of the Tongue: Implications for Speech.* Springfield, Ill.: Thomas, 1971.

23. Bowman, J. P. Lingual mechanoreceptive information I. An evoked potential study of the central projections of hypoglossal nerve afferent information. *J. Speech Hear. Res.* 25:348, 1982.

24. Bowman, J. P. Lingual mechanoreceptive information II. An evoked-potential study of the central projections of hypoglossal nerve afferent information. *J. Speech Hear. Res.* 25:357, 1982.

25. Buchwald, J. S. Basic mechanisms for motor learning. *J. Am. Phys. Ther. Assoc.* 45:314, 1965.

26. Catalanotto, F. A., and Moss, J. L. Manual and oral stereognosis in children with cleft palate, gonadal dysgenesis, pseudohypoparathyroidism, oral facial digital syndrome, and Kallman's syndrome. *Arch. Oral Biol.* 48: 1127, 1973.

27. Coleman, R. O., and Schliesser, H. F. Comment on "Articulation and stress/juncture production under oral anesthetization and masking." *J. Speech Hear. Res.* 15:669, 1972.

28. Cooper, S. Muscle spindles in the intrinsic muscles of the tongue. *J. Physiol.* 122:193, 1953.

29. Curtis, A. P., and Fucci, D. Sensory and motor changes during development and aging. *Speech and Language: Advances in Basic Research and Practice* 9:153, 1983.

30. Curtis, J. F. Segmenting the Stream of Speech. In J. Griffith and L. E. Miner (Eds.), *The First Lincolnland Conference on Dialectology.* University, Ala.: University of Alabama Press, 1970.

31. Daniloff, R., and Adams, M. Verbalizable knowledge of certain speech articulations. *J. Commun. Disord.* 8:343, 1975.

32. Daniloff, R., Percifield, P., Montgomery, A., and Hampton, J. Children's articulatory and auditory awareness of differences between vowel sounds. *J. Commun. Disord.* 8:335, 1975.

33. Daniloff, R., Schuckers, G., and Feth, L. *The Physiology of Speech and Hearing: An Introduction.* Englewood Cliffs, N.J.: Prentice-Hall, 1980.

34. Eldred, E. The dual sensory role of muscle spindles. *J. Am. Phys. Ther. Assoc.* 45:290, 1965. P. 306.

35. Fairbanks, G. Systematic research in experimental phonetics: 1: A theory of the speech mechanism as a servosystem. *J. Speech Hear. Disord.* 19:133, 1954.

36. Fletcher, S. G. Speech production and oral motor skill in an adult with an unrepaired palatal cleft. *J. Speech Hear. Disord.* 50:254, 1985.

37. Folkins, J. W. Issues in speech motor control and their relation to the speech of individuals with cleft palate. *Cleft Palate J.* 22:106, 1985.

38. Folkins, J. W., and Linnville, R. D. The effects of varying lower-lip displacement on upper-lip movements: Implications for the coordination of speech movements. *J. Speech Hear. Res.* 26:209, 1983.

39. Fucci, D., and Crary, M. A. Oral vibrotactile sensation and perception: State of the art. *Speech and Language: Advances in Basic Research and Practice* 2:321, 1979.

40. Fucci, D., Harris, D., and Petrocino, L. Threshold and suprathreshold correlations for the oral tactile sensory mechanism. *J. Speech Hear. Res.* 28:331, 1985.

41. Fucci, D., and Robertson, J. H. "Functional" defective articulation: An oral, sensorimotor disturbance. *Percept. Mot. Skills* 33:711, 1971.

42. Gammon, S. A., Smith, P. J., Daniloff, R. G., and Kim, C. W. Articulaton and stress/juncture production under oral anesthetization and masking. *J. Speech Hear. Res.* 14:271, 1971.

43. Gammon, S. A., Smith, P. J., Daniloff, R. G., and Kim, C. W. A reply to Coleman and Shliesser's "Comment on articulation and stress/juncture production under oral anesthetization and masking." *J. Speech Hear. Res.* 15:671, 1972.

44. Geldard, F. A. *The Human Senses.* New York: Wiley, 1953.

45. Gerber, A. *Goal Carryover: An Articulation Manual and Program.* Philadelphia: Temple University Press, 1973.

46. Gibson, J. J. Observations on active touch. *Psychol. Rev.* 69:477, 1962.

47. Gibson, J. J. *The Senses Considered as Perceptual Systems.* Boston: Houghton Mifflin, 1966.

48. Granit, R. *Receptors and Sensory Perception.* New Haven: Yale University Press, 1955.

49. Grossman, R. C., and Hattis, B. F. Oral Mucosal Sensory Innervation and Sensory Experience. In J. F. Bosma (Ed.), *Symposium on Oral Sensation and Perception.* Springfield, Ill.: Thomas, 1967.

50. Grossman, R. C., Hattis, B. F., and Ringel, R. L. Oral tactile experience. *Arch. Oral Biol.* 10:691, 1965.

51. Guyton, A. C. *Textbook of Medical Physiology* (6th ed.). Philadelphia: Saunders, 1981.

52. Hardcastle, W. J. Some aspects of speech production under controlled conditions of oral anesthesia and auditory masking. *J. Phonetics* 3:197, 1975.

53. Hardy, J. C. Development of Neuromuscular Systems Underlying Speech Production. In R. T. Wertz (Ed.), *Speech and the Dentofacial Complex: The State of the Art.* ASHA Reports No. 5. Washington, D.C.: American Speech and Hearing Association, 1970.

54. Harris, K. S. EMG and Fiberoptic Studies. In R. T. Wertz (Ed.), *Speech and the Dentofacial Complex: The State of the Art.* ASHA Reports No. 5. Washington, D.C.: American Speech and Hearing Association, 1970.

55. Hasan, Z. Receptors in Muscles and Joints. In J. B. Angevine and D. G. Stuart (Eds.), *Neurosciences Course Syllabus.* Tucson: College of Medicine, University of Arizona, 1985.

56. Henneman, E. Organization of the Motor Systems — A Preview. In V. B. Mountcastle (Ed.), *Medical Physiology*

(13th ed.). St. Louis: Mosby, 1974.

57. Hixon, T. J., and Hardy, J. C. Restricted motility of the speech articulators. *J. Speech Hear. Disord.* 29:293, 1964.

58. Hoch, L., Golding-Kushner, K., Siegel-Sadewitz, V. L., and Shprintzen, R. J. Speech Therapy. *Sem. Speech Lang.* 7:297, 1986.

59. Hochberg, I., and Kabcenell, J. Oral stereognosis in normal and cleft palate individuals. *Cleft Palate J.* 4:47, 1967.

60. Hodgson, W. R. Special Cases of Hearing Aid Assessment. In W. R. Hodgson (Ed.), *Hearing Aid Assessment and Use in Audiologic Rehabilitation* (3rd ed.). Baltimore: Williams & Wilkins, 1986.

61. Horii, Y., House, A. S., Ki, K., and Ringel, R. L. Acoustic characteristics of speech produced without oral sensation. *J. Speech Hear. Res.* 16:67, 1973.

62. Howard, I. P., and Templeton, W. B. *Human Spatial Orientation.* London: Wiley, 1966.

63. Hutchinson, J. M., and Putnam, A. H. B. Aerodynamic aspects of sensory deprived speech. *J. Acoust. Soc. Am.* 56:1612, 1974.

64. Johnson, A. F., Shelton, R. L., Arndt, W. B., and Furr, M. L. Factor analysis of measures of articulation, language, auditory processing, reading-spelling, and maxillofacial structure. *J. Speech Hear. Res.* 20:319, 1977.

65. Jordan, L. S., Hardy, J. C., and Morris, H. L. Performance of children with good and poor articulation on tasks of tongue placement. *J. Speech Hear. Res.* 21:429, 1978.

66. Kawamura, Y. A. Role of Oral Afferents for Mandibular and Lingual Movements. In J. F. Bosma (Ed.), *Second Symposium on Oral Sensation and Perception.* Springfield, Ill.: Thomas, 1970.

67. Kelso, J. A. S. Pattern Formation in Speech and Limb Movements Involving Many Degrees of Freedom. In H. Heuer and C. Fromm (Eds.), *Generation and Modulation of Action Patterns.* Experimental Brain Research Series; 15:105. Berlin: Springer-Verlag, 1986.

68. Kelso, J. A. S., and Tuller, B. "Compensatory articulation" under conditions of reduced afferent information: A dynamic formulation. *J. Speech Hear. Res.* 26:217, 1983.

69. Kennedy, J. G., III, and Abbs, J. H. Basic Neurophysiological Mechanisms Underlying Oral Communication. In N. J. Lass, L. V. McReynolds, J. L. Northern, and D. E. Yoder (Eds.), *Speech, Language, and Hearing* Vol. 1 *Normal Processes.* Philadelphia: Saunders, 1982.

70. Kent, R. D. Models of Speech Production. In N. J. Lass (Ed.), *Contemporary Issues in Experimental Phonetics.* New York: Academic Press, 1976.

71. Kent, R. D. Articulatory-Acoustic Perspectives on Speech Development. In R. Stark (Ed.), *Language Behavior in Infancy and Early Childhood.* New York: Elsevier, 1981.

72. Klein, R. M., and Posner, M. I. Attention to visual and kinesthetic components of skills. *Brain Res.* 71:401, 1974.

73. Kramer, M. B., Hoffman, P. R., Daniloff, R. G., and Wilcox, K. Effects of lingual anesthetization upon lingualabial coarticulation. *Phonetica* 39:83, 1982.

74. Kuehn, D. P., Folkins, J. W., and Cutting, C. B. Relationships between muscle activity and velar position. *Cleft Palate J.* 19:25, 1982.

75. Kuehn, D. P., Folkins, J. W., and Linnville, R. N. An electromyographic study of the musculus uvulae. *Cleft Palate J.* 25:348, 1988.

76. Landt, H., and Fransson, B. Oral ability to recognize forms and oral muscular coordination activity in dentulous and elderly adults. *J. Oral Rehab.* 2:125, 1975.

77. Lashley, K. S. The Problem of Serial Order in Behavior. In L. A. Jeffress (Ed.), *Cerebral Mechanism in Behavior* (the Hixon Symposium). New York: Wiley, 1951.

78. Lass, N. J., Bell, R. R., Simcoe, J. C., McClung, N. J., and Park, W. E. Assessment of Oral tactile perception: Some methodological considerations. *Cent. States Speech J.* 23:165, 1972.

79. Lass, N. J., and Clay, T. H. The effect of memory on subject peformance on a test of oral form discrimination. *West. Speech* 37:27, 1973.

80. Lass, N. J., Kotchek, C. L., and Deem, J. F. Oral two-point discrimination: Further evidence of asymmetry on right and left sides of selected oral structures. *Percept. Mot. Skills* 35:59, 1972.

81. Lass, N. J., and Park, W. E. Oral two-point discrimination: Consistency of two-point limens on selected oral sites. *Percept. Mot. Skills* 37:881, 1973.

82. Lass, N. J., Tekieli, M. E., and Eye, M. P. A comparative study of two procedures for assessment of oral tactile perception. *Cent. States Speech J.* 22:21, 1971.

83. Ling, D. *Speech and the Hearing Impaired Child: Theory and Practice.* Washington, D.C.: Alexander Graham Bell Association for the Deaf, 1976.

84. Locke, J. L. A methodological consideration in kinesthetic feedback research. *J. Speech Hear. Res.* 11:668, 1968.

85. Locke, J. L. Oral perception and articulation learning. *Percept. Mot. Skills* 26:1259, 1968.

86. Lowe, A. A. The neural regulation of tongue movements. *Prog. Neurobiol.* 15:295, 1981.

87. Lowe, A. A. Tongue movements — Brainstem mechanisms and clinical postulates. *Brain Behav. Evol.* 25:128, 1984.

88. Lubker, J. F. Some Teleological Considerations of Velopharyngeal Function. In R. G. Daniloff (Ed.), *Articulation Assessment and Treatment Issues.* Boston: College-Hill Press, 1984.

89. Luce, P. A., and Pisoni, D. B. Speech Perception: New Directions in Research, Theory and Applications. In H. Winitz (Ed.), *Human Communication and Its Disorders: A Review — 1987.* Norwood, N.J.: Ablex, 1987.

90. Luders, H., Lesser, R. P., Dinner, D. S., Hahn, J. F., Salanga, V., and Morris, H. H. The second sensory area in humans: Evoked potential and electrical stimulation studies. *Ann. Neurol.* 17:177, 1985.

91. MacNeilage, P. F. Motor control of serial ordering of speech. *Psychol. Rev.* 77:182, 1970.

92. MacNeilage, P. F. Speech Physiology. In J. H. Gilbert (Ed.), *Speech and Cortical Functioning.* New York: Academic Press, 1972.

93. MacNeilage, P. F., and MacNeilage, L. A. Central Processes Controlling Speech Production During Sleep and Waking. In F. A. McGuigan and R. A. Schoonover (Eds.), *The Psychophysiology of Thinking.* New York: Academic, 1973.

94. MacNeilage, P. F., Roots, T. P., and Chase, R. C. Speech production and perception in a patient with severe impairment of somesthetic perception and motor control. *J. Speech Hear. Res.* 10:449, 1967.

95. Madison, C. I., and Fucci, D. J. Speech-sound discrimination and tactile-kinesthetic discrimination in reference to speech production. *Percept. Mot. Skills* 33:831, 1971.

96. Mason, R. M. Studies of Oral Perception Involving Subjects with Alterations in Anatomy and Physiology. In J. F. Bosma (Ed.), *Symposium on Oral Sensation and Perception.* Springfield, Ill.: Thomas, 1967.

97. Matthews, P. B. C. *Mammalian Muscle Receptors and Their Central Actions.* London: Edward Arnold, 1972.

98. Matthews, P. B. C. Muscle afferents and kinesthesia. *Br. Med. Bull.* 33:137, 1977.

99. McCall, G. N., and Cunningham, N. M. Two-point discrimination: Asymmetry in spatial discrimination on the two sides of the tongue, a preliminary report. *Percept. Mot. Skills* 32:368, 1971.

100. McCroskey, R. L., Jr. The relative contribution of auditory and tactile cues to certain aspects of speech. *South. Speech J.* 24:84, 1958.

101. McCroskey, R. L., Jr., Corley, N. W., and Jackson, G. Some effects of disrupted tactile cues upon the production of consonants. *South. Speech J.* 25:55, 1959.

102. McDonald, E. T. *Articulation Testing and Treatment: A Sensory Motor Approach.* Pittsburgh: Stanwix House, 1964.

103. McDonald, E. T., and Aungst, L. F. Independence of Oral Sensory Functions and Articulatory Proficiency. In J. F. Bosma (Ed.), *Second Symposium on Oral Sensation and Perception.* Springfield, Ill.: Thomas, 1970.

103a. McDonald, R. *The Goodbye Look.* New York: Bantam.

104. McNutt, J. C. Assymmetry in two-point discrimination on the tongues of adults and children. *J. Commun. Disord.* 8:213, 1975.

105. McNutt, J. C. Oral sensory and motor behaviors of children with /s/ or /r/ misarticulations. *J. Speech Hear. Res.* 20:694, 1977.

106. McWilliams, B. J., Morris, H. L., and Shelton, R. L. *Cleft Palate Speech.* Philadelphia: Decker, 1984.

107. Moreau, V. K., and Lass, N. J. A correlational study of stimulability, oral form discrimination and auditory discrimination skills in children. *J. Commun. Disord.* 7:269, 1974.

108. Morley, M. E. *Cleft Palate and Speech* (2nd ed.). Edinburgh: Livingstone, 1951.

109. Moser, H., LaGourgue, J. R., and Class, L. Studies of Oral Stereognosis in Normal, Blind, and Deaf Subjects. In J. F. Bosma (Ed.), *Symposium on Oral Sensation and Perception.* Springfield, Ill.: Thomas, 1967.

110. Mountcastle, V. B. Neural Mechanisms in Somesthesis. In V. B. Mountcastle (Ed.), *Medical Physiology* (14th ed.). St. Louis: Mosby, 1980.

111. Netsell, R. *A Neurobiologic View of Speech Production and the Dysarthrias.* Boston: College-Hill Press, 1986.

112. Oliver, R. G. Oral form recognition with and without palatal coverage. *Br. J. Disord. Commun.* 20:201, 1985.

113. Oliver, R. G., Jones, M. G., and Smith, A. Oral stereognosis and diadochokinetic tests in children and young adults. *Br. J. Disord. Commun.* 20:271, 1985.

114. Oliver, R. G., Lewis, P., and Stokes, J. The relationship between oral stereognostic and diadochokinetic skills and oral morphology — a pilot study with groups of speech-handicapped and normal subjects. *J. Paediatr. Dent.* 2:67, 1986.

115. Perkins, W. H., and Kent, R. D. *Functional Anatomy of Speech, Language, and Hearing.* Boston: College-Hill Press, 1986.

116. Pressel, G., and Hochberg, I. Oral form discrimination of children with cleft palate. *Cleft Palate J.* 11:66, 1974.

117. Prosek, R. A., and House, A. S. Intraoral air pressure as a feedback cue in consonant production. *J. Speech Hear. Res.* 18:133, 1975.

118. Putnam, A. H. B., and Ringel, R. L. Some observations of articulation during labial sensory deprivation. *J. Speech Hear. Res.* 15:529, 1972.

119. Putnam, A. H. B., and Ringel, R. L. A cineradiographic study of two talkers with temporarily induced oral sensory deprivation. *J. Speech Hear. Res.* 19:247, 1976.

120. Putnam, A. H. B., Shelton, R. L., and Kastner, C. U. Intraoral air pressure and oral air flow under different bleed and bite-block conditions. *J. Speech Hear. Res.* 29:37, 1986.

121. Ringel, R. L., Oral Sensation and Perception: A Selective Review. In R. T. Wertz (Series Ed.) and J. E. Fricke (Project Dir.), *Speech and the Dentofacial Complex: The State of the Art.* ASHA Report No. 5. Washington, D.C.: American Speech and Hearing Association, 1970.

122. Ringel, R. L. Studies of Texture Perception by Oral Region Structures. In J. F. Bosma (Ed.), *Second Symposium on Oral Sensation and Perception.* Springfield, Ill.: Thomas, 1970.

123. Ringel, R. L. Oral Region Two-Point Discrimination in Normal and Myopathic Subjects. In J. F. Bosma (Ed.), *Second Symposium on Oral Sensation and Perception.* Springfield, Ill.: Thomas, 1970.

124. Ringel, R. L., Burke, K. W., and Scott, C. M. Tactile Perception: Form Discrimination in the Mouth. In J. F. Bosma (Ed.), *Second Symposium on Oral Sensation and Perception.* Springfield, Ill.: Thomas, 1970.

125. Ringel, R. L., and Ewanowski, S. J. Oral perception: I. Two-point discrimination. *J. Speech Hear. Res.* 8:389, 1965.

126. Ringel, R. L., and Fletcher, H. M. Oral perception: III. Texture discrimination. *J. Speech Hear. Res.* 10:642, 1967.

127. Ringel, R. L., House, A. S., Burk, K. W., Dolinsky, J. P., and Scott, C. M. Some relations between orosensory discrimination and articulatory aspects of speech sound production. *J. Speech Hear. Disord.* 35:3, 1970.

128. Ringel, R. L., Saxman, J. H., and Brooks, A. R. Oral perception: II. Mandibular kinesthesia. *J. Speech Hear. Res.* 10:637, 1967.

129. Ringel, R. L., and Steer, M. D. Some effects of tactile and auditory alterations on speech output. *J. Speech Hear. Res.* 6:369, 1963.

130. Rosenbek, J. C., Wertz, R. T., and Darley, F. L. Oral sensation and perception in apraxia of speech and aphasia. *J. Speech Hear. Res.* 6:369, 1973.

131. Ruscello, D. M. *Articulation Improvement and Oral Tactile Changes in Children.* Thesis, University of West Virginia, Morgantown, W. Va., 1972.

132. Ruscello, D. M. A selected review of palatal training procedures. *Cleft Palate J.* 19:181, 1982.

133. Ruscello, D. M., Moreau, V. K., and Sholtis, D. Awareness of certain articulatory gestures in normal-speaking and articulatory-defective children. *J. Commun. Disord.* 13:59, 1980.

134. Rutherford, D., and McCall, G. Testing Oral Sensation and Perception in Persons with Dysarthria. In J. F. Bosma (Ed.), *Symposium on Oral Sensation and Perception.* Springfield, Ill.: Thomas, 1967.

135. Schliesser, H. F. *Restricted Motility of the Speech Articulators and Selected Discriminative Modalities of Speech Defective Spastic Hemiplegic Children.* Dissertation, University of Iowa, Iowa City, 1965.

136. Schliesser, H. F., and Coleman, R. O. Effectiveness of certain procedures for alteration of auditory and oral

tactile sensation for speech. *Percept. Mot. Skills* 26:275, 1968.

137. Schmidt, R. F., Somatovisceral Sensibility: Cutaneous Senses, Proprioception, and Pain. In R. F. Schmidt and G. Thews (Ed.), *Human Physiology.* New York: Springer-Verlag, 1983.

138. Schuckers, G. H., Daniloff, R. G., Cieszkiewicz-Sciackitano, G., and Thompson, R. P. Children's verbal awareness of articulatory gestures. *J. Commun. Disord.* 7:239, 1974.

139. Schwartz, R. G. The Phonological System. In J. Costello (Ed.), *Speech Disorders in Children.* Boston: College-Hill Press, 1984.

140. Scott, C. M., and Ringel, R. L. Articulation without oral sensory control. *J. Speech Hear. Res.* 14:804, 1971.

141. Scott, C. M., and Ringel, R. L. The effects of motor and sensory disruptions on speech: A description of articulation. *J. Speech Hear. Res.* 14:819, 1971.

142. Semmes, J. Manual Stereognosis after Brain Injury. In J. F. Bosma (Ed.), *Symposium on Oral Sensation and Perception.* Springfield, Ill.: Thomas, 1967.

143. Semmes, J. Somesthetic Effects of Damage to the Central Nervous System. In A. Iggo (Ed.), *Handbook of Sensory Physiology* Vol. 2, *Somatosensory System.* New York: Springer-Verlag, 1973.

144. Shelton, R. L., Arndt, W. B., and Hetherington, J. J. Testing Oral Stereognosis. In J. F. Bosma (Ed.), *Symposium on Oral Sensation and Perception.* Springfield, Ill.: Thomas, 1967.

145. Shelton, R. L., Harris, K. S., Scholes, G. N., and Dooley, P. M. Study of Non-Speech Voluntary Palate Movements by Scaling and Electromyographic Techniques. In J. F. Bosma (Ed.), *Second Symposium on Oral Sensation and Perception.* Springfield, Ill.: Thomas, 1970.

146. Shelton, R. L., Beaumont, K. B., Trier, W. C., and Furr, M. L. Videopanendoscopic feedback in training velopharyngeal closure. *Cleft Palate J.* 15:6, 1978.

147. Shelton, R. L., Knox, A. W., Elbert, M., and Johnson, T. S. Palate Awareness and Non-Speech Voluntary Palate Movement. In J. F. Bosma (Ed.), *Second Symposium on Oral Sensation and Perception.* Springfield, Ill.: Thomas, 1970.

148. Shelton, R. L., and McCauley, R. J. Use of a hinge-type speech prosthesis. *Cleft Palate J.* 23:312, 1986.

149. Shelton, R. L., Paesani, A., McClelland, K. D., and Bradfield, S. S. Panendoscopic feedback in the study of voluntary velopharyngeal movements. *J. Speech Hear. Dis.* 40:232, 1975.

150. Shelton, R. L., and Ruscello, D. M. Palatal and articulation training in patients with velopharyngeal closure problems. Presented at the convention of the American Cleft Palate Association, San Diego, 1979.

151. Shelton, R. L., Willis, V., Johnson, A. F., and Arndt, W. B. Oral reform recognition training and articulation change. *Percept. Mot. Skills* 26:523, 1973.

152. Sherrick, C. E. Somesthetic senses. *Ann. Rev. Psychol.* 17:309, 1966.

153. Shprintzen, R. J., McCall, G. N., and Skolnick, M. L. A new therapeutic technique for the treatment of velopharyngeal incompetence. *J. Speech Hear. Disord.* 40:69, 1975.

154. Siegel, G. M., Pick, H. L., Jr., and Garber,S. R. Auditory feedback and speech development. *Adv. Child Dev. Behav.* 18:49, 1984.

155. Siegel-Sadewitz, V. L., and Shprintzen, R. J. Nasopharyngoscopy of the normal velopharyngeal sphincter:

An experiment in biofeedback. *Cleft Palate J.* 19:747, 1982.

156. Siegenthaler, B. M., and Hochberg, I. Reaction time of the tongue to auditory and tactile stimulation. *Percept. Mot. Skills* 21:387, 1965.

157. Skinner, P. H. Speech and Hearing in Communication. In P. H. Skinner and R. L. Shelton (Eds.), *Speech, Language and Hearing: Normal Processes and Disorders.* New York: Wiley, 1985.

158. Sommers, R. K., Cox, S., and West, C. Articulatory effectiveness, stimulability, and children's performances on perceptual and memory tasks. *J. Speech Hear. Res.* 15:579, 1972.

159. Sussman, H. M. What the tongue tells the brain. *Psychol. Bull.* 77:262, 1972.

160. Tueber, H. Formal discussion. In U. Bellugi and R. Brown (Eds.), The Acquisition of Language. *Monogr. Soc. Res. Child Dev.* 29:1, 1964.

161. Tiexeria, L. A., DeFran, R. H., and Nichols, A. C. Oral stereognostic differences between apraxics, dysarthrics, aphasics, and normals. *J. Commun. Disord.* 7:213, 1974.

162. Torrans, A., and Beasley, D. S. Oral stereognosis: Effect of varying form set, answer type, and retention time. *J. Psycholinguist. Res.* 2:159, 1975.

163. Van Riper, C. *Speech Correction: Principles and Methods* Englewood Cliffs, N.J.: Prentice-Hall, 1954.

164. Van Riper, C., and Irwin, J. V. *Voice and Articulation.* Englewood Cliffs, N.J.: Prentice-Hall, 1958.

165. Vaughn, G. R., and Clark, R. M. *Speech Facilitation: Extraoral and Intraoral Stimulation Technique for Improvement of Articulation Skills.* Springfield, Ill.: Thomas, 1979.

166. Vellutino, F. R., DeSetto, L., and Steger, J. A. Categorical judgment and the Wepman test of auditory discrimination. *J. Speech Hear. Dis.* 37:252, 1972.

167. Warren, D. W. Compensatory speech behaviors in cleft palate: A regulation/control phenomenon. *Cleft Palate J.* 23:251, 1986.

168. Weiffenbach, J. M. Infants with Clefts of Lip and Palate: Observations of Touch Elicited Oral Behavior. In J. F. Bosma (Ed.), *Third Symposium on Oral Sensation and Perception.* Springfield, Ill.: Thomas, 1972.

169. Weiffenbach, J. M., and Thach, B. T. Elicited Tongue Movements: Touch and Taste in the Newborn Human. In J. F. Bosma (Ed.), *Fourth Symposium on Oral Sensation and Perception.* U.S. Dept. of Health Education, and Welfare publication No. (NIH) 73-546, 1973.

170. Weinberg, B., Liss, G. M., and Hillis, J. A Comparative Study of Visual, Manual, and Oral Form Identification Skills in Speech Impaired and Normal Speaking Children. In J. F. Bosma (Ed.), *Second Symposium on Oral Sensation and Perception.* Springfield, Ill.: Thomas, 1970.

171. Weinberg, B., Lyons, M. J., and Liss, G. M. Studies of Oral, Manual, and Visual Form Identification Skills in Children and Adults. In J. F. Bosma (Ed.), *Second Symposium on Oral Sensation and Perception.* Springfield, Ill.: Thomas, 1970.

172. Welford, A. T. Introductory lecture to session IV on the sequencing of action. *Brain Res.* 71:381, 1974.

173. Wilhelm, C. L. *The Effects of Oral Form Recognition Training on Articulation in Children.* Dissertation, University of Kansas, Lawrence, 1971.

174. Williams, W. N., and LaPointe, L. L. Intra-oral recognition of geometric forms by normal subjects. *Percept. Mot. Skills* 32:419, 1971.

175. Witkop, C. J., Jr., Baldizon, G., Castro, O. R., and Umana, R. Auditory Memory Span and Oral Stereognosis in Children with Kwashiorkor. In J. F. Bosma (Ed.), *Second Symposium on Oral Sensation and Perception.* Springfield, Ill.: Thomas, 1970.

176. Woodford, L. D. *Oral Stereognosis.* Thesis, University of Illinois, Chicago, 1964.

177. Woodward, K. L., and Kenshalo, D. R., Jr. The recovery of sensory function following skin flaps in humans. *Plast. Reconstr. Surg.* 79:428, 1987.

178. Yairi, E., and Cavaness, D. Successive versus simultaneous presentation of forms in oral stereognostic testing. *Percept. Mot. Skills* 41:233, 1975.

CHAPTER 18

Directed Home Language Stimulation Program for Infants with Cleft Lip and Palate

Elise Hahn

The mother of a 7-year-old boy sought help in a speech clinic. The unintelligibility of the child's speech was not entirely related to his cleft condition. When asked if she ever helped him to say words, the mother replied, "We wouldn't dare. We might do something wrong. So we just tell him to point." A father visiting the clinic was frustrating his son by the say-it-right-or-you-don't-get-the-cookie method and then accepting the child's request composed only of nasalized vowels and glottal stops. A kindly family friend had shown another child how to make a /k/-like cough in the throat and had succeeded in starting the glottal substitution habit, which is difficult to correct.

It is one thing for the surgeon to suggest that speech training will not be necessary until the first grade, or for the orthodontist to indicate that speech work will only be wasted until he can bring the arches into alignment, and quite another thing to keep the parents from giving some kind of speech training during the early years. The anxious mother who encourages gestural language for communication, the father who is inconsistent in his demands, and the friend who actually teaches defective speech may be significant influences in starting behaviors that will interfere with the child's communication and will be difficult to correct later. Parents are going to teach speech and language consciously or unconsciously, whether or not they are advised; they need direction, information on normal language development, and specific suggestions on practical ways to start.

Because of the extreme differences in structure and function among the population of those with varying conditions of cleft, a program of language stimulation and early speech instruction must be individualized. The speech pathologist undertaking such counseling should be familiar with the initial anomaly, the time and type of surgical repair, and the general physical conditions of the baby. As the original case history is taken, tentative conclusions should also be recorded regarding the emotional stability of the father and mother, their intelligence and education, and the present state of their acceptance of a child with a problem that seems at first to make their baby so different from other children.

When the child is born, the parents usually have never seen such a condition; also they know little about the structure and function of their own speech mechanisms. Consequently, when the doctor delivering the baby or the surgeon operating on the lip explains the physical structures, the parents not only have no background for understanding the problems they will have to face, but they are also in an emotional state that interferes with the reception of information.

To these parents, plans for remediation must often seem far in the future, all to be accomplished by *other* people, by professionals with experience who will give directions but who will know little about the assets and needs of their particular child or their own desires to help their child. It is reassuring to such parents to be shown that they can become active members of the remediation team.

Consequently *the initial meeting between parents, baby, and speech pathologist should take place early, when the lip has been closed and the child is about 3 to 4 months of age.*

Unless such involvement is started early, parents may shift responsibility to the professionals, dutifully following the timetables for closure of the lip, closure of the palate, care of the ears and teeth, orthodontic correction, prosthodontic appliances, and possible secondary surgical procedures. The ability to speak effectively is then treated as an aftereffect of the physical remediation.

Actually, the desire and the need to communicate precede the physical correction of the structures. The baby, in order to develop within his environment, must have a means of announcing and defining his needs, of receiving information necessary to his understanding of his world, and of setting up the mutual exchange between adult and child that will direct and enhance his learning. Such a means is oral language. He must receive the messages spoken to him by his parents and achieve an understanding of those words; as he stores words, events, and meanings, he acquires concepts. Out of this fund of concepts he begins to initiate his own expressive use of words. This baby with the orofacial deformity must learn language in the same way as other children: through the early stimulation provided him by his parents.

The term *language* refers to a system of spoken symbols organized within the brain. Speech, the observable behavior involving production of articulated sounds, voice, and body action, makes use of language forms. The baby with the cleft condition may have later problems of articulating consonants and may have a nasal quality to his voice, but the language forms should not show a disturbance, provided his family has given him guidance. The ways and means of language training cannot be told to the parents in one or two meetings. Each encounter provides information and suggestions suitable to the age level of the infant, with advice on developmental stages immediately ahead.

THE FIRST MEETING

The speech specialist first welcomes the baby as a *baby,* not as a child with a defect, commenting on his responsiveness, his coloring, the shape of his head or whatever may be commended, touching the infant and talking directly to him in the short animated phrases that mothers often use. If the child will tolerate fondling, this follows. Such a demonstration is symbolic, indicating to the parents the acceptance of the child no matter how deviant his present appearance may be. The parents have already experienced stares and unthinking comments from strangers; this physical expression of acceptance of the infant relaxes much of the tension of the first visit.

The first step in involving the parents is an educational one, planned so that parents may understand the structure of the normal speech mechanism and its function during speech, their child's variation in structure, the vocal play that they must induce, the start of receptive language, and the beginning of babbling.

Taking into consideration the educational levels of both father and mother, the speech pathologist explains the working of the parents' own oral structures by means of drawings, a mirror for self-examination, simple anatomical illustrations in textbooks, and much verbal repetition. Even for a family of low economic and educational level, he can explain the arching of the palatal shelves, the positioning of the premaxilla, the action of the velum, the double sling functioning of muscles for the quick lifting of the soft palate, and the necessary contact between velum and pharyngeal wall to prevent nasal escape of breath. All of this can be presented simply, with the emphasis on normal functioning, while the parents examine their own mechanisms during speaking and swallowing. Technical words are omitted or explained simply; surely the speech therapist has no need to impress. An observer, if he were to open the door, would see the mother peering earnestly into her husband's mouth and the husband asking the speech clinician to say "ah" again as he holds the flashlight, the baby temporarily forgotten.

The speech specialist then calls attention to the ways in which their infant's structures differ from theirs, emphasizing the normality of the active tongue and the evidence of teeth erupting, while pointing out the present openness of the palate, the areas that after the operation will become a functioning velum, the possible division where a cleft exits through the alveolar ridge. The recent lip operation can be explained, although the surgeon may have done this; the parents now have a comparison with their own lip structure. They may ask why the tip of the nose is held down or why the nostrils flare. A simple explanation begins of the insufficiency of tissue and the malplacement of structures that occur with bilateral or unilateral cleft. Some clinicians show presurgical pictures at this time; these may produce comments of aversion and shock and quick statements that their baby is not like that. Such photographs probably should be saved until the parents have become more accepting of the condition. It suffices at this early date to explain the baby's own structures.

Pertinent facts can now be given: this lack of joining or breakdown in structures occurred when the embryo was between 6 and 8 weeks of age; the exact cause is not yet known and may never be known for *this* child. If some relative has such an anomaly, there is an indication that an hereditary trend exists, but the defect may not appear in every generation. If there is no evidence of inheritance, the occurrence is probably a chance factor. All this presentation has one purpose: any guilt felt by either father or mother must be modified. If need for information is indicated, the parents can be referred to their pediatrician for discussion of hereditary factors. The aim of the speech pathologist is to prevent this child from being constantly viewed as evidence of some mistake or sin committed by the parents. An individual with feelings of guilt will find it difficult to work cooperatively.

The parents at this time may or may not be able to word a common fear: does the orofacial deformity mean that the child will be mentally retarded? Great care should be taken in verbalizing a reply. If the 3- to 4-month old baby has been very responsive to the noise-making of the clinician, if he has examined objects in his hands or shown facial changes indicating recognition of his parents, if he reaches for interesting objects, the clinician comments on these behaviors with approval. If asked directly, the clinician states that an assessment of intelligence cannot be made at this time but that most of the babies with the cleft condition have normal intelligence. If this appears to be avoiding an answer, it is. The primary goal is to induce the parents to respond lovingly to the child, and to accept him as an individual who can profit by their help.

The first suggestions on language stimulation are now presented. The explanation that many behaviors must precede the expressive use of words suggests why parents may begin at once. The clinician describes random vocal play: vowel sounds ever changing in pitch and loudness while the baby is engaged in some physical activity, such as trying to wave his rattle or hit a ball tied on a thread that hangs in front of his face. If the speech pathologist is uninhibited in such noisy play, both he and the parents will notice at once that the infant is fascinated with such activity, particularly if the accompanying sound is high-pitched. When the adult stops, the baby will often obligingly try to continue the vocal play. He may not be imitating, but the broad spectrum of sounds has certainly suggested to him that this is pleasurable, satisfying behavior.

The mother is instructed to play in this way, making her face available to the baby so that he becomes used to the source of sound, allowing him to feel of her mouth if he wishes, as she makes the sounds loudly and vigorously to hold his attention.

When the baby indulges in vocal play while alone, the parents are instructed not to intrude. They can begin to keep a record of such noise-making, when it occurred, what the baby was doing, how long it lasted, etc. They are now involved in documentation of a reassuring kind. Their child is following normal development and they have evidence of it. Often at this step, the child, who may still look so different, becomes endearing, so that they can brag of his loudness and high pitch, his responsiveness and show of understanding.

The child's normal tendency to imitate action is discussed. He will not be able to duplicate adult sound-making, but he may clearly reproduce pitch changes or exaggerated facial expressions or hand play. The clinician points out that the vocal fluctuations in pitch and loudness will later act as signals to convey emotions and in a more subtle form will accompany words in adult speech. The changes in loudness and pitch in childhood are more extreme than those used by adults; therefore the parents, in this early training period, will exaggerate vocal behaviors. Body actions also act as signals of meaning: the obvious changes in facial expression, hand actions, and body positions must be brought into play, far more broad and exaggerated than those used in adult communication. The inhibited parent can hardly be effective as the baby's teacher; the speech clinician must demonstrate over and over how the baby responds to laughter, noisy play, and gesture, hoping that the parents will at least try. Often the baby's increased responsiveness will be the obvious reward.

Babbling is discussed, defined as a succession of syllables: consonant-vowel, consonant-vowel. When the father and mother have established some vocal play, they should then become loud babblers, connecting the repetition with physical action, repeating *bah-bah-bah* vigorously as they clap the child's hands or hit a toy. Because the palatal areas have not yet been closed, *ba-ba* resembles *ma-ma; da-da* is similar to *na-na*. This is explained to the parent. The quick strong movements and contact of the articulators are the goal rather than the orality of the tone at this time. Records should be kept of babbling that the baby does while lying alone in his crib.

The clinician describes the first consonant attempts that are likely to be recognized: /p/, /b/, /m/, /w/. Strong lip movement and closure of these sounds in babbled syllables is demonstrated, with the child held in a comfortable position while attention is directed to the mouth of the speaker. Imitation is often accomplished at this point. Both father and mother are shown how to hold the child while they play with him. Sometimes, after surgical closure of the lip, structures that have been made functionally adequate do not come into play in sound production or eating: the upper lip becomes immobile and, later, rigid and short. The lower lip, without its proper contact, grows flaccid and often everted. Any action that exercises the operated-on lip should therefore be helpful: pouting and drawing the lips back in making faces, popping the lips together in "fish talk," sucking around a small nipplelike object. The mother can stroke the infant's lip gently to encourage greater movement while she stimulates him with sounds.

The parents' use of strongly produced single words, such as *momma, daddy, up, down, no, dinner, potty,* and names of siblings or toys, all pronounced while the baby is watching or is engrossed in action, will start his receptive vocabulary. He will connect the word and the event, and gradually his recognition of the word alone will become evident.

Armed with all this information, the parent is ready to start work, knowing that he can report his successes or failures at the next meeting and receive further suggestions.

THE SECOND MEETING

The second meeting should take place when the child is between 7 and 12 months of age. The child's sound-making in the home is reviewed, with praise for results.

The period of naming begins in the attempt to build the child's receptive language, his recognition of the relationship between word and event, between the changes in the voice and the body signals of the speaker and the message that is being conveyed. The clinician begins with a demonstration, lining up small attractive objects just beyond the reach of the infant, playing the game of "Where's the *car?*" and "There's the *car.*" The word and the event must occur simultaneously: the word taught must be emphasized strongly by loudness, pitch rise, and increased duration, the facial expression must convey the pleasure of the experience rather than anxious teaching, and hand action must indicate location. Sometimes the parents will try the same teaching, saying, "Look at this cute little car over here," giving the key word no emphasis and burying it in detail, using the barest gesture. The teaching must be energetic and positive to gain the baby's attention and to leave a memory of the behaviors observed.

The words modeled for the child are not nouns only. A 1-year old child was walked down the hall while the clinician chanted, "Walk-walk. Walk-walk." When the parent asked what she was doing, the little girl pointed to the hall and announced "Walk." A verb can become the name of an event. The adjectives *big* and *little* can easily be acted out. Common nouns, verbs, and adjectives are thus given single-word production, never out of context but always closely related to the ongoing activity of the child. No attempt is made to demand the child's imitation; the purpose is to build a recognition vocabulary.

Teaching can take place in the car while driving or in the store while buying, but the most effective situations are those in which the child can touch and manipulate the object named. Picture books at this time seem to offer only the pleasure of ruffling the pages, while a collection of small durable animals offers a chance to name the animal, name his actions, and to attach any adjective to him. Handling, throwing, pounding, and mouthing all come into action as the child discovers the potentials of the object that the mother is naming repeatedly.

In this period just prior to the first word, the parents, ideally, will be engaging the child simultaneously in (1) vocal play, inducing lip and tongue-tip action in noisy sound-making, demonstrating broad pitch and loudness changes with considerable openness on vowels; (2) naming all objects that the baby touches or looks at, seeming by tone of voice and manner to invite participation; and (3) playing with the sounds of babbling, particularly the /p/, /b/, /m/, /t/, /d/, /n/, and even /l/. These consonants can be readily seen and often stimulate imitation.

The speech clinician may also suggest ways of increasing the child's range of experience; if he is taken to the store or on family outings, while the parents talk steadily of what is happening, he will be presented with a different vocabulary. He will also become an active participant in family affairs.

During the time when the child is learning to walk, he may become less vocal, as if he were quietly concentrating on the acquisition of this new skill. He will return to his sound-making as he achieves balance, particularly if his environment is widened.

The first words may start to appear any time between 12 and 18 months; often the child with the cleft will wait until the palate is closed. This delay is not alarming; he may have attempted words prior to the operation which could not be recognized because of the distortion of the consonants. Nasal emission of consonants and nasality on vowels are explained to the parents with helpful drawings of the oral structures involved.

After obtaining information from the surgeon, the speech pathologist now discusses the hoped-for effects of palatal closure: the functioning of the soft palate, its contact with the back throat wall, and the consequent direction of the airstream through the mouth. If expansion of the dental arch is planned in the near future — as it may be in severe cases — the possible effect on articulation will be made clear.

THE THIRD MEETING

The third meeting usually takes place 6 to 8 weeks after surgical closure of the palate. Any swelling should have subsided by this time. The parents can now review the operation, wording some of their fears and possible disappointments.

Additional sounds can be added to the child's repertoire. The parents can select objects whose names start with /k/ and /g/, such as *key* and *gum*. They are cautioned that the sound is not made in the throat but is produced by a quick contact between the raised back of the tongue and the posterior edge of the hard palate. The explosive release on all plosives is shown to the child by raising his hand up to the mother's mouth as she says single sounds, followed immediately by a word whose meaning is already established. Play with this explosive production while pushing the mo- *wells* torboat in the bathtub and guiding the little car across the table will introduce the child to representative sound-making. Competitions with the father in making a thin flexible piece of plastic or paper bend back from the mouth while the two of them are repeating, *pie, buy, tie, die, key, go*, should make the learning interesting.

A word of caution should be given to the parents: the child should not be taught or allowed to produce consonants with such tension that a grimace results. All sounds in adult speech are made lightly and quickly and blend into each other in the flow of movement within the phrase. The required blending of sounds for communicative speech must be taught at the start, not at a later time. If the child produces /k/ or /t/ with great force, too many muscles are brought into play; during the lengthened production the speech mechanism cannot proceed to the next sound with the steady smooth movement required. This excessive tension results from two ineffective methods of teaching: (1) the admonition to try harder, and (2) the teaching of single consonants isolated from context, so that the child may learn /k/ but cannot associate it with meaningful words or phrases.

The lower lip action of /f/ can be demonstrated in familiar words like *funny paper*; the contact must be light an quick and again the hand is held before the mouth to help the child to discover the air flow.

If the parents now find that /s/, /z/ and /ʃ/ are produced with the tongue protruding or made with the tongue retruded and spread in the back of the mouth, the speech specialist can explain that the sound will be improved if the back teeth are closed lightly. However, the teaching of a sibilant sounds can be postponed until the child is older, since these sounds are somewhat late in development for normally structured children. Production of the sibilants frequently needs the guidance of the trained speech pathologist, since their faulty produciton may be related to malocclusion, hearing loss, poor muscular control, or infantile distortion.

Other consonants that are frequently late in use — /tʃ/, /dʒ/, /θ/, /ð/, /v/, and /r/ — may be explained to the parents and the request made to avoid these in home training. Many kindergarten children are still in the process of acquiring these sounds.

As the child discovers the use of his newly reconstructed mechanism and achieves single words, the parents move into two-word structures — *go home, eat dinner, more cake, no candy* — all taught in context. The drive to imitate is now increasing; the child will try to copy a total phrase if it is associated with action in which he is involved and will carry the phrase back into private play situations. Speech is not always communicative; it can become a means of organizing one's own behavior, as in the monologue.

When the parents explain any event to the young child, they now use full sentences, simple in construction but containing many parts of speech. The child must become used to the rhythm of our language. When the mother announces, "We are going to the store," the child may repeat the key words, "Go store," which the mother accepts and, nodding, repeats after him, but she must lay the groundwork for the full sentence. Adults should listen to themselves occasionally, however, for they overload the listening situation and model sentences impossible to repeat or even translate, when they make such statements as "If you're really a good boy, mother might just take you to the store along with her." The cleft palate child, like any other, must have simple sentences modeled for him.

The use of speech in play-and-pretend situations starts early, although the child is usually not adept at role playing until he is about 3½ years of age. Parents making sounds for the toy dog or talking for the car, which logically says, "Here I come. Get out of my way," open up the normal play in which inanimate objects have life bestowed on them. The cleft palate child needs this pretend-play, which is always constructed and supported by language. Later, when the child ascribes roles to all toys, he can talk for them or tell them what to do. Role playing is a satisfying and effective practice period for oral language. The parents, as they watch the speech clinician demonstrate such play, will be challenged to create their own mutual play situations, rather than handing the child the toy and pointing to the play area.

As the words and phrases that the child uses in spontaneous communicaiton becomes more intelligible, parents often give rewards of candy or kisses. If the spoken idea fulfills some purpose of the child's — getting the parent to pick him up or reach him a toy or simply to give attention — these results are in themselves rewards. The child wants to communicate: acceptance and understanding of his message are sufficient reinforcement. Many children with cleft conditions, because of consistent failure to reach acceptance, lose their incentive to improve. Why go to all that effort to talk if no one responds appropriately? One of the main conbributions that the parents can make is to convince the child that he has something important to say, that he is a valued communicator whose listeners are actually waiting to know what he thinks. If the child arrives at the conclusion that he is valued at home, he will enter the social world of the school with greater confidence.

After this postoperative conference the family may be given an appointment 6 months or a year away; the time interval depends on the clinician's assessment of their eagerness to continue the home program.

LATER PRESCHOOL SESSIONS

In an additional session before the child is 3½ the speech clinician may suggest that he will profit from nursery school. He points out that the child needs the challenge of trying out language in peer group relationships. Sometimes parents may fear early persecution and ridicule: however, the 3- and 4-year-olds are far more accepting than older children. They themselves do not yet have the ability to formulate questions.

Eventually, before first grade, the child with the cleft must be taught by the parent that his physical difference exists, that he was born that way, that he has had an operation, and the "something more is going to be done," either surgically or orthodontically. Thus he will have a quick and ready answer always available. No one can prevent persecution, but the child's use of somewhat adult phrases or explanations can usually save him from verbal abuse. This realistic acceptance may be difficult for the parent; the clinician helps by sitting in front of a mirror with the child and quietly pointing out the differences between his lip and the child's, the alignment of his teeth or the structure of his nose, saying, "When you are bigger, the doctor will change you a little here and here," or "The dentist is going to straighten out these teeth." Children can explain the birth defect in their first-grade classes if the parents have laid the groundwork for a straightforward approach.

During the period following initial closure, the teeth may need special care and the condition of the ears may fluctuate. The speech specialist is often the one who reminds the parents about these special needs, relating this care to the improvement of the child's speech and often making the appropriate referrals.

By the time the child is ready for nursery school or kindergarten, he needs the highly trained care of the speech pathologist, who will give more specific practice.

Speech clinicians, in counseling this home training program, should exert some caution. Not every parent is emotionally equipped to help his child. One mother pursued the drill so relentlessly that the boy began to stutter. Another showed off her child's progress in language to the neighbors so frequently that the child learned to be quiet in the presence of adults. The emotional needs of the parents must not be fulfilled in demonstrations of sacrifice for the care of the child. The speech pathologist has to know when to tell the parents to do nothing, so that barriers will not be placed in the way of the child's future learning.

Usually the early program of language stimulation and guidance directly involves the parent in the child's development and lays the foundation for the child's belief in himself as an acceptable communicator. Motivation to communicate with others outside the family depends strongly on that early start in the home.

CHAPTER 19

Stimulating Language Development in Infants and Toddlers with Cleft Palate

Jane Scheuerle

The overall determiners of language skill acquisition for infants are considered to be (1) biological, (2) the cognitive level of the individual, (3) psychosocial adaptation within the family, and (4) the quality of the linguistic environment. Consistent data reported during the last 30 years seem to indicate that most infants born with isolated cleft lip or palate fall mainly within the normal distribution of cognitive, intellectual function. They can achieve good psychosocial adaptation before school age or later. Significant advances have been made in surgical and dental management for correcting the oral structure and the function of the peripheral hearing mechanism for children born with most forms of orofacial clefts. Such therapies continue to increase the adequacy of early biological structures for their adaptation in production for normal verbal language skills.

It is, therefore, the language environment of the child that must and can be addressed by the speech and language pathologist. We must interact with patients and their families, either by providing early therapy for the young patient with cleft palate or more often as members of interdisciplinary teams, by preventing further abnormal development. This chapter addresses three manageable environmental conditions which frequently affect adversely the more normal development of verbal communication skills of infants and toddlers born with cleft palate.

> ## CRITICAL ENVIRONMENTAL RISKS FOR LANGUAGE COMMUNICATION OF INFANTS BORN WITH CLEFT PALATE

This discussion encompasses three critical aspects of the birth defect and its impact on expected or anticipated routine daily life. The speech and language consultant on a cleft palate team should anticipate the following: (1) The baby's external environment will often contain negative reactions of caregivers and casual acquaintances to the infant and to the birth defect. Responses to the infant's orofacial cleft exert influences on behavior and attitudes of both the child and the respondent. (2) Adaptive interactive processes of the baby and caregivers must accommodate the orofacial difference for health care management from early feeding through the required series of staged early reconstructive surgeries. (3) The infant's own internal environment may confound aural function through conductive hearing loss due to middle ear effusion and otitis media.

During the first year after birth, any infant's learning of communication skills begins when the baby calms in response to voice or touch; is quieted when held, stroked, or fed [24, 51]. The success and repetition of the usual spontaneous infant behaviors, which elicit environmental change for the baby's comfort and thereby meet the infant's needs, are evidence of maturing individual traits and characteristics. According to Greenspan [17] the measure of developmental success which any infant realizes rests on the ability of the child to adapt to the environment but also on the environment's ablity to adapt to the needs of the infant. Absence or malfunction of that earliest interactive adaptive potential can disrupt normal progress and can entangle the various participants in very complex, and often counterproductive, interactions.

Since the mid-1970s, pediatric research among developmentally disabled children has repeatedly demonstrated that the most significant element in stabilization and maturation of "infants-at-risk" is the adaptability of the home environment to the evolving needs of the child [17]. That thought has special application to the infant born with cleft lip-palate. Unlike either the non-birth-defective baby or one with a developmental disability, acquisition of communication skills by the baby with an orofacial defect is at risk from unique multiple factors of both their internal and external environments. The need for mutual adaptability of both family and child is critical to the normalization of these infants within their families.

THE NEWBORN

Risks to communicative involvement of the neonate born with cleft lip-palate arise from a variety of environmental sources. These may relate to (1) the baby's appearance and the response of family members who see the cleft; (2) the level of oral malfunction which impedes feeding; and (3) the necessary introduction of many professional strangers with various types of expertise who will become part of the long-term team treatment process for this common birth defect.

Human neonates apparently utilize all external stimuli of the caregiver's voice, cuddling and stroking to achieve their initial internal stabilization. Reciprocal actions of calming and quieting when appropriate care is provided seem to be the earliest examples of infants expressing their needs and responding to fulfillment of those needs. Those early beginnings from tactile, visual, and auditory communication between the adults in the environment and the baby are at risk if there are factors which interfere with the capacity for mutual comforting [5]. The primary elements which appear and continue to disrupt the environment of the newborn infant with cleft lip-palate lie largely within the domain of early adaptive physical care.

Shock, the most universal reaction to the unexpected cleft lip-palate of the newborn, affects all the infants caregivers, both medical and nonmedical [14]. Parents appear early to adopt attitudes toward the cleft condition and toward their baby which they perceive are displayed by hospital personnel and cleft palate team members shortly after the baby's birth. While such attitudes may not diminish bonding or love of the parents for the infant, the resultant internal tensions can effect subtle changes in manner of touch, holding, cuddling, and stroking in the main caregivers' interactive behavior.

The presence of a cleft palate typically requires modifications of the elemental process of early feeding. That modification is sometimes negatively perceived as an imposition. In reality, the parent must manage to change a culturally generalized feeding procedure and provide a method to which the baby can successfully adapt the function of his deformed oral structures. The altered routine may increase fatigue and frustration even in the most loving parent. These and other sequelae resulting from the care of a new baby can generate negative feelings in the caregivers and new stresses within the family.

While the physical aspects of initial nutrition and hygiene are considered primarily medical and nursing concerns, the communicative aspects of these early interactions should not be neglected by the speech pathologist. It is within the first few months of life that critical linguistic receptive and expressive patterns are initiated and their neurological support established.

In the neonatal stage of life the infant with cleft lip-palate typically mediates the introduction of the family members to numerous strangers who are "experts" in diverse fields of allied health professions — the local cleft palate team. Those experts will become close acquaintances of the family and child over many years of treatment. The manner in which those introductions are made and the mutual sense of security and trust which the family and professionals may achieve are measures of the risks in each infant's communication environment. The available experts will have deeply rooted and long-lasting influences on the environment and the child and each family's adaptability to it.

Most immediately, preparation for the initial surgery to close the lip and insert pressure-equalizing (PE) tubes in the tympanic membranes must begin. That preparation may also introduce the family to the reality of the need for presurgical orthodontic models. The need for surgery for the new baby and the probable risk of hearing loss consequent on the cleft condition will be presented. Fears of strangulation from oral impression material, possible adverse effects of general anesthesia, concerns about pain and staying in the hospital, interacting with hospital personnel, possible poor outcomes of treatment, infection, postoperative care, and sundry other unfamiliar thoughts and feelings often surface to elevate the anxiety of or distract the parents. All too frequently, the urgency and significance of the actual physical management takes precedence over these nonmedical and surgical concerns of the family and baby. During those first weeks, vital and appropriate tactile, visual, and auditory stimulation can be postponed and accurate recognition and interpretation of the baby's responses distorted. Such distractons by this common birth defect may divert the parents from appropriate responses to and reinforcement of a baby's otherwise spontaneous communication behaviors, disrupting the foundation for healthy bonding and early normal auditory-oral symbolic communication behavior.

THE INFANT AND TODDLER

When closure of the cleft lip has been accomplished, babies with clefts of the primary palate or face achieve a more normal facial contour; the wound heals, the scar fades, and the daily care routine returns to the presurgical norm. The impact of the first experience with hospitalization of the baby establishes a reference point for the family's anticipation and endurance of subsequent surgical procedures for the infant. The individual

professionals, including the speech pathologist, may interact with the family in a variety of ways. Those interactions establish information and support resources for all later aspects of the infant's development. The risk to the infant's acquisition of normal communication abilities is affected by the extent of the family's inclusion in this earliest care process. While family participation in the infant's care depends largely on their adaptive abilities, successful interdisciplinary aspects of long-term management of cleft lip-palate care demand a broad range of modified involvement by parents. This is best realized when families are introduced to unfamiliar information and conditions by experienced, empathic professionals who are skilled in gauging both timeliness and manner of providing informaton and responding to inquiries.

All health professionals who serve on a cleft palate team, like family members, necessarily participate in the adaptable caregiving environment of the developing infant. Administrative, nursing, and medical members of hospital staffs are also a part of that environment at these crucial times when family and patient impressions and sensitivities are keenest. Especially significant is the skill of cleft palate team members to perform, demonstrate, and teach postoperative care to inexperienced parents. The level of skill and degree of comfort with which the parents care for the surgical result indicate and determine messages shared by them and the infant.

RISKS IN IDENTIFICATION AND REFERRAL

A major risk to the communication environment of both the newborn infant and the parents lies in the initial decision to postpone referral of the patient. This may happen where pediatric or surgical tradition holds that nothing can be done until the baby is more than 1 year to 4 years old.

Another risk to normal development of babies born with orofacial clefts may be related to the low incidence of this birth defect in a single practitioner's caseload. If referral is made to a surgeon who may have full academic and training credentials but limited experience in treatment of cleft lip-palate, or who does not work with an interdisciplinary team, the patient is not assured the best quality of care. In such circumstances, the energies of the family and patient tend to be focused only on the resolution of the biological defect to the neglect of concomitant responsibilities to the behavioral aspects of development.

Likewise, referral to and involvement of a family with a poorly coordinated multidisciplinary group cannot satisfy the family's needs. Disparate attitudes and approaches among experts who assume responsibility for a patient's cleft lip-palate care management often neglect the family's need and ability to comprehend and cope with developmental matters. Particularly harmful is the possibility of overloading parents with medical information without meeting their essential needs to provide adequately for the infant's linguistic environment.

Recurrent middle ear problems early in life can have profound effects on later language abilities [22, 45]. Reported phenomena of middle ear tissue masses present in newborn and older infants with cleft palates point to an unexplored concern for the auditory function. Frans and colleagues [16], like Stool and Randall [42], indicate that the traditional belief that otitis media is the only ear condition of concern in these patients also needs to be reexamined in view of new information.

Concurrent risks to communicative function not specifically related to or dependent on the cleft condition are suggested by the categorization of craniofacial anomalies [18] and the categorical aspects of cleft palate speech [10]. Examination of orofacial structures and spoken language behaviors in large numbers of patients with cleft lip-palate demonstrate the feasibility of their also having noncleft-related differences in (a) size and position of orofacial structures, (b) mass, contractile strength, and coordination of muscle, (c) neurological integration of the speech mechanism, and (d) intricate central neurological processing of language. Development of speech and language problems that are independent of the cleft condition may be reflected in the often repeated proportion (5–10%) of patients said to retain cleft palate speech.

LANGUAGE STIMULATION TRAINING AS EARLY DIRECT SPEECH THERAPY

Children with repaired cleft lip-palate, like children without clefts, exhibit a broad range of abilities in development of verbal communication skills. While some patients may experience expressive language problems related to the congenital anomaly and its sequelae, as a population they are expected to acquire the elements of verbal language according to the accepted chronology among the noncleft population. That is, when a cleft lip-palate patient who is 18 months of age or older continues to manipulate his or her environment primarily through gestural and intonational vocalizations, or when attempts at speech are unintelligible, that child should be considered a candidate for direct therapeutic intervention through a phonological and syntactic stimulation program.

Following primary surgery for cleft palate closure, some very young patients may still be experiencing velopharyngeal insufficiency. Dental malocclusions, mid-to-lower face disproportions, recurrent upper respiratory infections, otological disease, or significant hearing loss may also be present. Nonetheless, early evidence of the patient's normality is demonstrated best through developmental language skills. Through verbal communication the toddler establishes his or her individuality and potential for independence in the eyes of the family. Such environmental attitudes constitute a major consideration in the success of long-term treatment of the cleft lip-palate patient. Therefore, identification of the particular child or family or environment which needs direct therapeutic intervention must be a priority goal of the team speech pathologist. Therapy here means the process by which the clinician establishes an environment in which the client and family can and will change.

The results of recent grouped team evaluation reports of treatment success offer major clues to identification of the child who may need early individual phonological and syntactic stimulation. Those clues are readily restated in terms of purposes and goals for speech-language services and are expected to differ somewhat with each child. In general, the purposes of direct therapy for speech-language stimulation of the toddler and preschool child with cleft lip-palate may include:

1. Motivation for the child to acquire verbal communication skills commensurate with his or her age and abilities
2. Identification and development of acceptable compensatory verbal communication behaviors necessitated by phonological limits

imposed by the child's congenital orofacial anomaly and its physical management

3. Reduction of parental stress through learning to cope with the child's unintelligibility or immature communication behavior
4. Involvement of parents in creating and maintaining an appropriate language-saturated environment for the child
5. Recommendation for appropriate additional intervention such as secondary physical management, otological care, or educational placement

A program of direct phonological and syntactic stimulation in toddlers and preschool children with repaired cleft palates should be focused on the broad goal of normalization of the child's verbal communication. This goal includes development of appropriate use of receptive and expressive verbalization, through interacting with the clinical and home environments. Direct stimulation of verbal communication in young children with repaired cleft palates is often necessary for their achievement of normal language development.

The speech and language clinician should undertake the arduous task of organizing and managing an early childhood verbal communication program based on a thorough knowledge of normal child development. When the clinical setting and staff allow, enrollment of several children simultaneously in a preschool program can be applied. The individual clinical practitioner may choose to organize only individual sessions. However, careful scheduling can afford selected grouping. For example, sessions can be arranged for individual participants before and after a period of shared time. Experienced private practitioners who utilize this protocol report that the opportunity for parent interaction that it affords is a prime reason for its use. Initial ideal elements of a clinical preschool program of language stimulation include (1) individual and group sessions which are (2) informal, but structured around (3) child-oriented activities that (4) allow and encourage child-adult (and child-child) observation and interaction, and which (5) demonstrate procedures and techniques for use by the parent.

INDIVIDUAL AND GROUP SETTINGS

There is little doubt that the most intensive and specific phonoligical and syntactic stimulation is achieved in individual sessions. Two- and three-year-old children tend to participate in individual exploratory play. That developmental stage is most efficiently adapted to language stimulation when therapy is carried out in a one-to-one child-adult play setting. Experience of parallel play or coactivity in a group setting may be helpful in preventing or reducing negative ideas or attitudes of being different. Well-chosen and structured individual activities within the group setting can engender sharing, helping, and even competition among some young clients [8, 26, 41].

INFORMAL BUT STRUCTURED ENVIRONMENT

Play therapy can utilize carefully selected toys and materials that allow or require certain interactive behaviors. Both objects and potential play with them provide concrete references for stimulating selected phonological and syntactic utterances. Multimodal perception, gross and fine motor manipulation, and spontaneous exploration of space and objects contribute to essential semantic elements of language [31]. As a child engages in play, the clinician joins in and adds appropriate vocalization or verbalizations to clarify intent, to enhance the meaningfulness of the action, and to confirm or validate the child's communication. The inclination of young children to enjoy repetition can be used to involve the patient in production of selected verbalizations, and to involve the parent in reinforcement strategies and exercises in the clinic and at home.

CHILD CENTERED ACTIVITIES AND CHILD-ADULT INTERACTION

Perhaps the art of therapy lies in this element of a home stimulation program. The materials and activities, to be successful, must be appealing and within the particular child's abilities to explore and master. The clinician must be able to identify the child's level of function, understand the client's intent, provide acceptable and rewarding responses and reinforcement, and teach selected techniques to concerned family members. Because every child is different and every stage of development varies within each child, the experienced, empathic clinician will "tune in" to the best method of interacting, the need for change of activity or routine, the time for free play or for limiting freedom, and the reality of physiological limits. In such an environment the child will find an atmosphere conducive to participation in new adventures and the development of skills for verbal exchange.

DIRECTED PARENT INVOLVEMENT

The extent to which a parent becomes involved in stimulating the child's verbal communication is as different as the number of parents. The clinician recognizes that the child's predominant language environment is in the home, and that carry-over of newly acquired verbal skills is acknowledged to be the most difficult of the therapeutic steps. In managing a program of phonological and syntactic stimulation for the young child with repaired cleft palate, the clinician accepts the challenge to meet not only the clinical needs of the child, but also to identify the level of understanding, empathy, and attitudes of the parents in order to shape that matrix into a daily functioning resource to reinforce the child's verbal communication attempts.

As the child matures, behavioral displays should become more verbal and dependency on the mother reduced. The involved parent learns from concrete examples of communicative interaction through clinical demonstrations to apply, expand, and generalize those examples at home. Some parents, however, may fixate on a particular form or manner of verbalization, or confuse the timing or method of rewarding the child's efforts. The astute clinician will make time in each treatment session to listen to the parent, assess parent-child interaction, monitor the child's increase in spontaneous meaningful verbalizations, and encourage continuation of modification of at-home techniques as indicated. The check-recheck process serves to assure and encourage the parent and to ensure the confluence of clinical and home components of the stimulation program. It seems appropriate to consider next the two most frequent conditions of delayed verbal communication which may be encountered and which require modification of their communication environments: (1) the "reluctant" speaker, and (2) the "nonreluctant" but unintelligible speaker.

STIMULATION OF THE RELUCTANT SPEAKER

A phonological and syntactic language stimulation program is based on the hypothesis that normal emergent language skills can be acquired although its achievement is delayed due to factors related to cleft palate. In some cleft lip-palate patients delayed verbal development can be attributed to deprivation of stimulation in various modes, especially auditory [15]. Among a wide variety of potential differences, these patients experience, nearly universally, recurrence of otitis media. Conductive hearing loss during phonological acquisition age interferres with peripheral and central formation of necessary neurobiological networks, and general consequences of overprotection and low expectations of parenting family members.

Otologists and audiologists repeatedly warn that onset of a significant hearing loss can occur within a few hours. Frequent otoscopic and tympanometric monitoring is essential to maintain maximal hearing acuity. During periods of depressed auditory sensitivity, child behaviors differ. Parents must be apprised of this so they can recognize hearing-related changes. Such informed monitoring allows for the earliest possible remedial intervention. Also, the ongoing awareness of potential hearing deficits helps explain and support the need for enhanced auditory stimulation for the child with cleft lip-palate. In some severe cases use of low-gain acoustic amplification may be indicated.

An entirely different consideration of oral expressive language delay in infants and toddlers with cleft lip-palate finds the home environment of the child who is different remarkably altered from the norm. Some parents report that they do not or cannot talk with the child. Others demonstrate that they have altered their expectations of the child in a downward direction and are acting on or reacting to their own expectations. In cases where parental attitudes seem to underelie the lack of stimulation, the speech-language clinician will need both to demonstrate, and to involve the parents in, specific helpful language interactive activities so as to remedy the home language stimulation environment. Critical to that basic change is the parent's learning to observe, recognize, and report accurately and to maintain ongoing realistic acquaintance with the child's progress. Also of importance is the parent's adaptation to the time and rhythm of communication with the child [13, 39, 47]. In extreme cases, modifying the home communication environment may require assistance from a psychologist or a psychatric social worker.

Language stimulation activities should be carefully programmed to address the needs and level of function of each child [3, 12, 28]. Cautious planning prevents unnecessary confusion on the part of the child and serves to keep the parent's attention focused on specific short-range objectives. The long-standing axiom of therapy and learning, which supports proceeding from simple to complex language forms, is appropriate here. However, the level of complexity at which the treatment starts must be allowed to vary with the needs of each client.

STIMULATION AT THE
WORD AND PHRASE LEVEL

Perhaps the simplest form of phonological stimulation is naming of objects and actions observable in everyday experience. Consistent use of a single term for a single object or action provides the young child with auditory cues to match visible and tactile stimuli. Certainly all speakers within the home and clinical environment should adopt the same terminology for objects and activities found in the two environments. Consistent use of simple, meaningful phrases is also applicable to the child's interests and activities in both settings.

CHILD UTTERANCES
AND REACTIONS TO THEM

The initial attempts at verbalization by the young child who has a repaired orofacial cleft and delayed verbal communication skills may be minimally or totally unintelligible. The clinician's priority is to accept the child's speech attempts and to determine phonological variations of distortion, substitution, or omission. It is critical that those production errors be identified and the basic problem explained to the parents. Quite often the concept of individual phonemes as building blocks of words is unfamiliar to the parents. Appropriate and timely information about verbal language in general, and particularly that produced by their child enhances the parents' willingness to accept the child's attempted verbalizations. Meaningful interaction with utilization of verbal language assigns to the adult the role of providing both model and reinforcement while acting as discourse partner [39]. Each successful verbal exchange between child and adult demonstrates to the child the meaningfulness and purposefulness of his or her efforts. Whether the response to the child is adult verbalization, acquisition of a desired object, or change in circumstances or relative position, the child must realize

that his or her utterance was heard and understood. The long-accepted technique of adult repetition of the child's utterance and its inclusion in expanded verbalization indicate comprehension, approval, and appropriateness of the child's verbal communication.

During busy daily routines, family members may anticipate and even verbalize the child's intent or respond quickly to a gestured communication. With no evidence of a listener, the child experiences no need to talk. Evaluation of the child's communication behaviors will be complete only by including an analysis of the family communication setting. The evaluation must reflect any meaningful utterance used by the child even though that utterance may be a nonstandard form. Two case narratives presented by Philips [30] serve to demonstrate the application of various techniques of verbal communication stimulation in the minimally verbal child.

"NONRELUCTANT" BUT
UNINTELLIGIBLE SPEAKERS

A stimulation program should be based on developmental and preventive principles [6]. In younger children with repaired cleft palates, a primary consideration is production of intelligible speech without habituation of unacceptable compensatory behaviors. Even in the presence of physiological limitations, the child can achieve accurate production of many phonemes and the correct articulatory placement for others. Such physiological limits may be considered *functional* and *organic*.

Patients whose velopharyngeal insufficiency is a functional problem can sometimes learn muscular management of the palate and nasopharynx to obliterate hypernasal resonance and inappropriate nasal air emission during speech. In patients whose velopharyngeal insufficiency is an organic problem, that is, due to structural disproportion of the palate and pharynx or velar paralysis, therapeutic intervention through speech and language stimulation must be considered with caution. Because of the nature of the organic communication disorder, behavioral management cannot eliminate nasal emission of exhaled air during verbalization. To indicate otherwise is contrary to the American Speech-Language-Hearing Association (ASHA) Code of Ethics. In some cases, however, when the child's health and well-being or availability of surgical and prosthodontic assistance warrant, the responsible clinician can effectively instruct the young child in articulatory placement for more intelligible verbal communication. The goals of phonological and syntactic stimulation activities for the child with velopharyngeal insufficiency include identification and use of all speech sounds that can be correctly produced; development of acoustic production of speech sounds; use of correct productions in meaningful language; identification and treatment of any noncleft-related communication disorders; involvement of the parent in carry-over of learned verbal skills; and appropriate and timely referrals for physical or behavioral management.

Here again the clinician must apply knowledge of normal phonological development, and physiological processes utilized in normal verbal productions. From understanding of normal articulatory proficiency the clinician can analyze the jumble of meaningless sounds which the parent hears and reports. The initial analysis of a toddler's utterances and discussion of those findings with the parent may be the first indication to a distressed parent that the utterances are other than random sounds.

CORRECTLY PRODUCED PHONEMES

Review of articulatory acquisition studies indicates a fair agreement on sounds that should be well produced at various age levels. When no consonant is produced with consistent accuracy, selection of early target sounds in the stimulation program should begin with phonemes known to be produced by very young children, such as /m/, /b/, /n/, /h/, /p/, /ŋ/, /f/, and /j/ [33]. In addition to all vowels, vocal tract openness for production of /h/ invites its use in early work with toddlers; for younger children bilabials may be an appropriate starting place. Visual (facial expression and oral opening) or tactile (air flow) cues are easily provided to enhance initial production of /h/. Once acquired, /h/ lends itself to many appropriate combinations with vowels to generate useful vocabulary. It is easily recognized and accepted in *hi, high, ho, hoe, ha, hot, hop, how, who, hair, hat, here, hello, her, hurt.* It also supports effective dialogue in story games such as *The Three Little Pigs,* where the wolf huffs and puffs to blow the house down. Concentrating on and rewarding attempts at /h/ plus vowel productions diminishes the parents' critical reactions to the child's early errors of distortion or omission of other sounds in these words. For younger children, verbal communication exercises and protocols, as suggested

by Brookshire, Lynch, and Fox [7], are very helpful. Those involve not only phoneme production but also variations in syllabic pitch and stress.

The vocabulary utilized should relate to the environment of the young child, or the environment modified to provide appropriate referents. Demonstrations of the phoneme-combining technique help the parents become aware of individual sounds, the child's successful verbal productions, and the appropriateness of accepting approximations of newly acquired phonemes in words. The adult response serves as a very strong reinforcement for the child's verbal attempts.

ACQUIRING NEW SOUNDS

Articulation placement underlies correct production of speech-sound elements. Frequently simultaneous monitoring of the clinician's model and self-productions (in a mirror) leads to rapid success in achieving new articulatory placement. This is particularly true in anterior oral movements of the lips and tongue tip for /p/, /b/, /t/, /d/, /n/, and /l/. It is well for the clinician to investigate each client's oral motor coordination for noncleft-related differences. In some patients with congenital orofacial clefts, weak muscle tone or poor intraoral coordination may need to be addressed. Practice will be needed to habituate muscular contractions to achieve desired oral postures. The young child must be rewarded for each effort in this sometimes long and tedious series of postural approximations. Achievement of correct articulation placement frequently results in production of an acoustically correct phoneme. When this does not follow, selected activities and careful manipulation are needed to modify the sound toward the target.

Once the child has consistently achieved his or her best approximation of phoneme and/or consonant-initiated syllable production, introduction of the new sound into meaningful words and phrases should follow. Step-by-step treatment advances in complexity until correct use of target sounds in spontaneous discourse is achieved. Interaction between the clinician and child during this time must be meaningful and rewarding. Treatment results must show progress toward normalization of verbal communication. Philips [30] described selection and application of techniques and procedures used effectively in phonology and syntactic stimulation programs with a young unintelligible speaker with velopharyngeal insufficiency. That case narrative reflects speech-language treatment of a young child whose cleft palate surgery result provided oropharyngeal structures capable of achieving appropriate function for development of normal verbal communication. The goal of therapy was adaptation of the oral structure to perform habitually in acceptable articulatory placement. Additionally, the parent was encouraged to observe and assist in clinical procedures. Thus, the parent gained confidence to aid the child with carry-over of new phonological and syntactic skills into the home and other social settings. Clinicians who have worked with similar clients find ready acquisition and use of additional consonants once the initial target sound is habituated.

The "nonreluctant" but unintelligible young speaker may be a child whose abundant verbalization is diminished in usefulness because of inadequate structure or muscle strength in the velum and nasopharynx. Such an organic velopharyngeal configuraton may have one or more of the following: (a) short velum, (b) stiff or scarred velum, (c) excessive pharyngeal width, (d) expanded pharyngeal depth, or (e) palatal fistulae. Therapy goals for these children are limited to verbalization which utilizes correct articulatory placement with nasal air emission as the best production possible. The clinician must be certain that the parent recognizes and understands this aspect of treatment. To continue therapy in pursuit of further modification of the acoustic cue can only risk development of alternate undesirable speech habits and attitudes, or even delay in needed physical management of the organic problem.

Joey, 30 months old, exhibited (a) marked velopharyngeal insufficiency due to a short, almost immovable palate; (b) very poor intelligibility; (c) omission of most final consonants; (d) frequent use of glottal stops for initial and medial consonants; (e) hypernasality; and (f) obvious nasal air emission. Because of physical problems including upper respiratory disease, physical management of the structure had to be delayed. Agreement to initiate speech-language therapy was reached with the understanding that the goal was to improve intelligibility. Therapeutic foci were identified: (1) to facilitate appropriate intraoral coordination for correct articulatory placement; (2) to habituate appropriate production of currently omitted final consonant sounds; and (3) to reduce or eliminate use of gross substitution errors.

A treatment sequence involving Joey and his parents in play therapy was applied. Initial energies were focused on inclusion of omitted final sounds to give meaning to his many vowellike utterances. As articulatory placement and movements were identified and learned, speech intelligibility in the presence of nasal air emission enhanced Joey's verbal communication success. Successful use of articula-

tion skills encouraged the child to utilize his good speech in order to be understood. Reciprocal efforts of his improved verbal communication and his parents' positive response to it provided the reinforcement. Joey needed to master oral language skills within his physiological limitations. Likewise, early articulation skills management will be helpful in adapting surgically modified oral structures when Joey's health permits physical management of the velopharyngeal insufficiency.

Goal achievement in speech-language treatment for both functional and organic communication disorders reflects (a) accuracy of diagnosis, (b) efficiency of the clinical plan, (c) adaptability of the child for the tasks to be learned, and (d) involvement of the parents and home environment in the stimulation program. Realistic goal setting for the child with velopharyngeal insufficiency and for the family includes influential environmental factors and anticipates acceptance of the appropriate result.

ADVENT OF CRANIOFACIAL CENTERS

Since 1967, when the specialization of craniofacial surgery was inaugurated, a major change in the traditional concept of cleft palate management has evolved. Advances in physical management of orofacial clefts superseded the previous concept of team function, namely, evaluation, planning, and the rotation of patient assignment among attending professionals on the basis of their expressed interest in such cases. What evolved were what are now known as craniofacial centers where new parents and their babies with craniofacial birth defects are referred for care by a treatment team within the baby's first few days of life.

The treatment team, sometimes designated a "self-contained treatment team," is comprised of specialists in the fields similar to those found on traditional cleft lip-palate teams. However, these professionals typically share extended years of experience, specialized training, and backgrounds that incorporate research in their own fields and insight into tangential specializations to enhance their interaction and collective and collaborative service to the patient. A treatment team plans and carries out the staged long-term treatment and follow-up necessary for the care of the patient with an orofacial cleft.

THE TREATMENT TEAM COMMUNICOLOGIST

In applying advances in behavioral sciences, the treatment speech pathologist becomes what might be better termed a *communicologist*. He or she is involved in the task and opportunity to observe the newborn with cleft lip-palate and to interact with the new parents. Early acquaintance affords the opportunity to elicit their level of information and comprehension, acceptance, coping, and involvement with the baby as a person, with the birth defect and its sequelae as a reality.

From that beginning, the communicologist initiates an estimate of the infant's noncleft-related neurobiological integrity and the home communication environment, two determiners of language for that particular child. At that initial meeting the parents should be introduced to their role as a contributing part of the treatment team. Through their ability to care for the baby's physical needs, to cooperate with the multiple facets of long-term staged treatment, to interact with the baby's nonverbal expressions, and to provide appropriate tactile, visual, and auditory stimuli, the parents constitute the team's most continuous link to normalization of the child's verbal communication.

To encourage maximal patient benefits from family interrelationships, the initial meeting with the treatment team should establish for the family that they are accepted for what they are: the child with the orofacial deformity and the parents who produced that child. The attitude of the professionals must be accepting and should even be approving of the individuals involved. In handling the baby, the team members should reflect a pleasant comfort and sureness in the situation and demonstrate an open willingness to discuss any idea or concern, and answer any question or listen to whatever a family member needs to say. Even in this last quarter of the twentieth century, the team setting may be the first open invitation to talk that the parents have experienced since the birth of their baby [37].

The initial treatment team visit may be brief but it should be of sufficient length to introduce the family to the atmosphere of the setting, assure their welcome on return, and stabilize the idea of their significant role in the future program of care

for their baby. Regardless of what else is discussed, it is well to include two very important topics during that first visit: (1) feeding, and (2) stimulation.

The speech pathologist should utilize counseling skills of attending and listening to identify the extent to which information or suggestons are needed and which will be heard or accepted at that time. Feeding is important because of the biological need for the baby to give evidence of metabolizing its own body tissue. That evidence provides information on which judgments concerning timing for initial surgical intervention are based.

The act of feeding the baby is also important in stimulating the oral and facial mechanisms to develop and grow. That is, suckling and then sucking stimulate growth in the lower third of the face. These normal sequences of activity and development are a logical basis for discouraging use of nasogastric feeding tubes whenever possible, even in babies who have extreme orofacial dysmorphologies or very poorly functioning oral mechanisms. This belief in utilizing normal routines has led to the development of feeding techniques which are easily acquired, and selection of bottles which are readily available in ordinary and popular retail stores. Specifically, while feeding the infant, mothers are encouraged to monitor the movement of the lower jaw, the chin, and to become aware of the rhythm of that motion. Then, by using a pliable plastic bottle and a nipple with a crosscut opening, the mother can exert minimal pressure (squeeze) on the bottle to assist the infant in getting milk or formula from the bottle in a nearly normal manner. That is, the baby's jaw closure and the simultaneous manual pressure on the bottle by the caregiver squirts small amounts of liquid into the infant's mouth. The sucking-swallowing-breathing action usually experienced in infant feeding is simulated. By this method of feeding, it is possible to provide adequate nourishment for children with cleft lip-palate from birth and to provide physiological stimulation at the same time.

The activity of feeding also is very important communicatively in that during feeding the adult and child maintain the longest continous personal interaction during the day (or night) in early infancy. Managing this essential physical process with assurance and success allows the adult to transmit through touch and accompanying behaviors the stimulation essential to the continuum of caregiving causality through transactional influences, as described by Sameroff and Chandler [35]. That is, various combinations of events over time find the parents and child changing along a shared continuum. As the child matures, the forms of stimulation and response increase in complexity commensurate with the ability of the child and the parent and enhanced by the team's interactions with the parents.

During the first team visit, discussion of feeding techniques allows the parent not only to recheck technique and style but it opens the way for the communicologist to offer other assistance if it is obviously needed. Frequently, hospital nurses will have taught the parent good and efficient feeding techniques. Through observation of the parent's successful and comfortable feeding of the baby, the communicologist has an opportunity to praise the parent's skill and the baby's success and to encourage them to continue using the technique. It may be appropriate to tell the parent that activity of the oral mechanisms in feeding is important to growth and to developing coordination of muscles that will be used later in speech.

When either the parent or the infant is observed to be uncomfortable, unsuccessful, or unhappy (distressed) with the feeding procedure, the communicologist should offer assistance as needed. Frequently, a simple question about how things seem to be going will provide the parent a needed opportunity to state concerns, raise questions, and identify unresolved thoughts and impressions. Among other things, the communicologist may find that suggestions are appropriate in matters of infant positioning, or position and relaxation of the parent; applying pressure to the bottle to assist the infant in its sucking efforts; opening the end of the nipple with a crosscut instead of enlarging the round hole; and providing the infant with suitable visual and auditory stimuli during feeding.

Besides establishing mutual gaze and visual following, babies only a few weeks old imitate mouth positions and tongue protrusion. It is well-known that very young infants, only hours old, recognize faces as preferred patterns and very soon differentiate the mother's face from the rest. That selective attention is the first evidence of environmental differentiation. Babies with orofacial clefts need the same opportunity to do those exercises too, and their parents deserve the joy of recognizing the infant's participation. It is easy to demonstrate such child responses to parents. It is important that they learn the place of such interactions in normal development [8].

In the days of preparation for closure of the lip, which varies from 2 weeks to 2 months of age, parents and infant have the opportunity to establish the foundation of mutual trust, and the basis for normal affective development [52]. As they prepare for the hospital stay, parents and other caregivers should recognize the instances of mutual gaze and accompany them with vocalized intonation patterns and rhythmic sound sequences [1]. As the period of shared visual contact expands over the first few weeks, more specific aural stimulation can be offered, for example, nonspeech sounds, phonemes, syllables, words, and eventually even nursery rhymes and songs. Auditory stimulation without prior visual contact is introduced to gain attention and stimulate seeking behaviors. Such auditory stimuli initiate the formation of neurological pathways for later perception and discrimination of meaningful sounds.

MONITORING GROWTH AND DEVELOPMENT

The busy craniofacial center speech pathologist needs a protocol for monitoring the chronological progress of each infant's communication development. It is convenient and useful to utilize a screening procedure of the local pediatric community to facilitate sharing of data as treatment progresses. However, not all pediatricians maintain a standard chronology on each patient and the scale selected for use with cleft lip-palate patients will need to be reviewed to ensure that it addresses the development of language content, form, and use. The screening tool should follow multiple modes of perception and expression and extend from birth over several years.

A screening test has been preferred to an indepth test for use in the team setting because of the limited time required for administration. In the hands of an experienced clinician, even the brief form of screening can give clues to (a) developmental areas which need further evaluation; (b) any variation in rate of development for perception of various stimuli, especially acoustic, so that immediate assistance from team colleagues can be obtained to resolve problems, answer questions, or introduce new ideas to the family; (c) document prespeech communication and phonological and syntactic development; and (4) inform and guide the parents as they continue to work with and care for the child.

In-Depth Testing

Routine developmental screening using a standardized scale is one way to follow normal development across multiple modalities in each child, even for large caseloads. Thorough familiarity with the validity, reliability, and applications of the chosen scale, along with clinical observations, can alert the experienced examiner to content areas and modalities which need to be studied to a greater extent. Depending on the degree of urgency, the examination may take place during the same team visit, at a subsequent visit, or it may require a referral to a team consultant, a nonteam specialist, or a community agency.

Variations in Child Response

Although children are said to grow both physically and intellectually in spurts or stages, variations from the expected rate of development in a particular child require special attention. Notably this applies to acquisition of the various "milestones" of gross and fine motor coordination and to spontaneous responses to ordinary visual stimuli and particularly to auditory stimuli.

Figure 19-1. Phoneme frequency-by-type count for three groups: adult normal speakers (Voelker, 1934 [49]), 29- to 30-month-old noncleft palate toddlers (Irwin, 1947 [20]), and 22- to 30-month-old patients (TBCC) whose cleft palates were closed early (Barimo et al., 1987 [4]).

The speech-language clinician, with the audiologist, otologist, and pediatric neurologist, can prevent or identify, through early intervention, a broad array of developmental language disorders. Such intervention may be critical to normal phonological and syntactic development or to minimizing other communication disorders.

Documentation of Phonological Development

Developmental screening and astute clinical observation include documentation of spontaneous and elicited phonological productions from infant and toddler and recording of parent-reported child utterances. Direct observation of responses to auditory stimulation and interactive play, as well as parents' reports, yields a chronology of prespeech communication and sequential acquisition of verbal communication skills. Present evidence of normal linguistic communication development among infants and toddlers treated at craniofacial centers, unlike traditional expectations, reflects chronological norms based on the noncleft palate population as young as 12 to 18 months of age [34, 36].

Barimo and colleagues [4] reported a preliminary study of early phonological acquisition by 22- to 30-month-old children with cleft palate which closely resembled that reported for 20- to 30-month-old noncleft palate children [20, 49] and noncleft palate adults. Figure 19-1 shows the

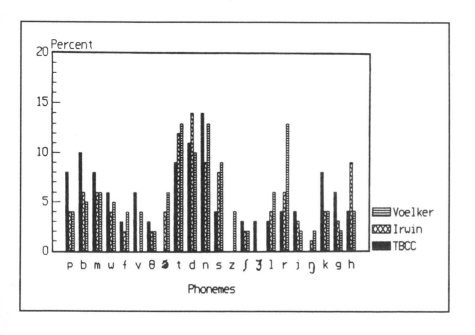

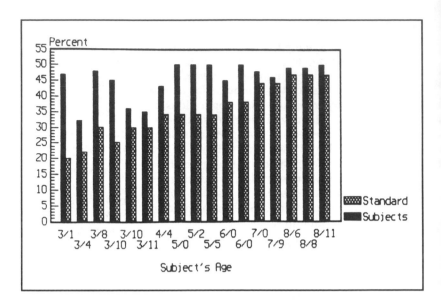

percentage of phonemes in utterances of those groups of speakers. These authors also presented evidence of articulatory proficiency among subjects 3 years, 1 month to 8 years, 11 months of age according to scores on the Templin-Darley Screening Test of Articulation [44]. Subjects' performances exceeded the cutoff scores for age as reflected in Figure 19-2. The crossed line indicates the sequence of cutoff scores listed in the test manual, while the continuous lines indicate the performance of individual subjects at the indicated age.

Sherman, Scheuerle, and Landis [40] reported on articulatory performance and velopharyngeal competency of preschoolers with orofacial clefts whose health care was managed by two protocols. Phonological analysis [10, 27] of responses to the Templin-Darley Screening Test of Articulation and the Iowa Pressure Test indicated that the subjects who had early intervention exhibited fewer incidences (5.9% of errors) of the speech characteristics usually associated with cleft palate than did the children whose health care management followed the protocol of the traditional team (10.6% of errors). Additionally, the speech of the former group contained no evidence of velar fricatives, pharyngeal fricatives, or glottal stops.

Informed Parents

Objective information about their child is very valuable to parents. It provides a basis for judging their observations and impressions and encourages them to continue to fulfill the parenting role.

Figure 19-2. Performance of subjects 1–3 and 8–11 years of age on the Templin-Darley Screening Test of Articulation and age-related cut-off scores (standard) provided in the technical manual for that test.

Most new parents are not well trained in child development. In some instances where the child's overall development as measured against normative data does not meet the parents' expectations or desires, the clinican has the opportunity to interact with the parents for the purpose of molding parental expectations or assisting the parents in maximizing their child's development. The communicologist especially is responsible for monitoring the developmental aspects of the child's language content, form, and use, while furnishing supportive directions to the family for the achievement of normal use of verbal communication. Especially valuable are opportunities to encourage activities that are supportive of the child's involvement with the environment, stimulation used in meaningful ways, and eradication of undesirable communicative behaviors.

Coaching Parents as the Child Progresses

Once the parents and patient are acquainted with the treatment team and have a grasp of the necessary information concerning cleft lip-palate management, their needs change. The type and manner of that change invites a professional-parent interactive style more like coaching than either teaching and informing or interviewing and answering questions. Coaching techniques acknowledge progress, achievements, strengths, and weaknesses with an eye to maintaining strengths and modifying weaknesses. Parents' awareness of present and coming events in the child's care is increased through the clinician's recognition of their understanding and attitudinal set, as well as through instruction, demonstrations, and anticipatory guidance.

In coaching, the professional avoids making assumptions but ascertains through listening and discussion the correctness and accuracy of parental observations and impressions. Although every effort is made to prevent misunderstandings and unrealistic expectations, these sometimes occur. Parents may present a view of the child which has little basis in fact, and display attitudes which have no relation to either the perceived cause or the effects of the attitude. Winnowing out the elements of such a puzzle requires astuteness and attention and is indeed rewarding to both the parents and professional.

Coaching also focuses on the parent as the primary model and teacher of the child. Various patterns of discourse are reflected in mother-to-child communication and differ with the verbal communication abilities of the child [13, 38]. Cleft palate patients, whose parents were coached on the importance and methods of communication from the time of the child's birth, have achieved age-normal scores on early language tests [25] and their parents use a range of discourse features similar to those of parents of noncleft palate, language-normal children [48].

EARLY SURGERY FOR CLEFT CLOSURE

The goals of proper function, normal speech, and appearance are apparently greatly enhanced through early (prior to 9 months) surgical closure of cleft lip and cleft palate. Application of surgical techniques include suturing of muscle segments across the cleft site, and realignment of abnormally attached muscles in the lip and soft palate [34]. Freed from osseous attachments, the tiny muscles gain in contractility and increase in strength and mass through the physiology of normal development and activity of daily living. Postoperative development following early closure apparently allows neurological patterning prior to the age of 2 years that is similar to that found in noncleft lip-palate infants. With appropriate stimulation, the modified structures are capable of adaptation for habituation of normal prespeech movements, postures, and sounds; and for the acquisition of phonological productions in the absence of hypernasal resonance and nasal air emission. Such patients reportedly do not need secondary surgical procedures for pharyngoplasty or for midface advancement [4, 37].

An added feature which must be noted relative to the early conclusion of surgical closure of the orofacial cleft is its impact on the family. This has many aspects but two seem to dominate. On the one hand, early closure allows the family to get on with its normal daily pursuits sooner than is the case when surgery is delayed until the baby's second year of life or later. On the other hand, acceptance of surgery for the very young baby is a difficult and even traumatic experience for parents. While they want the deformity treated, they must place their trust and their child in the hands of strangers. The traditional sociocultural status of the medical profession in the United States has been helpful in achieving parental compliance to available care plans for the needful child.

Today, two factors add to considerations for best available care for infants with cleft lip-palate: (1) Public awareness of birth defects and human differences is increasing through media programming and publications sponsored by national support organizations and professional associations. (2) Changes in delivery systems for medical services point to the need for review and considerations of traditional management protocols of care for patients with congenital craniofacial clefts. It may be that the future will find recognized regional centers where expert interdisciplinary treatment teams focus on care of babies with cleft lip-palate and their families. Advances in anesthetic and surgical techniques and equipment will be applied by experienced medical, surgical, dental, and nursing experts, and well trained pre- and postsurgical care staffs. Concomitantly, and with the assurance of adaptable biological outcomes, experts in behavioral sciences will initiate individualized programs of care from the time the child is born.

PRE- AND POSTSURGICAL PARENT TRAINING

Nurses on the treatment team participate intently in coaching parents throughout the infant's pre- and postsurgical care. Experienced nurses are the communicologist's best allies in addressing hospitalization concerns, both possible and probable. Most parents elect to stay in the hospital with their babies. For that purpose they need comfortable clothing, especially shoes, and a very few select "distraction" toys or play items for the child. Parents should not take valuable clothing or toys to the hospital. Personal items are often caught up in hospital materials and become permanently lost.

Parents are taught and encouraged to teach the infant before lip or palate surgery whatever modified feeding technique must be used to accomplish the task later when protecting the surgical wound and its sutures. Often such techniques require use of a modified syringe-type feeder with a short piece of tubing on the end. Babies and parents who are familiarized with the change before surgery seem to adapt better, and parents are more comfortable in meeting the demands of filling the device and delivering the food appropriately by applying assistive pressure to the plunger. Ease in management of the vital and time-consuming function of feeding the patient tends to help reduce stress and increase the opportunity for communication between the parent and the infant.

Parents must know about and understand the urgency of cleaning and lubricating the wound, and of maintaining the continuous use of arm restraints on the patient. Parents also seem comforted by the knowledge that the sutures dissolve and do not have to be removed. For cleft lip surgery they should be told to expect differences in the baby's appearance, due variously to the change in lip and face contour, the presence of a sutured wound, and paleness from the surgical experience. Also, under federal diagnosis-related grouping regulations (DRLs), most cleft lip-palate patients are discharged from the hospital within 24 to 36 hours following surgery, with the postoperative care continued at home.

Prior to hospitalization, the communicologist initiates open discussion of hospital facilities and personnel as well as the child's treatment and care. That exchange of information gives the family an opportunity to express and clarify thoughts and concerns about the anticipated experience. It likewise affords professionals on the team one more opportunity to trouble-shoot for the family so as to prevent surprises or misunderstandings, and to assure the parents that they may telephone a member of the treatment team for assistance or information while their child is in the hospital.

A preadmission visit to the hospital may be suggested or arranged. Fortunately, the craniofa-cial treatment team protocol generally finds that one family is rarely alone in the hospital at any given time. Comfort is derived from the presence of familiar faces of families met previously at the center — families that have shared similar experiences and information. Parents are exceedingly supportive of one another. With the help of hospital staff pediatric nurses who are experienced in the care of craniofacial cleft lip-palate patients, parents learn quickly how successfully they can care for their child in the postsurgery state.

Typically, within a few days, perhaps a week following surgery, the patient and family participate in the first follow-up team visit. Again, while the medical and surgical personnel concentrate on the biological progress of the child, the communicologist must view the family as a gestalt — an integrated progression toward normalization.

Sometimes parents and professionals tend to change the joy of communicating with a child into a job. Such constraints on parent-baby interaction are unnecessary and destructive. Treatment team clinicians seem to be highly successful in enjoying the babies, because they are babies, and they have potential to develop in all areas just as do babies without clefts. That is, from birth, and with monitoring of auditory function, babies whose orofacial clefts are closed in the first year can expect to follow a routine pediatric language development sequence. A very useful resource, which specifically targets the orofacial cleft population, is *A Parent-Child Cleft Palate Curriculum, Developing Speech and Language* by Brookshire and colleagues [7]. Another useful book is *Infant/Toddler, Introducing Your Child to the Joy of Learning* by Earladeen Badger [2].

An adaptive environment and adaptive infant behavior [17] establish a communicating inter-relationship between parent and infant. The following sequence may emerge: Parents introduce baby to environmental sound, melody, and rhythms accompanied by movement of objects and color. The baby cries, quiets, squeals, coos, babbles. Caregivers use real words, sounds of animals, machines, while within the visual field of the baby. They provide one-word names for items in the baby's essential world and use consistency in naming objects and actions. The baby hears, discriminates, imitates sounds and sound combinations. He or she attempts replication of the sounds in meaningful environmental context. Everyday language which the parents use in the baby's home environment must not be too complex. That language forms the psycholinguistic basis of the baby's understanding of his world and finding his place in it. Sharing picture books with very young babies is recommended [9, 46]. Beautiful illustrations expand the knowable world and stories stimulate the imagination.

Babies need to hear discrete units of sound in meaningful ways. Infants' first attempts at meaningful words may be phonemic or syllabic. Families may adopt the toddler's new "word" as a temporary term for some object or action. (Parents and babies tend to learn early that bah-bah means bottle.) The infant's first words of adult language tend to emerge around 12 months of age. What that first word is depends on the environment, reinforcement, and parents' recognition (or adoption) of the infant's utterance.

Watching the child's progression through auditory milestones [29] and phonological milestones [32, 33, 43] is very rewarding for the parent who understands some degree of the complex nature of verbal communication and its acquisition. For the communicologist, additional rewards are surfacing through parent-coaching for infant communication stimulation offered in treatment team settings. While little normative data on infant oral coordination for speech and infant central auditory processing are available, careful clinical assessment and follow-up of individual infants and toddlers has begun to differentiate skill levels in both language areas. The toddler with repaired cleft lip-palate whose speech is confounded with articulation errors in the absence of nasal air emission or hypernasality may present an oral motor profile of clumsiness or incoordination reflective of dyspraxias found in older children. Intervention through phonological stimulation during the early age of neurological plasticity may be effective in preventing articulation disorders or development of unacceptable compensatory phonological productions. Preliminary studies by Randall and colleagues [34] and Scheuerle and colleagues [36] support this hypothesis.

Monitoring of verbal communication development has yielded another interesting phenomenon in children whose cleft lips or palates were closed prior to the age of 1 year and who were provided an early stimulation program. In a study of expressive and receptive language of children with cleft lip-palate, cranial synostosis, and age-matched normal subjects, Letcher and colleagues [25] found no difference in performance among the three groups. That is, all subjects with cleft palates achieved age-equivalent or higher scores in both receptive and expressive language (Table 19-1). The tests utilized were the receptive-expressive emergent language test (REEL Scale) [11] and the Sequenced Inventory of Communication Development (SICD) [19]. Subsequent review of the test results for all the subjects in conjunction with their clinical data revealed interesting information. Most subjects earned higher scores in receptive tasks than in expressive skills.

Two 31-month-old subjects in the study, one male and one female with congenital complete bi-

TABLE 19-1. LANGUAGE PERFORMANCE OF TODDLERS WHO HAD EARLY INTERVENTION FOR CLEFT PALATE BY A TREATMENT TEAM

Age (mo.)	Cleft type	SICD		REEL	
		ECA	RCA	ECA	RCA
13	Bilateral L/P	20	20	11	14
22	Bilateral L/P	28	32	27	33
25	Bilateral L/P	30	32	29	33
27	Bilateral L/P	32	32	30	33
31	Bilateral L/P	48	36	36	36
31	Bilateral L/P	48	36	36	36
14	Unilateral L/P	12	16	11	16
14	Unilateral L/P	16	16	10	14
36	Unilateral L/P	40	36	36	36
31	Soft palate	48	48	36	36

Key: SICD = Sequenced Inventory of Communication Development; REEL = receptive-expressive emergent language; ECA = expressive communicative age; RCA = receptive communicative age; L/P = lip/palate.

lateral clefts, achieved the upper limits of the tests expressively (REEL Scale — 36 months, and SICD — 48 months), but unexpectedly did less well on the receptive scales. The male child moved away from the treatment team at the age of 3 years and was placed in a Headstart program near his new home. The female child was placed in an ongoing direct language stimulation program with specific recommendations for testing of receptive language processing, and for documenting and shaping her interactive behavior. After 3 months of diagnostic therapy twice a week, her progress was reviewed. While behavior in the clinical setting had greatly improved through acquisition of coping skills, several behaviors which remained reflected those described by Katz [21] and Keith [23] as typical of central auditory processing disorders. The child was referred for instrumental testing of retrocochlear and central auditory processing function [50] preparatory to appropriate preschool educational placement and family counseling. Recent parental reports indicate that she is doing well in a regular first-grade classroom where she has been on the principal's honor roll since entering school. Experience with this patient points to the potential for unprecedented early identification and intervention with noncleft-related communication disorders in individual patients with congenital orofacial clefts. Treatment for communication disorders prior to the age of 3 years blends well the modern concept of early intervention and continued behavioral management when indicated.

SUMMARY

This chapter discusses several aspects of prespeech by the very young child, first verbal communication of the infant and toddler, and the communication environment provided young children with cleft lip and palate. It introduces concepts of the modern approach to cleft lip-palate care management from birth by a self-contained treatment team which includes the parents, and the impact of very early physical and behavioral care management of the patient. In conclusion, it may be well to ask if current training programs are preparing speech-language pathologists and audiologists to fill the roles that are evident and emerging in team diagnosis and treatment of infants and toddlers with cleft lip and palate.

REFERENCES

1. Adamson, L., Als, H., Tronick, E., and Brazelton, T. B. Social interaction between a sighted infant and her blind parents. J. Am. Acad. Child Psychiatry 16:194–204, 1977.
2. Badger, E. Infant/Toddler, Introducing Your Child to the Joy of Learning. New York: McGraw-Hill, 1981.
3. Bangs, T. Language and Learning Disorders of the Pre-Academic Child with Curriculum Guide (2nd ed.). Englewood Cliffs, N.J.: Prentice-Hall, 1982.
4. Barimo, J., Habal, M. B., Scheuerle, J., and Ritterman, S. I. Postnatal palatoplasty, implications for normal speech articulation — a preliminary report. J. Reconstr. Surg. 21:139–143, 1987
5. Brazelton, T. B., Koslowski, B., and Main, M. The Origins of Reciprocity: The Early Mother-Infant Interaction. In M. Levine and L. Rosenblum (Eds.), The Effect of the Infant on Its Caregiver. New York: Wiley, 1977. Pp. 49–76.
6. Bricker, D., and Schiefelbusch, R. L. Infants at Risk. In L. McCormick and R. L. Schiefelbusch, Early Language Intervention. Columbus, Ohio: Charles E. Merrill, 1982.
7. Brookshire, B. L., Lynch, J. I., and Fox, D. A Parent-Child Cleft Palate Curriculum, Developing Speech and Language. Tegard, Ore.: C.C. Publications, 1980.
8. Bruner, J. From Communication to Language: A Psychological Perspective. In I. Markova (Ed.), The Social Context of Language. New York: Wiley. Pp. 17–48.
9. Butler, D. Babies Need Books. New York: Atheneum, 1980.
10. Bzoch, K. R. Measurement and Assessment of Categorical Aspects of Cleft Palate Speech. In K. R. Bzoch (Ed.), Communicative Disorders Related to Cleft Lip and Palate (2nd ed.). Boston: Little, Brown, 1979. Pp. 161–191.
11. Bzoch, K. R., and League, R. L. Assessing Language Skills in Infancy. Austin, Tex.: Pro Ed, 1978.
12. Cole, P. Language Disorders in Preschool Children. Englewood Cliffs, N.J.: Prentice-Hall, 1982.
13. Dore, J. Conditions for the Acquisition of Speech Acts. In I. Markova (Ed.), The Social Context of Language. New York: Wiley, 1978. Pp. 87–112.
14. Drotar, D., Baskiewicz, A., Irvin, N., Kennel, J., and Klaus, M. The adaptation of parents to the birth of an infant with a congenital malformation: A hypothetical model. Pediatrics 56:710–716, 1975.
15. Eilers, R. E., Gavin, E. J., and Wilson, W. R. Linguistic experience and phonemic perception in infancy: A cross-linguistic study. Child Dev. 50:14–18, 1979.
16. Frans, N., Scheuerle, J., Bequer, N., and Habal, M. B. Middle ear tissue mass and audiometric data from otologic care of infants with cleft palate. Cleft Palate J. 25:70–71, 1988.
17. Greenspan, S. I. Parenting in Infancy and Early Childhood. A Developmental Structuralist Approach to Delineating Adaptive and Maladaptive Patterns. In V. J. Sasserath (Ed.), Minimizing High-Risk Parenting. New Brunswick, N.J.: Johnson & Johnson, 1983. Pp. 79–86.

18. Habal, M. B., and Maniscalco, J. Categorization of craniofacial deformities based on our experiences with surgical manipulaton. *Ann. Plast. Surg.* 6:6–9, 1981.

19. Hedrick, D. L., Prather, E. M., and Tobin, A. R. *Sequenced Inventory of Communication Development.* Seattle: University of Washington Press, 1975.

20. Irwin, O. C. Development of speech during infancy: Curve of phonemic frequencies. *J. Exp. Psychol.* 37:187–193, 1947.

21. Katz, J. Phonemic Synthesis. In E. Z. Lasky and J. Katz (Eds.), *Central Auditory Processing Disorders: Problems of Speech, Language, Learning.* Baltimore: University Park Press, 1983. Pp. 269–296.

22. Kavanaugh, J. F. *Otitis Media and Child Development.* Parkton, Md.: York Press, 1986.

23. Keith, R. W. Audiological and Auditory Language Tests of Central Auditory Function. In R. W. Keith (Ed.), *Central Auditory and Language Disorders in Children.* Boston: College-Hill Press, 1981. Pp. 61–76.

24. Kroner, A. F., and Thoman, E. B. Relative efficacy of contact and vestibular stimulation on soothing neonates. *Child Dev.* 43:443–453, 1972.

25. Letcher, L., Scheuerle, J., Strange, W., and Habal, M. B. Receptive and expressive language in toddlers with and without craniofacial anomalies. Paper presented at the Annual Convention of the American Cleft Palate Association, San Antonio, Texas, 1987.

26. Lewis, M. The infant and its caregiver: The role of contingency. *Allied Health Behav. Sci.* 1:469–492, 1978.

27. Love, R. J. Phonological process analysis: Using three position tests. *Language, Speech and Hearing in the Schools* 17:72–79, 1981.

28. McCormick, L., and Schiefelbusch, R. L. *Early Language Intervention.* Columbus, Ohio: Charles E. Merrill, 1984.

29. Northern, J., and Downs, M. P. *Hearing in Children* (2nd ed). Baltimore: Williams & Wilkins, 1978.

30. Philips, B. J. Stimulating Syntactic and Phonological Development in Infants with Cleft Palate. In K. R. Bzoch (Ed.), *Communicative Disorders Related to Cleft Lip and Palate* (2nd ed.). Boston: Little, Brown, 1979. Pp. 304–311.

31. Piaget, J., and Inhelder, B. *The Psychology of the Child.* New York: Basic Books, 1969.

32. Poole, I. Genetic development in articulation of consonant sounds in speech. *Elementary English Rev.* 2:159–161, 1934.

33. Prather, E., Hedrich, D., and Kein, C. Articulation development in children aged two to four years. *J. Speech Hear. Disord.* 40:179–191, 1975.

34. Randall, P., LaRossa, D. D., Fakhraee, S. M., and Cohen, M. A. Cleft palate closure at three to seven months of age: A preliminary report. *Plast. Reconstr. Surg.* 71:5, 1983.

35. Sameroff, A., and Chandler, M. J. Reproductive Risk and the Continuum of Caretaking Causality. In F. D. Horowitz (Ed.), *Review of Child Development Research.* Chicago: University of Chicago Press, 1975. Pp. 187–244.

36. Scheuerle, J., Bollinger, A., Barimo, J., and Habal, M. B. Postnatal palatoplasty, early surgical correction and speech. Paper presented at the Fifth International Congress on Cleft Palate and Related Craniofacial Anomalies, Monte Carlo, 1985.

37. Scheuerle, J., Frans, N., and Habal, M. B. A developmental structuralist approach to normal speech and language development in patients with cleft lip/palate. Paper presented at Annual Convention of the American Cleft Palate Association, New York, 1986.

38. Searle, J. *An Essay in the Philosophy of Language.* London: Cambridge University Press, 1969.

39. Searle, J. Speech Acts and Recent Linguistics. In D. Aaronson and R. W. Riever (Eds.), *Minimizing High-Risk Parenting.* New Brunswick, N.J.: Johnson & Johnson, 1975. Pp. 44–50.

40. Sherman, A., Scheuerle, J., and Landis, P. An intercenter study of articulatory proficiency and velopharyngeal function in young children with repaired cleft palate. Paper presented at the Annual Convention of the American Cleft Palate Assn., Williamsburg, Va., 1988.

41. Stark, R. Infant speech production and communication skills. *Allied Health Behav. Sci.* 1:131–151, 1978.

42. Stool, S. E., and Randall, P. Unexpected ear disease in infants with cleft palate. *Cleft Palate J.* 4:99–103, 1967.

43. Templin, M. *Certain Language Skills in Children.* Child Welfare Monograph, No. 26. Minneapolis: University of Minnesota, 1957.

44. Templin, M., and Darley, F. L. *The Templin Darley Tests of Articulation* (2nd ed.). Iowa City: University of Iowa, Bureau of Educational Research and Service, 1969.

45. Trehub, S. E., Bull, D., and Schneider, B. A. Infant Speech and Non-Speech. In R. L. Schiefelbusch and D. D. Bricker (Eds.), *Early Language Acquisition and Intervention.* Baltimore: University Park Press, 1981. Pp. 9–50.

46. Trelease, J. *The Read-Aloud Handbook.* New York: Penguin Books, 1982.

47. Tronick, E. Infant Communication Intent. In A. P. Reilly (Ed.), *The Communication Game.* New Brunswick, N.J.: Johnson & Johnson, 1980, Pp. 4–10.

48. Turner, L. *Maternal Discourse Features with Children with Cleft Lip with or Without Cleft Palate.* Thesis, University of South Florida, Tampa, 1984.

49. Voelker, C. H. Phonetic distribution in formal American pronunciation. *J. Acoust. Soc. Am.* 5:242–246, 1934.

50. Willeford, J. Assessing Central Auditory Behavior in Children: A Test Battery Approach. In R. W. Keith (Ed.), *Central Auditory Dysfunction.* New York: Grune & Stratton, 1977.

51. Wolff, P. The causes, controls, and organization of behavior in the neonate. *Psychol. Issues* 5:1–99, 1966.

52. Wolff, P. The role of biological rhythms in early psychological development. *Bull. Menninger Clin.* 31:197–218, 1967.

CHAPTER 20

Modifying Velopharyngeal Closure Through Training Procedures

Dennis M. Ruscello

In simplified terms the velopharyngeal closure mechanism has been characterized as a valve [66, 68] whose actions act to separate the oral and nasal cavities. The valve functions in both speech and nonspeech activites; however, we are most interested in the operation of the valve during speech production. McWilliams, Morris, and Shelton [36] have described closure for speech as consisting of contact with the velum and posterior pharyngeal wall. The velum moves in an upward and backward direction to articulate with the posterior pharyngeal wall. In addition, many normal-speaking individuals exhibit midline excursion of the lateral pharyngeal walls during closure [74]. The achievement of closure enables a speaker to generate sufficient air pressure and flow for the production of certain consonant sounds and also allows for the production of voiced sounds without hypernasal resonance.

Persons who are unable to achieve velopharyngeal closure or show faulty timing of closure often exhibit problems with speech production [22]. Generally, surgical or prosthetic management is used to improve velopharyngeal closure for speech [36, 51, 57]; however, some speech-language pathologists have developed treatments aimed at improving velopharyngeal closure [23, 45]. Schneider and Shprintzen [48] summarized the findings of 592 speech-language pathologists who responded to a questionnaire concerning the diagnosis and management of velopharyngeal closure problems. Approximately 84 percent of the respondents indicated that they employed some form of palate training. A further analysis showed that 84 percent employed articulation therapy, 54 percent utilized nonspeech techniques such as blowing and sucking, and 48 per-

cent used some form of direct palatal stimulation. It should be noted that respondents could select more than one category if appropriate. It would appear that many speech-language pathologists utilize various speech or related methods in dealing with persons who demonstrate velopharyngeal closure deficits.

The purpose of this chapter is to discuss the use of palate training as a treatment for persons with velopharyngeal closure deficits. Important to the discussion are a number of issues that are inextricably related to the main topic and they are presented below:

1. What is the neurophysiological basis for palate training?
2. Has research data been generated on the use of palate training?
3. What are the results of palate training programs and what future recommendations might be made?
4. Are there any prognostic indicators which might be used to predict future success?

NEUROPHYSIOLOGY

The following discussion is a brief treatment of the neurophysiology of palate activity. Readers are referred to Shelton's comprehensive discussion in Chapter 17 of this book. Lubker [25] characterized velopharyngeal function in the production of nonnasal vowels and consonants as "very probably a predictably variable act." The speaker is trying to achieve a goal of "perceptually acceptable speech," thus indicating that motor programming of velopharyngeal activity is very important in overall speech production. It is clear that variations in closure occur [49], but information which might be used to predict variations is lacking. In this teleological characterization of velopharyngeal function, Lubker [26] theorized that the velopharyngeal mechanism assumes various articulatory positions requisite to the achievement of the proper acoustic signal. The effort employed is variable because different motor control commands are used to achieve a particular motor goal.

The theoretical position developed by Folkins [16] is that normal speakers formulate motor rules which enable them to produce acceptable speech. The rules are not tied into a specific phonetic construct such as the phone or syllable but are rather flexible holistic motor goals. The flexibility enables a speaker to make adjustments in a move ment pattern while meeting a particular motor goal. In addition to flexibility, Folkins also discusses plasticity in motor control systems. Speakers faced with certain types of speech adjustments might require a period of adaptation. During the period of adaptation, new motor command goals are formalized within a new rule system. Flexibility and plasticity are hypothesized as speech motor control strategies used by speakers to produce perceptually correct speech. In the former, adjustments are made within an existing rule system, while with the latter there is a modification of the rule system.

The construct of plasticity has great appeal in explaining perceptually correct speech with persons who exhibit closure deficits. Former discussions have referred to the compensatory movements of good cleft palate speakers [35]; however, plasticity would suggest that the speaker formulated new rules over time to achieve appropriate motor goals. That is, the motor pattern could reflect a rule reorganization on the part of the speaker. Karnell, Folkins, and Morris [20] studied oral and velar movements, voicing, and nasal resonance in four subjects who had repaired cleft palates. Previous clinical examinations indicated that two of the subjects were judged to have hypernasal speech while two were not. The two speakers without hypernasality exhibited velopharyngeal movements which differed from expected movement patterns. The findings prompted the investigators to speculate that good cleft pal-

ate speakers may restructure their motor systems because of structural deficits.

Feedback mechanisms were not a formal part of the control theories summarized herein, but descriptions of motor control [1, 39] and motor learning [46] do emphasize the use of sensory feedback. Wolf [71] has written that the anatomical and physiological factors underlying muscle feedback are complex and not completely understood. Nevertheless, pressure, touch, and vibratory stimuli can be used as stimulatory agents for individuals undergoing muscle training programs. The use of such stimuli acts to trigger reflex activity and provide a basis for continued retraining [8, 9].

Kuehn [22] has indicated that the oropharyngeal area contains sensory nerve endings which appear to lessen in number from anterior to posterior regions of the oropharynx. In addition, speech-related studies of oral sensory function indicate that sensory abilities diminish along the anterior-posterior dimension [61]. Dr. Shelton in Chapter 17 has written that somesthetic feedback includes "the senses of movement, position, touch-pressure, and pain and to muscle sense (awareness of muscle tension) and an associated sense of effort." Some sensory information is available for conscious introspection while other sensory information does not reach consciousness and cannot be utilized in such a fashion. It is implicitly presumed that sensory information that is available to speakers can be used in various speech therapy treatments. However, studies of sensory awareness [53, 54], anatomical evidence [22, 61], and information synthesized by Shelton (see Chap. 17) suggest that the employment of conscious somesthetic feedback for modifying velopharyngeal closure deficits may not be a viable therapeutic approach.

Investigators have provided a number of speculative explanations for positive results reported in palate training studies [23, 73] but the mechanisms responsible have not been identified. In order to examine this primary issue, it is important to consider the key variables — motor practice and anatomy and physiology. Shelton [50] has written that motor practice can be employed for a number of different purposes. Those purposes include strength development, extension of endurance, increasing range of motion, and skill formation. The training of oral articulation skills has been characterized as a skill-building process [21, 46], but application of such concepts to palate training is not a unitary process. It seems likely that strength development, increasing range of motion, and skill formation are legitimate goals of a palate training program. McWilliams and colleagues [36] have suggested that some individuals who improve closure for speech may do so through strength-building and resultant hypertrophy or the formation of skilled movement. Yet, others may benefit by increasing range of motion, and still others through a combination of the above.

Speculation concerning different purposes for engaging in motor practice is directly related to the treatment population. That is, subjects used in palate training studies are heterogeneous with respect to structural, physiological, and neurological status. Folkins [16] discussed the various structural and physiological problems that may present with cleft palate speakers and his excellent description is as follows:

In addition, structural disabilities in the speaker with repaired cleft palate may include a reduction in muscle strength, an inefficient alignment of muscular forces, or a change in the mechanical characteristics of the VP [velopharyngeal] tissue. There may be increases in elasticity, viscosity, or mass relative to the amount of active muscular force available. These factors may not only affect the range of motion for many structures, but they would also make it harder to move the structures within the range. One would expect that, in general, patients with a repaired palatal cleft would have some degree of mechanical disability when compared to speakers with a normal mechanism.

In summary, velopharyngeal closure for speech is an important aspect in developing perceptually correct speech. Two theoretical positions were presented which emphasized the speaker's utilization of different motor control commands to realize production goals. The variability in motor commands is a reflection of adjustments that a speaker must make. Commands must be flexible to enable such adjustments to be made within a motor rule system. In some instances a speaker is faced with speech adjustments that require potential motor rule changes, and the construct of plasticity may serve as an explanation. Plasticity might also be used to account for successful results in palate training programs. The speaker formulated a new set of motor command rules which facilitated good speech.

Finally, there are a number of different purposes for using motor practice techniques. The development of improved movement patterns may necessitate practice to build strength, range of motion, or motor skills, or a combination thereof. McWilliams and colleagues [36] feel that it is possible to teach individuals improved use of the palate for speech; however, any improvement would be limited by the structural and neurological conditions present. Although authors have discussed various hypotheses, the rationale underlying the completion of a successful palate training program has not been established.

PALATE TRAINING STUDIES

There have been a number of investigations which have examined palate training and they have differed with respect to the type of treatment, number of subjects, and dependent variable measures [8, 9, 45]. For ease of discussion, training techniques will be categorized as either indirect or direct palatal training procedures. A treatment in the former category would not involve formal palatal stimulation, but would be designed to influence palate activity. For example, articulation therapy might be provided and various measures of velopharyngeal closure for speech obtained to determine if the treatment had some effect on closure. Direct methods consist of stimulation or focus on the palate while engaged in some type of speech or nonspeech activity. A client who receives electrical stimulation to the palate while producing various speech sounds would be receiving a direct treatment. It should be noted that the use of the term *palate training* is employed herein. This was not done to minimize the contribution of pharyngeal wall movement in closure activity, but to provide a general discussion term. Where appropriate the review will include information concerning pharyngeal wall activity.

INDIRECT METHODS

Shelton and colleagues [52] examined the effect of articulation therapy on velopharyngeal closure. Nine patients served as experimental subjects and eight were controls. The experimental subjects received articulation training while the controls did not. Results indicated that articulation skills improved for the experimental group but there were no changes in closure or posterior pharyngeal wall movement.

DIRECT METHODS

Investigators have developed a number of direct treatments which have varied as a function of the type of activity or activities utilized. Consequently, they are subdivided into the following: investigations which examined the use of speech appliances to improve palatal activity; studies involving stimulation to the palate while subjects engaged in speech or nonspeech activities; and biofeedback studies which have furnished subjects with indices to palatal movement during speech production.

SPEECH APPLIANCE STUDIES

Blakeley [3] provided an initial report which suggested that a speech appliance might stimulate palate or pharyngeal wall activity, or both. The case study report described a youngster who was fitted with a speech appliance because of poor articulation skills. Following a 3-year period of wear, Blakeley found that articulation skills improved. In addition, it was necessary to remove the appliance because of a judged reduction in hypernasality. The author suggested that the appliance promoted increased excursion of the pharyngeal walls.

Other reports by Blakeley and his associates [4–6] provided clinical descriptions which supported the results presented initially. One such investigation [4] described a treatment for three cleft palate children who had initial surgical repair and lacked adequate velopharyngeal closure. They were fitted with speech appliances which were gradually reduced along the lateral and posterior margins without negative impact on speech production or resonance. Following the reduction program they underwent successful pharyngeal flap surgery.

Blakeley [5] provided a summary report of his clinical activities and indicated that 22 cases out of 100 that were fitted with speech appliances no longer needed them. Nasal flutter and listening tube judgments were negative for the 22 cases. The author felt that the appliances stimulated pharyngeal muscle development. The resulting hypertrophy created additional bulk and aided closure for speech.

The final report in this series was a case study of a youngster who exhibited velopharyngeal incompetency of some unknown neurological origin [6]. The boy was fitted with an appliance that was gradually reduced over a 31-month period.

Removal of the appliance did not result in any negative findings. Manometric readings were acceptable, nasal flutter negative, and use of listening tubes did not detect unwanted nasal air escape.

Similar to Blakeley, Weiss [70] summarized clinical data on 125 patients who were fitted with speech appliances and were subject to appliance reduction. Twenty-three patients (18%) were judged to have normal resonance quality following eventual removal of the appliances. The results are in agreement with those presented by Blakeley. An additional client report by Wong and Weiss [72] summarized the results of 40 patients who had been enrolled in an appliance reduction program. Twenty (50%) of the patients were able to eliminate appliance usage without adverse effect on speech production or vocal quality.

In contrast to the case study and retrospective research reports, Shelton and his research group carried out two investigations which systematically studied speech appliance reduction. In the first investigation, Shelton and colleagues [55] fitted three subjects with speech appliances. The appliances were custom-made and had removable pharyngeal sections. Subjects gradually had their appliances reduced in size, but there were no significant changes in the dependent variable measures. A companion study by Shelton and colleagues [56] used cinefluorography to examine the pharyngeal wall movements of 18 subjects who underwent appliance reduction. Subjects received one to three reductions in their appliances at periods of 4 to 6 weeks. Analysis of cinefluorographic films showed no difference between pre- and post-measurements.

PALATAL STIMULATION DURING SPEECH PRODUCTION

Yules and Chase [73] conducted an experiment wherein subjects received electrical stimulation to the velum and lateral pharyngeal walls. A total of 30 subjects with velopharyngeal closure deficits participated in the investigation. They were provided with electrical stimulations while producing the vowel /a/. Subjects also carried out home practice by stroking the posterior pharyngeal wall with cotton swabs. When assessment measures indicated reduced nasal air flow and velar elevation, practice shifted to continuous speech. The subjects were fitted with a device known as a Speechometer which contained oral and nasal microphones. Output from the microphones could be controlled by the experimenter to manipulate oral-nasal balance. The authors indicated that the treatment resulted in reduced nasal air flow for 24 subjects (80%), and 14 subjects of the 24 also eliminated their hypernasality.

A replication of the Yules and Chase study was done approximately a year later with 34 subjects [69]. The electrical and tactile stimulation procedures along with articulation therapy were implemented; however, the treatment did not significantly alter nasal air flow, hypernasality, or palatal movement in the group of subjects.

A study carried out by Tash and colleagues [65] examined the effectiveness of training pharyngeal wall movements. The subjects consisted of four normal-speaking children and two with velopharyngeal closure deficits in the absence of clefts. Two of the normal speakers served as controls while the other two normals and the defective speakers were given the treatment. The training sequence included lateral and posterior pharyngeal wall stimulation with cotton swabs and vowel phonation activities with observers noting pharyngeal wall excursion. Findings showed that speakers were able to develop pharyngeal wall movements but the movements did not significantly alter velopharyngeal closure in either treatment group.

Massengill, Quinn, and Pickrell [28] developed a prosthetic speech device called a palatal stimulator. The stimulator consisted of hard palate and soft palate sections and was kept in place with dental clasps. The authors suggested that the device facilitated posterior movement of the velum. Five patients who exhibited velum-posterior pharyngeal wall gaps from 3 to 13 mm wore the device for approximately 12 months. At the end of the period, cinefluorographic measures showed that velopharyngeal gaps were eliminated or reduced in size for all subjects.

PALATAL STIMULATION DURING NONSPEECH ACTIVITIES

Massengill and his research associates [27] evaluated the effectiveness of blowing, sucking, and swallowing exercises. The investigators employed lateral-view cinefluorography as the criterion measure. Thirteen subjects with closure deficits were assigned to one of three treatment groups. One group practiced blowing exercises with a manometer or other device, another group performed sucking exercises with a straw or used a meter which recorded pressure, and the final group engaged in swallowing exercises while noting thy-

roid excursion with their index finger. All subjects received articulation therapy in conjunction with their exercise program. Comparison of pre- and post-cinefluorographic studies showed that subjects who received swallow training improved velopharyngeal closure for speech.

A palatal exercise device was developed by Lubit and Larsen [24] in an attempt to improve velopharyngeal closure. The device was inserted orally and contained a bite-block and rubber bag which was inflated. The inflated bag acted to displace the palate posteriorly. The exercise device was employed with 28 subjects, but only a single case study was presented. The patient was said to have improved in all criterion measures except the rating of hypernasality.

Sucking exercises were implemented for an adult whose complaint was air leakage while playing musical instruments [29]. The subject practiced sucking through a straw during a 6-month training program. At the termination of the practice, the subject reported that he was able to play musical instruments without leakage of air through the nose.

Powers and Starr [43] employed a training regimen that included blowing, sucking, gagging, and swallowing exercises. The authors studied four subjects who had velum-posterior pharyngeal wall gaps of less than 8 mm. The training program lasted 6 weeks and subjects practiced all of the nonspeech activities. Judgments of nasality and x-ray measures of velar gap taken at the termination of the program did not differ from pretest findings.

The final investigation in this section was conducted by Peterson [41] who examined elevation of the soft palate in response to electrical or tactile stimulation. The electrical current and tactile force were measured for each trial. The 20 subjects included five who had closure deficits; another five with repaired clefts but acceptable closure; and 10 subjects with speech problems in the absence of a closure deficit. Subjects underwent cinefluorographic study before and during the stimulation trials. Tactile stimulation did not influence palatal movement; however, five subjects did exhibit some movement with electrical stimulation.

BIOFEEDBACK STUDIES

A number of treatments have been developed wherein the subject is provided with information concerning performance [12]. Some type of equipment is employed so that an individual is provided with information that is generally not available on a conscious level [17]. Basmajian [2] states that biofeedback "inserts a person's volition into the gaps of an open feedback loop. Once an individual has brought the behavior of interest under conscious control, the feedback technique is gradually faded to enable execution without instrumental monitoring." Fuller [17] feels that successful behavioral control through biofeedback is a function of motivation, reinforcement, and overlearning.

Fletcher [14] developed the TONAR and TONAR II instruments for the purpose of assessing hypernasal resonance; however, the author suggested that the instruments may also be useful in modifying nasality. Acoustic signals are isolated into oral and nasal components and a ratio between the two is automatically determined. Subjects could use the information in an attempt to change the oral-nasal ratio. Two different training experiments were reported by Fletcher. In the first, two subjects who wore speech appliances underwent a training program which progressively altered nasal-oral ratios, thus providing a series of progressive approximations to total elimination. Results indicated that the subjects did reduce the nasal component in their speech, but complete modification was not achieved. The second experiment used the same training procedure, but subjects consisted of seven individuals with surgically repaired clefts and closure deficits. Fletcher indicated that all subjects reduced the nasal component in their speech; however, they showed a great deal of variability in the degree of reduction.

An experiment conducted by Roll [44] examined the use of visual feedback. Two subjects with repaired clefts were fitted with a piezoelectric crystal from a contact microphone. The crystal was attached to the nares so that unwanted nasal vibration could be detected and presented via a light display. After a short training period, both subjects were able to produce isolated vowels without nasal vibration. Measures of generalization for vowels and other speech units were not conducted.

A case study carried out by Moller and colleagues [38] utilized a displacement transducer as a feedback device. The transducer was attached to a molar tooth and made contact with the velum. Movement of the velum during phonation of /u/ was displayed to the subject through tracings from an oscilloscope. The subject did show increases in palatal elevation, but there were no significant changes in the dependent variable measures of velopharyngeal gap and resonance judgments.

Daly and Johnson [11] used the TONAR instrumentation with three mentally retarded subjects who exhibited closure deficits. Two had repaired clefts and a single subject did not. Prior to training, each subject underwent articulation testing, intelligibility testing, and baseline TONAR assessment. Administration of the evaluation measures following TONAR training indicated that articulation, intelligibility, and resonance balance improved, but hypernasal resonance was not completely eliminated. That is, final testing showed that nasality was still present.

A palatal training device that sensed movement of the velum was constructed by Tudor and Selley [67]. The device included a palatal plate with dental clasps and a U-shaped bar that contacted the velum at rest. Movement of the palate from the bar deactivated a visual light display. Subjects were instructed to use the visual display as an indirect index to palatal movement. When the velum elevated during production trials, the light display provided immediate feedback. The device was used with 24 subjects; there were four cleft palate children, 11 noncleft children with closure deficits, and nine adults with dysarthria. The measurement variables in this investigation were not clear, but the authors stated that closure was established in some cases. The improvement noted during training did not generalize to other speaking contexts.

Direct observation of the velum and posterior pharyngeal walls for diagnosis and training of velopharyngeal deficits can be accomplished through the use of a nasal fiberscope [31, 37]. The device is inserted into the nasopharynx and the image is viewed on a television screen. An abstract of a study conducted by Nishio and colleagues [40] described the authors' visual feedback program. Nineteen subjects were first taught to blow while observing the velopharyngeal port. When closure was achieved for blowing, practice shifted to the production of various speech sounds. Nishio and associates indicated that closure for plosive and fricative sounds was achieved for all subjects in less than 1 month of training.

The use of progressive approximation in conjunction with a biofeedback procedure was used with four subjects who had closure deficits during speech, but not when whistling or blowing [64]. Initially, the subjects would whistle or blow simultaneously with speech production. A scape-

scope was inserted into a naris to detect unwanted nasal air escape. After subjects achieved
consistent closure during the simultaneous speech-
nonspeech activity, practice shifted to speech exclusively. The investigators indicated that two of
the four subjects achieved consistent closure for
speech following training. Of the remaining two,
one achieved inconsistent closure and the other
did not complete the program.

Ellis and colleagues [13] discussed their development of instrumentation to assess nasal air
flow. The patient is fitted with a mask and nasal air
flow is detected by an anemometer. The resultant
air flow rate is recorded along with a voicing signal on a graphic display. Although the paper was
devoted primarily to assessment, the authors discussed its use as a visual feedback device for closure modification. In addition, they cited a single
subject who did show improvement, but their
evaluation of improvement was unclear from
the paper.

Another visual feedback technique was employed by Shelton and his research group [58] in
the form of an oral endoscope. The instrument is
inserted into the oral cavity and the lens positioned to view the velopharyngeal port. Movement patterns are displayed to subjects via television. Shelton and colleagues [60] used the technique with two adult subjects who demonstrated
closure deficits. The subjects practiced isolated
vowels, syllables, and syllable repetitions while
observing movement of the velopharyngeal mechanism and receiving verbal feedback from one of
the experimenters. Judges viewed randomized
tapes of subject performance and rated closure
activity along a five-point open-closed scale. The
data showed increased movement during practice trials, but transfer was not observed on an
automatic basis.

Shelton and Ruscello [62] summarized the results of seven subjects who underwent various
palate training procedures. The subjects varied as
a function of articulation skills, chronological age,
and type of closure deficit. Five of the subjects
were furnished with nasal air flow information.
They observed tracings printed on an amplifier-
recorder or displayed via a storage oscilloscope.
One subject participated in videoendoscopy training, while a single subject engaged in both practice activities. Inspection of final testing results
indicated that only one subject demonstrated significant improvement. The subject, who has a sensorineural hearing loss without cleft palate, was

given visual feedback information through observation of air flow tracings.

Shprintzen and his research group have used
visual biofeedback training to modify the closure
pattern of a normal speaker (see Siegel–Sadewitz
and Shprintzen [47]), and they have also used the
procedure successfully with clinical cases (see
Hoch et al. [18]). Their clinical data are based on
nine subjects who underwent visual fiberscopic
training. Subjects observed closure activity while
practicing various speech materials. Results were
most promising in that six of nine patients achieved
closure, two improved their closure patterns prior
to secondary palatal surgery, and only one showed
no change. The subject demonstrating no change
was diagnosed as having pseudobulbar palsy. The
authors indicated that subjects readily adapted to
the training procedures and used the visual information to modify deficient performance after limited training.

RESULTS OF PALATAL TRAINING STUDIES

The palate training studies reviewed herein included numerous treatment programs which differed with respect to many factors. If one inspects
the data in relation to overall efficacy, the conclusion is that programs have not been successful in
modifying velopharyngeal closure for speech.
However, if one looks at the individual treatment
categories, there are some modest trends that
lend support to palate training as an alternative
treatment for some individuals.

INDIRECT METHODS

A single articulation study was reviewed and
the findings were not positive. Individuals with
closure deficits were found to improve articulation skills, but the acquisition of such skills did not
result in improved closure for speech [52]. Based
on the investigation, which employed very stringent experimental controls and measurement
procedures, it is concluded that indirect treatment is of little value in palate training.

DIRECT METHODS

The speech appliance studies were the first to furnish data suggesting that closure for speech was improved for a subset of individuals who wore the devices. The appliances were either reduced in size or completely eliminated in some cases. There are, however, some factors that need to be considered in an evaluation of speech appliance training. The first is that patient benefit would be difficult to predict on a case-by-case basis. Findings reported by Blakeley [5] and by Weiss [70] indicated that approximately 20 percent of their clinical cases were able to discontinue appliance wear. In both cases, the clinical populations contained large numbers of cases. Wong and Weiss [72] reported a slightly higher percentage of cases who were able to discard their appliances. Variables that were associated with successful results included age (younger patients had a better success rate than older patients); sex (more girls than boys were found in the successful group); cooperation (cases who cooperated and whose families cooperated were more successful); and anatomy (successful patients generally showed adequate velar length and pharyngeal wall movement). Despite the identification of some positive prognostic factors, individual prediction would still be very limited.

Another factor in employing speech appliances is that the duration of wear varied greatly among successful subjects. Some wore appliances for short periods of time, while others wore them for more than 6 years. The extreme variance in wear makes it difficult to establish a treatment effect [19]. There is certainly a group of individuals who would benefit from speech appliance wear [10, 32–34] in a clinical treatment plan. However, the routine selection and fitting of subjects who would eventually no longer need their appliances is not a viable palate training method.

The experimental treatments which involved palate pharyngeal wall excitation used a variety of stimuli. Electrical and tactile stimulation of various forms were presented to subjects while they engaged in various speech tasks, but improvements in velopharyngeal closure for speech were not obtained on a consistent basis. For example, studies by Yules and Chase [73] and Weber, Jobe, and Chase [69] used similar methods and were undertaken in the same laboratory, but the results were contradictory. Other treatments used stimulation agents such as cotton swabs and specially designed intraoral devices and the results were not promising. It appears that palate training programs which incorporate electrical or tactile stimulation are not effective in influencing closure patterns for speech.

The use of nonspeech activities to facilitate closure has been a recommended activity in the treatment of persons with closure deficits [7, 30]. The experimental applications reported herein have included blowing, sucking, swallowing, and electrical stimulation, but the utility of such procedures has not been established. Of particular interest in this section are investigations conducted by Peterson [41] and Powers and Starr [43]. They are examples of well-controlled studies which allowed systematic study of the experimental treatments. In both cases, the dependent variable measures showed that the treatments were ineffective.

The final subset of studies examined a number of diverse biofeedback procedures [12]. The biofeedback devices ranged from rather crude devices sensitive to nasal air flow [64], to visual fiberscopes [40] which allow direct visualization of the velopharyngeal port. Studies by Shprintzen, McCall, and Skolnick [64] and by Hoch and colleagues [18] have used nasal fiberscopic training and documented significant changes in velopharyngeal closure for speech. Results do not evince unequivocally biofeedback techniques in palate training; nevertheless, findings show promise and suggest that further research should continue. Until replication substantiates the method, biofeedback remains an area for research and not for use in routine clinical intervention.

IMPLICATIONS FOR FUTURE RESEARCH

In summarizing the results of palate training studies, it was proposed that the use of such treatments remains within the experimental domain. It was also proposed that future research be directed to further evaluation of biofeedback procedures. However, if the issue of palate training as a valid speech pathology treatment is to be resolved, investigations must be conducted in rigorous fashion. The material to follow suggests some considerations for future research. It is by no means an exhaustive analysis, but deals with some of the experimental issues.

SUBJECT ISSUES

Subject selection is one of the key issues that should be considered since past studies have included an extremely heterogeneous group. It is recommended that subjects display some potential for closure prior to participation in an experimental study. Investigators have also suggested that persons with closure deficits be evaluated to determine if there is potential for closure in speech or nonspeech contexts. Shelton, Hahn, and Morris [51] have proposed that speech pathologists probe clients in clinical evaluations for this purpose. Along the same lines, Cole [8, 9] has written that inconsistent hypernasality and nasal emission might serve as a positive prognostic sign.

Lotz and Netsell [23] evaluate their clinical cases to determine whether closure for speech is present in some context. Clients, identified as exhibiting some potential for closure, are enrolled initially for speech pathology training rather than surgical or prosthetic treatment. The authors' anecdotal descriptions suggest that closure has been established on a consistent basis for some of their patients. Particularly, individuals with phoneme-specific closure deficits generally eliminated the problem following enrollment in a behavioral training program.

Shprintzen and his associates (see Hoch et al. [18]) have found it useful to categorize subjects into groups that reflect closure activity and etiology. The categories include (1) subjects who display structural damage and consistently exhibit velopharyngeal gaps during speech; (2) subjects with neurological disease who show a consistent closure deficit; (3) subjects with inconsistent closure patterns and a palate defect of structural etiology; (4) subjects demonstrating inconsistent closure patterns in the presence of neurological disease; (5) subjects with inconsistent closure patterns who have no documented structural or neurological problems; and (6) subjects with variable closure in oral sound contexts who may have structural, neurological, or no observable problem. The authors feel that individuals in categories (3), (4), and (5) have the best potential for improvement; however, the outcome for category (4) patients would be guarded because of the neurological etiology. In each instance incon-

sistency is associated with a group thought to possess the potential for consistent closure.

In addition to inconsistent closure for speech, it is possible that closure in other activities may also serve some predictive value in subject selection. Shprintzen and colleagues [63] found that closure patterns for speech and such nonspeech activities as blowing and whistling show a similar configuration. Moreover, Shprintzen and colleagues [64] identified subjects who achieved closure during nonspeech tasks and paired the nonspeech activity with speech. Their results indicated that some patients did develop closure for speech. There is no guarantee that generalization will occur, but the issue of inconsistency deserves attention.

EXPERIMENTAL DESIGN ISSUES

The validation of a treatment effect is critical; consequently, it is important that dependent variable measures be sensitive to changes in the phenomenon of interest. Unfortunately, many studies in this area have used limited evaluation measures. Velopharyngeal closure is just one aspect of speech production and it is critical that it be studies in relation to the entire process [15]. Shelton and Trier [59] have expressed the position that multiple measurement procedures are necessary in trying to quantify closure patterns. Suffice to say that future studies should employ a number of dependent variable measures which will supply acoustic, physiological, and perceptual information.

In future experimental applications it is important that treatments be clearly specified, so replication may be undertaken. A number of treatments in the literature cannot be replicated because the treatment procedures are unclear. Plutchik [42] has written that replication of results enables the establishment of confidence in a treatment. The equivocal nature of palate training to date begets systematic study and replication.

Finally, the duration of treatment is an area of scrutiny because of the range noted in previous studies. Cole [9] felt that the upperbound limit of a palate training program was approximately 3 months. If improvement was not observed, it was unlikely that continued training would be beneficial. He further suggested that a successful person would probably show positive results after 1 month of training, if provided on a frequent basis.

McWilliams and colleagues [36] supported continued examination of biofeedback techniques, but also stated that a 3- to 6-month training period should be sufficient to document change. Subjects who receive training and do not show changes in closure for speech will probably not benefit by extending the training period. Hoch and colleagues [18] used a nasal fiberscope in their biofeedback training program; they suggested that if changes occur, they will do so after a limited amount of training. The time periods mentioned by the various authors are simply estimates; however, they do provide some guidance in planning an experimental regimen.

SUMMARY

At the present, palate training methods remain within the realm of experimental study because of the equivocal results generated to date. Some of the more recent studies have reported positive outcomes suggesting that continued research might substantiate palate training as a legitimate speech pathology treatment. The complex relationship between velopharyngeal closure and speech requires careful study and measurement in a variety of different ways. In this way experimenters might not only identify successful subjects, but they might also discover the mechanisms responsible for modifications of closure. The latter issue is very important, since we cannot explain precisely what happens when an individual improves closure for speech.

The clinical implications of this review are that most persons who exhibit closure deficits should be treated through surgical or prosthetic management. Speech-language pathologists should refrain from using various palate training methods unless they have the capabilities to carry out such procedures empirically. It is important to stress the recommendation since such methods have been advocated in one form or another for a long period of time, and speech-langauge pathologists currently use such methods despite the lack of empirical support.

REFERENCES

1. Abbs, J. H., and Kennedy, J. G. Neurophysiological Processes of Speech Movement Control. In N. J. Lass, L. V. McReynolds, J. L. Northern, and D. E. Yoder (Eds.), *Speech, Language, and Hearing.* Philadelphia: Saunders, 1982. Vol. 1.
2. Basmajian, J. V. Introduction: Principles and Background. In J. V. Basmajian (Ed.), *Biofeedback: Principles and Practice for Clinicans* (2nd ed.). Baltimore: Williams & Wilkins, 1983.
3. Blakeley, R. W. Temporary speech prostheses as an aid in speech therapy. *Cleft Palate Bull.* 10:63, 1960.
4. Blakeley, R. W. The complementary use of speech prostheses and pharyngeal flaps in palatal insufficiency. *Cleft Palate J.* 2:194, 1964.
5. Blakeley, R. W. The rationale for a temporary speech prosthesis in palatal insufficiency. *Br. J. Disord. Commun.* 4:134, 1969.
6. Blakeley, R. W., and Porter, D. R. Unexpected reduction and removal of an obturator in a patient with palate paralysis. *Br. J. Disord. Commun.* 6:33, 1971.
7. Buck, M., and Harrington, R. Organized speech therapy for cleft palate rehabilitation. *J. Speech Hear. Disord.* 14:43, 1949.
8. Cole, R. M. Direct Muscle Training for the Improvement of Velopharyngeal Function. In K. R. Bzoch (Ed.), *Communicative Disorders Related to Cleft Lip and Palate* (1st ed.). Boston: Little, Brown, 1971.
9. Cole, R. M. Direct Muscle Training for the Improvement of Velopharyngeal Function. In K. R. Bzoch (Ed.), *Communicative Disorders Related to Cleft Lip and Palate* (2nd ed.). Boston: Little, Brown, 1979.
10. Dalston, R. M. Prosthodontic management of the cleft palate patient: A speech pathologist's view. *J. Prosthet. Dent.* 37:190, 1977.
11. Daly, D. A., and Johnson, H. P. Instrumental modification of hypernasal voice quality in retarded children: Case reports. *J. Speech Hear. Disord.* 39:500, 1974.
12. Davis, S. M., and Drichta, C. E. Biofeedback: Theory and Application to Speech Pathology. In N. J. Lass (Ed.), *Speech and Language: Advances in Basic Research and Practice.* New York: Academic Press, 1980.
13. Ellis, R. E., Flack, F. C., Carle, H. J., and Selley, W. G. A system for assessment of nasal airflow during speech. *Br. J. Disord. Commun.* 13:31, 1978.
14. Fletcher, S. G. Contingencies for bioelectronic modification of nasality. *J. Speech Hear. Disord.* 37:329, 1972.
15. Folkins, J. W., and Kuehn, D. P. Speech Production. In N. J. Lass, L. V. McReynolds, J. L. Northern, and D. E. Yoder (Eds.), *Speech, Language and Hearing.* Philadelphia: Saunders, 1982. Vol. 1.
16. Folkins, J. W. Issues in speech motor control and their relation to the speech of individuals with cleft palate. *Cleft Palate J.* 22:106, 1985.
17. Fuller, G. D. *Projects in Biofeedback.* San Francisco: Biofeedback Press, 1980.
18. Hoch, L., Golding-Kushner, K., Siegel-Sadewitz, V. L., and Shprintzen, R. J. Speech therapy. *Semin. Speech Lang.* 7:313, 1986.
19. Hubbell, R. D. *Children's Language Disorders — An Integrated Approach.* Englewood Cliffs, N.J.: Prentice-Hall, 1981.
20. Karnell, M. D., Folkins, J. W., and Morris, H. Relationships between the perception of nasalization and speech movements in speakers with cleft palate. *J. Speech Hear. Res.* 28:63, 1985.
21. Kent, R. D., and Lybolt, J. T. Techniques of Therapy Based on Motor Learning Theory. In W. H. Perkins (Ed.), *Current Therapy of Communication Disorders: General Principles of Therapy.* New York: Thieme-Stratton, 1982.

22. Kuehn, D. V. Velopharyngeal anatomy and physiology. *Ear Nose Throat J.* 58:59, 1979.
23. Lotz, W. K., and Netsell, R. Treatment of velopharyngeal dysfunction. Short course presented at the Annual Convention of the American Speech-Language-Hearing Association, New Orleans, 1987.
24. Lubit, E. C., and Larsen, R. E. The Lubit Palatal Exerciser: A preliminary report. *Cleft Palate J.* 6:120, 1969.
25. Lubker, J. F. Normal velopharyngeal function in speech. *Clin. Plast. Surg.* 2:249, 1975.
26. Lubker, J. F. Some Teleological Considerations of Velopharyngeal Function. In R. G. Daniloff (Ed.), *Articulation Assessment and Treatment Issues.* Boston: College-Hill Press, 1984.
27. Massengill, R., Quinn, G. W., Pickrell, K. L., and Levinson, C. Therapeutic exercise and velopharyngeal gap. *Cleft Palate J.* 5:44, 1968.
28. Massengill, R., Quinn, G. W., and Pickrell, K. L. The use of a palatal stimulator to decrease velopharyngeal gap. *Ann. Otol. Rhinol. Laryngol.* 80:135, 1971.
29. Massengill, R., and Quinn, G. Adenoidal atrophy, velopharyngeal incompetence and sucking exercises; a 2-yr follow-up case report. *Cleft Palate J.* 11:196, 1974.
30. Massengill, R., and Phillips, P. P. *Cleft Palate and Associated Characteristics.* Lincoln, Neb.: Cliffs Notes, 1975.
31. Matsuya, T., Yamaoka, M., and Miyazaki, T. A fiberscopic study of velopharyngeal closure in patients with operated cleft palates. *Plast. Reconstr. Surg.* 63:497, 1979.
32. Mazaheri, M. Indications and contraindications for prosthetic speech appliances in cleft palate. *Plast. Reconstr. Surg.* 30:663, 1962.
33. Mazaheri, M., and Mazaheri, E. H. Correction of palatal defects: A prosthodontist's viewpoint. *J. Oral Surg.* 73:913, 1973.
34. Mazaheri, M., and Mazaheri, E. H. Prosthodontic aspects of palatal elevation and palatopharyngeal stimulation. *J. Prosthet. Dent.* 35:319, 1976.
35. McWilliams, B. J. Speech Problems Associated with Craniofacial Anomalies. In J. M. Costello (Ed.), *Speech Disorders in Children.* Boston: College-Hill Press, 1984.
36. McWilliams, B. J., Morris, H. L., and Shelton, R. L. *Cleft Palate Speech.* Philadelphia: Decker, 1984.
37. Miyazaki, T., Matsuya, T., and Yamaoka, M. Fiberscopic methods for assessment of velopharyngeal closure during various activities. *Cleft Palate J.* 12:107, 1975.
38. Moller, K. T., Path, M., Werth, L. J., and Christiansen, R. L. The modification of velar movement. *J. Speech Hear. Disord.* 38:323, 1973.
39. Netsell, R. Speech Motor Control: Theoretical Issues with Clinical Impact. In W. Berry (Ed.), *Clinical Dysarthria.* Boston: College-Hill Press, 1982.
40. Nishio, J., Yamaoka, M., Matsuya, T., and Miyazaki, T. How to exercise the velopharyngeal movement by the velopharyngeal fiberscope. *Jpn. J. Oral Surg.* 20:450, 1974 [Abstracted in *Cleft Palate J.* 13:310, 1976].
41. Peterson, S. J. Electrical stimulation of the soft palate. *Cleft Palate J.* 11:72, 1974.
42. Plutchik, R. *Foundations of Experimental Research.* New York: Harper & Row, 1968.
43. Powers, G. L., and Starr, C. D. The effects of muscle exercises on velopharyngeal gap and nasality. *Cleft Palate J.* 11:28, 1974.
44. Roll, D. J. Modification of nasal resonance in cleft palate children by informative feedback. *J. Appl. Behav. Anal.* 6:397, 1973.
45. Ruscello, D. M. A selected review of palatal training

procedures. *Cleft Palate J.* 19:181, 1982.
46. Ruscello, D. M. Motor Learning as a Model for Articulation Instruction. In J. Costello (Ed.), *Speech Disorders in Children.* Boston: College-Hill Press, 1984.
47. Siegel–Sadewitz, V. L., and Shprintzen, R. J. Nasopharyngoscopy of the normal velopharyngeal sphincter: An experiment of biofeedback. *Cleft Palate J.* 19:194, 1982.
48. Schneider, E., and Shprintzen, R. J. A survey of speech pathologists: Current trends in the diagnosis and management of velopharyngeal insufficiency. *Cleft Palate J.* 17:249, 1980.
49. Seaver, E., and Kuehn, D. P. Cineradiographic and electromyographic investigation of velar positioning in non-nasal speech. *Cleft Palate J.* 17:216, 1980.
50. Shelton, R. L. Therapeutic exercise and speech pathology. *ASHA* 5:855, 1963.
51. Shelton, R. L., Hahn, E., and Morris, H. Diagnosis and Therapy. In D. C. Spriestersbach and D. Sherman (Eds.), *Cleft Palate and Communication.* New York: Academic Press, 1968.
52. Shelton, R. L., Chisum, L., Youngstrom, K. A., Arndt, W. B., and Elbert, M. Effect of articulation therapy on palatopharyngeal closure, movement of the pharyngeal wall, and tongue posture. *Cleft Palate J.* 6:440, 1969.
53. Shelton, R. L., Knox, A. W., Elbert, M., and Johnson, T. S. Palate Awareness and Nonspeech Voluntary Palate Movement. In J. F. Bosma (Ed.), *Second Symposium on Oral Sensation and Perception.* Springfield, Ill.: Thomas, 1970.
54. Shelton, R. L., Harris, K. S., Sholes, G. N., and Dooley, P. M. Study of Nonspeech Voluntary Palate Movements by Scaling and Electromyographic Techniques. In J. F. Bosma (Ed.), *Second Symposium on Oral Sensation and Perception.* Springfield, Ill.: Thomas, 1970.
55. Shelton, R. L., Lindquist, A. F., Knox, A. W., Wright, V. L., Arndt, W. B., Elbert, M., and Youngstrom, K. A. The relationship between pharyngeal wall movements and exchangeable speech appliance sections. *Cleft Palate J.* 8:145, 1971.
56. Shelton, R. L., Lindquist, A. F., Arndt, W. B., Elbert, M., and Youngstrom, K. A. Effect of speech bulb reduction on movement of the posterior wall of the pharynx and posture of the tongue. *Cleft Palate J.* 8:10, 1971.
57. Shelton, R. L., Morris, H., and McWilliams, B. J. Assessment of Speech. In *Speech, Language, and Psychosocial Aspects of Cleft Lip and Cleft Palate: The State of the Art.* ASHA Reports No. 9. Washington, D.C.: American Speech and Hearing Association, 1973.
58. Shelton, R. L., Paesani, A., McClelland, K. D., and Bradfield, S. S. Panendoscopic feedback in the study of voluntary velopharyngeal movements. *J. Speech Hear. Disord.* 40:232, 1975.
59. Shelton, R. L., and Trier, W. C. Issues involved in the evaluation of velopharyngeal closure. *Cleft Palate J.* 13:127, 1976.
60. Shelton, R. L., Beaumont, K., Trier, W. C., and Furr, M. L. Videoendoscopic feedback in training velopharyngeal closure. *Cleft Palate J.* 15:6, 1978.
61. Shelton, R. L. Oral Sensory Function in Speech Production and Remediation. In K. R. Bzoch (Ed.), *Communicative Disorders Related to Cleft Lip and Palate* (2nd ed.). Boston: Little, Brown, 1979. Pp. 120–147.
62. Shelton, R. L., and Ruscello, D. M. Palatal and articulation training in patients with velopharyngeal closure problems. Paper presented at Annual Convention of the American Cleft Palate Association, San Diego, 1979.

63. Shprintzen, R. J., Lencione, R. M., McCall, G. N., and Skolnick, M. L. A three dimensional cinefluoroscopic analysis of velopharyngeal closure during speech and nonspeech activities in normals. *Cleft Palate J.* 11:412, 1974.
64. Shprintzen, R., McCall, G. M., and Skolnick, L. A new therapeutic technique for the treatment of velopharyngeal incompetence. *J. Speech Hear. Disord.* 40:69, 1975.
65. Tash, E. L., Shelton, R. I., Knox, A. W., and Michel, J. F. Training voluntary pharyngeal wall movements in children with normal and inadequate velopharyngeal closure. *Cleft Palate J.* 8:277, 1971.
66. Thompson, A. E., and Hixon, T. J. Nasal airflow during normal speech production. *Cleft Palate J.* 16:412, 1979.
67. Tudor, C., and Selley, W. G. A palatal training appliance and a visual aid for use in the treatment of hypernasal speech. *Br. J. Disord. Commun.* 9:117, 1974.
68. Warren, D. W. Aerodynamics of Speech. In N. J. Lass, L. V. McReynolds, J. L. Northern, and D. E. Yoder (Eds.), *Speech, Language and Hearing.* Philadelphia: Saunders, 1982. Vol. 1.
69. Weber, J., Jobe, R. P., and Chase, R. A. Evaluation of muscle stimulation in the rehabilitation of patients with hypernasal speech. *Plast. Reconstr. Surg.* 46:173, 1970.
70. Weiss, C. E. Success of an obturator reduction program. *Cleft Palate J.* 6:291, 1971.
71. Wolf, S. L. Neurophysiological Factors in Electromyographic Feedback for Neuromotor Disturbances. In J. V. Basmajian (Ed.), *Biofeedback: Principles and Practices for Clinicians* (2nd ed.). Baltimore: Williams & Wilkins, 1983.
72. Wong, L. P., and Weiss, C. E. A clinical assessment of obturator wearing cleft palate patients. *J. Prosthet. Dent.* 27:632, 1972.
73. Yules, R. B., and Chase, R. A. A training method for reduction of hypernasality in speech. *Plast. Reconstr. Surg.* 43:180, 1969.
74. Zwitman, D. H., Sonderman, J. C., and Ward, P. H. Variations in velopharyngeal closure assessed by endoscopy. *J. Speech Hear. Disord.* 39:366, 1974.

Key to Phonetic Symbols

Frequent reference is made to specific distinctive sound elements of our language generally referred to as *phonemes*. The broadest definition possible, including all references to articulating speech sound elements or distinguishing distinctive sound units in speech, was used to standardize and simplify this material for our readers from many different backgrounds. Such sound units have been set off in slashes throughout — for example, /p/. Syllables have been set off in brackets — for example, [pi-pi-pi]. Listed below are the symbols used and a common key word; the sound is indicated by the portion of the key word underlined.

/ʔ/	glottal stop	/h/	as in horse	/ŋ/	as in sing	/ð/	as in this
/ɑ/	as in father	/hw/	as in when	/o/	as in open	/θ/	as in thin
/æ/	as in cat	/i/	as in see	/p/	as in pie	/ʊ/	as in cook
/b/	as in boy	/ɪ/	as in hit	/r/	as in rose	/u/	as in cool
/d/	as in do	/j/	as in yes	/s/	as in sun	/ʌ/	as in cup
/dʒ/	as in jump	/k/	as in cat	/ʃ/	as in shoe	/v/	as in vase
/ɛ/	as in get	/l/	as in love	/ʒ/	as in television	/w/	as in we
/f/	as in fun	/m/	as in me	/t/	as in tie	/z/	as in zoo
/g/	as in gun	/n/	as in no	/tʃ/	as in chair		

INDEX

Index

An italicized page number denotes a figure; the abbreviation *t* denotes a table.

625-6367   Jen
825-9052   Lisa